Stedman's

ORGANISMS & INFECTIOUS DISEASE

WORDS

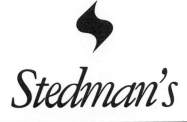

Stedman's

ORGANISMS &
INFECTIOUS DISEASE
WORDS

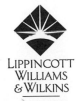

LIPPINCOTT
WILLIAMS
&WILKINS

Publisher: Rhonda M. Kumm
Senior Manager: Julie K. Stegman
Associate Managing Editor: Trista A. DiPaula
Associate Managing Editor: William A. Howard
Art Director: Jennifer Clements
Production Manager: Julie K. Stegman
Production Coordinator: Kevin Iarossi
Typesetter: Peirce Graphic Services, Inc.
Printer & Binder: Malloy Litho

2002

Library of Congress Cataloging-in-Publication Data

Stedman's organisms & infectious diesase words.
    p. cm
    ISBN 0-7817-3351-0 (alk. paper)
    1. Communicable diseases—Terminology. 2. Medical microbiology—
Terminology. I. Title: Stedman's organisms and infectious disease words.
II. Stedman, Thomas Lathrop, 1853–1938.

RC112 .S69 2001
616'.001'4—dc21

                              2001050348

                        02 03
              2 3 4 5 6 7 8 9 10

Contents

Acknowledgments

An important part of our editorial process is the involvement of medical transcriptionists—as advisors, reviewers, and/or editors.

We extend special thanks to Ellen Atwood for editing the manuscript, helping resolve many difficult questions, and contributing material for the appendix sections. We also extend thanks to Jeanne Bock, CSR, MT, for assisting with the editing of the manuscript.

Special thanks also goes to our Editorial Advisory Board members, including Mary O'Connor; Natasha Brown; Kathryn C. Mason, CMT; Peg Nelson, CMT; and Susan Bartolucci, CMT, who were instrumental to the development of this reference. They recommended sources and provided valuable judgment, insights, and perspectives.

We also extend thanks to Catherine Baxter; Lin Harvell; Robin Koza; and Kathryn C. Mason, CMT, for working on the appendix sections, as well as to Helen Littrell, CMT, for performing the final prepublication review. Other important contributors to this edition include Donna C. Brosmer, CMT; Shemah Fletcher; Kathleen M. Gavin, CMT; Sheila Hatch; and Mary Chiara Zaratkiewicz

Barb Ferretti played an integral role in the process by reviewing the content files for format, updating the database, and providing a final quality check.

As with all our *Stedman's* word references, this resource incorporates the suggestions and expertise of our many contacts in the medical transcriptionist community. Thanks to all of our advisory board participants, reviewers, and editors; AAMT meeting attendees; and others who have written us with requests and comments—keep talking, and we'll keep listening.

Editor's Preface

Antony von Leeuwenhoek's poking around in rainwater, teeth scrapings, bits of dirt and wood, and hair containing ever-present lice started a revolution three centuries ago. His documented discovery of the "wretched beasties" led to miracles taken for granted in this century: pasteurized milk, antisepsis, preventing infectious disease, eradication of smallpox.

Contagious and vector-borne diseases like camp fever; massively infected wounds; and gangrenous limbs claimed more soldiers' lives before World War II than did the battlefields. Fleming's recognition in 1928 that a contaminating mold on a Petri dish eradicated resident colonies of bacteria, and the 1932 discovery that a chemical variation of a red dye also had antibacterial properties led to the first antimicrobials effectively administered to humans, saving and restoring to health countless wounded soldiers. Now maligned in some medical and lay circles, antibiotics were the first natural medicines to consistently cure infectious diseases.

After the war, research and development of more antibiotics, coupled with Salk's polio vaccine saving a generation of children from death and paralysis, led to medical authorities proclaiming victory in the war against microbes. Human genius and industry had overpowered Nature. Medical students were advised not to pursue a career in infectious disease, because it was evident there would be no jobs for them in that field upon completion of their studies. Immense, probably justified, pride supported the belief that no mere bug could ever again threaten humanity. The intellectual curiosity necessary to stimulate research all but disappeared—after all, everything to now had already been discovered, and vaccines could be whipped up on the spot!

All the while, microbes and other organisms were engaging in covert ops, counterattacks and defensive moves, right under the experts' noses. While Watson and Crick were unraveling the mystery of DNA, which would lead to understanding viruses and the Human Genome Project, microbes were already swapping their DNA and specialized molecules, not only with their own but also across species. Nature's imperative of survival stimulated processes unrecognized by humans, and the microorganisms fought back.

Until, that is, antibiotic resistant organisms started turning hospitals back into a dangerous place for sick people. Until, that is, the AIDS epidemic reached startling proportions. Until, that is, a ubiquitous bacteria "borrowed" the toxin-producing genes from a dangerous variety, discovered when kids started dying from eating hamburgers. Until Gulf War veterans' mysterious ailments renewed the fear of biological weaponry, and bioterrorism was no longer just a nifty plot for suspense novels.

Fortunately for us all, the complacency exhibited after microorganisms were supposedly vanquished is long gone. The worldwide impact of AIDS, superbly healthy Navajo young men and women dropping dead from a virus with no name (Sin Nombre), West Nile fever in New York city—all these and more have served to reignite the flame of passionate inquiry of the world of microscopic organisms.

This renewed interest is good news, and one of the reasons for our resurrecting books published nearly a decade ago, combining four separate references into one comprehensive one. In the process, some fascinating things were discovered.

Everybody knows that *Pneumocystis carinii* is a protozoan parasite, right? Guess again. It's been reclassified as a fungus. Then there are fungi that have been "promoted" to bacteria and vice versa, with some species being claimed by both mycologists and bacteriologists. Mycosis is a disease caused by a fungus, but mycosis fungoides is a lymphoma and mycosis intestinalis is a gastroenteric form caused by the deadly anthrax bacillus. Humans in search of a beauty lift are now routinely injected with the equally deadly toxin that causes botulism when ingested. Everybody knew that bacteria couldn't possibly survive in the incredibly high temperatures and pressures of the deep ocean thermal vents. Guess again, there are now dozens of new genera and species of microorganisms recovered from areas previously out of our reach. Everybody knows that malaria was banished from the United States decades ago. Guess who's back?

While fascinating to an inveterate dictionary diver, all these changes in nomenclature and taxonomy can be more than confusing to medical transcriptionists and others who need accurate information and a quick way to find it. When the previous editions of reference materials were reviewed, they were found wanting. Combining disparate groups of organisms; updating their names; identifying the obsolete but still used and separating them from the obsolete and unimportant; and verifying Latin genus and species spellings presented a variety of challenges.

We hope that the resulting product, *Stedman's Organisms and Infectious Disease Words,* will demonstrate a comprehensive approach to taxonomic nomenclature, as well as provide current drugs, procedures, tests, and commonly used terms associated with the newly important medical specialty, Infectious Disease.

Special thanks to Barb Ferretti for making magic with the database, and to Catherine Baxter, my coeditor, for her attention to current style and associated critical issues. Jeanne Bock deserves special recognition for her timely help and excellent attention to detail.

We are also grateful to the many Medical Transcriptionists who have provided feedback, opinions, participated in surveys, and helped in so many other ways by contributing time and information to assist in the creation of this first edition combining relevant information from *Stedman's ASP Parasite Names; Stedman's ATCC Fungus Names; Stedman's Bergey's Bacteria Words;* and *Stedman's ICTV Virus Words.*

The vision for and driving force behind this edition was provided by Beverly Wolpert, former Series Editor for the Stedman's Word Books, who left to pursue her dream of an advanced degree before the product was completed. All the good parts herein are in her honor.

Ellen Atwood
August 30, 2001

Publisher's Preface

Stedman's Organisms & Infectious Disease Words offers an authoritative assurance of quality and exactness to the wordsmiths of the health-care professions—medical transcriptionists, medical editors and copyeditors, health information management personnel, court reporters, and the many other users and producers of medical documentation.

In *Stedman's Organisms & Infectious Disease Words,* users will find thousands of words as they relate to the bacteria, viruses, parasites, and fungi. Users will also find infectious disease terms, diagnostic and therapeutic procedures, new techniques, and lab tests, as well as equipment names, and abbreviations with their expansions. The appendix sections provide illustrations with useful captions and labels, lists of poisonous and hazardous organisms, lists of simplified virus categories, sample reports, common terms by assessment, and drugs by indication.

This compilation of more than 75,000 entries, fully cross-indexed for quick access, was built from a base vocabulary of approximately 45,000 medical words, phrases, abbreviations, and acronyms. The extensive A-Z list was developed from manufacturers' literature, scientific reports, books, journals, CDs, and web sites (please see list of References on page xxii)

We at Lippincott Williams & Wilkins strive to provide you with the most up-to-date and accurate word references available. Your use of this word book will prompt new editions, which we will publish as often as updates and revisions justify. We welcome your suggestions for improvements, changes, corrections, and additions—whatever will make this *Stedman's* product more useful to you. Please complete the postpaid card at the back of this book, and send your recommendations care of "Stedman's" at Lippincott Williams & Wilkins.

Explanatory Notes

Medical transcription is an art as well as a science. Both approaches are needed to correctly interpret the dictation of a physician, whose language is a product of education, training, and experience. This variety in medical language means that there are several acceptable ways to express certain terms, including jargon. *Stedman's Organisms & Infectious Disease Words* provides variant spellings and phrasings for many terms. These elements, in addition to complete cross-indexing, make *Stedman's Organisms & Infectious Disease Words* a valuable resource for determining the validity of terms as they are encountered.

Alphabetical Organization

Alphabetization of main entries is letter by letter as spelled, ignoring punctuation, spaces, prefixed numbers, or other special characters. For example:

insulinotardic
insulinotropin
insulin-producing cell
insulin promoter factor 1
insulin-receptor antibody

Terms beginning with Greek letters show the Greek letters spelled out and listed alphabetically. For example:

beta, β
        b. corynebacteriophage
        b. gene
        b. hemolysin

In subentry alphabetization, the abbreviated singular form or the spelled-out plural form of the noun main entry word is ignored.

Format and Style

All main entries are in **boldface** to expedite locating a sought-after term, to enhance distinction between main entries and subentries, and to relieve the textual density of the pages.

Irregular plurals and variant spellings are shown on the same line as the singular or preferred form of the word. For example:

baterium, pl. bacteria
Cnemidocoptes, Knemidocoptes

Hyphenation

As a rule of style, multiple eponyms (e.g., Mears-Rubash approach) are hyphenated. Also, hyphens have been added between a manufacturer and one or more eponyms (e.g., Vital-Metzenbaum dissecting scissors). Please note that in many cases, hyphenation is a question of style, not of accuracy, and thus is a matter of choice.

Possessives

Possessive forms have been dropped in this reference for the sake of consistency and conformance with the guidelines of the American Association for Medical Transcription (AAMT) and other groups. Please note, however, that in many cases, retaining the possessive, like hyphenating, is a question of style, not of accuracy, and thus is a matter of choice. To form the possessive of a word, simply add the apostrophe or apostrophe "s" to the end of the word.

Cross-indexing

The word list is in an index-like main entry-subentry format that contains two combined alphabetical listings:

(1) A *noun* main entry-subentry organization, which is typical of the A-Z section of medical dictionaries like *Stedman's*:

neck
    n. of pancreas
    webbed n.

fluid
    amniotic f.
    bloody f.

(2) An *adjective* main entry-subentry organization, which lists words and phrases as you hear them. The main entries are the adjectives or modifiers in a multiword term. The subentries are the nouns around which the terms are constructed and to which the adjectives or modifiers pertain:

red
    r. blood cell (RBC)
    r. bone marrow

hypoplastic
    h. gland
    h. mandible

This format provides the user with more than one way to locate and identify a multiword term. For example:

benign
    b. nodular goiter

goiter
    benign nodular g.

anterior
    a. pituitary lobe

lobe
    anterior pituitary l.

net
    n. calcium absorption

absorption
    net calcium a.

It also allows the user to see together all terms that contain a particular descriptor, as well as all types, kinds, or variations of a noun entity. For example:

receptor
    estrogen r. (ER)
    r. expression
    extracellular r.

thyroid
    t. axis.
    t. biopsy
    black t.

Wherever possible, abbreviations are separately defined and cross-referenced. For example:

SPA
    single-photon absorptiometry

single-photon
    s.-p. absorptiometry (SPA)

absorptiometry
    single-photon a. (SPA)

Identification of Organisms: Type Style and Labeling

Classes Higher Than Genus
Classifications higher than genus are presented in normal (Roman) typeface with an initial capital letter. Although rarely used in medical reports, on occasion, a Phylum, Class, Order, or Family name is dictated and thus many of the more common ones are included in the A-Z portion of the

book. The rules for nomenclature are not consistent across all disciplines. Please see our list of References on page xxii to find more information on scientific nomenclature.

Genus and Species
Genus, species, and genus/species names are italicized; the genus name is in initial caps, and the species name is in lowercase.

Staphylococcus aureus

Many genera of organisms also have a commonly used name, identical to the formal Latin name, which is presented in Roman type, lowercase:

staphylococcus

Genus
Initial capital letter, italics, and singular when specific to the term or its usage:

Staphylococcus food poisoning

Lowercase, Roman type when used in a general sense, depending on type of report, or when plural:

staphylococcus food poisoning
staphylococci food poisoning

Labels
Genus names are labeled with a one-letter abbreviation, limited to bacteria, fungi, parasites, and viruses:

(b)=bacterium
(f)=fungus
(p)=parasite
(v)=virus

Tags are located after the genus name:

> *Leishmania* (p)
>> *L. aethiopica*
>> *L. braziliensis*
>> *L. donovani*
>> *L. mexicana*

If there is only one species for a genus, the tag will appear after the combined genus and species names.

> *Acetoanaerobium noterae* (b)

Spelling Variations

In this wordbook, there are several terms with spellings that are very similar to each other. Please note that closely spelled species names are organism-specific and are not variants to each other, as in this example:

> *Borrelia brasiliensis*   a bacterium

but

> *Leishmania braziliensis*   a parasite
> *Coemansia braziliensis*   a fungus

Other similarly spelled terms include:

> *brasilense*
>> *Azospirillum b.*
> *brasiliense*
>> *Elytrosporangium b.*

We have taken care to select proper spellings from only approved lists.

As a subentry to a species, the genus name does not carry a tag. To find the tag for the genus, look at the alphabetical listing of the genus name:

> *Azospirillum* (b)
>> *A. amazonense*
>> *A. brasilense*
>> *A. doebereinerae*

Parasites and Organisms Loosely Associated with Diseases

The A-Z portion of the book also lists the Latin names of many organisms that are involved in diseases, but that are not the actual causes of diseases. We have tagged only the actual parasite known to cause a disease. We have not tagged any of the vectors, hosts, reservoirs, or other genus/species loosely associated but critical to the life cycle of the parasite.

For example, the actual cause of malaria is a protozoan parasite. The genus will be tagged:

> *Plasmodium* (p)
> *P. falciparum*
> *P. malariae*

but the vector that transmits the disease, and without which humans would not be affected, will not be tagged:

> *Anopheles*
> *A. albimanus*
> *A. albitarsus*

This example shows only a genus of mosquitoes. There are many other untagged genus/species names from all classes of organisms, including but not limited to flies, snails, ticks, and mites, listed in this book. Please check the list of references on page xxii for help in determining the type of organism.

Changes in Taxonomy and Other Classifications

The names of some organisms have undergone changes, and in some cases, previously used synonyms have been discarded. One well known example is the yeast, *Candida,* formerly named *Monilia,* which also has half a dozen or more other previously used synonyms. We have kept the most common ones, simply listed alphabetically in the A-Z portion as usual.

Other organisms have been reclassified completely, and in some instances, the former discipline sometimes still refers to the organism as belonging to its area of interest. We have chosen to tag these organisms with their current classifications. Examples include:

> *Pneumocystis* (f)
> formerly considered to be a protozoan parasite
> *Actinomadura* (b)
> formerly considered to be a fungus

References

In addition to the manufacturers' literature we gather at various medical meetings, scientific reports from hospitals, and the lists of our MT Editorial Advisory Board members from their daily transcription work, we used the following sources for new terms in *Stedman's Organisms & Infectious Disease Words:*

Books

Cohen PT, Sande MA, Volberding PA, Osmond DH, Feinberg MB, Deeks S, Safrin S, Kaplan LJ, Gerberding JL. The AIDS Knowledge Base: A Textbook on HIV Disease from the University of California, San Francisco and San Francisco Genera, Third Edition. Baltimore: Lippincott Williams & Wilkins, 1999.

Fields BN, Knipe DM, Howley PM, Chanock RM, Melnick JL, Monath TP, Roizman B, Straus SE. Fields Virology, Third Edition, Volumes 1 and 2. Baltimore: Lippincott Williams & Wilkins, 1996.

Folks T. AIDS 2000 — A Year in Review. Baltimore: Lippincott Williams & Wilkins, 2000.

Foster S, Caras R. A Field Guide to Venomous Animals & Poisonous Plants, North America, North of Mexico. New York: Houghton Mifflin Company, 1998.

Gorbach SL, Mensa J, Gatell, J. 1999 Pocket Book of Antimicrobial Therapy and Prevention, Second Edition. Baltimore: Lippincott Williams & Wilkins, 1999.

Isada CM, Kasten BL, Goldman MP, Gray LD, Aberg JA. Infectious Diseases Handbook, Including Antimicrobial Therapy & Diagnostic Tests/Procedures. Cleveland: Lexi-Comp, 2001.

Johnson RT. Viral Infections of the Nervous System, Second Edition. Baltimore: Lippincott Williams & Wilkins, 1998.

Knipe DM, Howley PM, Griffin DE, Lamb RA, Martin MA, Roizman B, Straus SE. Fields Virology, Fourth Edition, Volumes 1 and 2. Baltimore: Lippincott Williams & Wilkins, 2001.

Koneman EW, Allen SD, Janda WM, Schreckenberger PC, Winn Jr. WC. Color Atlas and Textbook of Diagnostic Microbiology, Fifth Edition. Baltimore: Lippincott Williams & Wilkins, 1997.

Lance LL. 2001 Quick Look Drug Book. Baltimore: Lippincott Williams & Wilkins, 2001.

Mandell GL, Bennett JE, Dolin R. Mandell, Douglas, and Bennett's Principles and Practice of Infectious Diseases, Fifth Edition, Volumes 1 and 2. New York: Churchill Livingstone, 2000.

Markell EK, John DT, Krotoski WA. Markell and Voge's Medical Parasitology, Eighth Edition. Philadelphia: Saunders, 1999.

Nathanson N, Ahmed R, Gonzalez-Scarano F, Griffin DE, Holmes KV, Murphy FA, Robinson HL. Viral Pathogenesis. Baltimore: Lippincott Williams & Wilkins, 1996.

Powderly WG. Manual of HIV Therapeutics, Second Edition. Baltimore: Lippincott Williams & Wilkins, 2000.

Reese RE, Betts RF. A Practical Approach to Infectious Diseases, Fourth Edition. Baltimore: Lippincott Williams & Wilkins, 1997.

Rom WN, Garay, SM. Tuberculosis. Baltimore: Lippincott Williams & Wilkins, 1995.

Stedman's Concise Medical Dictionary for the Health Professions, Illustrated Fourth Edition. Baltimore: Lippincott Williams & Wilkins, 2001.

Stedman's Medical Dictionary, 27th Edition. Baltimore: Lippincott Williams & Wilkins, 2000.

Sugar AM, Lyman CA. A Practical Guide to Medically Important Fungi and the Diseases They Cause. Baltimore: Lippincott Williams & Wilkins, 1997.

Sun T. Parasitic Disorders, Second Edition. Baltimore: Lippincott Williams & Wilkins, 1998.

Wenzel RP. Prevention and Control of Nosocomial Infections, Third Edition. Baltimore: Lippincott Williams & Wilkins, 1997.

Yu V, Merigan T, Barriere S. Antimicrobial Therapy and Vaccines. Baltimore: Lippincott Williams & Wilkins, 1998.

CDs

Koneman EW, Sutton DA, Fothergill AW, Rinaldi MG, Tsieh S, Straus SE. LWW's Organism Central CD-ROM for Windows. Baltimore: Lippincott Williams & Wilkins, 2001.

Journals

JAIDS: Journal of Acquired Immune Deficiency Syndromes. Baltimore: Lippincott Williams & Wilkins, 1999–2001.

Journal of Human Virology. Baltimore: Lippincott Williams & Wilkins, 1999–2001.

Journal of Immunotherapy. Baltimore: Lippincott Williams & Wilkins, 1999–2001.

Journal of Medical Microbiology. Baltimore: Lippincott Williams & Wilkins, 1999–2001.

Journal of Microbiology, Immunology and Infection. Baltimore: Lippincott Williams & Wilkins, 1999–2001.

Sexually Transmitted Diseases. Baltimore: Lippincott Williams & Wilkins, 1999–2001.

Websites

http://medic.med.uth.tmc.edu/path/00001458.htm

http://vm.cfsan.fda.gov/~mow/bactoc.html

http://vm.cfsan.fda.gov/~mow/intro.html

http://www.bacterio.cict.fr/

http://www.bacterio.cict.fr/buchanan.html

http://www.entomology.wisc.edu

A
    A and D Ointment
    A virus
A1
    Coxsackie virus A1
019/6-A
    Gaeumannomyces graminis virus -
        A. (GgV-019/6A)
3A
    Yersinia enterocolitica biogroup 3A
4A
    parainfluenza type 4A
17-1A
    glycoprotein 17-1A
A19 virus
A1-Dat virus
alpha-2
    rLFN–alpha-2
A-200 Shampoo
A23 virus
A25 virus
A-4 virus
A5/A6 virus
A6 virus
AA-1 virus
AAC
    antibiotic-associated colitis
AAD
    antibiotic-associated diarrhea
A-a gradient
aalborgi
    Brachyspira a.
aaseri
    Candida a.
AAV
    adenoassociated virus
        avian AAV
AAV 1–5
    adenoassociated virus 1–5
abacavir (ABC)
abactoclasticum
    Anaeroplasma a.
abattoir
abattoir-associated pneumonia
Abbott
    A. LCx LCR
    A. LCx ligase chain reaction
ABC
    abacavir
ABCD
    amphotericin B colloid dispersion
    asymmetry, border, color, and diameter
ABD
    autologous blood donation

abdelmalekii
    Ectothiorhodospira a.
    Halorhodospira a.
abdominal
    a. actinomycosis
    a. angiostrongyliasis
    a. anthrax
    a. infection
    a. paracentesis
    a. paragonimiasis
    a. trauma
    a. tuberculosis
    a. typhoid
    a. ultrasound
ABE
    acute bacterial endocarditis
Abel bacillus (*See Klebsiella ozaenae*)
Abelcet
Abenol
aberrant cysticercus
ABG
    arterial blood gas
ABI AnIDENT panel
abidjanum
    Eupenicillium a.
abietaniphila
    Pseudomonas a.
abikoense
    Streptoverticillium a.
abikoensis
    Streptomyces a.
Abiotrophia (b)
    A. adiacens
    A. balaenopterae
    A. defectiva
    A. elegans
ablative chemotherapy
ABMV
    Abu Mina virus
abnormality
    cardiac a.
abominator
    Culex a.
aboriginis
    Aedes a.
abortion
    clonal a.
abortive poliomyelitis
abortus
    Bacillus a.
    a. bacillus
    Brucella a.
    Chlamydophila a.

ABPA
  allergic bronchopulmonary aspergillosis
Abras virus (ABRV)
abruptio placentae
ABRV
  Abras virus
abscess
  adnexal a.
  amebic brain a.
  amebic liver a.
  bacterial peritonsillar a.
  brain a.
  breast a.
  Brodie a.
  circumcision wound a.
  cold a.
  conglobate a.
  crypt a.
  cryptococcal a.
  cutaneous a.
  eosinophilic a.
  epidural a.
  follicular a.
  gonococcal scalp a.
  hepatic a.
  intraabdominal a.
  intraepidermal a.
  intrarenal a.
  ischiorectal a.
  lacrimal a.
  liver a.
  loculated a.
  mediastinal a.
  mixed aerobic and anaerobic a.
  Munro a.
  mycobacterial a.
  Mycobacterium chelonae a.
  Nocardia brain a.
  orbital a.
  pancreatic a.
  parafrenal a.
  Pautrier a.
  periapical a.
  periappendiceal a.
  perinephric a.
  periodontal a.
  periurethral a.
  prostatic a.
  psoas a.
  pulmonary amebic a.
  pyogenic liver a.
  recurrent cutaneous a.
  recurrent pyogenic a.
  retroperitoneal a.
  retropharyngeal a.
  scrotal a.
  spinal epidural a.

  staphylococcal a.
  stellate a.
  sterile a.
  subdiaphragmatic a.
  subepidermal a.
  subhepatic a.
  subphrenic a.
  subungual a.
  sudoriparous a.
  tuberculous a.
  tuboovarian a. (TOA)
  verminous a.
  visceral a.
  worm a.
abscess-granulomatous reaction
abscessus
  Mycobacterium a.
  Mycobacterium chelonae subsp. *a.*
  Nocardia a.
absent bowel sounds
abserratus
  Aedes a.
Absidia (f)
  A. coerulea
  A. corymbifera
  A. cylindrospora
  A. glauca
  A. spinosa
absolute
  atmosphere a. (ATA)
  a. CD4 cell count
  a. CD4 lymphocyte count
  a. neutrophil count (ANC)
  a. plasma concentration (APC)
absonum
  Clostridium a.
absorbent
Absorbine
  A. Antifungal Foot Powder
  A. Jock Itch
  A. Jr. Antifungal
absorptiometry
  dual-energy x-ray a. (DEXA)
absorption
  fluorescent treponemal antibody a.
    (FTA-ABS, FTA-Abs)
abstinens
  Brettanomyces a.
abstriction
ABT-378/r
Abu
  A. Hammad virus (AHV)
  A. Mina virus (ABMV)
aburaviensis
  Streptomyces a.
ABV
  Aransas Bay virus

A

ABVD
Adriamycin, bleomycin, vinblastine,
dacarbazine
abyssalis
Idiomarina a.
abyssi
Pyrodictium a.
ABZ
albendazole
AC
Guaituss AC
Mytussin AC
A-C
Robitussin A-C
AC-17
carbazochrome sodium sulfonate
AC-1 virus
ACA
acrodermatitis chronica atrophicans
Acado virus (ACDV)
acalculous cholecystitis
acanthamebiasis
acanthamebic
a. keratitis
a. uveitis
Acanthamoeba (p)
A. astronyxis
A. castellanii
A. comandoni
A. culbertsoni
disseminated A.
A. griffini
A. hatchetti
A. keratitis
A. lenticulata
A. medium
A. palestinensis
A. polyphaga
A. rhysodes
A. royreba
A. terricola
A. tubiashi
acanthamoebae
Parachlamydia a.
Acanthamoebidae
Acanthaster planci
acanthella
Acanthocephala
A. compressipes
A. confraterna
A. terminalis
A. thomasi

acanthocephala
acanthocephaliasis
Acanthocephalus
A. anguillae
A. bufonis
A. rauschi
Acanthocheilonema (*See* **Mansonella**)
A. viteae
acanthoma
Acanthopodina
acanthopodium, pl. **acanthopodia**
acanthor
acanthosis
extreme a.
acanthotorynus
Anopheles acanthotorynus
acanthuri
Acara virus (ACAV)
acarayense
Simulium a.
Acari
acariasis
demodectic a.
psoroptic a.
sarcoptic a.
acaricide
acarid
acaridan, acaridean, acaridian
acaridiasis
acarine dermatosis
acarinosis
acarodermatitis
acaroid
Acaroidea
acarology
acatalasemia
ACAV
Acara virus
accessory cholera enterotoxin (ace)
accidental
a. host
a. myiasis
a. parasite
accole form
accolens
Corynebacterium a.
accomplice
AccuProbe
AccuProbe *Campylobacter* Culture
AccuProbe *Campylobacter* Culture
Identification Test

NOTES

AccuProbe *(continued)*
    AccuProbe Culture Confirmation
      Test
    AccuProbe *Gonorrhoeae* Culture
      Confirmation
AccuSite
Accu-Staph test
Accutane
ACDV
    Acado virus
ace
    accessory cholera enterotoxin
Acel-Imune
acellular
    a. pertussis vaccine
    a. vaccine
acelom
acelomate
acephaline
acephalocyst
Acephen
acerina
    Centrospora a.
    Mycocentrospora a.
acervulina
    Eimeria a.
Aceta
Acetab
Acet-Am Expectorant
acetamide utilization test
acetamidolyticum
    Mycobacterium fortuitum subsp. *a.*
acetaminophen
    a. and dextromethorphan
    a., dextromethorphan, and
      pseudoephedrine
    phenyltoloxamine,
      phenylpropanolamine, and a.
Acetasol HC Otic
acetate
    cortisone a.
    Cortone A.
    depot medroxyprogesterone a.
    (DMPA)
    Hydrocortone A.
    mafenide a.
    m-cresyl a.
    medroxyprogesterone a. (MPA)
    megestrol a.
    octreotide a.
    paramethasone a.
    retinyl a.
    a. utilization test
Acetazolam
acetazolamide
acetethylicum
    Halanaerobium a.

acetexigens
    Desulfuromonas a.
aceti
    Acetobacter a.
    Anguillula a.
    Turbatrix a.
acetic
    a. acid
    a. acid, propylene glycol diacetate,
      and hydrocortisone
aceticum
    Clostridium a.
aceticus
    Acidilobus a.
acetigena
    Natroniella a.
acetigenum
    Thermoanaerobium a.
acetiphilus
    Denitrovibrio a.
acetireducens
    Clostridium a.
Acetitomaculum ruminis (b)
Acetivibrio (b)
    A. cellulolyticus
    A. cellulosolvens
    A. ethanolgignens
acetivorans
    Desulfurella a.
    Methanosarcina a.
acetoacetate
Acetoanaerobium noterae (b)
Acetobacter (b)
    A. aceti
    A. aceti subsp. *liquefaciens*
    A. aceti subsp. *orleanensis*
    A. aceti subsp. *xylinum*
    A. diazotrophicus
    A. estunensis
    A. europaeus
    A. hansenii
    A. indonesiensis
    A. intermedius
    A. methanolicus
    A. oboediens
    A. orleanensis
    A. pasteurianus
    A. pasteurianus subsp. *ascendens*
    A. pasteurianus subsp. *estunensis*
    A. pasteurianus subsp. *lovaniensis*
    A. pasteurianus subsp. *paradoxus*
    A. peroxydans
    A. pomorum
    A. tropicalis
    A. xylinus subsp. *sucrofermentans*
    A. xylinus subsp. *xylinus*
Acetobacteraceae

Acetobacterium (b)
    A. bakii
    A. carbinolicum
    A. fimetarium
    A. malicum
    A. paludosum
    A. tundrae
    A. wieringae
    A. woodii
acetobutylicum
    Clostridium a.
acetoethylicus
    Halobacteroides a.
    Thermoanaerobacter a.
    Thermobacteroides a.
Acetofilamentum rigidum (b)
Acetogenium kivui (b)
Acetohalobium arabaticum (b)
acetohydroxamic acid
acetoin production test
Acetomicrobium (b)
    A. faecale
    A. flavidum
acetone-alcohol
Acetonema longum (b)
Acetothermus paucivorans (b)
acetotolerans
    Lactobacillus a.
acetowhitening
acetoxidans
    Desulfobacca a.
    Desulfotomaculum a.
    Desulfuromonas a.
Acetoxyl
aceturate
    diminazene a.
acetyl
    a. phosphate
    sulfisoxazole a.
acetylandromedol
acetylcholine
    a. receptor
    a. receptor-inducing activity (ARIA)
acetylcysteine
N-acetylcysteine
acetylenicus
    Pelobacter a.
N-acetylglucosamine
acetylicum
    Brevibacterium a.
    Exiguobacterium a.

ACH
    air changes per hour
Achaetomium (f)
Acherontia atropas virus
Aches-N-Pain
Acheta domestica densovirus (AdDNV)
achlorhydria
achlorophyllous
Acholeplasma (b)
    A. axanthum
    A. brassicae
    A. cavigenitalium
    A. entomophilum
    A. equifetale
    A. florum
    A. granularum
    A. hippikon
    A. laidlawii
    A. modicum
    A. morum
    A. multilocale
    A. oculi
    A. palmae
    A. parvum
    A. phage L2 virus
    A. phage MV L51 virus
    A seiffertii
    A. vituli
Acholeplasmataceae
Acholeplasmatales
Achorion (f)
Achromatium oxaliferum (b)
achromic macular skin lesion
Achromobacter (b)
    A. piechaudii
    A. ruhlandii
    A. xylosoxidans
    A. xylosoxidans subsp. denitrificans
    A. xylosoxidans subsp. xylosoxidans
achromogenes
    Aeromonas salmonicida subsp. a.
    Azotobacter nigricans subsp. a.
    Streptomyces achromogenes subsp. a.
Achromycin
    A. Ophthalmic
    A. Topical
    A. V
acid
    acetic a.
    acetohydroxamic a.
    N-acetylgalactosaminouronic a.

NOTES

acid *(continued)*
    N-acetylmuramic a.
    a. agglutination
    aluminum acetate and acetic a.
    amino a.
    aminosalicylic a.
    arachidonic a.
    ascorbic a.
    azelaic a.
    benzoic acid and salicylic a.
    bichloracetic a.
    boric a.
    a. buffer
    carbolic a.
    casamino a.
    9-*cis*-retinoic a.
    clavulanic a.
    coal tar and salicylic a.
    delta-aminolevulinic a. (ALA)
    deoxyribonucleic a. (DNA)
    domoic a.
    ethylenediaminetetraacetic a.
    a. fastness
    folinic a.
    free fatty a. (FFA)
    fusidic a.
    glacial acetic a.
    hypochlorous a.
    ibotenic a.
    lipoteichoic a.
    liquefied carbolic a.
    a. milieu
    mycolic a.
    mycophenolic a. (MA)
    nalidixic a.
    neomycin/polymyxin/nalidixic a.
    octulosonic a.
    okadaic a.
    omega-3 fatty a.
    oxolinic a.
    paraaminosalicylic a. (PAS)
    peracetic a.
    a. phosphatase test
    phosphonoformic a. (PFA)
    podophyllin and salicylic a.
    a. reflux
    retinoic a.
    ribonucleic a. (RNA)
    ribosomal ribonucleic a. (rRNA)
    salicylic acid and lactic a.
    silver oxide/trichloroisocyanuric a.
    sucrose-phosphate-glutamic a. (SPG)
    sulfur and salicylic a.
    teichoic a.
    tetrodonic a.
    trichloroacetic a.
    tuberculostearic a.

    uric a.
    viral nucleic a.
Acidaminobacter hydrogenoformans (b)
Acidaminococcus fermentans (b)
acidaminophila
    Anaeromusa a.
acidaminophilum
    Eubacterium a.
acidaminovorans
    Dethiosulfovibrio a.
    Selenomonas a.
    Thermanaerovibrio a.
    Thermococcus a.
acid-base balance
acidemia
acid-fast
    a.-f. bacillus (AFB)
    a.-f. bacteria
    a.-f. microscopy
    a.-f. smear
    a.-f. stain
Acidianus (b)
    A. ambivalens
    A. brierleyi
    A. infernus
acidifaciens
    Bacteroides a.
acidificum
    Flavobacterium a.
acidigallici
    Pelobacter a.
acidilactici
    Pediococcus a.
Acidilobus aceticus (b)
Acidimicrobium ferrooxidans (b)
Acidiphilium (b)
    A. acidophilum
    A. aminilyticum
    A. angustum
    A. cryptum
    A. facile
    A. multivorum
    A. organovorum
    A. rubrum
acidiphilum
    Ferroplasma a.
acidipiscis
    Lactobacillus a.
acidipropionici
    Propionibacterium a.
acidiscabies
    Streptomyces a.
acidisoli
    Clostridium a.
Acidisphaera rubrifaciens (b)
Acidithiobacillus (b)
    A. albertensis
    A. caldus

A. *ferrooxidans*
A. *thiooxidans*
acidiurici
    Clostridium a.
Acidobacterium capsulatum (b)
acidocaldarius
    Alicyclobacillus a.
    Bacillus a.
    Sulfolobus a.
Acidocella (b)
    A. *aminolytica*
    A. *facilis*
acidometric test
acidominimus
    Streptococcus a.
Acidomonas methanolica (b)
acidophila
    Rhodopseudomonas a.
acidophilum
    Acidiphilium a.
    Thermoplasma a.
acidophilus
    Hydrogenobacter u.
    Lactobacillus a.
    Sulfobacillus a.
    Thiobacillus a.
acidosis
    lactic a.
aciduterrestris
    Alicyclobacillus a.
    Bacillus a.
Acidothermus cellulolyticus (b)
acidovorans
    Comamonas a.
    Delftia a.
    Pseudomonas a.
    Sporomusa a.
Acidovorax (b)
    A. *anthurii*
    A. *avenae* subsp. *avenae*
    A. *avenae* subsp. *cattleyae*
    A. *avenae* subsp. *citrulli*
    A. *defluvii*
    A. *delafieldii*
    A. *facilis*
    A. *konjaci*
    A. *temperans*
acid-Schiff
    periodic a.-S. (PAS)
    a.-S. reagent
acidurans
    Flavobacterium a.

aciduric
Acinetobacter (b)
    A. *baumannii*
    A. *calcoaceticus*
    A. *calcoaceticus-baumannii* complex
    A. *haemolyticus*
    A. *johnsonii*
    A. *junii*
    A. *lwoffii*
    A. *radioresistens*
acinonychis
    Helicobacter a.
ACIP
    Advisory Committee on Immunization
    Practices
aclometasonc dipropionate cream
Aclovate Topical
acne
    a. rosacea
    a. vulgaris
acneiform pustule
acnes
    Propionibacterium a.
Acnex
acnitis
Acnomel
    A. Acne Mask
    A. BP 5
Acomatacarus australiensis (p)
acoustic nerve damage
acquired
    a. immune deficiency syndrome
    (AIDS)
    a. immunity
    a. immunodeficiency syndrome
    (AIDS)
    a. toxoplasmosis in adults
Acremonium (f)
    A. *alabamense*
    A. *atrogriseum*
    A. *blochii*
    A. *curvulum*
    A. *falciforme*
    A. *hyalinulum*
    A. *kiliense*
    A. *murorum*
    A. *potronii*
    A. *recifei*
    A. *roseogriseum*
    A. *spinosum*
    A. *strictum*
acremonium

NOTES

acridine
  a. ester-labeled nucleic acid probe
  a. orange (AO)
  a. orange stain
Acridine-Orange Leukocyte Cytospin Test
acrimycini
  Streptomyces a.
acrivastine and pseudoephedrine
Acrocarpospora (b)
  A. corrugata
  A. macrocephala
  A. pleiomorpha
acrochordon
acrocyanosis
Acrocylindrium (f)
acrodermatitis
  a. chronica atrophicans (ACA)
  a. continua
  a. enteropathica
  infantile papular a.
  papular a.
  a. papulosa infantum
  a. perstans
  a. pustolosa continua
  a. pustolosis hiemalis
  pustular a.
  recalcitrant pustular a.
  a. vesiculosa tropica
Acrodontium salmoneum (f)
acrogenous
acropetal
Acrophialophora fusispora (f)
acropleurogenous
Acrosporium (f)
Acrostalagmus (*See* **Verticillium alboatrum**)
Acrotheca (*See* **Pleurophragmium**)
acrotheca
acrylicus
  Desulfovibrio a.
ACT
  adenylate cyclase toxin
act
  Infant Formula A.
Actagen
  A. Syrup
  A. Tablet
Actagen-C
ACTG
  AIDS Clinical Trials Group
  ACTG classification
  ACTG staging system
Acthar
ActHIB
ACTH test
Acticin Cream
Acticort Topical

Actidione
Actifed
  A. Allergy Tablet (Day)
  A. Allergy Tablet (Night)
  A. 12 Hour
Actinoalloteichus cyanogriseus (b)
actinobacillosis
Actinobacillus (b)
  A. actinomycetemcomitans
  A. capsulatus
  A. delphinicola
  A. equuli
  A. hominis
  A. indolicus
  A. lignieresii
  A. minor
  A. muris
  A. pleuropneumoniae
  A. porcinus
  A. rossii
  A. scotiae
  A. seminis
  A. succinogenes
  A. suis
  A. ureae
Actinobaculum (b)
  A. schaalii
  A. suis
Actinobispora (b)
  A. alaniniphila
  A. aurantiaca
  A. xinjiangensis
  A. yunnanensis
Actinocorallia (b)
  A. aurantiaca
  A. glomerata
  A. herbida
  A. libanotica
  A. longicatena
actinodermatitis
actinohematin
actinoides
  Thysanosoma a.
Actinokineospora (b)
  A. diospyrosa
  A. globicatena
  A. inagensis
  A. riparia
  A. terrae
Actinomadura (b), (f)
  A. africana
  A. atramentaria
  A. aurantiaca
  A. carminata
  A. citrea
  A. coerulea
  A. coeruleofusca
  A. coeruleoviolacea

A. *cremea* subsp. *cremea*
A. *cremea* subsp. *rifamycini*
A. *echinospora*
A. *fastidiosa*
A. *ferruginea*
A. *fibrosa*
A. *flava*
A. *flexuosa*
A. *formosensis*
A. *fulvescens*
A. *glomerata*
A. *helvata*
A. *hibisca*
A. *kijaniata*
A. *latina*
A. *libanotica*
A. *livida*
A. *longicatena*
A. *longispora*
A. *luteofluorescens*
A. *macra*
A. *madurae*
A. *malachitica*
A. *nitritigenes*
A. *oligospora*
A. *pelletieri*
A. *polychroma*
A. *pusilla*
A. *recticatena*
A. *roseola*
A. *roseoviolacea*
A. *rubra*
A. *rubrobrunea*
A. *rugatobispora*
A. *salmonea*
A. *spadix*
A. *spiralis*
A. *turkmeniaca*
A. *umbrina*
A. *verrucosospora*
A. *vinacea*
A. *viridilutea*
A. *viridis*
A. *yumaensis*
actinomorphic
actinomycelial
Actinomyces (b)
A. *bernardiae*
A. *bovis*
A. *bowdenii*
A. *canis*
A. *catuli*

A. culture
A. *denticolens*
A. *europaeus*
A. *funkei*
A. *georgiae*
A. *gerencseriae*
A. *graevenitzii*
A. *hordeovulneris*
A. *howellii*
A. *humiferus*
A. *hyovaginalis*
A. *israelii*
A. *marimammalium*
A. *meyeri*
A. *naeslundii*
A. *neuii* subsp. *anitratus*
A. *neuii* subsp. *neuii*
A. *odontolyticus*
A. *pyogenes*
A. *radicidentis*
A. *radingae*
A. *slackii*
A. *suimastitidis*
A. *suis*
A. *turicensis*
A. *urogenitalis*
A. *viscosus*
Actinomycetaceae
Actinomycetales
actinomycete
　microaerophilic a.
actinomycetemcomitans
　Actinobacillus a.
　Haemophilus a.
actinomycetes
actinomycetoma
actinomycin D
actinomycoma
actinomycosis
　abdominal a.
　cervicofacial a.
　pelvic a.
　pulmonary a.
　thoracic a.
actinomycotic
　a. lesion
　a. mycetoma
Actinomyxidia
Actinoplanaceae
Actinoplanes (b)
　A. *armeniacus*
　A. *auranticolor*

NOTES

Actinoplanes (continued)
A. *brasiliensis*
A. *caeruleus*
A. *campanulatus*
A. *capillaceus*
A. *consettensis*
A. *cyaneus*
A. *deccanensis*
A. *derwentensis*
A. *digitatis*
A. *durhamensis*
A. *ferrugineus*
A. *friuliensis*
A. *globisporus*
A. *humidus*
A. *italicus*
A. *lobatus*
A. *minutisporangius*
A. *missouriensis*
A. *palleronii*
A. *philippinensis*
A. *rectilineatus*
A. *regularis*
A. *utahensis*
Actinopoda
Actinopolymorpha *singaporensis* (b)
Actinopolyspora (b)
A. *halophila*
A. *iraqiensis*
A. *mortivallis*
Actinopycnidium *caeruleum* (b)
actinosclerus
Hymenobacter a.
Actinosporangium (b)
A. *violaceum*
A. *vitaminophilum*
Actinosynnema (b)
A. *mirum*
A. *pretiosum* subsp. *auranticum*
A. *pretiosum* subsp. *pretiosum*
Actinothyriaceae
Actiprofen
activated
a. partial thromboplastin time (aPTT)
a. sludge
a. sludge method
activation
cell sorting fluorescence a.
activation-induced cell death
activator
urokinase plasminogen a. (uPA)
active
a. brucellosis
a. immunity
a. immunization
a. immunoprophylaxis
a. sarcoidosis

a. sensitization
a. specific immunotherapy (ASI)
a. syphilis
activity
acetylcholine receptor-inducing a. (ARIA)
AM1155 a.
antispirochetal a.
bactericidal a.
cytotoxic T-lymphocyte a.
percent of the periphery that has ciliary a. (PPCA)
serum antibacterial a.
serum inhibitory a.
serum lethal a.
time-dependent bactericidal a.
Acuariidae
Acuariinae
Acuarioidea
acuity
visual a.
aculeate
aculeatus
Aspergillus a.
aculeolatus
Streptomyces a.
acuminata
Dinophysis a.
verruca a.
acuminatum
condyloma a.
Fusarium a.
Trichopyton a.
acupuncture
acute
a. acquired toxoplasmosis
a. adnexitis
a. African sleeping sickness
a. alveolitis
a. amebic dysentery
a. angle-closure glaucoma
a. anterior poliomyelitis
a. atrophic oral candidiasis
a. attack
a. bacterial endocarditis (ABE)
a. bacterial exacerbation
a. bulbar poliomyelitis
a. cholecystitis
a. contagious conjunctivitis
a. cutaneous leishmaniasis
a. diffuse otitis externa
a. disseminated encephalomyelitis
a. enteritis
a. epidemic conjunctivitis
a. epidemic leukoencephalitis
a. exacerbation
a. febrile lymphadenitis
a. febrile tracheobronchitis

a. follicular conjunctivitis
a. glomerulonephritis (AGN)
a. gonococcal salpingitis
a. hemorrhagic encephalitis
a. hemorrhagic glomerulonephritis
a. hemorrhagic leukoencephalitis
a. herpes zoster
a. herpetic gingivostomatitis
a. HIV-1 infection (AHI)
a. infectious mononucleosis
a. infectious nonbacterial
   gastroenteritis
a. inflammation (AI)
a. interstitial nephritis
a. invasive aspergillosis
a. laryngotracheobronchitis
a. malaria
a. mastoiditis
a. meningococcemia
a. monarticular arthritis
a. myositis
a. necrotizing encephalitis
a. necrotizing ulcerative gingivitis
a. neuritis
a. neurologic disease
a. nonbacterial infectious
   gastroenteritis
a. obstructive cholangitis
a. otitis media (AOM)
a. pharyngitis
a. phase reactant
a. phase reaction (APR)
a. physiology and chronic health
   evaluation score (APACHE II
   score)
a. poststreptococcal
   glomerulonephritis
a. primary hemorrhagic
   meningoencephalitis
a. promyelocytic leukemia
a. pulmonary histoplasmosis
a. respiratory disease (ARD)
a. retinal necrosis (ARN)
a. retroviral syndrome (ARS)
a. rheumatic fever (ARF)
a. salivary adenitis
a. scalp cellulitis
a. septicemic melioidosis
a. sinusitis
a. suppurative cholangitis
a. suppurative otitis
a. symmetric polyarthropathy

a. toxic syndrome
a. transverse myelopathy (ATM)
a. trypanosomiasis
a. tubular necrosis (ATN)
a. tubulointerstitial nephritis
a. urethral syndrome
a. viral gastroenteritis
a. viral rhinitis
acycloguanosine
acyclovir crystalluria
acyclovir-resistant
   a.-r. disease
   a.-r. herpes
acyltrehaloses
AD
   adenoid degeneration
adamantanamine hydrochloride
adansonian classification
ADAP
   AIDS Drug Assistance Program
adapalene
ADC
   AIDS dementia complex
ADCC
   antibody-dependent cellular cytotoxicity
   antibody-directed cellular cytotoxicity
addiction
   alcohol a.
   drug a.
AdDNV
   Acheta domestica densovirus
adecarboxylata
   Escherichia a.
   Leclercia a.
adefovir (PMEA)
   a. dipivoxil (ADV)
adelaidensis
   Legionella a.
Adelaide River virus (ARV)
Adeleorina
adematous hyperplasia
Aden
   A. fever
   A. ulcer
adenine
   a. arabinoside (ARA-A)
   a. arabinoside monophosphate (Ara-
      AMP)
adeninivorans
   Arxula a.
adenitis
   acute salivary a.

NOTES

adenitis *(continued)*
    cervical a.
    mesenteric a.
adenoassociated
    a. virus (AAV)
    a. virus 1–5 (AAV 1–5)
    a. virus group
adenocarcinoma
    mucin-secreting a.
adenoeides
    Eimeria a.
adenoidal hypertrophy
adenoid degeneration (AD)
adenoidectomy
adenoiditis
    tuberculous a.
adenolymphangitis
adenolymphocele
adenopathy
    axillary a.
    cervical a.
    generalized a.
    hilar a.
    inguinal a.
    localized a.
    mediastinal a.
    mesenteric a.
    necrotizing inguinal a.
Adenophorasida
Adenophorea
adenosine
    a. deaminase
    a. triphosphatase (ATPase)
    a. triphosphate (ATP)
adenoviral
    a. pneumonia
    a. vector
Adenoviridae
adenoviruria
adenovirus
    avian a.
    Bos a. 1–10 (bos 1–10)
    bovine a. 1–9
    caprine a. 1 (cap1)
    enteric a.
    fowl a. 1
    Galius a. 1–2 (gal 1–2)
    human a. 1–47 (h 1–47)
    mammalian a.
    Meleagris a. 1–3 (mel 1–3)
    Mus a. 1–2 (mus 1–2)
    ovine a. 1–6 (ovi 1–6)
    porcine a. 1–6
    simian a. 1–27 (sim 1–27)
adenovirus-like
adenovirus-mediated gene transfer

adenylate
    a. cyclase
    a. cyclase toxin (ACT)
adetum
    Ancalomicrobium a.
adextromethorphan
adhaerans
    Hyphomonas a.
adhaerens
    Ensifer a.
adhaesiva
    Sphingomonas a.
adherent discharge
adhesin
    pneumococcal surface a. A
adhesion molecule
adhesive arachnoiditis
adiacens
    Abiotrophia a.
    Granulicatella a.
adiaspiromycosis
adiaspore
Adinida (p)
adipica
    Desulfovirga a.
adipose
adiposity
    central a.
adjacens
    Streptococcus a.
adjunctive
adleri
    Mycoplasma a.
Adlone Injection
administration
    Food and Drug A. (FDA)
    Occupational Safety and Health A.
    (OSHA)
admirandus
    Micavibrio a.
admixture
ADNase-B
    antideoxyribonuclease-B
adnexal
    a. abscess
    a. mass
adnexitis
    acute a.
adolescentis
    Bifidobacterium a.
adonitol fermentation test
adoptive
    a. cellular immunotherapy
    a. cellular therapy
    a. immunotherapy (AIT)
adrenal
    a. crisis
    a. insufficiency

Adrenalin Chloride
adrenalitis
    CMV a.
adrenocortical axis testing
adrenocorticotrophin hormone
Adriamycin, bleomycin, vinblastine,
  dacarbazine (ABVD)
adriatica
    Rhodopseudomonas a.
adriaticum
    Rhodovulum a.
adriaticus
    Rhodobacter a.
ADRV
   adult diarrhea rotavirus
adsorbed
    anthrax vaccine, a.
    rabies vaccine a. (RVA)
    a. tetanus toxoid
adsorption
    fluorescent treponemal antibody a.
    (FTA-ABS, FTA-Abs)
ADSV
   Arboledas virus
adult
    acquired toxoplasmosis in a.'s
    a. diarrhea rotavirus (ADRV)
    a. respiratory distress syndrome
    (ARDS)
    a. T-cell leukemia (ATL)
    a. T-cell leukemia/lymphoma
    (ATLL)
    a. T-cell lymphoma (ATL)
    a. tuberculosis
aduncum
    Hysterothylacium a.
ADV
   adefovir dipivoxil
Advanced Formula Oxy Sensitive Gel
advance directive
advanced-stage disease
Advantage 24
Advera
adverse
    a. drug reaction
Advil Cold & Sinus Caplets
Advisory Committee on Immunization
  Practices (ACIP)
AE-2 virus
Aedes
    A. aboriginis
    A. abserratus

A. aegypti
A. africanus
A. albopictus
A. albopictus cell fusing agent
A. aloponotum
A. atlanticus
A. atropalpus
A. aurifer
A. australis
A. berlini
A. bieristatus
A. bimaculatus
A. brelandi
A. burgeri
A. campestris
A. canadensis
A. cantator
A. cataphylla
A. churchillensis
A. cinereus
A. communis
A. dasyorrhus
A. decticus
A. deserticola
A. diantaeus
A. dorsalis
A. dupreei
A. euedes
A. excrucians
A. fitchii
A. flavescens
A. fulvus
A. fulvus fulvus
A. fulvus pallens
A. grossbecki
A. hemiteleus
A. hendersoni
A. hexodontus
A. impiger
A. implicatus
A. increpitus
A. infirmatus
A. intrudens
A. mariae
A. mediovittata
A. melanimon
A. mercurator
A. mitchellae
A. monticola
A. muelleri
A. nevadensis
A. nigripes

NOTES

Aedes *(continued)*
>A. *nigromaculis*
>A. *niphadopsis*
>A. *papago*
>A. *phoeniciae*
>A. *pionips*
>A. *polynesiensis*
>A. *portoricensis*
>A. *provocans*
>A. *pullatus*
>A. *punctodes*
>A. *punctor*
>A. *purpureipes*
>A. *rempeli*
>A. *riparius*
>A. *scapularis*
>A. *schizopinax*
>A. *scutellaris*
>A. *serratus*
>A. *sierrensis*
>A. *sollicitans*
>A. *spencerii*
>A. *squamiger*
>A. *sticticus*
>A. *stimulans*
>A. *taeniorhynchus*
>A. *thelcter*
>A. *thibaulti*
>A. *togoi*
>A. *tormentor*
>A. *tortilis*
>A. *triseriatus*
>A. *trivittatus*
>A. *varipalpus*
>A. *ventrovittis*
>A. *vexans*
>A. *vittatus*
>A. *zammitii*
>A. *zoosophus*

aegaeus
>*Thermococcus* a.

aegypti
>*Aedes* a.

aegyptia
>*Natrialba* a.

Aegyptianella pullorum (b)

aegyptius
>*Haemophilus* a.
>*Haemophilus influenzae* biogroup *a.*
>*Thermicanus* a.

Aeh-2 virus

aerata
>*Microbispora* a.
>*Microbispora rosea* subsp. *a.*

aeria
>*Curvularia lunata* var. *a.*

aerial mycelium

aerius
>*Cryptococcus* a.

aerobactin

aerobe
>gram-negative a.
>gram-positive a.
>obligate a.

aerobia
>*Naegleria* a.

aerobic
>a. bone marrow culture
>a. facultatively anaerobic organism
>a. microbial flora

aerobically

aerobioscope

aerobiosis

aerobiotic

Aerococcus (b)
>A. *christensenii*
>A. *sanguinicola*
>A. *urinae*
>A. *urinaehominis*
>A. *viridans*

Aerococcus-like organism (ALO)

aerocolonigenes
>*Lechevalieria* a. subsp.
> *aerocolonigenes*
>*Saccharothrix* a.
>*Saccharothrix aerocolonigenes*
> subsp. *a.*
>*Streptomyces* a.

aerodenitrificans
>*Microvirgula* a.

aerofaciens
>*Collinsella* a.
>*Eubacterium* a.

aerogen

aerogenes
>*Enterobacter* a.
>*Pasteurella* a.
>*Vibrio* a.

aerogenesis

aerogenic

Aerolate
>A. III
>A. JR, SR

Aeromicrobium (b)
>A. *erythreum*
>A. *fastidiosum*

aeromonad

Aeromonadaceae

Aeromonas (b)
>A. *allosaccharophila*
>A. *bestiarum*
>A. *caviae*
>A. *encheleia*
>A. *enteropelogenes*
>A. *eucrenophila*

A. *hydrophila* subsp. *anaerogenes*
A. *hydrophila* subsp. *hydrophila*
A. *hydrophila* subsp. *proteolytica*
A. *ichthiosmia*
A. *jandaei*
A. *media*
A. *popoffii*
A. *punctata* subsp. *caviae*
A. *punctata* subsp. *punctata*
A. *salmonicida* subsp. *achromogenes*
A. *salmonicida* subsp. *masoucida*
A. *salmonicida* subsp. *pectinolytica*
A. *salmonicida* subsp. *salmonicida*
A. *salmonicida* subsp. *smithia*
A. *schubertii*
A. *sobria*
A. *trota*
A. *veronii*
aeronauticum
    Desulfotomaculum a.
aerophil
aerophila
    Capillaria a.
aerophilic
aerophilum
    Pyrobaculum a.
    Thialkalimicrobium a.
aerophilus
    Thominx a.
aeroplankton
Aeropyrum (b)
    A. *pernix*
aerosaccus
    Enhydrobacter a.
Aeroseb-Dex
Aeroseb-HC Topical
aerosol
    a. transmission of *Mycobacterium*
        tuberculosis
    Virazole A.
aerosolization
aerosolized
    a. interferon-gamma
    a. pentamidine
Aerosporin
aerotolerance
aerotolerans
    Clostridium a.
aeruginosa
    Pseudomonas a.
aeschlimannii
    Rickettsia a.

aespoeensis
    Desulfovibrio a.
Aessosporon (f)
aesta
    Deleya a.
aestiva
    Paregle a.
aestivoautumnal fever
aestivum
    Simulium a.
aestuarianus
    Vibrio a.
aestuarii
    Desulfovibrio desulfuricans subsp. *a.*
    Hyphomicrobium a.
    Prosthecochloris a.
aestus
    Alcaligenes a.
aethiopica
    Leishmania a.
    Leptopsylla a.
AF
    222 AF
    SSD AF
AFA fixative
A.F. Anacin
AFB
    acid-fast bacillus
    AFB culture
afermentans
    Corynebacterium afermentans subsp.
        a.
affinis
    Ixodes a.
    Pegomya a.
affinity chromatography
afghaniensis
    Streptomyces a.
Afipia (b)
    A. *broomeae*
    A. *clevelandensis*
    A. *felis*
aflatoxicosis
aflatoxin
    a. B1
    a. B2
    a. G1
    a. G2
AFLP
    amplicon fragment length polymorphism
AFP
    serum alpha-fetoprotein

NOTES

Africa
  subSaharan A.
africae
  Rickettsia a.
African
  A. American
  A. furuncular myiasis
  A. hemorrhagic fever
  A. histoplasmosis
  A. horse sickness virus (AHSV)
  A. horse sickness virus 1–9
    (AHSV 1–9)
  A. sleeping sickness
  A. tick virus
  A. trypanosomiasis
africana
  Actinomadura a.
  Limnatis a.
  Microtetraspora a.
  Nocardia a.
  Nocardiopsis a.
  Nonomuraea a.
  Spirochaeta a.
  Stenotrophomonas a.
africanum
  Mycobacterium a.
africanus
  Aedes a.
  Desulfovibrio a.
  Linognathus a.
  Paragonimus a.
  Pedobacter a.
  Thermosipho a.
Afrin
  A. Children's Nose Drops
  A. Nasal solution
Afrinol
Aftate
  A. for Athlete's Foot
  A. for Jock Itch
afzelii
  Borrelia a.
AG 1549
Ag
  antigen
  silver
agalactiae
  Mycoplasma a.
  Streptococcus a.
agamete
agamic
agammaglobulinemia
  congenital a.
  X-linked a.
agamocytogeny
Agamofilaria streptocerca
agamogenesis
agamogenetic

agamogony
Agamomermis (p)
agamont
agamous
aganoensis
  Aminobacter a.
agar
  BCYE a.
  bile esculin a.
  bile salt a.
  bismuth sulfite a.
  blood a.
  Bordet-Gengou potato blood a.
  brain-heart infusion a.
  Brucella sheep blood a.
  buffered charcoal yeast extract a.
  camp blood a.
  Centers for Disease Control and
    Prevention anaerobe a.
  charcoal a.
  chocolate a.
  cholera a.
  cornmeal a.
  Czapek solution a.
  deoxycholate a.
  Difco blood a.
  a. diffusion assay
  a. diffusion test
  a. dilution test
  a. disk elution
  EMB a.
  Endo a.
  eosin methylene blue a.
  fastidious anaerobe a.
  a. gel diffusion
  a. gel diffusion technique
  Hektoen a.
  kanamycin-vancomycin laked
    blood a.
  Kirby-Bauer a.
  KVLB a.
  Lowenstein-Jensen a.
  MacConkey a.
  Mueller-Hinton a.
  mycobiotic a.
  mycosel a.
  Novy and MacNeal blood a.
  nutrient a.
  oatmeal-tomato paste a.
  rice-Tween a.
  Sabouraud a.
  Schaedler a.
  serum a.
  TCBS a.
  thiosulfate citrate bile salts
    sucrose a.
  Tindale a.
  triple sugar iron a.

A

trypticase soy a.
TSI a.
yeast extract a.
agaradhaerens
    Bacillus a.
agaric
    deadly a.
    fly a.
Agaricaceae
Agaricales
agarici
    Pseudomonas a.
agaricidamnosum
    Janthinobacterium a.
Agaricus (f)
    A. arvensis
    A. bisporus
    A. meleagris
agarolyticus
    Alterococcus a.
agarose gel electrophoresis
agarovorans
    Cytophaga a.
    Marinilabilia a.
agassizii
    Mycoplasma a.
agency
    Environmental Protection A. (EPA)
    A. for Health Care Policy and
      Research
    A. for Toxic Substances and
      Disease Registry, Airborne
      Pathogens
Agenerase
agent
    Aedes albopictus cell fusing a.
    Amulree a.
    anticholinergic a.
    antidiarrheal a.
    antimalarial a.
    antimicrobial a.
    antimotility a.
    antineoplastic a.
    antipyretic/analgesic a.
    antiretroviral a.
    caustic a.
    chemofluorescent optical
      brightening a.
    chemotherapeutic a.
    cockle a.
    dideoxynucleoside a.
    Ditchling a.

Eaton a. (*See Mycoplasma pneumoniae*)
etiologic a.
F a.
fertility a.
filterable a.
foamy a.
Hawaii a.
lipid-lowering a.
luminal a.
Marin County a.
Montgomery County a.
Moorcroft a.
narrow-spectrum a.
nephrotoxic a.
nonsteroidal antiinflammatory a.
  (NSAIA)
Norwalk a.
Norwalk-like a.
Otofuke a.
Paramatta a.
picorna-parvo-like a.
Pittsburgh pneumonia a.
preferred a.
reovirus-like a.
Sapporo a.
sclerosing a.
Snow Mountain a.
sulfonylurea a.
Taunton a.
TRIC a.
viral a.
virus-like infectious a. (VLIA)
Wollan a.
agglomerans
    Enterobacter a.
    Pantoea a.
agglutinate
agglutinating antibody
agglutination
    acid a.
    bacteriogenic a.
    cold a.
    cross a.
    Cryptococcus latex antigen a.
    diagnostic particle a.
    false a.
    group a.
    immune a.
    indirect a.
    lactoferrin latex bead a. (LFLA)
    latex a. (LA)

NOTES

agglutination *(continued)*
    latex particle a. (LPA)
    mixed a.
    monoclonal antibody-based latex a. (MAb-LA)
    nonimmune a.
    passive a.
    reversed passive latex a.
    reversed passive latex particle a. (RPLA)
    spontaneous a.
    tube a. (TA)
    ultrasound-enhanced latex a.
    ultrasound-enhanced particle a.
agglutinative
agglutinin
    blood group a.
    chief a.
    cold a.
    cross-reacting a.
    febrile a.
    flagellar a.
    group a.
    H a.
    immune a.
    incomplete a.
    major a.
    minor a.
    O a.
    partial a.
    plant a.
    saline a.
    serum a.
    somatic a.
    warm a.
    Yersinia pseudotuberculosis a.
aggregans
    Chloroflexus a.
    Eubacterium a.
    Flexibacter a.
    Methanocorpusculum a.
    Methanogenium a.
    Thermococcus a.
    Thermosphaera a.
aggregata
    Stappia a.
aggregate
    IgG-RF-complement a.
aggregation substance
aggregatus
    Blastobacter a.
    Blastococcus a.
aggressive monoclonal lymphoma
agile
    Anaerofilum a.
    Methylomicrobium a.
agilis
    Arthrobacter a.

    Azomonas a.
    Giardia a.
    Lactobacillus a.
    Methylobacter a.
    Micrococcus a.
    Xanthobacter a.
aging
    clonal a.
agitata
    Dechloromonas a.
Agitococcus lubricus (b)
AGN
    acute glomerulonephritis
    poststreptococcal AGN
AgNO$_3$
    silver nitrate
agonist-antagonist
Agonomycetaceae
Agonomycetales
agouti
agranular PMN
agranulocytosis
agreste
    Thermocrispum a.
agrestis
    Buttiauxella a.
agri
    Bacillus a.
    Brevibacillus a.
    Mycobacterium a.
Agrobacterium (b)
    A. *atlanticum*
    A. *ferrugineum*
    A. *gelatinovorum*
    A. *larrymoorei*
    A. *meteori*
    A. *radiobacter*
    A. *rhizogenes*
    A. *rubi*
    A. *stellulatum*
    A. *tumefaciens*
    A. *vitis*
Agrococcus (b)
    A. *citreus*
    A. *jenensis*
Agromonas oligotrophica (b)
Agromyces (b)
    A. *bracchium*
    A. *cerinus* subsp. *cerinus*
    A. *cerinus* subsp. *nitratus*
    A. *fucosus* subsp. *fucosus*
    A. *fucosus* subsp. *hippuratus*
    A. *luteolus*
    A. *mediolanus*
    A. *ramosus*
    A. *rhizosphaerae*
ags
Aguacate virus (AGUV)

A

AGUV
  Aguacate virus
AG1746V
AHI
  acute HIV-1 infection
Ahrensia (b)
    A. kielensis
AHSV
  African horse sickness virus
AHSV 1–9
  African horse sickness virus 1–9
AHV
  Abu Hammad virus
AI
  acute inflammation
aichiense
    Mycobacterium a.
aichiensis
    Gordonia a.
    Rhodococcus a.
Aid
    Congest A.
aid-in-dying
AIDS
  acquired immune deficiency syndrome
  acquired immunodeficiency syndrome
    AIDS blood culture
    AIDS cholangiopathy
    clinical AIDS
    AIDS Clinical Trials Group
      (ACTG)
    AIDS Clinical Trials Group staging
      system
    AIDS dementia complex (ADC)
    dementia complex of AIDS
    AIDS Drug Assistance Program
      (ADAP)
    full-blown AIDS
    AIDS Link to Intravenous
      Experiences (ALIVE)
    AIDS Link to Intravenous
      Experiences study
    AIDS lymphoma
    person with AIDS (PWA)
    AIDS registry
    AIDS Vaccine Evaluation Group
      (AVEG)
    AIDS wasting syndrome (AWS)
AIDS-associated
    AIDS-a. BCBL
    AIDS-a. lymphoma
AIDS-defining illness

AIDS-related
    AIDS-r. complex (ARC)
    AIDS-r. cryptococcosis
    AIDS-r. Kaposi sarcoma
    AIDS-r. lymphoma
    AIDS-r. virus (ARV)
AIHA
  autoimmune hemolytic anemia
air
    a. changes per hour (ACH)
    a. embolism
    a. filtration machine
    high-efficiency particulate a.
      (HEPA)
airborne
    a. spore
    a. transmission
Airbron
air-conditioner lung
Airet
airport malaria
airspace ground-glass infiltrate
AIT
  adoptive immunotherapy
ajelloi
    Keratinomyces a.
    Trichophyton a.
Ajellomyces (f)
    A. capsulatus
    A. dermatitidis
AK
  amebic keratitis
Akabane virus (AKAV)
akagii
    Clostridium a.
akamushi
    a. disease
akari
    Rickettsia a.
AKAV
  Akabane virus
AK-Chlor Ophthalmic
AK-Cide Ophthalmic
akhurstii
    Photorhabdus luminescens subsp. *a.*
akinetic mutism
AK-Mycin
Akne-Mycin Topical
AK-Neo-Dex Ophthalmic
AK-Poly-Bac Ophthalmic
AK-Spore
    AK-S. H.C. Ophthalmic Ointment

NOTES

AK-Spore *(continued)*
  AK-S. H.C. Ophthalmic Suspension
  AK-S. H.C. Otic
  AK-S. Ophthalmic Solution
AK-Sulf Ophthalmic
Ak-Tate
AKTob Ophthalmic
AK-Tracin Ophthalmic
AK-Trol
ALA
  delta-aminolevulinic acid
  ALA porphyrin test
alabamense
  Acremonium a.
alabamensis
  Eimeria a.
alachua
  Culicoides a.
Ala-Cort Topical
alactolyticum
  Eubacterium a.
alactolyticus
  Pseudoramibacter a.
  Streptococcus a.
alactosus
  Lactobacillus casei subsp. a.
Alajuela virus
alanine
  a. aminotransferase (ALT)
  a. aminotransferase level
  a. transaminase
alaniniphila
  Actinobispora a.
alanosinicus
  Streptomyces a.
Alaria (p)
  A. americana
  A. arisaemoides
  A. marcianae
Alariinae
Ala-Scalp Topical
alaskensis
  Culicoides a.
  Culiseta a.
  Sphingomonas a.
alataceus
  Aspergillus a.
alba
  Amanita phalloides var. a.
  Amycolatopsis a.
  Bactoderma a.
  Beggiatoa a.
  Brevundimonas a.
  Nocardiopsis a.
  Planomonospora a.
  Thermobifida a.
  Thermomonospora a.

albaduncus
  Streptomyces a.
albatum
  Kibdelosporangium a.
albendazole (ABZ)
albensis
  Prevotella a.
  Vibrio a.
Albenza
albertensis
  Acidithiobacillus a.
albertis
  Thiobacillus a.
albertoi
  Anopheles evansae a.
albiaxialis
  Streptomyces a.
Albibacter methylovorans (b)
albicans
  Candida a.
  Procandida a.
  Syringospora a.
albiceps
  Chrysomyia a.
albicinctum
  Simulium a.
albida
  Kutzneria a.
  Lentzea a.
  Spirillospora a.
albidocapillata
  Lentzea a.
  Saccharothrix a.
albidochromogenes
  Streptomyces a.
albidoflavus
  Amycolatopsis a.
  Streptomyces a.
albidosimilis
  Cryptococcus a.
albidum
  Brevibacterium a.
  Curtobacterium a.
  Streptosporangium a.
albidus
  Cryptococcus a.
  Cryptococcus albidus var. a.
albilineans
  Xanthomonas a.
albilineatum
  Simulium a.
albimanus
  Anopheles a.
albipictus
  Dermacentor a.
albipuncta
  Hydrotaea a.

albipunctata
> Clogmia a.

albipunctatus
> Telmatoscopus a.

albireticuli
> Streptomyces a.
> Streptoverticillium a.

albirubida
> Nocardiopsis dassonvillei subsp. a.

albitarsis
> Anopheles a.
> Anopheles albitarsis a.

ALBI trial

alboatrum
> Verticillium a.

albofaciens
> Streptomyces a.

alboflavus
> Streptomyces a.

albogriseolus
> Streptomyces a.

albohirtum
> Dermolepida a.

albolongus
> Streptomyces a.

albomaculatus
> Haemagogus a.

albomarginata
> Candida a.

alboniger
> Streptomyces a.

albopictum
> Simulium a.

albopictus
> Aedes a.

alboraceum
> Melittangium a.

alborubida
> Nocardiopsis a.

albospinus
> Streptomyces a.

albosporeus
> Streptomyces a.
> Streptomyces albosporeus subsp. a.

albosporum
> Streptoverticillium cinnamoneum
> subsp. a.

albosporus
> Streptomyces cinnamoneus subsp. a.

alboverticillatum
> Streptoverticillium a.

alboverticillatus
> Streptomyces a.

albovinaceus
> Streptomyces a.

alboviridis
> Streptomyces a.

Albuginaceae

albulus
> Streptomyces a.

album
> Cylindrocarpon a.
> Engyodontium a.
> Methylomicrobium a.
> Streptosporangium a.
> Streptoverticillium a.
> Thermoleophilum a.

albumin
> ampicillin-human serum a. (AMP-
> HSA)
> serum a.

albumin-to-globulin ratio

albuminuria

albus
> Arthrobacter a.
> Bulleromyces a.
> lichen a.
> Marinococcus a.
> Methylobacter a.
> Nocardioides a.
> Ruminococcus a.
> Streptomyces albus subsp. a.

albuterol

alcalescens
> Veillonella a.
> Veillonella alcalescens subsp. a.

alcalifaciens
> Providencia a.

Alcaligenaceae

Alcaligenes (b)
> A. aestus
> A. aquamarinus
> A. cupidus
> A. defragrans
> A. denitrificans
> A. eutrophus
> A. faecalis subsp. *faecalis*
> A. faecalis subsp. *homari*
> A. latus
> A. pacificus
> A. paradoxus
> A. piechaudii
> A. ruhlandii

NOTES

Alcaligenes (*continued*)
   A. *venustus*
   A. *xylosoxidans*
   A. *xylosoxidans* subsp. *denitrificans*
alcaligenes
   Pseudomonas a.
alcaliphila
   Pseudomonas a.
alcaliphilum
   Halanaerobium a.
   Methanobacterium a.
alcaliphilus
   Paracoccus a.
   Thermococcus a.
alcalophilus
   Bacillus a.
Alcanivorax borkumensis (b)
alclometasone
alcohol
   a. addiction
   ethyl a.
   isopropyl a.
   methyl a.
   polyvinyl a. (PVA)
alcohol-glycerin fixative
alcohol-induced cardiomyopathy
alcoholivorans
   Desulfovibrio a.
alcoholophila
   Pichia a.
Alcomicin
Aldara
aldolase
aldosterone biosynthesis
aldovae
   Yersinia a.
aldrichii
   Clostridium a.
Alectorobius (p) (*See* **Ornithodoros**)
Alenquer virus (ALEV)
aleurioconidium
aleuriospore
Aleurisma (*See* **Trichoderma**)
Aleurostrongylus (p)
ALEV
   Alenquer virus
Aleve
alexanderi
   Culicoides a.
   Leptospira a.
alfa
   epoetin a.
alfa-2a
   interferon a.-2a
alfa-2b
   interferon a.-2b
   recombinant interferon a.-2b

alfacon-1
   interferon a.
Alfamovirus (v)
alfa-n3
   interferon a.-n3
Alfate
Alferon
   A. N
alfreddugesi
   Eutrombicula a.
   Trombicula a.
Alfuy virus
ALG
   antilymphocytic globulin
alga, pl. **algae**
   blue-green algae
   planktonic algae
   Shewanella algae
algal
algens
   Gelidibacter a.
algerae
   Nosema a.
algicola
   Cellulophaga a.
   Roseobacter a.
   Ruegeria a.
algidicarnis
   Clostridium a.
algidixylanolyticum
   Clostridium a.
algid malaria
algidus
   Lactobacillus a.
alginate
   calcium a.
alginolytica
   Beneckea a.
alginolyticus
   Bacillus a.
   Paenibacillus a.
   Vibrio a.
algorithm
Alicyclobacillus (b)
   A. *acidocaldarius*
   A. *acidoterrestris*
   A. *cycloheptanicus*
   A. *hesperidum*
A-like non-A non-B hepatitis
alimentarium
   Brachybacterium a.
alimentarius
   Lactobacillus a.
aliphatic
aliquot
alirioi
   Simulium a.
Alishewanella fetalis (b)

alitretinoin gel
ALIVE
   AIDS Link to Intravenous Experiences
   ALIVE study
alkalescens
   Mycoplasma a.
Alkalibacterium olivapovliticus (b)
alkalica
   Spirochaeta a.
alkalicus
   Nitrobacter a.
alkaline
   a. buffer
   a. phosphatase
   a. tide
alkaline-encrusted cystitis
alkalinization
alkaliphilum
   Desulfotomaculum a.
Alkaliphilus transvaalensis (b)
alkaloid
   pyrrolizidine a.
alkalosis
   respiratory a.
alkanivorans
   Gordonia a.
alkanoclasticus
   Planococcus a.
Alka-Seltzer Plus Flu & Body Aches
   Non-Drowsy Liqui-Gels
alkenifer
   Paracoccus a.
allantoin
Allantospora (*See **Cylindrocarpon***)
alleghenense
   Spiroplasma a.
Allegra
allele
allelocatalysis
allelocatalytic
Allercon tablet
Allerdryl
Allerest
   A. 12 Hour Nasal solution
   A. Maximum Strength
Allerfrin
   A. Syrup
   A. Tablet
   A. w/Codeine
Allergan Ear Drops

allergic
   a. bronchopulmonary aspergillosis
   (ABPA)
   a. bronchopulmonary fusariosis
   a. conjunctivitis
   a. laryngeal edema
   a. reaction
   a. rhinitis
allerginae
   Cytophaga a.
allergy
   Benylin for A.'s
   drug a.
   A. Elixir
   skin test for penicillin a.
Allerphed syrup
Allescheria (*See **Pseudallescheria***)
Allexivirus (v)
alliaceus
   Aspergillus a.
alligatoris
   Mycoplasma a.
allii
   Embellisia a.
alloantibody
Allochromatium (b)
   A. minutissimum
   A. vinosum
   A. warmingii
Allocreadiidae
Allocreadioidea
Allodermanyssus sanguineus
allogeneic BMT
allograft reaction
Alloiococcus otitis (b)
Allolevivirus (v)
Allomonas enterica (b)
allopurinol
Allorhizobium undicola (b)
allosaccharophila
   Aeromonas a.
allotransplantation
Almeida disease
Almeirim virus (AMRV)
Almpiwar virus (ALMV)
almquistii
   Streptomyces a.
ALMV
   Almpiwar virus
alni
   Amycolata a.
   Brenneria a.

NOTES

alni (continued)
> *Erwinia a.*
> *Frankia a.*
> *Pseudonocardia a.*

ALO
> *Aerococcus*-like organism

alocis
> *Filifactor a.*
> *Fusobacterium a.*

Alocort
Alomide Ophthalmic
alopecia
aloponotum
> *Aedes a.*

Alora Transdermal
alpha
> a. antigen
> a. gene
> a. hemolysin
> a. hemolysis
> a. hemolytic streptococcus
> interferon a.
> a. 1-proteinase inhibitor
> recombinant tumor necrosis
> factor a. (rTNFα)
> *Streptomyces griseus* subsp. *a.*
> thymosin a.

2-alpha
> IFN-alpha 2-a.
> interferon-alpha 2-alpha
> interferon-alpha 2-a. (IFN-alpha 2-
> alpha)

alpha-agonist
alpha₁-antitrypsin deficiency
alpha-carotene
Alphacryptovirus (v)
alpha-fetoprotein
> serum a.-f. (AFP)

alpha-galactosidase test
Alphaherpesvirinae
alpha-IFN
> alpha-interferon

alpha-interferon (alpha-IFN)
alpha-2-interferon
alpha-lipoproteinase
Alphanodavirus (v)
Alpharetrovirus (v)
alpha-thalassemia
alpha-tocopherol
alpha-toxin
Alphatrex Topical
Alphaviridae
Alphavirus (v)
alphavirus
alpica
> *Balneatrix a.*

alpicalis
> *Culex a.*

alpinus
> *Microanthomyces a.*

alprazolam
ALPS
> autoimmune lymphoproliferative
> syndrome

alsatica
> *Bartonella a.*

Alsiphene
ALT
> alanine aminotransferase
> serum ALT

Altamira virus (ALTV)
altered mentation
alterfunditum
> *Carnobacterium a.*

alternans
> pulsus a.

Alternaria (f)
> *A. alternata*
> *A. chartarum*
> *A. chlamydospora*
> *A. dianthicola*
> *A. geophilia*
> *A. infectoria*
> *A. longipes*
> *A. mold*
> *A. stemphyloides*
> *A. tenuissima*

alternata
> *Alternaria a.*
> *Psychoda a.*

alternative
Alterococcus agarolyticus (b)
Alteromonas (b)
> *A. atlantica*
> *A. aurantia*
> *A. carrageenovora*
> *A. citrea*
> *A. colwelliana*
> *A. communis*
> *A. denitrificans*
> *A. distincta*
> *A. elyakovii*
> *A. espejiana*
> *A. fuliginea*
> *A. haloplanktis*
> *A. hanedai*
> *A. luteoviolacea*
> *A. macleodii*
> *A. nigrifaciens*
> *A. phage PM2 virus*
> *A. putrefaciens*
> *A. rubra*
> *A. tetraodonis*
> *A. undina*
> *A. vaga*

althioticus
    Streptomyces a.
altroolivaceus
ALTV
    Altamira virus
alum
    ammonium a.
    potassium a.
aluminum
    a. acetate and acetic acid
    a. hydroxide
ALV
    avian leukosis virus
alvei
    Bacillus a.
    Hafnia a.
    Mycobacterium a.
    Paenibacillus a.
alveolar
    a. cyst disease
    a. hydatid cyst
    a. hydatid disease
    a. macrophage
    a. proteinosis
alveolar-arterial
    a.-a. oxygen gradient
alveolar-to-arterial oxygen difference
    ($D_{A-a}O_2$)
alveolitis
    acute a.
    cryptogenic fibrosing a.
alvi
    Mycoplasma a.
alvinipulli
    Brachyspira a.
    Serpulina a.
ALV-related virus
Alysiella (b)
    A. filiformis
Alzheimer disease
AM1155 activity
amakusaensis
    Streptomyces a.
amalonatica
    Levinea a.
amalonaticus
    Citrobacter a.
Amanita (f)
    A. bisporigera
    A. cothurnata
    A. muscaria var. formosa

    A. muscaria var. muscaria
    A. ocreata
    A. pantherina
    A. phalloides
    A. phalloides var. alba
    A. suballiacea
    A. tenuifolia
    A. verna
    A. virosa
Amanitaceae
amanitin
amantadine hydrochloride
amapae
    Candida a.
Amapari virus (AMAV)
amarae
    Gordonia a.
    Nocardia a.
Amaricoccus (b)
    A. kaplicensis
    A. macauensis
    A. tamworthensis
    A. veronensis
amastigote
    a. laden
    a. proliferation
Amauroascus (f)
AMAV
    Amapari virus
amazonense
    Azospirillum a.
amazonensis
    Leishmania a.
    Shewanella a.
amazonicum
    Microsporum a.
    Simulium a.
amazonicus
    Goeldichironomus a.
amazonius
    Culicoides a.
AmB
    L AmB
        liposomal amphotericin B
Ambenyl Cough syrup
Ambi 10
Ambien
ambifaria
    Burkholderia a.
ambigua
    Gyromitra a.

NOTES

ambiguus
    Muscor a.
    Passalurus a.
AmBisome
ambivalens
    Acidianus a.
    Desulfurolobus a.
Amblyomma (p)
    A. americanum
    A. brasiliense
    A. cajennense
    A. hebraeum
    A. maculatum
    A. striatum
    A. variegatum
Amblyomminae
Ambrosiozyma cicatricosa (f) (*See* **Pichia**)
ambulatory patient
AMBV
    Anhembi virus
amcinonide
Amcort Injection
amdinocillin
ameba, amoeba, pl. **amebae**
    soil a.
amebacide
amebiasis, amoebiasis
    cutaneous a.
    a. cutis
    extraintestinal a.
    hepatic a.
    invasive a.
    pleuropulmonary a.
    a. serological test
amebic
    a. brain abscess
    a. colitis
    a. dysentery
    a. keratitis (AK)
    a. liver abscess
    a. meningoencephalitis
    a. pseudotumor
    a. vaginitis
amebicidal
amebicide
amebiform
amebiosis
amebism
amebocyte
ameboid
ameboma, amoeboma
amebula
amebule
amelibiosum
    Leuconostoc a.
amelioration
amenorrhea

America
    Society for Healthcare
      Epidemiology of A. (SHEA)
    Society for Hospital Epidemiology
      of A.
Americaine
American
    A. eel virus (EVA)
    A. leishmaniasis
    A. tarantula
    A. trypanosomiasis
    A. Type Culture Collection
      (ATCC)
americana
    Alaria a.
    Cochliomyia a.
    Cuterebra a.
    Ewingella a.
    Haematopota a.
    Heterobilharzia a.
    Phialophora a.
    Uncinaria a.
americanum
    Amblyomma a.
    Pedomicrobium a.
americanus
    Necator a.
    Syrphus a.
amerism
ameristic
Amersol
Ames test
A-methaPred Injection
amethystogenes
    Microbispora a.
    Streptosporangium a.
    Streptosporangium amethystogenes
      subsp. *a.*
Amgenal Cough syrup
AMI
    antibody-mediated immunity
amicalis
    Gordonia a.
amicrobic
amictus
    Anopheles a. amictus
amide
    pyrazinoic acid a.
amidon fermentation test
Amidostomum (p) (*See* **Strongylus**
  vulgaris)
amifloxacin
amikacin
    a. level
    a. sulfate
Amikin Injection
aminacrine hydrochloride

amine
    a. odor
    a. test
    vasoactive a.
aminilyticum
    Acidiphilium a.
amino
    a. acid
    a. acid sequence variation
    a. penicillin
Aminobacter (b)
    A. aganoensis
    A. aminovorans
    A. niigataensis
Aminobacterium (b)
    A. colombiense
    A. mobile
aminobenzylpenicillin
aminocyclitol
3′-amino-3′-deoxythymidine (AMT)
aminoglycoside
aminolytica
    Acidocella a.
Aminomonas paucivorans (b)
aminopenicillin
aminopeptidase
    leucine a. (LAP)
aminophilum
    Clostridium a.
aminophilus
    Desulfovibrio a.
    Paracoccus a.
    Streptomyces a.
aminophylline
aminosalicylate sodium
aminosalicylic acid
aminotransferase
    alanine a. (ALT)
    aspartate a. (AST)
    serum alanine a.
    serum aspartate a.
aminovalericum
    Clostridium a.
aminovorans
    Aminobacter a.
    Methylobacterium a.
    Paracoccus a.
    Pseudomonas a.
amiodarone HCl
Ami-Tex LA
amitriptyline
amlexanox

ammoniagenes
    Brevibacterium a.
    Corynebacterium a.
Ammonifex degensii (b)
Ammoniphilus (b)
    A. oxalaticus
    A. oxalivorans
ammonium
    a. alum
    a. urate
amnesic shellfish poisoning (ASP)
amnigena
    Desulforhabdus a.
amnigenus
    Enterobacter a.
amniocentesis
amnionitis
amniotic
    a. fluid infection
    a. membrane
amodiaquine
Amoeba (*See Entamoeba*)
amoeba (*var. of* ameba)
amoebapore
amocbiasis (*var. of* amebiasis)
Amoebida
Amoebobacter (b)
    A. pedioformis
    A. pendens
    A. purpureus
    A. roseus
amoeboma (*var. of* ameboma)
Amoebotaenia sphenoides (p)
amorphae
    Mesorhizobium a.
Amorphosporangium (b)
    A. auranticolor
    A. globisporum
amorphous material
amoxicillin
    a. and clavulanate potassium
    a. trihydrate
Amoxil
Amp
    Jaa A.
ampelina
    Xanthomonas a.
ampelinus
    Xylophilus a.
amphetamine
Amphibacillus (b)
    A. xylanus

NOTES

amphid
Amphimerus pseudofelineus
amphistome
amphixenosis
Amphocin
ampholytic compound
Amphotec
amphotericin
    a. B
    a. B cholesteryl sulfate complex
    a. B colloidal dispersion
    a. B colloid dispersion (ABCD)
    a. B (conventional)
    a. B deoxycholate
    a. B level
    a. B lipid complex injection
    a. B liposomal
    a. B liposomal formulation
    a. B lozenge
    a. B oral suspension
    liposomal a. B (L AmB)
AMP-HSA
    ampicillin-human serum albumin
ampicillin
    a. and probenecid
    a. sodium
    sulbactam and a.
    a. and sulbactam
    a. trihydrate
ampicillin-human serum albumin (AMP-HSA)
Ampicin Sodium
Ampilean
amplication
    transcription-mediated a. (TMA)
amplicon fragment length polymorphism (AFLP)
Amplicor
    A. *Chlamydia trachomatis* test
    A. HCV Detection Kit
    A. HIV-1 Monitor Ultra Sensitive Specimen Preparation Protocol Ultra Direct Assay
    A. *Mycobacterium tuberculosis* test
    A. PCR
    A. testing
amplification
    a. assay
    nucleic acid a.
    nucleic acid sequence-band a. (NASBA)
    nucleic acid sequence-based a. (NASBA, NAS-BA)
    Qbeta probe a.
    a. refractory mutation system (ARMS)
    sequence-independent single primer a. (SISPA)
    spin a.
    strand displacement a. (SDA)
    transcription-based a.
Amplified *Mycobacterium tuberculosis* Direct Test
amplifier host
amprenavir (APV)
ampulla, pl. ampullae
Ampullariella (b)
    A. campanulata
    A. digitata
    A. lobata
    A. regularis
amputation
AMRV
    Almeirim virus
Amsacta moorei
Amsel criteria
amstelodami
    Eurotium a.
AMT
    3′-amino-3′-deoxythymidine
AMTV
    Arumowot virus
Amulree agent
Amycolata (b)
    A. alni
    A. autotrophica
    A. hydrocarbonoxydans
    A. saturnea
Amycolatopsis (b)
    A. alba
    A. albidoflavus
    A. azurea
    A. coloradensis
    A. fastidiosa
    A. japonica
    A. mediterranei
    A. methanolica
    A. orientalis subsp. *lurida*
    A. orientalis subsp. *orientalis*
    A. rubida
    A. rugosa
    A. sacchari
    A. sulphurea
    A. thermoflava
amycolatum
    Corynebacterium a.
amygdali
    Pseudomonas a.
amyl
    A. Nitrate Vaporole
    a. nitrite
    A. Nitrite Aspirols
amylase
    pancreatic a.
    salivary a.

amyloidosis
    renal a.
amylolentus
    Cryptococcus a.
amyloliquefaciens
    Bacillus a.
amylolytica
    Succinimonas a.
amylolyticus
    Bacillus a.
    Lactobacillus a.
    Natronococcus a.
    Paenibacillus a.
amylophilus
    Bacteroides a.
    Lactobacillus a.
    Ruminobacter a.
amylovora
    Erwinia a.
amylovorum
    Treponema a.
amylovorus
    Lactobacillus a.
amyotrophic lateral sclerosis
AN25S-1 virus
ANA
    antinuclear antibody
    ANA test
Anabaena
anabolic
    a. block
    a. steroid
Anacin
    A.F. A.
Anacin-3
Anadrol
anadromous
Anaeroarcus burkinensis (b)
Anaerobacter polyendosporus (b)
Anaerobaculum thermoterrenum (b)
anaerobe
    facultative a.
    obligate a.
anaerobic
    a. bacteria
    a. bacterial arthritis
    a. cellulitis
    a. culture
    a. infection
    a. microbial flora
    a. susceptibility testing
anaerobically

anaerobiosis
Anaerobiospirillum (b)
    A. succiniciproducens
    A. thomasii
anaerobium
    Asteroleplasma a.
anaerobius
    Azoarcus a.
    Peptostreptococcus a.
    Staphylococcus aureus subsp. *a.*
Anaerobranca (b)
    A. gottschalkii
    A. horikoshii
Anaerococcus (b)
    A. hydrogenalis
    A. lactolyticus
    A. octavius
    A. prevotii
    A. tetradius
    A. vaginalis
Anaerofilum (b)
    A. agile
    A. pentosovorans
anaerogenes
    Aeromonas hydrophila subsp. *a.*
anaerogenic
Anaeromusa acidaminophila (b)
anaerophyte
Anaeroplasma (b)
    A. abactoclasticum
    A. bactoclasticum
    A. intermedium
    A. varium
Anaeroplasmataceae
Anaeroplasmatales
Anaerorhabdus furcosa (b)
Anaerosinus glycerini (b)
Anaerovibrio (b)
    A. burkinabensis
    A. glycerini
    A. lipolyticus
Anaerovorax odorimutans (b)
anal
    a. cancer
    a. crypt
    a. fissure
    a. HPV infection
    a. intraepithelial neoplasia
    a. sphincter swab
    a. squamous intraepithelial lesion
    a. stenosis
    a. tuberculosis

NOTES

analgesia
analgesic
analgesic-antipyretic
anal human papilloma virus infection
analog, analogue
    BrdU nucleoside a.
    bromodeoxyuridine nucleoside a.
    nucleoside a.
    nucleotide a.
    thymidine a.
analogous
analysis, pl. analyses
    directed heteroduplex a. (DHDA)
    DNA hybridization a.
    dual-fluorescence a.
    electrophoretic mobility shift a.
    (EMSA)
    fatty acid a.
    flow cytometric a.
    heteroduplex a.
    immunofluorescence a.
    isoenzyme a.
    mass spectrometric a.
    multilocus enzyme
      electrophoresis a.
    nucleic acid hybridization a.
    nucleotide sequence a.
    PCR fragment a.
    PCR-RFLP a.
    peripheral blood lymphocyte a.
    plasmid a.
    plasmid pattern a. (PPA)
    quantitative immunoglobulin a.
    radioimmunoprecipitation a.
    restriction endonuclease a. (REA,
      READ)
    restriction enzyme a. (REA)
    reverse transcriptase primer
      extension a.
    rRNA sequence a.
    RTPE a.
    SAS software for statistical a.
    sequencing a.
    Southern blot a.
    spinal fluid a.
    videomicroscope image a.
analyzer
    Electra 1000C coagulation a.
    Malvern a.
anamariae
    Simulium a.
Anamine syrup
anamnestic
anamorph
ananas
    Erwinia a.
ananassae
    Drosophila a.

ananatis
    Pantoea a.
anandii
    Streptomyces a.
Ananindeua virus (ANUV)
anaphylactic
anaphylactica
    enteritis a.
anaphylactoid
anaphylaxin
anaphylaxis
Anaplasma (b)
    A. caudatum
    A. centrale
    A. marginale
    A. ovis
Anaplasmataceae
anaplastic large cell lymphoma
Anaplex Liquid
Anapolon
Anaport
Anaprox
anasarca
Anaspaz
anastomosis
    end-to-end a.
anatina
    Coenonia a.
anatinum
    Simulium a.
anatipestifer
    Moraxella a.
    Riemerella a.
anatis
    Cochlosoma a.
    Eimeria a.
    Mycoplasma a.
    Pasteurella a.
anatolicum
    Hyalomma a.
anatomiae
    Candida a.
Anatrichosoma cutaneum (p)
Anatube
Anatuss DM
Anbesol
    A. Baby
    A. Maximum Strength
    Maximum Strength A.
ANC
    absolute neutrophil count
Ancalochloris perfilievii (b)
Ancalomicrobium adetum (b)
Ancef
anchoratus
    Dactylogyrus a.
anchovy sauce pus
Ancobon level

ancoratus
    Pedicinus a.
Ancotil
ancudensis
    Candida a.
Ancylobacter aquaticus (b)
Ancylostoma (p)
    A. *braziliense*
    A. *caninum*
    A. *ceylanicum*
    A. *ceylonicum*
    A. *duodenale*
    A. *tubaeforme*
ancylostoma dermatitis
ancylostomatic
Ancylostomatidae
Ancylostomatinae
Ancylostomatoidea
ancylostomiasis
    cutaneous a.
    a. cutis
Andasibe virus (ANDV)
andersoni
    Dermatocentor a.
andersonii
    Brevinema a.
andresi
    Bothriocephalus a.
Androderm Transdermal System
Androlaelaps glasgowi
Andro-L.A. Injection
Androlone
Androlone-D
andropogonis
    Burkholderia a.
    Pseudomonas a.
Andropository Injection
ANDV
    Andasibe virus
anecdotal
anechoic
anemia
    aplastic crisis in hemolytic a.
    autoimmune hemolytic a. (AIHA)
    brickmaker's a.
    congenital a.
    Coombs-negative hemolytic a.
    Diamond-Blackfan a.
    diphyllobothrium a.
    fish tapeworm a.
    ground itch a.
    hemolytic a.

    hookworm a.
    hypochromic a.
    immune hemolytic a.
    iron-deficiency a.
    macrocytic hyperchromic a.
    malarial a.
    megaloblastic a.
    myelophthisic a.
    normocytic normochromic a.
    pernicious a.
    sickle cell a.
    transfusion-dependent a.
    transient aplastic a.
    tropical a.
anenterous
anergic leishmaniasis
anergy skin test battery
anesthesia
    epidural a.
Aneurinibacillus (b)
    A. *aneurinilyticus*
    A. *migulanus*
    A. *thermoaerophilus*
aneurinilyticus
    Aneurinibacillus a.
aneurinolyticum
    Trichosporon a.
aneurinolyticus
    Bacillus a.
aneurysm
    aortic a.
    dissecting aortic a.
    mycotic a.
    Rasmussen a.
Ang-2
    angiopoietin-2
angiitis
    cerebral a.
    choroidal a.
    Churg-Strauss a.
    granulomatous a.
    hypersensitivity a.
    necrotizing a.
angina
    herpetic a.
    Ludwig a.
    Vincent a.
anginosus
    Streptococcus a.
angioaccess
angioblastoma
angiocatheter

NOTES

Angiococcus (b)
    A. disciformis
angioedema
    migrating a.
angiogenesis
angiogenic cytokine
angiography
angioimmunoblastic lymphadenopathy
angiokeratoma
angiolipoma
angioma
    spider a.
angiomatoid
angiomatosis
    bacillary a. (BA)
    bacillary epithelioid a.
    epithelioid a.
angiomatosis-peliosis
    bacillary a.-p.
angiopoietin-2 (Ang-2)
angiospora
    Micropolyspora a.
    Microtetraspora a.
    Nonomuraea a.
angiostatin
angiostrongyliasis
    abdominal a.
    cerebral a.
Angiostrongylidae
angiostrongylosis
Angiostrongylus (p)
    A. cantonensis
    A. costaricensis
    A. vasorum
angiotensin-converting enzyme inhibitor
Angiozyme
angrense
    Simulium a.
anguillae
    Acanthocephalus a.
anguillarum
    Listonella a.
    Vibrio a.
anguillimortifera
    Edwardsiella a.
anguilliseptica
    Pseudomonas a.
Anguillula (p)
    A. aceti
angular cheilitis
angulatum
    Bifidobacterium a.
Angulomicrobium tetraedrale (b)
angusta
    Pichia a.
    Pseudallescheria a.
angustifolia
    Echinacea a.

angustifrons
    Cuterebra a.
angustmyceticus
    Streptomyces hygroscopicus subsp.
      a.
angustum
    Acidiphilium a.
    Eubacterium a.
    Photobacterium a.
Anhanga virus (ANHV)
Anhembi virus (AMBV)
ANHV
    Anhanga virus
anhydrotetrodotoxin 4-epitetrodotoxin
ani (*pl. of* anus)
Anichkov (*var. of* Anistchkow)
anicteric
    a. leptospirosis
    a. virus hepatitis
An-IDENT system
anilini
    Desulfobacterium a.
animal botulism
animalcule
animalis
    Bifidobacterium a.
    Fusobacterium nucleatum subsp. *a.*
    Lactobacillus a.
    Neisseria a.
animation
    suspended a.
anips
    Culex a.
anisa
    Legionella a.
anisakiasis
Anisakidae
anisakid nematode
anisakidosis
    extragastrointestinal a.
    gastric a.
    intestinal a.
    intraperitoneal a.
    luminal a.
Anisakinae
anisakine larva
Anisakis simplex (p)
Anisolpidiaceae
anisomycin
anisonucleosis
    hepatocyte a.
anisopliae
    Metarhizium a.
Anisopodidae
Anisopus fenestralis
Anistchkow, Anichkov
    A. myocyte

A

anitratus
    Actinomyces neuii subsp. *a.*
Anixiopsis (f)
ankle arthrogram
ankylosing spondylitis
ankylosis
Ankylostoma (*See* **Ancylostoma**)
ankylostomiasis
Ankylostomum
Ann Arbor stage
Annelida
annelids
annellide
annelloconidium
annua
    Artemisia *a.*
annulare
    granuloma *a.*
annulata
    Culiseta *a.*
annulatus
    Boophilus *a.*
annulipalpis
    Anopheles *a.*
Anocentor nitens (p)
anogenital
    a. herpes
    a. neoplasm
    a. wart
anomala
    Dekkera *a.*
    Hansenula *a.*
    Pichia *a.*
Anomala cuprea
anomalophyllus
    Anopheles *a.*
anomalous atrioventricular excitation
anomalum
anomalus
    Brettanomyces *a.*
    Hoplopsyllus *a.*
anomaly
    Pelger-Huet *a.*
Anopheles
    A. A, B virus
    A. acanthotorynus
    A. albimanus
    A. albitarsis
    A. albitarsis albitarsis
    A. albitarsis domesticus
    A. amictus amictus
    A. amictus hilli

A. annulipalpis
A. anomalophyllus
A. antunesi
A. apicimacula
A. aquasalis
A. argyritarsis
A. argyritarsis sawyeri
A. atropos
A. aztecus
A. bambusicolus
A. barberi
A. barbirostris
A. bellator
A. benarrochi
A. bifoliata
A. boliviensis
A. bonnei
A. bradleyi
A. braziliensis
A. bustamentei
A. canorii
A. crucians
A. cruzii
A. cruzii cruzii
A. cruzii laneanus
A. darlingi
A. davisi
A. earlei
A. eiseni
A. eiseni eiseni
A. eiseni geometricus
A. evandroi
A. evansae
A. evansae albertoi
A. evansae arthuri
A. evansae evansae
A. evansae lloydi
A. evansae ramosi
A. farauti
A. fausti
A. fluminensis
A. franciscanus
A. franciscanus franciscanus
A. franciscanus levicastilloi
A. franciscanus neghmei
A. franciscanus noei
A. franciscanus patersoni
A. freeborni
A. gabaldoni
A. galvaoi
A. gambiae
A. georgianus

NOTES

Anopheles *(continued)*
- A. *gilesi*
- A. *gomezdelatorrei*
- A. *grabhami*
- A. *guarao*
- A. *hectoris*
- A. *homunculus*
- A. *ininii*
- A. *intermedius*
- A. *judithae*
- A. *kompi*
- A. *lanei*
- A. *lutzii*
- A. *maculipes*
- A. *mattogrossensis*
- A. *mediopunctatus*
- A. *melas*
- A. *merus*
- A. *minor*
- A. *neivai*
- A. *neomaculipalpus*
- A. *nigritarsis*
- A. *nimbus*
- A. *noroestensis*
- A. *nuneztovari*
- A. *occidentalis*
- A. *oiketorakras*
- A. *oswaldoi*
- A. *parapunctipennis guatemalensis*
- A. *parapunctipennis parapunctipennis*
- A. *parvus*
- A. *perplexens*
- A. *peryassui*
- A. *pictipennis*
- A. *pseudomaculipes*
- A. *pseudopunctipennis*
- A. *pseudotibiamaculatus*
- A. *punctimacula*
- A. *punctipennis*
- A. *punctulatus*
- A. *quadrimaculatus*
- A. *rachoui*
- A. *rangeli*
- A. *rivadeneirai*
- A. *rondoni*
- A. *sanctielii*
- A. *shannoni*
- A. *squamifemur*
- A. *thomasi*
- A. *tibiamaculatus*
- A. *triannulatus*
- A. *triannulatus davisi*
- A. *triannulatus triannulatus*
- A. *vargasi*
- A. *vestitipennis*
- A. *walkeri*
- A. *xelajuensis*

anophelicide
anophelifuge
Anophelinae
anopheline
- a. mosquito
- a. vector

Anophelini
anophelism
Anoplocephala perfoliata (p)
Anoplocephalidae
Anoplocephalinae
Anoplura
anorectal
- a. gonorrhea
- a. junction

anorexia
anoscopic aspirate
anoscopy
Anoxybacillus (b)
- A. *flavithermus*
- A. *pushchinoensis*

ansamycin
Ansatospora
anserina
- Borrelia a.
- Podospora a.

anseris
- Mycoplasma a.

Anspor
ant
- fire a.
- harvester a.
- velvet a.

antacid
antagonism
- bacterial a.

antagonist
- histamine-2-receptor a.
- 5-HT3 receptor a.

antagonistic
antarctica
- Candida a.
- Friedmanniella a.
- Nocardiopsis a.
- Pseudoalteromonas a.
- Psychromonas a.

antarcticum
- Desulfotomaculum a.
- Sphingobacterium a.

antarcticus
- Cryptococcus a.
- Micrococcus a.
- Octadecabacter a.
- Rhodoferax a.

Antarctobacter heliothermus (b)
antecubital
antemortem
antenatal

antenatally
Antennulariellaceae
antepartum
Antequera virus (ANTV)
anterior
    a. chamber aspiration
    a. uveitis
anthelmintic, anthelminthic
Antheraea eucalypti virus
antheridium
anthocyanicus
    Streptomyces a.
Anthomyia
    A. facialis
    A. liturata
    A. mimetica
    A. nigriceps
    A. obscuripennis
    A. ochripes
    A. oculifera
    A. pluvialis
    A. procellaris
Anthomyiidae
anthonyi
    Crassicauda a.
Anthopsis delthoidea (f)
anthracis
    Bacillus a.
anthracoid
anthracycline
    liposomal encapsulated a.
anthramucin
anthrax
    abdominal a.
    cutaneous a.
    gastrointestinal a.
    inhalation a.
    oropharyngeal a.
    pulmonary a.
    respiratory a.
    a. vaccine
    a. vaccine, adsorbed
anthraxin skin test
anthropi
    Ochrobactrum a.
anthropii
    Ochromobactrum a.
anthropoid
anthropometry
anthropomorphic

anthroponotic
    a. cutaneous leishmaniasis
    a. genotype
anthropophaga
    Cordylobia a.
anthropophilic
anthropophthera
    Trachipleistophora a.
anthropozoonosis
anthurii
    Acidovorax a.
Anti-Acne
    A.-A. Control Formula
    A.-A. Formula for Men
    A.-A. Spot Treatment
antiadherent
antiagglutinin
anti-A isohemagglutinin
antianaerobic
antiangiogenic
antiarrhythmic
antibacterial
    a. therapy
Antiben
antibiogram
antibiosis
antibiotic
    antistaphylococcal a.
    antitumor a.
    beta-lactam a,
    broad-spectrum a.
    empiric a.
    a. enterocolitis
    fluoronaphthyrodine a.
    home intravenous a.
    intramuscular a.
    A. Ointment
    parenteral a.
    peptide a.
    prophylactic a.
    a. prophylaxis
    a. protein
    a. selection
    a. sensitivity
    a. sensitivity testing
    a. treatment
antibiotica
    Chainia a.
    Planomonospora parontospora
    subsp. *a.*
antibiotic-associated
    a.-a. colitis (AAC)

NOTES

antibiotic-associated *(continued)*
    a.-a. colitis toxin test
    a.-a. diarrhea (AAD)
AntibiOtic Otic
antibiotic-related colitis
antibiotic-resistant
antibioticus
    Lysobacter a.
    Streptomyces a.
Antibiotique Onguent
anti-B isohemagglutinin
antibody
    agglutinating a.
    anti-*Bordetella pertussis* a.
    anticapsular a.
    anti-CD3 a.
    anticytomegalovirus a.
    anti-double-stranded DNA a.
    anti-*Escherichia coli*-derived
      protein a.
    anti-GM1 a.
    anti-HAV a.
    anti-HBe a.
    anti-HIV-1 a.
    antimitochondrial a.
    antinuclear a. (ANA)
    anti-*Paracoccidioides brasiliensis* a.
    antiparvovirus B19 IgG a.
    antiparvovirus B19 IgM a.
    antiphospholipid a.
    antiplatelet a.
    anti-rhIL-3 a.
    anti-tat a.
    anti-*Toxoplasma gondii* a.
    anti-V3 a.
    anti-von Willebrand factor a.
    anti-vWF a.
    basement membrane a.
    beta-lactam IgE a.
    bispecific monoclonal a. (BiMAB)
    Bordetella pertussis a.
    bullous pemphigoid a.
    a. capture immunoassay
    cell-bound a.
    CF a.
    cold a.
    complement-fixing a.
    cross-reacting a.
    dermatitis herpetiformis a.
    a. detection
    direct fluorescent a. (DFA)
    endocardium, vascular structures,
      interstitium of striated muscle a.
    EVI a.
    fluorescein-conjugated polyclonal a.
    Forssman a.
    Francisella tularensis a.
    heat shock protein a.

    hepatitis B core a.
    a. to hepatitis B core antigen
    a. to hepatitis B e antigen
    hepatitis B surface a. (anti-HBs)
    a. to hepatitis B surface antigen
    herpes simplex a.
    heterophil a.
    HHV-8 latent IgG a.
    HHV-8 lytic IgG a.
    HSV-2 a.
    HTLV-I/II a.
    human immunodeficiency virus
      DNA a.
    IgA a.
    IgA immunofluorescent a. (IgA-
      IFA)
    IgE a.
    IgG hepatitis E a.
    IgG HEV a.
    IgG nuclear a.
    IgM anti-GM1 a.
    IgM immunofluorescent a. (IgM-
      IFA)
    immune fluorescent a. (IFA)
    immunofluorescent a. (IFA)
    indirect fluorescent a. (IFA)
    indirect immunofluorescent a. (IFA)
    intercellular antibody basement
      membrane a.
    intrathecal *Treponema pallidum* a.
      (ITPA)
    KSHV latent IgG a.
    KSHV lytic IgG a.
    LE a.
    Legionella pneumophila a.
    Legionnaires disease a.
    liver/kidney microsomal a.
    Lyme borreliosis a.
    maternal a.
    measles a.
    monoclonal a.
    OKT3 murine monoclonal a.
    parvovirus B19 IgG a.
    parvovirus B19 IgM a.
    pemphigus a.
    Plasmodium-opsonizing a.
    poliovirus a.
    polyclonal a.
    a. production
    quantitative human herpesvirus 6
      IgG a.
    quantitative human herpesvirus 6
      IgM a.
    rabbit fever a.
    rabies neutralizing a.
    rubella a.
    serum antinuclear a.
    serum-neutralizing a.

smooth muscle a.
Sporothrix a.
teichoic acid a.
a. test
a. titer
toxoplasmosis a.
TP a.
tube precipitin a.
viral direct detection by
  fluorescent a.
antibody-dependent
  a.-d. cell-mediated cytotoxicity
  a.-d. cellular cytotoxicity (ADCC)
**antibody-directed cellular cytotoxicity
(ADCC)**
antibody-mediated immunity (AMI)
antibody-secreting cell (ASC)
anti-*Bordetella pertussis* antibody
anticapsular antibody
anti-CD3 antibody
anticholinergic agent
anticoagulant
  lupus a.
anticonvulsant
anticytokine vaccination
anticytomegalovirus
  a. antibody
  a. immunoglobulin
Anti-Dandruff
  Neutrogena Healthy Scalp A.-D.
  Satinique A.-D.
  A.-D. Shampoo
antideoxyribonuclease-B (ADNase-B)
antidepressant
  tricyclic a. (TCA)
antidiarrheal agent
anti-DNase-B titer
antidote
  H-F A.
anti-double-stranded DNA antibody
antiemetic
antienterotoxin
anti-Epstein-Barr virus
**anti-*Escherichia coli*-derived protein
antibody**
antifolate
antifungal
  Absorbine Jr. A.
  azole a.
  Breezee Mist A.
  a. susceptibility testing
  a. therapy

anti-g209
antigen (Ag)
  alpha a.
  antibody to hepatitis B core a.
  antibody to hepatitis B e a.
  antibody to hepatitis B surface a.
  Australia a.
  bacterial a.
  blood group P a.
  capsular K a.
  carbohydrate a.
  carcinoembryonic a. (CEA)
  cardiolipin-cholesterol-lecithin a.
  Casoni a.
  circulating anodic a. (CAA)
  circulating cathodic a. (CCA)
  colonization factor a. (CFA)
  a. 85 complex
  CPS a.
  cross-reactive a.
  a. detection
  direct *Helicobacter pylori* a.
  EB nuclear a.
  EBV capsid a.
  EBV early a.
  Epstein-Barr nuclear a. (EBNA)
  flagellar H a.
  GAS a.
  hepatitis A a. (HAA)
  hepatitis-associated a. (HAA)
  hepatitis B a. (HBAg)
  hepatitis B core a.
  hepatitis B e a. (HBeAg)
  hepatitis B surface a. (HBsAg,
    HbsAg)
  heterogenic endobacterial a.
  Histoplasma capsulatum a. (HAG)
  Histoplasma capsulatum antibody
    and a.
  Histoplasma capsulatum
    polysaccharide a. (HPA)
  HIV core a.
  HIV p24 a.
  HLA-B27 histocompatibility a.
  human leukocyte a. (HLA)
  human leukocyte a.-A24 (HLA-
    A24)
  immune complex-dissociated p24 a.
    (ICD p24)
  Ki67 a.
  latency-associated nuclear a.
    (LANA)

NOTES

antigen *(continued)*
    latent nuclear a. (LNA)
    a. load
    lymphocyte detected membrane a. (LDMA)
    metacercarial a.
    mumps skin test a.
    mycelia-derived a.
    p24 a.
    parainfluenza virus a.
    pneumococcal capsular polysaccharide a.
    pneumococcal surface a. A
    prostate-specific a. (PSA)
    protective a. (PA)
    recombinant a.
    RSV a.
    secretory-excretory a.
    skin test a.
    somatic O a.
    streptococcal M a.
    streptococcal protein preabsorbing a.
    Streptococcus M a.
    surface protein a.
    Toxoplasma a.
    Treponema pallidum a.
    tumor a.
    tumor-associated a. (TAA)
    urine *Legionella* a.
    Vi a.
    viral a.
    viral capsid a. (VCA)
    W a.
antigen-absorption
    fluorescent treponemal a.-a.
antigen-antibody system
antigenemia
    a. assay
    CMV a.
    negative a.
    p24 a.
    pp65 a.
    viral a.
antigenic
    a. drift
    a. shift
antigen-positive
    hepatitis B e a.-p.
antigen-presenting cell (APC)
antigen-reactive T cell
antigen-specific
    a.-s. T cell
    a.-s. TCR
antigenuria
    Legionella a.
anti-*Giardia* IgM
antiglobulin

antiglomerular basement membrane glomerulonephritis
anti-GM1 antibody
anti-HAV antibody
anti-HBe antibody
anti-HBs
    hepatitis B surface antibody
anti-hepatitis E virus (anti-HEV)
anti-HEV
    anti-hepatitis E virus
antihistamine
anti-HIV-1 antibody
antihuman parvovirus immunoglobin G
antihyaluronidase
antihypertensive
antiinfective
antiinflammatory
    nonsteroidal a.
antiinterferon-alpha immunization
antiintrinsic
anti-LFLA test
antillancae
    Candida a.
antillarum
    Simulium a.
antilymphocyte
antilymphocytic globulin (ALG)
antimalarial
    a. agent
    a. drug
antimetabolite
antimicrobial
    a. agent
    a. dosing regimen
    a. level
    a. prophylaxis
    a. removal device (ARD)
    a. susceptibility testing
    a. therapy
antimicrobial-resistant *Salmonella*
antimicrobica
    Pseudomonas a.
Antiminth
antimitochondrial antibody
antimonate
    meglumine a.
antimonial
    pentavalent a.
antimotility agent
antimycobacterial susceptibility testing
antimycotic resistance
antimycoticus
    Streptomyces a.
antineoplastic
    a. agent
    a. chemotherapy
    a. drug
    a. therapy

antinicotinamide adenine dinucleotidase
antinuclear antibody (ANA)
antioxidant
    a. supplement
    a. therapy
anti-*Paracoccidioides brasiliensis* antibody
antiparasitic
antiparvovirus
    a. B19 IgG antibody
    a. B19 IgM antibody
    a. B19 immunoglobulin G
    a. B19 immunoglobulin M
    a. B19-specific IgM
antipedicular
antipediculotic
Anti-Pelliculaire
    Shampooing A.-P.
antiperiodic
antipertussis acellular vaccine
antiphospholipid antibody
antiplatelet antibody
antiproliferative
antiprotease therapy
antiprotozoal therapy
antiprotozoan
antipruritic
antipseudomonad penicillin
antipyretic
antipyretic/analgesic agent
antipyrine and benzocaine
antirabies
    a. serum (ARS)
    a. serum (equine)
antiretroviral (ARV)
    a. agent
    a. pregnancy registry
    a. triple combination therapy
antiretroviral-exposed mother
anti-Rh(D) immune globulin
anti-rhIL-3 antibody
anti-RT chemotherapy
antischistosomal
antisecretory
antisense
    a. oligonucleotide viral therapy
    a. riboprobe
antisepsis
    skin a.
antiseptic
    Dettol a.
antiserum, pl. antisera
    FITC-conjugated polyvalent a.

    hyperimmune group B-specific a.
    Lancefield grouping a.
    Lancefield group-specific a.
antispirochetal activity
antistaphylococcal antibiotic
antistreptococcal DNase-B titer
antistreptokinase
antistreptolysin
    a. O (ASO)
    a. O titer
anti-tat
    a.-t. antibody
    a.-t. IgG
anti-TB cellular immunity
antithymocyte globulin (ATG)
antithyroglobulin autoantibody
antitoxin
    bivalent gas gangrene a.
    botulinal a.
    botulinum a.
    botulism a.
    bovine a.
    Crotalus a.
    despeciated a.
    diphtheria a.
    dysentery a.
    gas gangrene a.
    normal a.
    pentavalent gas gangrene a.
    polyvalent gas gangrene a.
    a. rash
    scarlet fever a.
    staphylococcus a.
    tetanus a. (TAT)
anti-*Toxoplasma*
    IgA a.-*T.*
anti-*Toxoplasma gondii*
    a. antibody
    a. antibody secretion assay
antitoxoplasmosis therapy
antitreponemal antibody test
antitrichomonal therapy
antitrypsin
    fecal alpha$_2$-a.
antituberculosis therapy
antituberculous
antitumor
    a. antibiotic
    a. necrosis factor-based therapy
    a. response
Anti-Tuss Expectorant
antityphoid

NOTES

anti-V3 antibody
antivenin
    a. Crotalidae polyvalent
    a. *Micrurus fulvius*
antiviral
    a. chemotherapy
    a. drug
    a. immunity
    a. protein
    a. therapy
anti-von
    a.-v. Willebrand factor (anti-vWF)
    a.-v. Willebrand factor antibody
anti-vWF
    anti-von Willebrand factor
    anti-vWF antibody
antonii
    Simulium a.
antranikianii
    Thermus a.
antunesi
    Anopheles a.
    Simulium a.
ANTV
    Antequera virus
anular lesion
anulata
    Pilimelia a.
anulatus
    Streptomyces a.
anulus
    Aquaspirillum a.
anuria
anus, pl. **ani**
    pruritus ani
Anusol
    A. HC-1 Topical
    A. HC-2.5% Topical
ANUV
    Ananindeua virus
anxiety
anxiolytic
    benzodiazepine a.
AO
    acridine orange
    AO stain
AOM
    acute otitis media
Aonchotheca
aorta, pl. **aortae**
aortic
    a. aneurysm
    a. regurgitation
    a. stenosis
    a. valve
aotearoense
    Thermoanaerobacterium a.
AP50 virus

Apacet
APACHE II score
apathetic
apathy
apatite
APC
    absolute plasma concentration
    antigen-presenting cell
APEUV
    Apeu virus
Apeu virus (APEUV)
apex, pl. **apices**
    ventricular a.
Aphanoascus (f)
    A. fulvescens
Aphanocladium (f)
aphasia
aphasmid
Aphasmidia
Aphelenchoidea
Aphelenchoides cocophilus
aphidicola
    Buchnera a.
    Erwinia a.
aphid lethal paralysis virus
Aphodius
aphrophilus
    Haemophilus a.
aphtha, pl. **aphthae**
    oropharyngeal aphthae
Aphthasol
aphthous
    a. stomatitis
    a. ulcer
    a. ulceration
Aphthovirus (v)
    A. Asia 1
    A. A virus
    A. C
    A. O
    A. SAT1
    A. SAT2
    A. SAT3
Aphyllophorales
API
    API 20NE nonenteric identification system
    API Rapid 20E System
    API Rapid STREP
    API Rapid Strep test
    API Staph-IDENT test
    API STAPH test
apiarius
    Paenibacillus a.
apical complex
apicalis
    Culex a.
apices (*pl. of* apex)

apicimacula
    Anopheles a.
apicola
    Candida a.
Apicomplexa
apicomplexan parasite
apiculate
apiculatus
    Chondromyces a.
apiculus
apii (f)
    Cercospora a.
apingens
    Streptomyces thermoviolaceus subsp.
     a.
apiospermum
    Scedosporium a.
apiostomum
    Oesophagostomum a.
Apiotrichum (p)
apis
    Candida a.
    Spiroplasma a.
apista
    Pandoraea a.
aplasia
    marrow a.
    pure red cell a. (PRCA)
    red cell a.
aplastic
    a. crisis
    a. crisis in hemolytic anemia
Aplisol
Aplitest
Apo-Acetazolamide
Apo-Amoxi
Apo-Ampi Trihydrate
Apo-ASA
Apo-Cefaclor
Apo-Cephalex
Apo-Chlorax
Apo-Cimetidine
Apo-Cloxi
apocrine region
Apo-Doxy Tabs
Apo-Erythro E-C
Apo-Famotidine
Apo-Fluconazole
Apo-Gain
apogamia
Apo-Ibuprofen

APOIV
    Apoi virus
Apoi virus (APOIV)
apollinis
    Coniosporium a.
Apo-Metronidazole
Apo-Minocycline
apomixia
Apo-Napro-Na
Apo-Naproxen
Apo-Nitrofurantoin
Apo-Nizatidine
Apo-Norflox
Apo-Oflox
Apo-Pen VK
Apophysomyces elegans (f)
Apo-Prednisone
Apo-Propranolol
apoptosis
Apo-Ranitidine
Apo-Salvent
Aposphaeria fuscidula (f)
Apostain assay
Apo-Sulfamethoxazole
Apo-Sulfatrim
Apo-Tetra
Apo-Theo LA
Apo-Zidovudine
apparatus
    Golgi a.
    pyriform a.
AP-PCR
    arbitrary-primed PCR
    PCR with arbitrary primer
appearance
    corkscrew a.
    cushingoid a.
    grape cluster a.
    hypervascular a.
    moth-eaten a.
    soap bubble a.
    verrucous a.
appendage
    auricular a.
appendectomy
appendicitis
    Bifidobacterium a.
    bilharzial a.
    verminous a.
appendicitis-like syndrome
appendicular

NOTES

appendiculare
>   *Trichosporon a.*

appendiculatum
>   *Distomum a.*

appendiculatus
>   *Rhipicephalus a.*

appetite stimulant

APPG
>   aqueous procaine penicillin G

applique form

approach
>   Jennerian a.

appropriate culture

APR
>   acute phase reaction

apri
>   *Metastrongylus a.*

aprica
>   *Cytophaga a.*
>   *Flammeovirga a.*

Aprodine
>   A. Syrup
>   A. Tablet
>   A. w/C

apronophorus
>   *Ixodes a.*

Apscaviroid (v)

apsheronum
>   *Desulfomicrobium a.*

aPTT
>   activated partial thromboplastin time

APV
>   amprenavir

Aquabacterium (b)
>   *A. citratiphilum*
>   *A. commune*
>   *A. parvum*

Aquabacter spiritensis (b)

Aquacort

aquaeductuum
>   *Fusarium a.*

aquaeolei
>   *Arhodomonas a.*
>   *Marinobacter a.*

aquaesulis
>   *Thiobacillus a.*

aquamarina
>   *Deleya a.*
>   *Halomonas a.*

aquamarinus
>   *Alcaligenes a.*

Aquamicrobium defluvii (b)

Aquaphyllin

Aquareovirus (v)
>   A. A (ARV-A)
>   A. B (ARV-B)
>   A. C (ARV-C)
>   A. D (ARV-D)

A. E (ARV-E)
A. F (ARV-F)

aquasalis
>   *Anopheles a.*

Aquasol AD

aquaspersa
>   *Rhinocladiella a.*

Aquaspirillum (b)
>   *A. anulus*
>   *A. aquaticum*
>   *A. arcticum*
>   *A. autotrophicum*
>   *A. bengal*
>   *A. delicatum*
>   *A. dispar*
>   *A. fasciculus*
>   *A. giesbergeri*
>   *A. gracile*
>   *A. itersonii* subsp. *itersonii*
>   *A. itersonii* subsp. *nipponicum*
>   *A. magnetotacticum*
>   *A. metamorphum*
>   *A. peregrinum* subsp. *integrum*
>   *A. peregrinum* subsp. *peregrinum*
>   *A. polymorphum*
>   *A. psychrophilum*
>   *A. putridiconchylium*
>   *A. serpens*
>   *A. sinuosum*

AquaTar

aquatic

aquatica
>   *Budvicia a.*
>   *Leifsonia a.*

aquaticum
>   *Aquaspirillum a.*

aquaticus
>   *Ancylobacter a.*
>   *Cryptoccus a.*
>   *Gordius a.*
>   *Microcyclus a.*
>   *Nocardioides a.*
>   *Thermus a.*

aquatile
>   *Flavobacterium a.*

aquatilis
>   *Cytophaga a.*
>   *Gemmobacter a.*
>   *Rahnella a.*
>   *Sphingomonas a.*

aqueduct of Sylvius

aqueous
>   a. cocaine
>   a. crystalline penicillin G
>   a. epinephrine
>   a. extract
>   a. formaldehyde
>   a. humor

penicillin a.
a. procaine penicillin G (APPG)
a. solution
a. testosterone
a. vaccine
Aquest
Aquifex pyrophilus (b)
aquimarina
    Sporosarcina a.
Aquitaine cohort
aquosa
    cachexia a.
AR
    Axid AR
Ar-577 virus
Ar-578 virus
ARA-A
    adenine arabinoside
Ara-AMP
    adenine arabinoside monophosphate
arabaticum
    Acetohalobium a.
arabicus
    Streptomyces a.
arabinogalactanolyticum
    Aureobacterium a.
    Microbacterium a.
arabinoglactan
arabinose fermentation test
arabinoside
    adenine a. (ARA-A)
arabinosyl hypoxanthine
arachidonic acid
Arachnia propionica (b)
arachnid
Arachnida
arachnidism
    necrotic a.
Arachniotus (f)
arachnoid
arachnoiditis
    adhesive a.
Arachnomyces nodososetosus (f)
araffinosus
    Lactobacillus aviarius subsp. *a.*
araguata
    Stenella a.
Aralen
    A. HCl
    A. Phosphate With Primaquine
       Phosphate
Araneae

araneism
Aransas Bay virus (ABV)
aranti
    Simulium a.
araucae
    Thioploca a.
Arbia virus (ARBV)
arbitrary-primed PCR (AP-PCR)
Arboledas virus (ADSV)
arbophilicum
    Methanobacterium a.
arborescens
    Microbacterium a.
arboricola
    Culicoides a.
    Xanthomonas a.
arboriphilicus
    Methanobrevibacter a.
arboris
    Propionispira a.
    Sinorhizobium a.
arboroid
arboviral infection
arbovirus group A, B
arbuta
    Dipetalonema a.
ARBV
    Arbia virus
ARC
    AIDS related complex
arcachonense
    Sulfurospirillum a.
arcanobacterial pharyngitis
Arcanobacterium (b)
    A. *bernardiae*
    A. *haemolyticum*
    A. *phocae*
    A. *pluranimalium*
    A. *pyogenes*
Archaeobacteria
Archaeoglobaceae
Archaeoglobales
Archaeoglobus (b)
    A. *fulgidus*
    A. *profundus*
    A. *veneficus*
Archangiaceae
Archangium gephyra (b)
archeologic excavation
Archiacanthocephala
archibaldi

NOTES

Arcobacter (b)
    A. *butzleri*
    A. *cryaerophilus*
    A. *nitrofigilis*
    A. *skirrowii*
arctica
    Desulfotalea a.
arcticum
    Aquaspirillum a.
    Clostridium a.
    Simulium a.
arcticus
    Octadecabacter a.
arcuata
    Gymnodia a.
arcuatum
    Monostoma a.
arcuatus
    Chortoglyphus a.
ARD
    acute respiratory disease
    antimicrobial removal device
ardeae
    Giardia a.
ardesiacus
    Streptomyces diastaticus subsp. *a.*
ARDS
    adult respiratory distress syndrome
ardum
    Streptoverticillium a.
ardus
    Streptomyces a.
area
    body surface a. (BSA)
areactive tuberculosis
areflexia
arenae
    Streptomyces a.
arenaria
    Meloidogyne a.
Arenaviridae
Arenavirus (v)
arenavirus
arenicola
    Leptotrombidium a.
ARF
    acute rheumatic fever
Argas (p)
    A. *brumpti*
    A. *cooleyi*
    A. *miniatus*
    A. *persicus*
    A. *radiatus*
    A. *reflexus*
    A. *sanchezi*
    A. *vespertillionis*
argasid
Argasidae

argentatum
    Simulium a.
argenteolus
    Streptomyces a.
argentina
    Babesia a.
Argentine
    A. hemorrhagic fever
    A. hemorrhagic fever virus
argentinense
    Clostridium a.
argentinensis
    Haloarcula a.
argentinum
    Leuconostoc a.
argentoratense
    Corynebacterium a.
Argesic-SA
arginine test
arginini
    Mycoplasma a.
argon laser therapy
argus
    Simulium a.
Argyll Robertson pupil
argyritarsis
    Anopheles a.
argyrostoma
    Liopygia a.
    Sarcophaga a.
Arhodomonas aquaeolei (b)
ARIA
    acetylcholine receptor-inducing activity
aridum
    Kibdelosporangium aridum subsp. *a.*
arisaemoides
    Alaria a.
aristata
    Tetraploa a.
Aristocort
    A. A Topical
    A. Forte Injection
    A. Intralesional Injection
    A. Oral
Aristospan
    A. Intra-articular Injection
    A. Intralesional Injection
arizonae
    Salmonella a.
Arizona hinshawii (b) (*See* **Salmonella**
   arizonae)
arizonensis
    Culex a.
    Culicoides a.
    Lactobacillus a.
Arkonam virus (ARKV)
ARKV
    Arkonam virus

arlettae
    Staphylococcus a.
Arm-a-Med
    A.-a-M. Isoetharine
    A.-a-M. Isoproterenol
armamentarium
armed rostellum
armeniaca
    Bullera a.
armeniacus
    Actinoplanes a.
    Azotobacter a.
    Streptomyces a.
armillatus
    Armillifer a.
    Porocephalus a.
Armillifer
    A. armillatus
    A. moniliformis
ARMS
    amplification refractory mutation system
ARN
    acute retinal necrosis
Arnium leporinum (f)
arnoglossi
    Hysterothylacium a.
AROAV
    Aroa virus
Aroa virus (AROAV)
aromatica
    Thauera a.
aromaticivorans
    Sphingomonas a.
aromaticivorum
    Novosphingobium a.
arprinocid
Arp virus
Arracacha
    A. A virus (AVA)
    A. B virus (AVB)
    A. latent virus
    A. Y virus
arrangement
    birds-in-flight a.
arrhizus
    Rhizopus a.
arrhythmia
ARS
    acute retroviral syndrome
    antirabies serum
arsenaticum
    Pyrobaculum a.

arsenatis
    Chrysiogenes a.
arsenical
    organic a.
arsenic-fast
arseniciselenatis
    Bacillus a.
arsenophilum
    Sulfurospirillum a.
Arsenophonus nasoniae (b)
ART
    automated reagin test
artemether
artemidis
    Selenomonas a.
Artemisia
    A. annua
    A. salina
artemisinin derivative
arterial
    a. blood gas (ABG)
    a. embolization
    a. line culture
arteriolitis
arteriopathy
    coronary a.
arteriosclerosis
arteriosclerotic
arteriovenous (AV)
    a. conduction disturbance
    a. fistula (AVF)
    a. shunt infection
arteritis
    retinal a.
    temporal a.
Arterivirus (v)
artery
    intercostal a.
    internal mammary a. (IMA)
artesunate
Artha-G
Arthobotrys oligospora (f)
arthralgia
Arthrinium (f)
    A. phaeospermum
    A. phaeospermum var. indicum
Arthrisin
arthriticum
    erythema a.
arthritidis
    Mycoplasma a.
arthritis, pl. **arthritides**

NOTES

arthritis *(continued)*
    acute monarticular a.
    anaerobic bacterial a.
    bacterial a.
    Candida a.
    candidal a.
    chronic inflammatory a.
    chronic monarticular a.
    destructive gonococcal a.
    gonococcal a.
    gonorrheal a.
    herpes simplex virus a.
    infectious a.
    juvenile rheumatoid a.
    nongonococcal septic a.
    polyarticular a.
    postenteritis reactive a.
    psoriatic a.
    purulent gonococcal a.
    reactive a.
    rheumatoid a.
    Salmonella a.
    septic a.
    syphilitic a.
    tuberculous a.
    Yersinia a.
arthritis-dermatitis
Arthrobacter (b)
    A. agilis
    A. albus
    A. atrocyaneus
    A. aurescens
    A. chlorophenolicus
    A. citreus
    A. creatinolyticus
    A. crystallopoietes
    A. cumminsii
    A. duodecadis
    A. flavescens
    A. flavus
    A. globiformis
    A. histidinolovorans
    A. ilicis
    A. luteolus
    A. mysorens
    A. nicotianae
    A. nicotinovorans
    A. oxydans
    A. pascens
    A. picolinophilus
    A. polychromogenes
    A. protophormiae
    A. psychrolactophilus
    A. radiotolerans
    A. ramosus
    A. rhombi
    A. siderocapsulatus
    A. simplex

    A. sulfureus
    A. terregens
    A. tumescens
    A. uratoxydans
    A. ureafaciens
    A. variabilis
    A. viscosus
    A. woluwensis
Arthrobacteraceae
arthrocentesis
arthroconidium
Arthroderma (f)
    A. benhamiae
    A. cajetani
    A. cookiellum
    A. corniculatum
    A. flavescens
    A. fulvum
    A. gertleri
    A. gloriae
    A. grubyi
    A. gypseum
    A. incurvatum
    A. insingulare
    A. lenticularum
    A. obtusum
    A. otae
    A. persicolor
    A. quadrifidum
    A. racemosum
    A. simii
    A. uncinatum
    A. vanbreuseghemii
arthrogram
    ankle a.
    elbow a.
    hip a.
    knee a.
    shoulder a.
    temporomandibular joint a.
    wrist a.
Arthrographis (f)
    A. cuboidea
    A. kalrae
Arthropan
arthropathy
    HTLV-1-associated a. (HAAP)
arthroplasty
    hip a.
arthropod
    a. identification
    a. vector
Arthropoda
arthropod-borne
    a.-b. viral arthritis and rash
    a.-b. viral disease
    a.-b. viral encephalitis

a.-b. viral hemorrhagic fever
a.-b. virus
arthropodiasis
arthropodic
Arthropsis hispanica (f)
arthroscopic
arthrosia
exanthesis a.
arthrospore
arthuri
Anopheles evansae a.
Arthus
A. hypersensitivity
A. reaction
articular
a. leprosy
a. tuberculosis
artifactual
artificial
a. rupture of membranes
a. valve endocarditis
Artria
Artritol
Artyfechinostomum mehrai (p)
Aruac virus (ARUV)
arubae
Culicoides a.
Arumowot virus (AMTV)
arupensis
Bartonella vinsonii subsp. a.
ARUV
Aruac virus
ARV
Adelaide River virus
AIDS-related virus
antiretroviral
ARV-A
Aquareovirus A
ARV-B
Aquareovirus B
ARV-C
Aquareovirus C
ARV-D
Aquareovirus D
ARV-E
Aquareovirus E
arvensicola
Cytophaga a.
arvensis
Agaricus a.
ARV-F
Aquareovirus F

arvum
Cryptosporangium a.
arxii
Cladophialophora a.
Arxiozyma (f)
Arxula adeninivorans (f)
arylamidase
pyrrolidonyl a. (PYR)
arylsulfatase activity test
A.S.
Crysticillin A.S.
AS-1 virus
ASA
MSD Enteric Coated ASA
A.S.A.
asaccharolytica
Porphyromonas a.
Pseudonocardia a.
Sphingomonas a.
asaccharolyticus
Bacteroides a.
Peptococcus a.
Peptoniphilus a.
Peptostreptococcus a.
asaccharovorans
Chelatococcus a.
asadai
Centrocestus a.
Asadrine
asahii
Trichosporon a.
Asaia (b)
A. bogorensis
A. siamensis
asaii
Gluconobacter a.
Asamycin
Asaphen
Asbolisiaceae
asburiae
Enterobacter a.
ASC
antibody-secreting cell
ascariasis
biliary a.
ascaricide
ascarid
Ascaridae
ascaridata
Ascaridia galli (p)
Ascaridida
Ascarididae

NOTES

Ascaridinae
Ascaridoidea
Ascaris (p)
    A. lumbricoides
    A. suum
Ascaroidea
ascaron
Ascarops strongylina (p)
ascended healing
ascendens
    Acetobacter pasteurianus subsp. *a.*
ascending
    a. gonococcal infection
    a. polyradiculitis
Aschelminthes
Aschiza
Aschoff nodule
asci (*pl. of* ascus)
ascites
    culture-negative neutrocytic a. (CNNA)
    a. fluid tap
    infected a.
    malignant a.
    transudative a.
    tuberculous a.
ascitic
    a. fluid
    a. fluid cytology
Ascobolaceae
ascocarp
Ascocorticiaceae
Ascodichaenaceae
ascogenous
ascogonium
Ascomycetes
ascomycetous
Ascomycota
Ascomycotina
ascorbata
    Kluyvera a.
ascorbic acid
Ascosphaeraceae
Ascosphaerales
ascospore
Ascotrichosporon (f)
Ascovirus (v)
Ascriptin
ASCT
    autologous stem cell transplantation
ASCUS
    atypical squamous cells of uncertain significance
    atypical squamous cells of undetermined significance
ascus, pl. **asci**
ASD
    atrial septal defect

aseptate
aseptic
    a. meningitis
    a. meningitis syndrome
asexual
    a. generation
    a. reproduction
Asfivirus (v)
ASHD
    atherosclerotic heart disease
ASI
    active specific immunotherapy
Asian taeniasis
Asiatic
    A. cholera
    A. schistosomiasis
asiatica
    Natrialba a.
    Raillietina a.
    Spirochaeta a.
asiaticum
    Mycobacterium a.
asigna
    Thosea a.
asini
    Enterococcus a.
    Haematopinus a.
asinigenitalis
    Taylorella a.
Asmalix
Asmavent
ASO
    antistreptolysin O
    Pseudomonas species ASO
asoensis
    Streptomyces cacaoi subsp. *a.*
asomatognosis
ASP
    amnesic shellfish poisoning
aspartate
    a. aminotransferase (AST)
    a. aminotransferase level
A-Spas S/L
aspergilloma
    pulmonary a.
aspergillosis
    acute invasive a.
    allergic bronchopulmonary a. (ABPA)
    chronic necrotizing a.
    cutaneous a.
    invasive a. (IA)
    obstructing bronchial a.
    saprophytic a.
    superficial a.
Aspergillus (f)
    A. aculeatus
    A. alataceus

A. *alliaceus*
A. *atroviolaceus*
A. *avenaceus*
A. *caesiellus*
A. *candidus*
A. *carneus*
A. *chevalieri*
A. *clavato-nanicus*
A. *clavatus*
A. *conicus*
A. *conidia*
A. *deflectus*
A. endophthalmitis
A. *fisherianus*
A. *flavipes*
A. *flavus*
A. *fumigatus*
A. fungus ball
A. *glaucus*
A. *granulosus*
A. *hollandicus*
A. IgG titer
A. immunodiffusion
A. *janus*
A. *japonicus*
A. *nidulans*
A. *niger*
A. *niger* var. >awamori
A. *niveus*
A. *ochraceus*
A. *oryzae*
A. osteomyelitis
A. *penicilloides*
A. *reptans*
A. *restrictus*
A. *rubrobrunneus*
A. *sclerotiorum*
A. *sejunctus*
A. *spinosus*
A. *sydowii*
A. *tamarii*
A. *terreus*
A. *tetrazonus*
A. *thermomutatus*
A. *tubingensis*
A. *unguis*
A. *ustus*
A. *versicolor*
***Aspergillus*-specific IgE**
Aspergum
asperula
    Scopulariopsis a.

asperum
    Trichocladium a.
asphyxia
asphyxiation
Aspiculuris tetraptera (p)
aspidieticola
    Phome a.
Aspidogaster conchicola (p)
Aspidogastrea
aspirate
    anoscopic a.
    bone marrow a.
    bronchial a.
    fine-needle a.
    gastric a.
    joint a.
    nasopharyngeal a.
    pleural a.
    protected catheter a. (PCA)
    tracheal a.
    transthoracic pulmonary a.
    transtracheal a.
    tympanic membrane a.
aspiration
    anterior chamber a.
    a. biopsy
    bone marrow a.
    closed joint a.
    endotracheal a. (EA)
    fine-needle a.
    a. of gastric contents
    joint a.
    nasotracheal a.
    percutaneous needle a.
    a. pneumonia
    recurrent a.
    suprapubic a.
    translaryngeal a.
    transtracheal a. (TTA)
    vitreous a.
aspirin
    Bayer A.
    A. Plus Stomach Guard
Aspirols
    Amyl Nitrite A.
asplenia
    congenital a.
asplenic
asplenii
    Pseudomonas a.
asporogenous
asporous

NOTES

asporulate
Assam fever
assassin bug
assay
    agar diffusion a.
    Amplicor HIV-1 Monitor Ultra
      Sensitive Specimen Preparation
      Protocol Ultra Direct A.
    amplification a.
    antigenemia a.
    anti-*Toxoplasma gondii* antibody
      secretion a.
    Apostain a.
    bDNA a.
    Bio-EnzaBead A.
    BioStar *Chlamydia* OIA a.
    blocking a.
    Borrelia burgdorferi DNA a.
    branched DNA a.
    Captia IgM a.
    checkerboard a.
    chemiluminescence a.
    Chlamydia trachomatis Probe
      Competition A.
    chromatographic a.
    chromium-release a.
    Clostridium difficile toxin a.
    CMV-Vue a.
    colorimetric a.
    Color Vue *Cryptosporidium* a.
    ^{51}Cr release a.
    cytokine a.
    cytotoxic a.
    direct a.
    direct fluorescence a. (DFA)
    direct fluorescent a. (DFA)
    dot blot a.
    drug susceptibility a.
    electrophoretic mobility shift a.
      (EMSA)
    ELISPOT a.
    endpoint dilution a.
    enzyme-linked immunosorbent a.
      (ELISA)
    enzyme-linked immunospot a.
      (ELISPOT)
    Enzymun-Test DNA Detection A.
    FlashTrack DNA Probe a.
    functional proliferative a.
    GENIE HIV 1/2 a.
    genotypic a.
    Gen-Probe PACE a.
    GHOST cell a.
    glutathione-*S*-transferase pull-
      down a. (GST pull-down assay)
    glycoprotein-based enzyme-linked
      immunosorbent a. (gpELISA)
    GST pull-down a.
    glutathione-*S*-transferase pull-down
      assay
    HAG a.
    hepatitis B viral DNA a.
    heteroduplex mobility a. (HMA)
    high-performance liquid
      chromatography a.
    HIVCHEK-1/2 a.
    HIV-1 culture a.
    HIV DNA amplication a.
    HIV viral load a.
    HPLC a.
    Hybrid Capture a.
    IgM enzyme-linked
      immunosorbent a.
    immune complex a.
    immune-electrophoresis a.
    immunoblot a.
    immunochromatographic a.
    immunoenzymatic a.
    immunofluorescence a. (IFA)
    immunofluorescent antibody a.
      (IFA)
    immunosorbent agglutination a.
      (ISAGA)
    indicator cell a.
    indirect hemagglutination a. (IHA)
    indirect hemagglutination
      serologic a.
    indirect hemagglutinin a. (IHA)
    Kirby-Bauer type a.
    LANA antibody a.
    LCR a.
    LCx *Chlamydia trachomatis*
      LCR a.
    Legionella a.
    limulus amoebocyte lysate a.
    line probe a. (LIPA, LiPA)
    LiPA strip a.
    Luminetics ATP a.
    lymphocyte proliferation a. (LPA)
    lymphocytic proliferation a. (LPA)
    lymphoproliferative a.
    microhemagglutination a.
    Murex CMV DNA hybrid
      capture a.
    NASBA HIV-1 RNA QT a.
    nucleic acid probe a.
    opsonophagocytosis a.
    OrthoProbe a.
    PEIA a.
    PERT a.
    Phenosense a.
    phenotypic a.
    plaque reduction neutralization a.
    Premier *Helicobacter pylori* a.
    proliferation a.

A

ProSpect *Cryptosporidium*
  microtiter a.
pseudomembranous colitis toxin a.
pulldown a.
qualitative RNA PCR a.
Quantiplex HCV-RNA A.
Quantiplex HIV-1 RNA a.
quantitative a.
radioimmunoblot a. (RIBA)
Recombigen HIV 1/2 a.
recombinant immunoblot a. (RIBA)
recombinant virus a. (RVA)
replication-competent retrovirus a.
restriction endonuclease a.
reverse passive hemagglutination a.
RNA-based a.
serologic a.
serum p24 HIV-1 antigen a.
slot-blot a.
strychnine antagonist a.
SUDS-1 a.
tissue culture a. (TCA)
Treponema pallidum
  hemagglutination a. (TPHA)
ultrasensitive viral load a.
in vitro pull-down a.
WB a.
Western blot a.
Western immunoblot a.
associate
  microbial a.'s
association
  cell a.
AST
  aspartate aminotransferase
astemizole
Asterinaceae
asterixis
asteroid body
asteroides
  Bifidobacterium a.
  Trichosporon a.
Asteroleplasma anaerobium (b)
asterosporus
  Streptomyces a.
asthenia
AsthmaHaler Mist
AsthmaNefrin
Asticcacaulis (b)
  A. biprosthecium
  A. excentricus
Astigmata

astimazole
Astraeaceae
astringent
  Clean & Clear Deep Cleaning A.
astrocyte
  gemistocytic a.
astrocytic gliosis
astrogliosis
  reactive a.
astronyxis
  Acanthamoeba a.
Astroviridae
Astrovirus (v)
astrovirus
  bovine a. 1–2
  human a. serotype 1-7 (HAstV-1-7)
  porcine a. 1–11
asymbiotica
  Photorhabdus a.
asymmetric nasopharyngeal lymphoid hyperplasia
asymmetry, border, color, and diameter (ABCD)
asymptomatic
  a. bacteriuria
asystole
ATA
  atmosphere absolute
Atabrine
Atarax
Atasol
ataxia
  cerebellar a.
ATCC
  American Type Culture Collection
atchleyi
  Culicoides a.
atelectasis
  basilar a.
  segmental a.
  subsegmental a.
ater
  Cryptococcus a.
ATG
  antithymocyte globulin
Atherigona orientalis
Atherix
  A. lantha
  A. pachypus
  A. variegata
atheromatous plaque

NOTES

51

atherosclerosis
  peripheral a.
atherosclerotic
  a. cardiovascular disease
  a. heart disease (ASHD)
athetosis
athlete's foot
Ativan
ATL
  adult T-cell leukemia
  adult T-cell lymphoma
  cutaneous ATL
atlantae
  Moraxella (Moraxella) a.
atlantica
  Alteromonas a.
  Candida a.
  Pseudoalteromonas a.
  Ruegeria a.
atlanticum
  Agrobacterium a.
atlanticus
  Aedes a.
ATLL
  adult T-cell leukemia/lymphoma
ATM
  acute transverse myelopathy
atmosphaerica
  Candida a.
atmosphere absolute (ATA)
ATN
  acute tubular necrosis
Atolone Oral
atomic force microscopy
atopic dermatitis
Atopobacter phocae (b)
Atopobium (b)
  A. fossor
  A. minutum
  A. parvulum
  A. rimae
  A. vaginae
atorvastatin
atovaquone
  a. and proguanil
  proguanil and a.
  a. suspension
ATP
  adenosine triphosphate
ATPase
  adenosine triphosphatase
atramentaria
  Actinomadura a.
atramentarius
atratus
  Culex a.
  Streptomyces a.
  Tabanus a.

atresia
  biliary a.
  esophageal a.
atrial septal defect (ASD)
Atridox
atrioventricular
  a. node
  a. septal defect
atroaurantiacus
  Streptomyces a.
atrobrunneum
  Chaetomium a.
atrocyaneus
  Arthrobacter a.
atrogriseum
  Acremonium a.
atro-olivaceus
  Pithomyces a.-o.
atroolivaceus
  Streptomyces a.
atropalpus
  Aedes a.
atrophaeus
  Bacillus a.
atrophic
  a. candidiasis
  a. gastritis
  a. rhinitis
atrophicans
  acrodermatitis chronica a. (ACA)
atrophicus
  lichen sclerosus et a.
atrophy
  intrinsic muscular a.
  iris a.
  testicular a.
atropine sulfate
atropos
  Anopheles a.
Atrosept
atroseptica
  Erwinia carotovora subsp. *a.*
atrosepticum
  Pectobacterium carotovorum subsp.
    a.
atrovinosus
  Catenuloplanes a.
atroviolaceus
  Aspergillus a.
atrovirens
  Rhinocladiella a.
  Streptomyces a.
atrum
  Coniosporium a.
A/T/S Topical
attack
  acute a.
  transient ischemic a.

attenuated
    a. fever response
    a. human rotavirus
attenuatus
    Chironomus a.
Attenuvax
attributable
atypia
    cellular a.
atypica
    koilocytotic a.
    Veillonella a.
    Veillonella parvula subsp. *a.*
atypical
    a. immune-mediated
      thrombocytopenia
    a. lymphocytosis
    a. manifestation
    a. mycobacteria
    a. mycobacterial colonization
    a. pneumonia
    a. squamous cells of uncertain
      significance (ASCUS)
    a. squamous cells of undetermined
      significance (ASCUS)
auburnensis
    Eimeria a.
Auchmeromyia (p)
    A. luteola
    A. senegalensis
auctum
    Hysterothylacium a.
audiogram
auditory brain-stem response testing
audouinii
    Microsporum a.
auensis
    Tolumonas a.
Auerbach plexus
Auer rod
Augmentin
Aulographaceae
Auralgan
aural myiasis
auramine
    a. fluorochrome stain
    a. O stain
auramine-phenol stain
auramine-rhodamine acid-fast stain
aurantia
    Alteromonas a.
    Frateuria a.

    Pelczaria a.
    Pseudoalteromonas a.
    Spirochaeta aurantia subsp. *a.*
aurantiaca
    Actinobispora a.
    Actinocorallia a.
    Actinomadura a.
    Brevundimonas a.
    Cytophaga a.
    Kineosporia a.
    Methylomonas a.
    Micromonospora a.
    Micromonospora carbonacea subsp.
      a.
    Pseudomonas a.
    Stigmatella a.
aurantiacum
    Dactylosporangium a.
    Exiguobacterium a.
    Microbacterium a.
aurantiacus
    Chloroflexus a.
    Flexibacter a.
    Herpetosiphon a.
    Kineococcus a.
    Marmoricola a.
    Rhodococcus a.
    Streptomyces a.
    Thermoascus a.
aurantibutyricum
    Clostridium a.
auranticolor
    Actinoplanes a.
    Amorphosporangium a.
auranticum
    Actinosynnema pretiosum subsp. *a.*
aurantiogriseus
    Streptomyces a.
aurantius
    Hypomyces a.
AURAV
    Aura virus
Aura virus (AURAV)
aurease
aurelia
    Paramecium a.
Aureobacterium (b)
    A. arabinogalactanolyticum
    A. barkeri
    A. esteraromaticum
    A. flavescens
    A. keratanolyticum

NOTES

Aureobacterium (continued)
A. *liquefaciens*
A. *luteolum*
A. *resistens*
A. *saperdae*
A. *schleiferi*
A. *terrae*
A. *terregens*
A. *testaceum*
A. *trichothecenolyticum*
Aureobasidium pullulans (f)
aureocirculatus
Streptomyces a.
aureofaciens
Pseudomonas a.
Streptomyces a.
Aureomycin
aureorectus
Streptomyces a.
aureoversile
Streptoverticillium a.
aureoversilis
Streptomyces a.
aureoverticillatus
Streptomyces a.
aurescens
Arthrobacter a.
aureum
Polyangium a.
Simulium a.
aureus
epidemic methicillin-resistant
Staphylococcus a. (EMRSA)
glycopeptide-intermediate
Staphylococcus a. (GISA)
glycopeptide-resistant
Staphylococcus a. (GRSA)
methicillin-resistant
Staphylococcus a. (MRSA)
methicillin-susceptible
Staphylococcus a. (MSSA)
mupirocin-resistant, methicillin-resistant Staphylococcus a. (MMRSA)
mupirocin-resistant
Staphylococcus a.
mutiresistant Staphylococcus a.
oxacillin-resistant Staphylococcus a. (ORSA)
Staphylococcus a.
Staphylococcus aureus subsp. a.
vancomycin-resistant
Staphylococcus a. (VRSA)
Aureusvirus (v)
auriantica
Hyphelia a.
auricle
auricular appendage

auricularis
Staphylococcus a.
aurifer
Aedes a.
auringiensis
Candida a.
auripellitum
Simulium a.
auripigmentum
Desulfotomaculum a.
auris
Corynebacterium a.
Mycoplasma a.
auriscanis
Corynebacterium a.
auristriatum
Simulium a.
Aurodex
Aurolate
aurothioglucose
Auroto
aurum
Microbacterium a.
Mycobacterium a.
austini
Culicoides a.
Australia antigen
australicum
Desulfotomaculum a.
Pedomicrobium a.
australiensis
Acomatacarus a.
Bipolaris a.
Cochliobolus a.
Naegleria a.
Saccharothrix a.
Tetrasphaera a.
australis
Aedes a.
Leptospira interrogans serovar a.
Rickettsia a.
Streptococcus a.
austriacum
Coniothecium a.
austroafricanum
Mycobacterium a.
Austrobilharzia variglandis (p)
austromarina
Candida a.
autecic
autistic parasite
autoagglutinin
cold a.
autoamputation of penis
autoantibody
antithyroglobulin a.
cold a.
autoblast

autochthonous
    a. malaria
    a. parasite
autoclave
autocrine-paracrine growth loop
autofluorescence test
autogamous
autogamy
autogenesis
autogenetic
autogenous vaccine
autoimmune
    a. chronic hepatitis
    a. disease
    a. disorder
    a. encephalomyelitis
    a. hemolysis
    a. hemolytic anemia (AIHA)
    a. lymphoproliferative syndrome
    (ALPS)
    a. thyroiditis
autoimmunity
autoinfection
autoinoculation
autologous
    a. blood donation (ABD)
    a. melanoma
    a. stem cell transplantation (ASCT)
    a. tumor vaccine
autolysis
automated reagin test (ART)
autonomic
autoradiography
autoreinfection
autosepticemia
autosplenectomized
autosplenectomy
autotomy
autotroph
autotrophic
autotrophica
    Amycolata a.
    Nocardia a.
    Pseudonocardia a.
autotrophicum
    Aquaspirillum a.
    Desulfobacterium a.
    Trichophyton equinum var. *a.*
autotrophicus
    Streptomyces a.
    Xanthobacter a.

autumn
    a. fever
    a. skullcap mushroom
autumnale
    Phormidium a.
autumnal fever
autumnalis
    Galerina a.
    Leptospira interrogans serovar *a.*
    Musca a.
    Neotrombicula a.
    Trombicula a.
AU virus
auxanogram
auxanographic method
auxanography
Auxarthron (f)
auxiliaris
    Chorizagrotis a.
    Euxoa a.
auxotroph
auxotrophic
    a. mutant
    a. strain
auxotype
auxotyping
Auzduk disease virus
AV
    arteriovenous
AV-1 virus
AVA
    Arracacha A virus
Avalon virus (AVAV)
Avant Garde Shampoo
avara
    Vahlkampfia a.
avascular necrosis (AVN)
AVAV
    Avalon virus
AVB
    Arracacha B virus
AVC
    AVC Cream
    AVC Suppository
Aveeno Cleansing Bar
AVEG
    AIDS Vaccine Evaluation Group
avellanae
    Pseudomonas a.
avellaneus
    Streptomyces a.
Avelox

NOTES

avenaceus
    Aspergillus a.
avenae
    Acidovorax avenae subsp. *a.*
    Drechslera a.
    Pseudomonas avenae subsp. *a.*
Avenavirus (v)
AVF
    arteriovenous fistula
Aviadenovirus (v)
avian
    a. AAV
    a. adenovirus
    a. diphtheria
    a. encephalomyelitis virus
    a. erythroblastosis virus
    a. infectious bronchitis virus (IBV)
    a. infectious encephalomyelitis
    a. infectious laryngotracheitis
    a. infectious laryngotracheitis virus
    a. influenza
    a. influenza virus
    a. leukosis virus (ALV)
    a. lymphomatosis virus
    a. myeloblastosis virus
    a. orthoreovirus
    a. paramyxovirus virus 1–9 (PMV 1–9)
    a. rotavirus
    a. type C retrovirus group
aviarius
    Lactobacillus aviarius subsp. *a.*
Avibirnavirus (v)
avidinii
    Streptomyces a.
avidum
    Propionibacterium a.
Avihepadnavirus (v)
Avipoxvirus (v)
Avirax
aviremia
avirulent
Avita
avium
    Bordetella a.
    Brevibacterium a.
    Enterococcus a.
    Haemophilus a.
    Mycobacterium avium subsp. *a.*
    Pasteurella a.
    Trypanosoma a.
avium-intracellulare
    Mycobacterium a.-i. (MAI)
Avlosulfon
AVN
    avascular necrosis
avoparcin
Avsunviroidae (v)

awamori
    Aspergillus niger var. *a.*
AWS
    AIDS wasting syndrome
axanthum
    Acholeplasma a.
axei
    Rhabditella a.
    Trichostrongylus a.
axenic medium
axes (*pl. of* axis)
axetil
    cefuroxime a.
axial filament
Axid
    A. AR
axilla, pl. **axillae**
axillaris
    trichomycosis a.
    trichonocardiosis a.
axillary adenopathy
axiopodium
axis, pl. **axes**
    HPG a.
    hypothalamic-pituitary-gonadal a.
    a. of symmetry
axoneme
axonopodis
    Xanthomonas a.
axopodium
axostyle
Axsain
Ayercillin
azacoluta
    Streptomyces cinnamoneus subsp. *a.*
Azactam
azar
    kala a.
azatadine maleate
azathioprine
azatica
    Kitasatospora a.
azaticus
    Streptomyces a.
azelaic acid
Azelex
3′-azido-3′-deoxythymidine (AZT, ZDV)
azidothymidine (AZT, ZDV)
    a. monophosphate (AZTMP)
    a. triphosphate (AZTTP)
azithromycin dihydrate
Azlin
azlocillin
Azmacort Oral Inhaler
Azo
    A. Gantanol
    A. Gantrisin

Azoarcus (b)
  A. *anaerobius*
  A. *communis*
  A. *evansii*
  A. *indigens*
  A. *toluclasticus*
  A. *tolulyticus*
  A. *toluvora*
Azobacteraceae
azole
  a. antifungal
  a. drug
  a. resistant
  systemic a.
  a. treatment
Azomonas (b)
  A. *agilis*
  A. *insignis*
  A. *macrocytogenes*
Azomonotrichon macrocytogenes (b)
Azonexus fungiphilus (b)
azoospermia
azorensis
  Thermothrix a.
Azorhizobium caulinodans (b)
Azorhizophilus paspali (b)
azoricus
  Stygiolobus a.
Azospira (b)
  A. *oryzae*
Azospirillum (b)
  A. *amazonense*
  A. *brasilense*
  A. *doebereinerae*
  A. *halopraeferens*
  A. *irakense*
  A. *largimobile*
  A. *lipoferum*
azo-sulfisoxazole
azotemia
azothioprine
Azotobacter (b)
  A. *armeniacus*
  A. *beijerinckii*

  A. *chroococcum*
  A. *macrocytogenes*
  A. *nigricans* subsp. *achromogenes*
  A. *nigricans* subsp. *nigricans*
  A. *salinestris*
  A. *vinelandii*
azotocaptans
  Gluconacetobacter a.
azotofixans
  Bacillus a.
  Paenibacillus a.
azotoformans
  Bacillus a.
  Pseudomonas a.
  Rhodobacter a.
Azovibrio restrictus (b)
AZT, ZDV
  3'-azido-3'-deoxythymidine
  azidothymidine
    AZT monotherapy
    AZT + 3TC
aztecus
  Anopheles a.
AZTMP
  azidothymidine monophosphate
aztreonam
AZTTP
  azidothymidine triphosphate
azul
Azulfidine
  A. EN-tabs
azurea
  Amycolatopsis a.
  Pseudonocardia a.
  Saccharomonospora a.
azure II stain
azureus
  Couchioplanes caeruleus subsp. *a.*
  Streptomyces a.
azyma
  Candida a.
Azymocandida
Azymoprocandida (f) (*See* **Candida**)

NOTES

B

B cell
B cell epitope
B lymphocyte
B symptom
B virus

B1

aflatoxin B1
B1 cell

1B

rhinovirus 1B

B2

aflatoxin B2

2B

Uvitex 2B

3B

Yersinia enterocolitica biogroup 3B

4B

parainfluenza type 4B

B6-250
B12

B12 deficiency
B12 virus

B19

B19 DNA
parvovirus B19
B19 virus

B291

monoclonal antibody B291

2b

interferon-alpha 2b

B11-M15 virus
B6 virus
B7-positive tumor cell
B7 virus
BA

bacillary angiomatosis

baarnense

Eupenicillium b.

baarnensis

Streptomyces b.

baarsii

Desulfovibrio b.

BAAV

bovine AAV virus

Babahoya virus (BABV)
Babanki

Sindbis virus subtype B.
B. virus

Babee Teething
Babesia (p)

B. argentina
B. bigemina
B. bovis
B. caballi

B. canis
B. divergens
B. major
B. microti

Babesiella
Babesiidae
babesiosis

human b.

BABV

Babahoya virus

baby

Anbesol B.
B. Liquid
B. Nighttime
B. Orajel

Baby's Own Ointment
bacampicillin

b. hydrochloride

bacarum

Candida b.

Bace

Neo B.

Baciguent Topical
Bacigvent
Baci-IM Injection
Bacillaceae
bacillar
Bacillariophta
Bacillariophyta diatoms
bacillaris

Streptomyces b.

bacillary

b. angiomatosis (BA)
b. angiomatosis-peliosis
b. dysentery
b. epithelioid angiomatosis
b. peliosis (BP)

bacille Calmette-Guérin (BCG)
bacilli (*pl. of* bacillus)
bacilliferous
bacilliform
bacilliformis

Bartonella b.

bacillin
bacillisporum

Ophiostoma b.

bacillomyxin
bacillosum

Thiodictyon b.

bacilluria
Bacillus (b)

B. abortus
B. acidocaldarius
B. acidoterrestris
B. agaradhaerens

B

Bacillus *(continued)*
- *B. agri*
- *B. alcalophilus*
- *B. alginolyticus*
- *B. alvei*
- *B. amyloliquefaciens*
- *B. amylolyticus*
- *B. aneurinolyticus*
- *B. anthracis*
- *B. arseniciselenatis*
- *B. atrophaeus*
- *B. azotofixans*
- *B. azotoformans*
- *B. badius*
- *B. benzoevorans*
- *B. borstelensis*
- *B. brevis*
- *B. carboniphilus*
- *B. centrosporus*
- *B. cereus*
- *B. chitinolyticus*
- *B. chondroitinus*
- *B. choshinensis*
- *B. circulans*
- *B. clarkii*
- *B. clausii*
- *B. coagulans*
- *B. cohnii*
- *B. curdlanolyticus*
- *B. cycloheptanicus*
- *B. dipsosauri*
- *B. edaphicus*
- *B. ehimensis*
- *B. fastidiosus*
- *B. firmus*
- *B. flexus*
- *B. formosus*
- *B. fumarioli*
- *B. fusiformis*
- *B. galactophilus*
- *B. gibsonii*
- *B. globisporus*
- *B. globisporus* subsp. *marinus*
- *B. glucanolyticus*
- *B. gordonae*
- *B. halmapalus*
- *B. haloalkaliphilus*
- *B. halodenitrificans*
- *B. halodurans*
- *B. halophilus*
- *B. horikoshii*
- *B. horti*
- *B. infernus*
- *B. insolitus*
- *B. jeotgali*
- *B. kaustophilus*
- *B. kobensis*
- *B. laevolacticus*

- *B. larvae*
- *B. laterosporus*
- *B. lautus*
- *B. lentimorbus*
- *B. lentus*
- *B. licheniformis*
- *B. macerans*
- *B. macquariensis*
- *B. marinus*
- *B. marismortui*
- *B. megaterium*
- *B. methanolicus*
- *B. migulanus*
- *B. mojavensis*
- *B. mucilaginosus*
- *B. mycoides*
- *B. naganoensis*
- *B. oleronius*
- *B. pabuli*
- *B. pallidus*
- *B. pantothenticus*
- *B. parabrevis*
- *B. pasteurii*
- *B. peoriae*
- *B. polymyxa*
- *B. popilliae*
- *B. pseudalcaliphilus*
- *B. pseudofirmus*
- *B. pseudomycoides*
- *B. psychrophilus*
- *B. psychrosaccharolyticus*
- *B. pulvifaciens*
- *B. pumilus*
- *B. reuszeri*
- *B. salexigens*
- *B. schlegelii*
- *B. selenitrireducens*
- *B. silvestris*
- *B. simplex*
- *B. siralis*
- *B. smithii*
- *B. sphaericus*
- *B. sporothermodurans*
- *B. stearothermophilus*
- *B. subtilis* subsp. *spizizenii*
- *B. subtilis* subsp. *subtilis*
- *B. thermoaerophilus*
- *B. thermoamylovorans*
- *B. thermocatenulatus*
- *B. thermocloacae*
- *B. thermodenitrificans*
- *B. thermoglucosidasius*
- *B. thermoleovorans*
- *B. thermoruber*
- *B. thermosphaericus*
- *B. thiaminolyticus*
- *B. thuringiensis*
- *B. tusciae*

B. *validus*
B. *vallismortis*
B. *vedderi*
B. *vulcani*
B. *weihenstephanensis*
bacillus, pl. **bacilli**
Abel b. (*See Klebsiella ozaenae*)
abortus b.
acid-fast b. (AFB)
Bang b. (*See Brucella abortus*)
Battey b. (*See Mycobacterium intracellulare*)
blue pus b.
Bordet-Gengou b. (*See Bordetella pertussis*)
Calmette-Guérin b. (BCG)
cholera b.
coliform b.
colon b.
comma b.
corroding b.
diphtheroid b.
Döderlein b. (*See Lactobacillus acidophilus*)
Ducrey b.
dysentery b.
Eberth b. (*See Salmonella typhi*)
enteric gram-negative b.
Flexner b.
Friedländer b.
gas b.
Ghon-Sachs b. (*See Clostridium septicum*)
glanders b.
gram-negative b.
gram-positive b.
Hansen b.
hay b.
Hofmann b.
influenza b.
Johne b.
Klebs-Loeffler b. (*See Corynebacterium*)
Koch b. (*See Mycobacterium tuberculosis*)
Koch-Weeks b. (*See Haemophilus aegyptius*)
lactic acid b.
leprosy b. (*See Mycobacterium leprae*)
Loeffler b.
mist b.

Morgan b. (*See Morganella morganii*)
necrosis b.
nonmotile pleomorphic b.
paracolon b.
paradysentery b.
paratyphoid b. (*See Salmonella enteritidis*)
Pfeiffer b. (*See Haemophilus influenzae*)
plague b.
Preisz-Nocard b. (*See Corynebacterium pseudotuberculosis*)
Schmorl b. (*See Fusobacterium necrophorum*)
Shiga b. (*See Shigella dysenteriae*)
Shiga-Kruse b. (*See Shigella dysenteriae*)
tap water b.
timothy hay b.
tubercle b.
typhoid b.
Vincent b.
Weeks b. (*See Haemophilus aegyptius*)
Welch b. (*See Clostridium perfringens*)
Whitmore b.
Bacimyxin
Bacitin
bacitracin
    b., neomycin, polymixin B, and lidocaine
    b., neomycin, and polymyxin B
    b., neomycin, polymyxin B, and hydrocortisone
    b. and polymyxin B
    b. susceptibility test
Back-Ese M
Backusia (f)
bacoti
    Liponyssus b.
    Ornithonyssus b.
BacT/Alert blood culture
Bactcard *Candida* test
BACTEC
    BACTEC blood culture
    BACTEC 9440/9120 Blood Culture System
    BACTEC radiometric system

B

NOTES

bacteremia
    catheter-associated b. (CAB)
    catheter-related b.
    community-acquired b.
    enterococcal b.
    Enterococcus avium b.
    Enterococcus faecalis b.
    gram-negative b.
    gram-positive b.
    Haemophilus influenzae b.
    MAI b.
    meningococcal b.
    Mycoplasma hominis b.
    nontyphi *Salmonella* b.
    nosocomial b.
    pneumococcal b.
    polymicrobial b.
    postpartum b.
    primary occult b.
    Pseudomonas aeruginosa b.
    staphylococcal b.
    Streptococcus mitis b.
    unimicrobial b.
bacteremia/fungemia
    catheter-related b.
bacteremic epididymitis
bacteria (*pl. of* bacterium)
bacteria-free stage of bacterial
    endocarditis
bacterial
    b. antagonism
    b. antigen
    b. arthritis
    b. bronchopneumonia
    b. capsule
    b. conjunctivitis
    b. contamination
    b. corneal culture
    b. disease
    b. endarteritis
    b. endocarditis (BE)
    b. endophthalmitis
    b. enteritis
    b. exotoxin
    b. food poisoning
    b. gastroenteritis
    b. hemolysin
    b. infection
    b. interference
    b. keratitis
    b. macromolecule
    b. morphotype
    b. motility
    b. peritonitis
    b. peritonsillar abscess
    b. phagocytosis test
    b. plaque
    b. pneumococcal pneumonia

    b. pyogenic meningitis
    b. septicemia
    b. smear
    b. superinfection
    b. synergistic gangrene
    b. toxin
    b. vaccine
    b. vaginosis (BV)
    b. virus
bactericidal, bacteriocidal
    b. activity
    b. concentration (MBC)
bacteriocide, bactericide
bacteriocin factor
bacteriocinogen
bacteriocinogenic plasmid
bacteriocins
bacteriofluorescin
bacteriogenic agglutination
bacteriogenous
bacterioid
bacteriologic
bacteriologist
bacteriology
    systematic b.
bacteriolysis
bacteriolytic
bacteriolyze
Bacterionema matruchotii (b)
bacteriopexy
bacteriophage
    defective b.
    b. plaque
    b. typing
bacteriophagology
bacteriophytoma
bacterioprotein
bacteriosis
bacteriostasis
bacteriostat
bacteriostatic
bacteriotoxic
bacteriotropic
bacteriotropin
bacteriotrypsin
Bacteriovorax (b)
    B. starrii
    B. stolpii
bacteriovorus
    Bdellovibrio b.
bacterium, pl. **bacteria**
    acid-fast bacteria
    anaerobic bacteria
    blue-green b.
    cell wall-defective bacteria
    Chauveau b.
    coliform bacteria
    coryneform b.

diplococcoid b.
endoteric b.
enteric b.
exoteric b.
facultative bacteria
Gram-variable bacteria
herbicola-lathyri bacteria (*See*
  Enterobacter agglomerans)
lysogenic b.
multidrug-resistant bacteria
nocardioform bacteria
non-spore-forming bacteria
paratyphoid bacteria (*See*
  Salmonella enteritidis)
prokaryotic bacteria
pyogenic b.
red mouth b.
bacteriuria
  asymptomatic b.
  urease-positive b.
bacteriuric
bacteroid
Bacteroidaceae
Bacteroides (b)
  B. acidifaciens
  B. amylophilus
  B. asaccharolyticus
  B. bivius
  B. buccae
  B. bucculis
  B. caccae
  B. capillosus
  B. capillus
  B. cellulosolvens
  B. coagulans
  B. corporis
  B. denticola
  B. disiens
  B. distasonis
  B. eggerthii
  B. endodontalis
  B. forsythus
  B. fragilis
  B. furcosus
  B. galacturonicus
  B. gingivalis
  B. gracilis
  B. helcogenes
  B. heparinolyticus
  B. hypermegas
  B. intermedius
  B. levii

B. loescheii
B. macacae
B. melaninogenicus
B. melaninogenicus subsp.
  intermedius
B. melaninogenicus subsp. *macacae*
B. melaninogenicus subsp.
  melaninogenicus
B. merdae
B. microfusus
B. multiacidus
B. nodosus
B. ochraceus
B. oralis
B. oris
B. oulorum
B. ovatus
B. pectinophilus
B. pentosaceus
B. pneumosintes
B. polypragmatus
B. praeacutus
B. putredinis
B. pyogenes
B. ruminicola subsp. *brevis*
B. ruminicola subsp. *ruminicola*
B. salivosus
B. splanchnicus
B. stercoris
B. succinogenes
B. suis
B. tectus
B. termitidis
B. thetaiotaomicron
B. uniformis
B. ureolyticus
B. veroralis
B. vulgatus
B. xylanolyticus
B. zoogleoformans
bacteroides
  Brevundimonas b.
  Caulobacter b.
BactiCard *Neisseria*
Bacticort Otic
Bactigen *Haemophilus influenzae* **type B
  test**
Bactine Hydrocortisone
Bacto-agar medium
Bactocill
bactoclasticum
  Anaeroplasma b.

B

NOTES

Bactoderma (b)
  B. alba
  B. rosea
Bacto *Entamoeba* medium
Bactopen
BactoShield Topical
Bactrim DS
Bactroban Nasal
Bac-T Screen
baculata
  Heliorestis b.
baculatum
  Desulfomicrobium b.
baculatus
  Desulfovibrio b.
Baculoviridae
baculovirus
  b. expressed
  nonoccluded b.
  occluded b.
Badhamia utricularis (f)
badius
  Bacillus b.
  Streptomyces b.
Badnavirus (v)
Baermann
  B. concentration
  B. fecal extraction technique
baffinense
  Simulium b.
Bagaza virus (BAGV)
BAGV
  Bagaza virus
bahamensis
  Culex b.
Bahig virus (BAHV)
BAHV
  Bahig virus
baiense
  Simulium b.
bailii
  Saccharomyces b.
Bairnsdale ulcer
Bakau virus (BAKUV)
bakii
  Acetobacterium b.
  Desulfuromusa b.
BAKUV
  Bakau virus
  Baku virus
Baku virus (BAKUV)
BAL
  bronchoalveolar lavage
  BAL in Oil
balaenopterae
  Abiotrophia b.
  Granulicatella b.

Balamuth aqueous egg yolk infusion medium
Balamuthia mandrillaris (p)
balance
  acid-base b.
balanitis
  Candida b.
  circinate b.
  b. circumscripta plasma cellularis
  erosive *Candida* b.
  Follman b.
  plasma cell b.
  b. xerotica oliterans
  b. of Zoon
balanoposthitis
  streptococcal b.
balantidial dysentery
balantidiasis
Balantidiidae
balantidiosis
Balantidium (p)
  B. coli
  B. suis
balantidium infection
baldaccii
  Streptomyces b.
  Streptoverticillium b.
balearica
  Ferrimonas b.
  Pseudomonas b.
ball
  Aspergillus fungus b.
  fungus b.
balloon
  intrabladder b.
ballum
  Leptospira interrogans serovar b.
Balminil
  B. Decongestant
  B. DM
  B. DM D
  B. Expectorant
Balneatrix alpica (b)
Balnetar
Balpred
Balsamiaceae
Balsulph
BALT
  bronchus-associated lymphoid tissue
baltazardii
  Borrelia b.
baltica
  Cellulophaga b.
  Hirschia b.
  Shewanella b.
balticum
  Desulfotignum b.

balustinum
    Chryseobacterium b.
    Flavobacterium b.
balzeri
    Trichosporon b.
Bam35 virus
bambergiensis
    Streptomyces b.
bambusicolus
    Anopheles b.
banana
    b., white rice, apple, and white
      toast (BRAT)
    b., white rice, apple, and white
      toast diet
bancrofti
    Wuchereria b.
bancroftian filariasis
bancroftiasis
band
    neutrophil b.
    oligoclonal b.
Bandia virus (BDAV)
banding
Bang
    B. bacillus (*See Brucella abortus*)
    B. disease
bangense
    Natronorubrum b.
Bangoran virus (BGNV)
Bangui virus (BGIV)
banhegyii
    Paratorulosis b.
Banna virus (BAV)
Bannwarth syndrome
Banocide
Banophen Decongestant Capsule
Banthine
bantiana
    Cladophialophora b.
BANV
    Banzi virus
Banzi virus (BANV)
bar
    Aveeno Cleansing B.
    chromatoidal b.
    Fostex B.
    HI-CAL VM b.
    PanOxyl B.
    ZNP B.
barati
    Clostridium b.

Barbados leg
barbae
    folliculitis b.
    sycosis b.
    tinea b.
    trichophytosis b.
barbatipes
    Simulium b.
barbatus
    Bothriocephalus b.
barberi
    Anopheles b.
barber's itch
Barbidonna
barbiero
barbirostris
    Anopheles b.
barbiturate
barbosai
    Culicoides b.
barbotage
Barbour-Stoenner-Kelly medium
Barc Liquid
barium
    b. sulfate suspension
    b. swallow
barkeri
    Aureobacterium b.
    Clostridium b.
    Eubacterium b.
    Methanosarcina b.
    Microbacterium b.
Barmah Forest virus (BFV)
Barnavirus (v)
barnesae
    Gallicola b.
    Peptostreptococcus b.
barnesii
    Sulfurospirillum b.
barophilus
    Thermococcus b.
Barranqueras virus (BQSV)
barrier
    blood-brain b. (BBB)
    blood-cerebrospinal fluid b.
    b. contraceptive
Barriere-HC
Bartholin gland
bartholinitis
Bartlett grading system
Bartonella (b)
    B. alsatica

B

NOTES

Bartonella (continued)
    B. bacilliformis
    B. birtlesii
    B. clarridgeiae
    B. doshiae
    B. elizabethae
    B. grahamii
    B. henselae
    B. henselae detection
    B. koehlerae
    B. peromysci
    B. quintana
    B. talpae
    B. taylorii
    B. tribocorum
    B. vinsonii subsp. *arupensis*
    B. vinsonii subsp. *berkhoffii*
    B. vinsonii subsp. *vinsonii*
Bartonellaceae
bartonellosis
Barur virus (BARV)
BARV
    Barur virus
basal
    b. body
    b. body temperature
    b. cell carcinoma
    b. corpuscle
    b. cortisol level
    b. ganglion
    b. granule
    b. nucleus
    b. rod
    b. subarachnoid space
basaloid proliferation
base
    erythromycin b.
baseline
basement membrane antibody
basic fuchsin stain
basicola
    Thielaviopsis b.
Basidiobiolaceae
basidiobolae
    entomophthoramycosis b.
Basidiobolus ranarum (f)
Basidiomycetes
basilar
    b. atelectasis
    b. skull fracture
basilensis
    Ralstonia b.
basin
    lymph node b.
basipetal
Basipetospora rubra (f)
basis
    compassionate-use b.

Basisporium (*See* *Nigrospora sphaerica*)
basket nucleus
basophilic
    b. halo of Nevinny
    b. stippling
bassiana
    Beauveria b.
bat
    vampire b.
Batai virus (BATV)
Batama virus (BMAV)
bataviae
    Leptospira interrogans serovar b.
bath
    ice-water b.
Batken virus
Batson plexus
battery
    anergy skin test b.
    multipuncture b.
    b. of tests
    TORCH serology b.
Battey bacillus (*See* **Mycobacterium intracellulare**)
BATV
    Batai virus
baueri
    Culicoides b.
Bauer-Kirby susceptibility test
Bauline virus (BAUV)
baumannii
    Acinetobacter b.
    imipenem-resistant *Acinetobacter b.*
    Oceanimonas b.
baumgartneri
    Caulochora b.
BAUV
    Bauline virus
BAV
    Banna virus
    BeAr 328208 virus
bavaricum
    Methanocorpusculum b.
bavaricus
    Lactobacillus b.
Baxedin
bayanus
    Saccharomyces b.
Bayer
    B. 205
    B. Aspirin
    B. Select Chest Cold Caplets
Baylisascaris (p)
    B. columnaris
    B. procyonis
Bayou virus (BAYV)
BAYV
    Bayou virus

Bazin
    erythema induratum of B.
BB
    creatinine kinase BB
BBB
    blood-brain barrier
BBOV
    Bimbo virus
BBV
    black beetle virus
BCBL
    body cavity-based lymphoma
        AIDS-associated BCBL
BCCV
    Black Creek Canal virus
B-cell
    B-c. chronic lymphocytic leukemia
    B-c. function
    B-c. hybridoma
    B-c. lymphoma
    B-c. memory
    B-c. receptor
BCG
    bacille Calmette-Guérin
    Calmette-Guérin bacillus
        BCG host resistance gene
        BCG organism
        TICE BCG
        BCG vaccine
B-chronic lymphocyte leukemia (B CLL)
B-CLL
    B-chronic lymphocyte leukemia
BCM
    body cell mass
BCP
    birth control pill
BCV
    Bunyip Creek virus
BCYE
    BCYE agar
BDAV
    Bandia virus
Bdellomicrovirus (v)
Bdellovibrio (b)
    B. bacteriovorus
    B. phage virus
    B. starrii
    B. stolpii
BDI
    Beck Depression Inventory
bDNA
    branched chain DNA

branched DNA
    bDNA assay
    quantitative bDNA
BDV
    border disease virus
    Borna disease virus
BE
    bacterial endocarditis
BE/1 virus
beaded rod
beadlet
    enteric coated b.
bean-shaped
    kidney b.-s.
BeAnV-157575
    BeAn 157575 virus
BeAn 157575 virus (BeAnV-157575)
beard
    ringworm of b.
BeAr 328208 virus (BAV)
beaupertuyi
    Simulium b.
Beauveria bassiana (f)
beaveri
    Brugia b.
    Euparyphium b.
bebaru virus (BEBV)
Bcben
BEBV
    bebaru virus
beckae
    Culicoides b.
Beck Depression Inventory (BDI)
beclomethasone
bedbug
beddingii
    Xenorhabdus b.
    Xenorhabdus nematophila subsp. b.
beechii
    Candida b.
beefy red
Beepen-VK
BEFV
    bovine ephemeral fever
Beggiatoa alba (b)
Beggiatoaceae
Beggiatoales
beggiatoides
    Vitreoscilla b.
behavior
    drug-seeking b.

NOTES

behavioral
  b. risk factor
  B. Risk Factor Surveillance System
    (BRFSS)
Behçet disease
beigelii
  Trichosporon b.
Beijerinckia (b)
  B. derxii subsp. *derxii*
  B. derxii subsp. *venezuelae*
  B. fluminensis
  B. indica subsp. *indica*
  B. indica subsp. *lacticogenes*
  B. mobilis
beijerinckii
  Azotobacter b.
  Clostridium b.
  Oceanospirillum beijerinckii subsp.
    b.
  Pseudomonas b.
Beijing virus
bekefii
  Planctomyces b.
Belascaris procyonis
Belem virus (BLMV)
Belgrade virus
belkini
  Culicoides b.
Bellatal
bellator
  Anopheles b.
belli
  Isospora b.
bellii
  Rickettsia b.
Bell palsy
bellus
  Streptomyces b.
belly
  Delhi b.
Belmont virus (BELV)
Belterra virus (BELTV)
BELTV
  Belterra virus
BELV
  Belmont virus
Benadryl Decongestant Allergy tablet
Ben-Aqua
benarrochi
  Anopheles b.
bendigoensis
  Tessaracoccus b.
Beneckea (b)
  B. alginolytica
  B. campbellii
  B. gazogenes
  B. harveyi
  B. natriegens

  B. nereida
  B. nigrapulchrituda
  B. parahaemolytica
  B. pelagia
  B. splendida
  B. vulnifica
benedekii
  Pullularia fermentans var. *b.*
benedeni
  Moniezia b.
Benevides virus (BENV)
Benfica virus (BENV)
bengal
  Aquaspirillum b.
  Vibrio cholerae O139 B.
benhamiae
  Arthroderma b.
benign
  b. lymphadenopathy
  b. syphilis
  b. tertian fever
  b. tertian malaria
benjamini
  Fannia b.
Benoxyl
benthica
  Shewanella b.
bentonite flocculation test (BFT)
bentoquatam
BENV
  Benevides virus
  Benfica virus
Benylin
  B. for Allergies
  B. Codeine
  B. Cold
  B. Cough syrup
  B. Decongestant
  B. DM
  B. DM-D
  B. DM-E
  B.-E
  B. Expectorant
  B. Pediatric
Benyvirus (v)
Benzac
  B. AC Gel
  B. AC Wash
  B. W Gel
  B. W Wash
Benzagel
5-Benzagel
10-Benzagel
benzalkonium chloride (BZK)
benzamide
Benzamycin
Benzashave Cream

B

benzathine
    b. penicillin
    penicillin G b.
    b. penicillin G
benzene hexachloride
benzethonium chloride
benzocaine
    antipyrine and b.
Benzocol
Benzodent
benzodiazepine anxiolytic
benzoevorans
    Bacillus b.
benzoic acid and salicylic acid
benzoin
benzonatate
benzoyl
    b. peroxide
    b. peroxide and hydrocortisone
benztropine
benzylpenicillin
    b. potassium
    procaine b.
benzylpenicilloyl (BPO)
bepridil
bercovleri
    Yersinia b.
bergeri
    Gemella b.
Bergeyella zoohelcum (b)
berghei
    Plasmodium b.
bergi
    Culicoides b.
berkhoffii
    Bartonella vinsonii subsp. *b.*
berlini
    Aedes b.
bermudensis
    Culicoides b.
Berna
    Vivotif B.
bernardiae
    Actinomyces b.
    Arcanobacterium b.
Berne virus (BEV)
berrensis
    Thermohalobacter b.
Berrimah virus (BRMV)
bertae
    Candida b.

berthetii
    Candida b.
bertholletiae
    Cunninghamella b.
Bertia
    B. satyri
    B. studeri
Bertiella
    B. mucronata
    B. studeri
bertiellosis
Bertioga virus
Besnoitiidae
bestiarum
    Aeromonas b.
beta
    b. blocker
    b. carotene
    b. corynebacteriophage
    b. cryptoxanthin
    b. gene
    b. hemolysin
    b. hemolysis
    b. hemolytic
    b. hemolytic strep culture
    b. hemolytic streptococci infection
    b. hemolytic streptococcus
    b. phage
    b. toxin
beta-*N*-acetylglucosaminidase production test
beta-adrenergic receptor
Betachron
Betacort
Betacryptovirus (v)
Betaderm
Betadine
    B. First Aid Antibiotics +
    Moisturizer
betae
    Corynebacterium b.
beta-galactosidase test
Betagel
beta-globin
beta-HCG
    beta-human chorionic gonadotropin
Betaherpesvirinae
beta-human chorionic gonadotropin (beta-HCG)
beta-lactam
    b.-l. antibiotic

NOTES

beta-lactam *(continued)*
    b.-l. IgE antibody
    b.-l. ring
beta-lactamase
    b.-l. inhibitor
    b.-l. production test
beta-lactamase-mediated resistance
beta-lactam-beta-lactamase
    b.-l.-b.-l. combination
    b.-l.-b.-l. inhibitor
Betalene Topical
betamethasone
    b. and clotrimazole
    b. (systemic)
    b. (topical)
beta$_2$-microglobulin
Betanodavirus (v)
Betapen-VK
Betaretrovirus (v)
Betasept
Betatetravirus (v)
Betatrex Topical
Beta-Val Topical
betavasculorum
    Erwinia carotovora subsp. *b.*
    Pectobacterium carotovorum subsp.
      b.
beteli
    Pseudomonas b.
Bethesda
    B. classification
    B. classification system
Bethesda-Ballerup Group
beticola
    Corynebacterium b.
Betnesol
Betnovate
bettyae
    Pasteurella b.
betulinum
    Trimmatostroma b.
Beutenbergia (b)
    B. cavernae
BEV
    Berne virus
bezziana
    Chrysomyia b.
BFP
    biologic false positive
BFT
    bentonite flocculation test
BFV
    Barmah Forest virus
BG
    Bordet-Gengou
      BG medium
BGIV
    Bangui virus

BGNV
    Bangoran virus
Bhanja virus
BHI
    brain-heart infusion
bhutanensis
    Cryptococcus b.
BIA
    bioelectric impedance
    bioimpedance
biacutus
    Desulfococcus b.
biapenem
BIAV
    Bobia virus
Biavax
Biaxin
    B. Filmtabs
    B. XL
biazotea
    Cellulomonas b.
bicarbonate
    sodium b.
Bichat fat pad
bichloracetic acid
Bicillin
    B. C-R
    B. C-R 900/300 injection
    B. L-A
    B. L-A injection
bickleyi
    Culicoides b.
bicoloratum
    Simulium b.
bicompartmental
bicorne
    Simulium b.
bicuspidatus
    Cyclops b.
bidet
bidimensional
bieneusi
    Enterocytozoon b.
bieristatus
    Aedes b.
bifermentans
    Clostridium b.
    Lactobacillus b.
bifidalatum
    Hysterothylacium b.
Bifidobacterium (b)
    B. adolescentis
    B. angulatum
    B. animalis
    B. appendicitis
    B. asteroides
    B. bifidum
    B. boum

B. *breve*
B. *catenulatum*
B. *choerinum*
B. *coryneforme*
B. *cuniculi*
B. *denticolens*
B. *dentium*
B. *gallicum*
B. *gallinarum*
B. *globosum*
B. *indicum*
B. *infantis*
B. *inopinatum*
B. *lactis*
B. *longum*
B. *magnum*
B. *merycicum*
B. *minimum*
B. *pseudocatenulatum*
B. *pseudolongum* var. *globosum*
B. *pseudolongum* var. *pseudolongum*
B. *pullorum*
B. *ruminantium*
B. *saeculare*
B. *subtile*
B. *suis*
B. *thermacidophilum*
B. *thermophilum*
bifidum
    Bifidobacterium b.
bifidus factor
biflagellated trophozoite
biflexa
    Leptospira b.
bifoliata
    Anopheles b.
bifonazole
biforme
    Eubacterium b.
bifurcation
    bronchial b.
bifurcum
    Oesophagostomum b.
big
    b. laughing mushroom
    b. spleen disease
bigemina
    Babesia b.
bigeminum
    Coccidium b.
biguttatus
    Culicoides b.

bikiniensis
    Streptomyces b.
bilateral retinochoroiditis
bile
    b. duct obstruction
    b. esculin
    b. esculin agar
    b. salt
    b. salt agar
    b. solubility test
bilharzial
    b. appendicitis
    b. dysentery
    b. granuloma
bilharziasis
    urinary b.
Bilharziella polonica (p)
bilharzioma
bilharziosis
biliary
    b. ascariasis
    b. atresia
    b. cryptosporidiosis
    b. pancreatitis
    b. pseudolithiasis
    b. scintigraphy
    b. sepsis
    b. tract
    b. tract infection
    b. tract surgery
bilious
    b. remittent malaria
    b. typhoid of Griesinger
bilirubin elevation
bilis
    Helicobacter b.
billingiae
    Erwinia b.
biloma
Bilophila wadsworthia (b)
Biltricide
BiMAB
    bispecific monoclonal antibody
bimaculatus
    Aedes b.
bimanual examination
Bimbo virus (BBOV)
Bimiti virus (BIMV)
bimodal
BIMV
    Bimiti virus

NOTES

B

binary
  b. combination
  b. fission
  b. nomenclature
Binax
binocular dissecting microscope
binomial
bioassay
  L-929 b.
Bio-bag
bioburden
Biocef
biocenosis
biochemical
  b. differentiation
  b. profiling
biocidal
bioclimatology
Bioderm
bioelectric impedance (BIA)
Bio-EnzaBead Assay
biogroup
  Enterobacter amnigenus b. 1, 2
biohazard
bioimpedance (BIA)
biologic
  b. control
  b. false positive (BFP)
  b. hemolysis
  b. vector
biological response modifier (BRM)
Biolog Microplate Identification System
bioluminescence
Biomox
Biomphalaria
  B. glabrata
  B. haranensis
biophage
biophagism
biophagous
biophagy
biopsy
  aspiration b.
  blind liver b.
  bone marrow aspiration and b.
  bone marrow trephine b.
  brush b.
  cold-knife cone b.
  b. culture
  cutaneous b.
  cystoscopic b.
  endobronchial b.
  excisional b.
  b. forceps
  gastric mucosal b.
  immunofluorescence skin b.
  incisional b.
  liver b.

  lung b. tissue
  lymph node b.
  muscle b.
  needle aspiration b.
  percutaneous liver b.
  percutaneous needle aspiration b.
  punch b.
  shave b.
  skeletal muscle b.
  synovial b.
  tissue b.
  tonsillar b.
  transbronchial b.
  b. urease test
biosafety
  b. cabinet (BSC)
  b. level (BSL)
biospeleology
BioStar *Chlamydia* **OIA assay**
biosynthesis
  aldosterone b.
Bio-Tab Oral
biotechnology
  Molecular Genetics Unit of the
    Institute of B. (ITQB)
biotherapy
  IL-2-based b.
Biothrax
biotic
  b. community
  b. factor
biotin-avitin
biotope
Biot spot
biotype
  Haemophilus influenzae b. III, IV
  Pseudomonas putida b. B
  Vibrio cholerae serotype O1 of El
    Tor b.
biotyping
biovar
  Fusobacterium necrophorum subsp.
    necrophorum b. C
  Yersinia enterocolitica b. 1
biparasitism
biparental
bipartite dsRNA mycovirus group
biphasic
biphenylol
bipolar
Bipolaris (f)
  B. australiensis
  B. spicifera
biprosthecium
  Asticcacaulis b.
bipunctata
  Macromonas b.
Birao virus (BIRV)

birds-in-flight arrangement
birefringent
birminghamensis
    Legionella b.
Birnaviridae
birth control pill (BCP)
birtlesii
    Bartonella b.
BIRV
    Birao virus
bisegmented dsRNA virus group
biseptata
    Drechslera b.
Bismatrol
Bismed
bismuth
    b. salt
    b. subsalicylate (BSS)
    b. subsalicylate, metronidazole, and
      tetracycline
    b. sulfite agar
Bismylate
bispecific monoclonal antibody (BiMAB)
Bis-POM PMEA
bispora
    Microbispora b.
    Pichia b.
    Thermobispora b.
bisporigera
    Amanita b.
bisporus
    Agaricus b.
    Saccharomyces b.
bisulfite
    sodium b.
bite
    cat b.
biting louse
bitolterol
bitropic
biundulant
bivalent gas gangrene antitoxin
Bivens Arm virus
biverticillatum
    Streptoverticillium b.
biverticillatus
    Streptomyces b.
bivia
    Prevotella b.
Bivitellobilharzia nairi
bivittatum
    Simulium b.

bivius
    Bacteroides b.
bizzozeronii
    Helicobacter b.
BJ5-T virus
BK
    polyomavirus BK
    BK virus
BKV human polyomavirus
BL
    borderline lepromatous
Blac
    Linctus Codeine B.
black
    b. beetle virus (BBV)
    B. Creek Canal virus (BCCV)
    b. fever
    b. piedra
    b. sickness
    b. spore
    b. tarantula
    b. widow spider
black-dot ringworm
blackwater fever
bladder
    b. contractility
    fibrotic b.
    hyperreflexic b.
    hypertrophic b.
    kidneys, ureters and b. (KUB)
    b. neck obstruction
    neurogenic b.
    b. schistosomiasis
    superficial transitional cell
      carcinoma of the b.
    uninhibited b.
    unstable b.
bladderworm
blakei
    Cheyletiella b.
blakesleeana
    Cunninghamella b.
blancasi
    Simulium b.
blanket
    cooling b.
blankii
    Candida b.
blantoni
    Culicoides b.
blast
blastic

NOTES

blastica
    Rhodopseudomonas b.
blasticus
    Rhodobacter b.
blastmyceticum
    Streptoverticillium b.
blastmyceticus
    Streptomyces b.
Blastobacter (b)
    B. *aggregatus*
    B. *capsulatus*
    B. *denitrificans*
    B. *henricii*
    B. *natatorius*
Blastochloris (b)
    B. *sulfoviridis*
    B. *viridis*
Blastocladiaceae
Blastocladiales
Blastococcus aggregatus (b)
blastoconidium, pl. **blastoconidia**
    Candida blastoconidia
Blastocystis hominis (p)
blastocystosis
blastocytosis
Blastodendrion (*See* **Candida**)
blastoderm
Blastomonas (b)
    B. *natatoria*
    B. *ursincola*
Blastomyces dermatitidis (f)
Blastomycetes
blastomycetica
    erosio interdigitalis b.
blastomycetic dermatitis
blastomycin
Blastomycoides (f)
blastomycosis
    cutaneous b.
    b. immunodiffusion
    keloidal b.
    North American b.
    South American b.
blastophore
Blastoschizomyces capitatus (f)
blastospore
Blatta
Blattabacterium cuenoti (b)
blattae
    Escherichia b.
Blattella
    B. *germanica*
    B. *lituricollis*
blatticola
    Methanomicrococcus b.
bleb
blebbing
bleb-related

B/LEE/40 virus
bleeding
    intermenstrual b.
    intracranial b.
BlemErase Lotion
Blemish Control
blennophthalmia
blennorrhea
    inclusion b.
Blenoxane
Blephamide Ophthalmic
blepharitis
    marginal b.
    mixed seborrheic-staphylococcal b.
    tuberculous b.
blepharoconjunctivitis
blepharoplast
blepharospasm
Bleph-10 Ophthalmic
BLE virus
B-like non-A non-B hepatitis
blinding
    b. river disease
blind liver biopsy
blindness
    river b.
blister
    fever b.
    fly b.
blistering distal dactylitis
Blis-To-Sol
BLMV
    Belem virus
blochii
    Acremonium b.
block
    anabolic b.
    complete atrioventricular b.
    complete heart b.
    motor conduction b.
    tobramycin-impregnated polymethyl
      methacrylate spacer b.
blockade
    neuromuscular b.
    reticuloendothelial b.
blocker
    beta b.
    calcium channel b.
    selective serotonin receptor b.
blocking assay
Blomia tropicalis
blood
    b. agar
    b. agar hemolysis
    b. Amikin level
    b. cell profile
    cord b.
    b. count

b. Fungizone level
b. gas
b. group agglutinin
b. group P antigen
b. IgE
kanamycin-vancomycin laked b. (KVLB)
b. lysis tube
occult b. (OB)
semiquantitative occult b.
b. smear for malarial parasites
b. Sporanox level
b. urea nitrogen (BUN)
b. urea nitrogen/creatinine (BUN/Cr)
b. Vancocin level
b. Vancoled level
b. viral load
bloodborne
blood-brain barrier (BBB)
blood-cerebrospinal fluid barrier
bloodstream infection (BSI)
bloodworm
blot
dot b.
Southern b.
Western b. (WB)
blowfly
blue
b. disease
b. dye
eosin methylene b. (EMB)
b. fever
lactophenol cotton b. (LPCB)
methenamine, phenyl salicylate, atropine, hyoscyamine, benzoic acid, and methylene b.
methylene b.
b. pus bacillus
Selsun B.
Urolene B.
blue-green
b.-g. algae
b.-g. bacterium
bluensis
Streptomyces b.
bluetongue virus 1–24 (BLUV 1–24, BTV 1–24)
BLUV 1–24
bluetongue virus 1–24
BLV
bovine leukemia

BM
bone marrow
BMAV
Batama virus
BMI
body mass index
BMS-232632
BMT
bone marrow transplant
bone marrow transplantation
allogeneic BMT
BMTU
bone marrow transplant unit
BMV
Buenaventura virus
Bobaya virus (BOBV)
Bobia virus (BIAV)
bobili
Streptomyces b.
BOBV
Bobaya virus
Bodo
B. caudatus
B. saltans
B. urinarius
Bodonidae
BodPod
BodPod plethysmography
BodPod testing
body
asteroid b.
basal b.
brassy b.
b. cavity-based lymphoma (BCBL)
b. cavity fluid cytology
b. cell mass (BCM)
chromatin b.
Councilman b.
cyanobacterium-like b.
cytoplasmic keratohyalin inclusion b.
Dohle b.
Donovan b.
elementary b. (EB)
eosinophilic nuclear inclusion b.
fruiting b.
gamma-Gandy b.
Guanieri b.
herpetic inclusion b.
Howell-Jolly b.'s
inclusion b.
L-D b.

B

NOTES

body *(continued)*
    Leishman-Donovan b.
    b. louse
    b. mass index (BMI)
    Masson b.
    Medlar b.
    metachromatic b.
    Miyagawa b.
    Mooser b.
    Negri b.
    nodular b.
    parabasal b.
    b. plasma viral load
    psittacosis inclusion b.
    rest b.
    reticulate b. (RB)
    ringworm of b.
    Russell b.
    sclerotic b.
    segmenting b.
    b. surface area (BSA)
    T b.
    vaccine b.
    vertebral b.
Boeck and Drbohlav Locke-egg-serum medium
boevrei
    Moraxella b.
bogorensis
    Asaia b.
Bogoriella caseilytica (b)
bogoriensis
    Candida b.
    Rhodobaca b.
boharti
    Culex b.
bohemica
    Verpa b.
bohemicum
    Mycobacterium b.
boidinii
    Candida b.
boil
    Madura b.
bois
    pian b.
Bolbosoma
boleticola
    Candida b.
boletus
    Melittangium b.
Boletus piperatus (f)
Boletus virus X (BolVX)
Bolivian hemorrhagic fever
boliviensis
    Anopheles b.
BolVX
    Boletus virus X

bombayensis
    Methanolobus b.
bombi
    Candida b.
bombicola
    Candida b.
bombycis
    Nosema b.
bone
    b. demineralization
    b. infection
    b. and joint tuberculosis
    b. marrow (BM)
    b. marrow aspirate
    b. marrow aspiration
    b. marrow aspiration and biopsy
    b. marrow culture
    b. marrow fungus culture
    b. marrow iron stain
    b. marrow mycobacteria culture
    b. marrow sampling
    b. marrow suppression
    b. marrow transplant (BMT)
    b. marrow transplantation (BMT)
    b. marrow transplant unit (BMTU)
    b. marrow trephine biopsy
    b. scan
    b. scan with flow
    b. scintigraphy
    b. sialoprotein
    b. spicule
bongori
    Salmonella b.
    Salmonella choleraesuis subsp. *b.*
bonnei
    Anopheles b.
    Phaneropsolus b.
BOOP
    bronchiolitis obliterans-organizing pneumonia
Boophilus annulatus (p)
boopis
    Crassicauda b.
boppii
    Cladophialophora b.
Boraceia virus (BORV)
boranensis
    Demodema b.
borax
borborygmus
bordai
    Simulium b.
border
    b. disease
    b. disease virus (BDV)
borderline
    b. lepromatous (BL)

b. leprosy
b. tuberculoid (BT)
Bordetella (b)
  B. avium
  B. bronchiseptica
  B. hinzii
  B. holmesii
  B. parapertussis
  B. pertussis
  B. pertussis antibody
  B. pertussis serology
  B. pertussis titer
  B. petrii
  B. trematum
Bordet-Gengou (BG)
  B.-G. bacillus (*See Bordetella pertussis*)
  B.-G. potato blood agar
borealis
  Paenibacillus b.
boreopolis
  Pseudomonas b.
boreus
  Subtercola b.
borgpetersenii
  Leptospira b.
boric acid
borinquense
  Halogeometricum b.
borkumensis
  Alcanivorax b.
Borna
  B. disease
  B. disease virus (BDV)
Bornavirus (v)
bornavirus retinitis
Bornholm
  B. disease
  B. disease virus
Borofax Topical
Borrelia (b)
  B. afzelii
  B. anserina
  B. baltazardii
  B. brasiliensis
  B. burgdorferi
  B. burgdorferi DNA assay
  B. burgdorferi sensu lato
  B. burgdorferi sensu stricto
  B. caucasica
  B. coriaceae
  B. crocidurae

B. dugesii
B. duttonii
B. garinii
B. graingeri
B. harveyi
B. hermsii
B. hispanica
B. japonica
B. latyschewii
B. lusitaniae
B. mazzottii
B. miyamotoi
B. parkeri
B. persica
B. recurrentis
B. tanukii
B. theileri
B. tillae
B. turdi
B. turicatae
B. valaisiana
B. venezuelensis
borrelial
  b. infection
  b. lymphocytoma
borreliosis
  Lyme b.
  b. serology
  tick-borne b.
borstelensis
  Bacillus b.
  Brevibacillus b.
BORV
  Boraceia virus
Borzia
Bos
  Bos adenovirus 1–10 (bos 1–10)
bos
  Psorergates b.
bos 1–10
  Bos adenovirus 1–10
Bosch yaw
Bosea thiooxidans (b)
bot
  ox b.
  sheep b.
Botambi virus (BOTV)
Boteke virus (BTKV)
botfly
  head b.
  human b.

NOTES

B

botfly *(continued)*
    skin b.
    warble b.
bothria
bothriocephaliasis
Bothriocephalidae
Bothriocephalus (p)
    B. *andresi*
    B. *barbatus*
    B. *clavibothrium*
    B. *claviceps*
    B. *funiculus*
    B. *gregarius*
    B. *scorpii*
bothrium
Botkins disease
Botryodiplodia theobromae (f) (*See Lasiodiplodia theobromae*)
botryoides
Botryomyces caespitosus (f)
botryosa
    Veronaea b.
Botryosphaeriaceae
Botryosphaeria rhodina (f)
Botrytis (f)
Botrytoides
bottimeri
    Culicoides b.
bottropensis
    Streptomyces b.
botulibranchium
    Simulium b.
botulin
botulinal
    b. antitoxin
    b. toxin
botulinogenic
botulinum
    b. antitoxin
    Clostridium b.
    b. neurotoxin
    b. toxoid pentavalent vaccine
botulism
    animal b.
    b. antitoxin
    fermented food b.
    foodborne b.
    human b.
    infant b.
    intestinal toxemia b.
    neonatal b.
    wound b.
botulismotoxin
botulogenic
BOTV
    Botambi virus
Bouboui virus (BOUV)
Boudierella (f) (*See Conidiobolus*)

boueti
    Leptocimex b.
boullardii
    Microsporum b.
boum
    Bifidobacterium b.
bound coagulase
bouquet fever
bourgense
    Methanogenium b.
bourgensis
    Methanoculleus b.
boutonneuse fever
BOUV
    Bouboui virus
Bovicola (p)
    B. *bovis*
    B. *caprae*
    B. *equi*
    B. *ovis*
bovicus
    Macrococcus b.
bovienii
    Xenorhabdus b.
    Xenorhabdus nematophila subsp. b.
bovifelis
    Sarcocystis b.
bovigenitalium
    Mycoplasma b.
bovina
    Candida b.
bovine
    b. AAV virus (BAAV)
    b. adenovirus 1–9
    b. antitoxin
    b. astrovirus 1–2
    b. brucellosis
    b. coronavirus
    b. enterovirus 1–2
    b. ephemeral fever (BEFV)
    b. herpes mammillitis
    b. herpesvirus 1–5
    b. heterograft
    b. immunodeficiency
    b. immunodeficiency virus
    b. leukemia (BLV)
    b. leukemia virus
    b. mammalitis
    b. mastitis
    b. papular stomatitis (BPSV)
    b. parvovirus
    b. respiratory syncytial virus
    b. rhinovirus
    b. rhinovirus 1–2
    b. rotavirus stain
    b. spongiform encephalopathy
    b. ulcerative mammillitis

b. vaccinia mammillitis
b. viral diarrhea virus (BVDV)
bovirhinis
    Mycoplasma b.
bovis
    Actinomyces b.
    Babesia b.
    Bovicola b.
    Chorioptes b.
    Corynebacterium b.
    Cysticercus b.
    Damalina b.
    Demodex b.
    Eimeria b.
    Hypoderma b.
    Methylococcus b.
    Moraxella (Moraxella) b.
    Mycobacterium b.
    Mycoplasma b.
    Schistosoma b.
    Staphylococcus saprophyticus subsp.
     b.
    Streptococcus b.
bovistum
    Thiobacterium b.
bovoculi
    Mycoplasma b.
bowdenii
    Actinomyces b.
bowel
    b. fissure
    b. perforation
Bowen disease
bowenoid papulosis
boxcar shaped
boydii
    Pseudallescheria b.
    Shigella b.
bozemaii
    Legionella b.
bozemanae
    Fluoribacter b.
bozemanii
    Legionella b.
Bozo virus
BP
    bacillary peliosis
BPD
    bronchopulmonary dysplasia
BPF
    Brazilian purpuric fever

BPO
    benzylpenicilloyl
BPSV
    bovine papular stomatitis
BQSV
    Barranqueras virus
braakii
    Citrobacter b.
bracchium
    Agromyces b.
brachial
    b. neuritis
    b. plexus neuropathy
Brachiola (p)
    B. connori
    B. vesicularum
brachioradialis
brachy
    Eubacterium b.
Brachybacterium (b)
    B. alimentarium
    B. conglomeratum
    B. faecium
    B. nesterenkovii
    B. paraconglomeratum
    B. rhamnosum
    B. tyrofermentans
Brachybasidiaceae
Brachybasidiales
Brachycera
Brachycladium (p)
brachycladum
    Simulium b.
Brachymonas denitrificans (b)
Brachyspira (h)
    B. aalborgi
    B. alvinipulli
    B. hyodysenteriae
    B. innocens
    B. pilosicoli
brachyspora
    Curvularia b.
Brachysporium (f)
Bracovirus (v)
bracteatum
    Simulium b.
bradleyi
    Anopheles b.
bradyarrhythmia
bradycardia
bradykinin

B

NOTES

Bradyrhizobium (b)
  B. elkanii
  B. japonicum
  B. liaoningense
bradyzoite form
brain
  b. abscess
  b. toxoplasmosis
  tuberculosis of the b.
  b. viral culture
Brainerd diarrhea
brain-heart
  b.-h. infusion (BHI)
  b.-h. infusion agar
  b.-h. infusion broth
brainstem dysfunction
branched
  b. chain DNA (bDNA)
  b. DNA (bDNA)
  b. DNA assay
branching
  false b.
branchiophilum
  Flavobacterium b.
branderi
  Mycobacterium b.
Branhamella catarrhalis (b)
brasilense
  Azospirillum b.
brasiliana, braziliana
  bubas b.
brasiliense
  Amblyomma b.
  Trichosporon b.
brasiliensis
  Actinoplanes b.
  Borrelia b.
  Nocardia b.
  Paracoccidioides b.
  Planctomyces b.
  Streptomyces b.
  Triatoma b.
brassicacearum
  Pseudomonas b.
brassicae
  Acholeplasma b.
brassy body
BRAT
  banana, white rice, apple, and white toast
  BRAT diet
braulti
  Enantiothamnus b.
brauni
  Digramma b.
  Multiceps b.
  Taenia b.
brazilensis

Brazilian
  B. hemorrhagic fever
  B. purpuric fever (BPF)
braziliana (*var. of* brasiliana)
braziliense
  Ancylostoma b.
braziliensis
  Anopheles b.
  Leishmania b.
BrdU
  BrdU nucleoside analog
  BrdU uptake
breakbone fever
breast
  b. abscess
  b. infection
breath H₂ testing
breathing
  intermittent positive-pressure b.
  (IPPB)
Breda
  B. disease
  B. virus
Breezee Mist Antifungal
brelandi
  Aedes b.
brennaborense
  Treponema b.
brennerae
  Buttiauxella b.
Brenneria (b)
  B. alni
  B. nigrifluens
  B. paradisiaca
  B. quercina
  B. rubrifaciens
  B. salicis
Breonesin
brequinar
Brettanomyces (f)
  B. abstinens
  B. anomalus
  B. bruxellensis
  B. claussenii
  B. custerianus
  B. custesii
  B. intermedius
  B. lambicus
  B. naardenensis
breve
  Bifidobacterium b.
  Flavobacterium b.
  Gymnodinium b.
brevetoxin
Brevibacillus (b)
  B. agri
  B. borstelensis
  B. brevis

B. *centrosporus*
B. *choshinensis*
B. *formosus*
B. *laterosporus*
B. *parabrevis*
B. *reuszeri*
B. *thermoruber*
Brevibacteriaceae
Brevibacterium (b)
B. *acetylicum*
B. *albidum*
B. *ammoniagenes*
B. *avium*
B. *casei*
B. *citreum*
B. *divaricatum*
B. *epidermidis*
B. *fermentans*
B. *frigoritolerans*
B. *fuscum*
B. *halotolerans*
B. *imperiale*
B. *incertum*
B. *iodinum*
B. *linens*
B. *liquefaciens*
B. *luteum*
B. *lyticum*
B. *mcbrellneri*
B. *otitidis*
B. *oxydans*
B. *protophormiae*
B. *pusillum*
B. *saperdae*
B. *stationis*
B. *testaceum*
B. *vitarumen*
brevicatena
Micropolyspora b.
Nocardia b.
Sporichthya b.
brevicaulis
Brevidensovirus (v)
brevifurcatum
Simulium b.
Brevinema andersonii (b)
brevis
Bacillus b.
Bacteroides ruminicola subsp. *b.*
Brevibacillus b.
Demodex b.
Empedobacter b.

Janibacter b.
Lactobacillus b.
Prevotella b.
Prevotella ruminicola subsp. *b.*
Sulfitobacter b.
Trichostrongylus b.
Brevoxyl Gel
Brevundimonas (b)
B. *alba*
B. *aurantiaca*
B. *bacteroides*
B. *diminuta*
B. *intermedia*
B. *subvibrioides*
B. *variabilis*
B. *vesicularis*
BRFSS
Behavioral Risk Factor Surveillance
System
brickmaker's anemia
briensis
Nitrosospira b.
brierleyi
Acidianus b.
Sulfolobus b.
briggsae
Caenorhabditis b.
brilliant green
Brill-Zinsser disease
brim
pelvic b.
Briosia (f)
britovi
Trichinella b.
brizae
Drechslera b.
BRM
biological response modifier
BRMV
Berrimah virus
broad-spectrum
b.-s. antibiotic
b.-s. penicillin
broad waxy cast
Brochothrix (b)
B. *campestris*
B. *thermosphacta*
brockianus
Thermus b.
brockii
Pyrodictium b.

NOTES

brockii (continued)
>*Thermoanaerobacter brockii* subsp.
>b.
>*Thermoanaerobium b.*

Brodie abscess
broegbernensis
>*Pseudoxanthomonas b.*

Brolene Drop
Bromanate DC
Bromanyl Cough Syrup
Brome
>B. mosaic virus group

bromi
>*Xanthomonas b.*

bromide
>ethidium b.

bromii
>*Ruminococcus b.*

bromocriptine
bromodeoxyuridine nucleoside analog
bromodiphenhydramine and codeine
Bromotuss w/Codeine Cough syrup
Bromovirus (v)
Bromphen DC w/Codeine
brompheniramine, phenylpropanolamine,
and codeine
bronchial
>b. aspirate
>b. bifurcation
>b. brush
>b. epituberculosis
>b. washing

bronchialis
>*Gordonia b.*
>*Rhodococcus b.*

bronchiectasis
bronchiolitis
>fulminant b.
>b. obliterans-organizing pneumonia
>(BOOP)

bronchiseptica
>*Bordetella b.*

bronchitis
>chronic b.
>infectious avian b.

bronchoalveolar
>b. lavage (BAL)
>b. lavage fluid
>b. washing

bronchoalveolitis
bronchodilator
bronchogram
Broncho-Grippol-DM
bronchohepatic fistula
bronchomycosis
Bronchopan DM
bronchopleural fistula

bronchopneumonia
>bacterial b.
>eosinophilic b.
>interstitial b.

bronchopulmonary
>b. dysplasia (BPD)
>b. lavage

bronchoscopic *Legionella* **culture**
bronchoscopy
>diagnostic b.
>fiberoptic b. (FOB)
>flexible b.

bronchospasm
bronchus-associated lymphoid tissue
(BALT)
Bronitin Mist
Bronkaid Mist
Bronkometer
Bronkosol
Brontex
>B. Liquid
>B. Tablet

brood capsule
brookmani
>*Culicoides b.*

broomeae
>*Afipia b.*

broomeanus
>*Hypomyces b.*

Broomeiaceae
broth
>brain-heart infusion b.
>b. culture
>b. dilution test
>b. microdilution
>Mueller-Hinton b.
>b. susceptibility test
>tryptophan b.

Broviac catheter
Broviac-type catheter
brown
>B. & Hopps Gram stain
>b. recluse spider

Brown-Brenn stain
brucei
>*Trypanosoma b.*
>*Trypanosoma brucei b.*

Brucella (b)
>B. abortus
>B. canis
>B. card test
>B. melitensis
>B. melitensis peritonitis
>B. neotomae
>B. ovis
>B. sheep blood agar
>B. suis

Brucellaceae

brucellar endocarditis
brucellosis
    active b.
    bovine b.
    cardiovascular b.
    inactive b.
Bruconha virus
Brudzinski sign
Brugia (p)
    B. beaveri
    B. buckleyi
    B. ceylonensis
    B. guyanensis
    B. lepori
    B. malayi
    B. pahangi
    B. putei
    B. timori
    B. tupaiae
brugian filariasis
brumae
    Mycobacterium b.
brumata
    Opherophtera b.
brumpti
    Argas b.
brumptii
    Candida b.
    Tritirachium b.
Brumpt white mycetoma
brunensis
    Legionella b.
brunescens
    Lysobacter b.
Brunn
    nest of von B.
brunnea
    Micromonospora b.
brush
    b. biopsy
    bronchial b.
    cytology b.
    flexible fiberoptic bronchoscopy
      with protected b. (FFPB)
    Kruse b.
    protected specimen b. (PSB)
bruxellensis
    Brettanomyces b.
    Dekkera b.
bruxism
bryantii
    Clostridium b.

    Methanobacterium b.
    Prevotella b.
    Syntrophospora b.
    Treponema b.
BSA
    body surface area
BSBV
    Bushbush virus
BSC
    biosafety cabinet
BSI
    bloodstream infection
BSL
    biosafety level
BSQV
    Bussuquara virus
BSS
    bismuth subsalicylate
BT
    borderline tuberculoid
BTKV
    Boteke virus
BTV 1–24
    bluetongue virus 1–24
bubakii
    Phialophora b.
bubas
    b. brasiliana
bubble diffusion
bubo, pl. buboes
    chancroidal b.
    inguinal b.
    virulent b.
bubonic plague
bubulus
    Campylobacter sputorum subsp. *b.*
buccae
    Bacteroides b.
    Prevotella b.
buccal
    b. membrane
    b. mucosa
buccale
    Mycoplasma b.
    Treponema socranskii subsp. *b.*
buccalis
    Bacteroides b.
    Leptotrichia b.
    Prevotella b.
buccata
    Cuterebra b.
Buchnera aphidicola (b)

NOTES

buchneri
    Lactobacillus b.
buckle
    scleral b.
buckleyi
    Brugia b.
Buckley's
    B. DM
    B. DM Decongestant
buck moth caterpillar
bud
budayi
    Eubacterium b.
Budd-Chiari syndrome
budding
    nonsynchronous b.
buderi
    Chromatium b.
    Isochromatium b.
budesonide
Budvicia aquatica
Buenaventura virus (BMV)
buetschlii
    Iodamoeba b.
buffalo hump
buffalopox virus
buffer
    acid b.
    alkaline b.
buffered charcoal yeast extract agar
BufferGel
Bufferin
buffy
    b. coat
    b. coat concentration
    b. coat viral culture
bufonis
    Acanthocephalus b.
bug
    assassin b.
    harvest b.
    kissing b.
    reduviid b.
    triatomid b.
    Woodburg b.
Buggy Creek virus
buinensis
    Candida b.
Bujaru virus
Bukalasa bat virus
bulbar
    b. conjunctiva
    b. poliomyelitis
bulbillosum
    Cladorrhinum b.
bulbous skin lesion
bulgaricus
    Kluyveromyces b.

    Lactobacillus b.
    Lactobacillus delbrueckii subsp. *b.*
bulge-eye
bulging
    b. eye disease
    b. tympanic membrane
Bulinus
    B. globosus
    B. truncatus
bulla, pl. **bullae**
    hemorrhagic b.
bullata
    Mycoplana b.
Bulleidia extructa (b)
Bullera (f)
    B. armeniaca
    B. crocea
    B. dendrophila
    B. globispora
    B. myagiana
    B. oryzae
    B. pseudoalba
    B. sinensis
    B. variabilis
Bulleromyces albus (f)
Bulletin of World Health Organization
bullet-shaped virus group
bull neck
bullosa
    impetigo contagiosa b.
    Pseudostertagia b.
bullosus
    herpes circinatus b.
bullous
    b. disease
    b. erythema multiforme
    b. impetigo
    b. myringitis
    b. pemphigoid
    b. pemphigoid antibody
bull's-eye maculopathy
BUN
    blood urea nitrogen
BUN/Cr
    blood urea nitrogen/creatinine
bung-eye
bungoensis
    Streptomyces b.
bungpagga
Bunostominae
Bunostomum (p)
BUNV
    Bunyamwera virus
Bunyamwera
    B. fever
    B. supergroup
    B. *virus* (BUNV)
Bunyaviridae

Bunyavirus (v)
bunyavirus
    b. encephalitis
Bunyip Creek virus (BCV)
bupropion
burden
    leukemic b.
    plasma viral b.
    tumor b.
    viral b.
Burdwan fever
burgdorferi
    Borrelia b.
burgeri
    Aedes b.
Burkholderia (b)
    B. umbifaria
    B. andropogonis
    B. caledonica
    B. caribensis
    B. caryophylli
    B. cepacia
    B. cocovenenans
    B. fungorum
    B. gladioli
    B. glathei
    B. glumae
    B. graminis
    B. kururiensis
    B. mallei
    B. multivorans
    B. norimbergensis
    B. phenazinium
    B. pickettii
    B. plantarii
    B. pseudomallei
    B. pyrrocinia
    B. solanacearum
    B. stabilis
    B. thailandensis
    B. ubonensis
    B. vandii
    B. vietnamiensis
burkinabensis
    Anaerovibrio b.
burkinensis
    Anaeroarcus b.
    Desulfovibrio b.
Burkitt-like lymphoma
Burkitt lymphoma
burnetii
    Coxiella b.

burrow
burrowing ulcer
bursa
    Liponyssus b.
    Ornithonyssus b.
bursaria
    Paramecium b.
bursitis
    infectious b.
    olecranon b.
    septic b.
burtonensis
    Psychroserpens b.
burtonii
    Endomycopsis b.
    Methanococcoides b.
    Pichia b.
Buruli ulcer
Buschke disease
Buschke-Löwenstein tumor
Bushbush virus (BSBV)
Bushley medium
bush yaw
buski
    Fasciolopsis b.
buspirone
Bussuquara virus (BSQV)
bustamentei
    Anopheles b.
busulfan
buswellii
    Syntrophus b.
butcher's wart
butenafine hydrochloride
buteonis
    Mycoplasma b.
butleri
    Culicoides b.
butoconazole nitrate
butorphanol
butoxide
    pyrethrins and piperonyl b.
butterfly distribution
Buttiauxella (b)
    B. agrestis
    B. brennerae
    B. ferragutiae
    B. gaviniae
    B. izardii
    B. noackiae
    B. warmboldiae
Buttonwillow virus (BUTV)

B

NOTES

BUTV
Buttonwillow virus
butylicus
Hyperthermus b.
butyri
Candida b.
butyricum
Clostridium b.
Butyrivibrio (b)
B. crossotus
B. fibrisolvens
butyrophenone
butyrous
butzleri
Arcobacter b.
Campylobacter b.
BV
bacterial vaginosis

BV-araU
BVDV
bovine viral diarrhea virus
Bwamba virus (BWAV)
BWAV
Bwamba virus
Bydramine Cough syrup
byersi
Culicoides b.
Bymovirus (v)
byrdii
Trichosporon b.
byssina
Dendrostilbella b.
Byssoascus (f)
Byssochlamys (f)
BZK
benzalkonium chloride

C

C complex strain of *Chlamydia trachomatis*
C group virus
C peptide concentration
C16 virus
C1q immune complex detection
C-1 virus
CAA
circulating anodic antigen
CAB
catheter-associated bacteremia
caballi
Babesia c.
Pasteurella c.
Cabassou virus
cabinet
biosafety c. (BSC)
cabrerai
Cathaemasia c.
cacaoi
Candida c.
Streptomyces c.
Streptomyces cacaoi subsp. *c.*
caccae
Bacteroides c.
cachectic
c. fever
Cache Valley virus (CVV)
cachexia
c. aquosa
malarial c.
Cacipacore virus (CPCV)
CaCo-2 cell
cacticida
Erwinia c.
Pectobacterium c.
cacticola
Culicoides c.
cadaveric
cadaverina
Cynomya c.
cadaveris
Clostridium c.
caddis worm
Caddo Canyon virus
cadmium
Cadophora (*See* **Phialophora**)
CAE
cefuroxime axetil suspension
Caedibacter (b)
C. caryophilus
C. paraconjugatus
C. pseudomutans

C. taeniospiralis
C. varicaedens
caelestis
Streptomyces c.
Caenorhabditis (p)
C. briggsae
C. dolichura
C. elegans
C. rara
caeruleum
Actinopycnidium c.
caeruleus
Actinoplanes c.
Couchioplanes caeruleus subsp. *c.*
Streptomyces c.
caesiellus
Aspergillus c.
caespitosus
Botryomyces c.
Streptomyces c.
café-au-lait spot
caffeine
hydrocodone, chlorpheniramine, phenylephrine, acetaminophen, and c.
CAH
chronic active hepatitis
CAI
catheter-associated infection
Caimito virus (CAIV)
CAIV
Caimito virus
cajennense
Amblyomma c.
cajetani
Arthroderma c.
Calabar swelling
Calanolide A
calcarea
Nocardia c.
calcareous corpuscle
Calchaqui virus (CQIV)
calcification
cystic c.
calcipotriol
calcitrans
Stomoxys c.
calcium
c. alginate
c. alginate swab
c. carbonate stone
c. channel blocker
c. gluconate
c. ionophore (CI)
c. magnesium ammonium phospate

C

87

calcium *(continued)*
  mupirocin c.
  c. oxalate crystal
  c. phosphate stone
calcium-mediated toxicity
Calcivirus
calcivirus
  human c.
  porcine enteric c.
calcoaceticus
  Acinetobacter c.
calcofluor
  c. white
  c. white solution
  c. white stain
calculus
  c. formation
  renal c.
  staghorn c.
caldaria
  Spirochaeta c.
CaldeCort
  C. Anti-Itch Topical Spray
  C. Topical
Calderobacterium hydrogenophilum (b)
Caldesene Topical
Caldicellulosiruptor (b)
  C. kristjanssonii
  C. lactoaceticus
  C. owensensis
  C. saccharolyticus
Caldivirga marquilingensis (b)
caldoxylosilyticus
  Saccharococcus c.
caldus
  Acidithiobacillus c.
  Thiobacillus c.
caledonense
  Simulium c.
caledonica
  Burkholderia c.
calexicanus
  Culicoides c.
Calgiswab
Caliciviridae
Calicivirus (v)
calicivirus
  feline c.
California
  C. encephalitis
  C. encephalitis virus (CEV)
  C. harbor seal poxvirus
californica
  Hansenula c.
californicum
  Mycoplasma c.

californicus
  Streptomyces c.
  Zygowilliopsis c.
californiensis
  Culicoides c.
  Lentzea c.
  Thelazia c.
call
  fungus c.
callanderi
  Eubacterium c.
callidus
  Ruminococcus c.
callipaeda
  Thelazia c.
Calliphora (p)
  C. terraenovae
  C. uralensis
  C. vicina
  C. viridescens
  C. vomitoria
Calliphoridae
Callitroga (p) (*See* **Cochliomyia**)
  C. hominivorax
  C. macellaria
callunae
  Corynebacterium c.
Callus Salve
Calmers
  Robitussin Cough C.
  Sucrets Cough C.
Calmette-Guérin
  bacille C.-G. (BCG)
  C.-G. bacillus (BCG)
Calmette test
Calmylin
  C. #1, 2, 3
  C. Codeine D-E
  C. Expectorant
  C. Pediatric
Calodium
Calonectria (*See* **Fusarium**)
calor
Caloramator (b)
  C. coolhaasii
  C. fervidus
  C. indicus
  C. proteoclasticus
calorimetry
  indirect c.
Calospora (f)
Calostomataceae
calotermitidis
  Diplocalyx c.
  Pillotina c.
calvarial tuberculosis
calvum
  Intrasporangium c.

calvus
>Streptomyces *c.*

calyces (*pl. of* calyx)

Calycophora dermatitis

Calymmatobacterium granulomatis (b)

Calypterae

calyx, pl. calyces

CAM
>cellular adhesion molecule

Camallanina

camerostome

camini
>Marinitoga *c.*

Camoquin

CAMP
>Christie, Atkins, and Munch-Petersen
>CAMP factor
>CAMP test

camp
>c. blood agar

campanulata
>Ampullariella *c.*

campanulatus
>Actinoplanes *c.*

campbellii
>Beneckea *c.*
>Vibrio *c.*

campestris
>Aedes *c.*
>Brochothrix *c.*
>Xanthomonas *c.*

campinasensis
>Paenibacillus *c.*

campisalis
>Halomonas *c.*

camporealensis
>Corynebacterium *c.*

Campylobacter (b)
>C. *butzleri*
>C. *cinaedi*
>C. *coli*
>C. *concisus*
>C. *cryaerophilus*
>C. *curvus*
>C. *enteritis*
>C. *fennelliae*
>C. *fetus* subsp. *fetus*
>C. *fetus* subsp. *venerealis*
>C. *gastroenteritis*
>C. *gracilis*
>C. *helveticus*
>C. *hominis*

>C. *hyoilei*
>C. *hyointestinalis* subsp.
>hyointestinalis
>C. *hyointestinalis* subsp. *lawsonii*
>C. *jejuni*
>C. *jejuni* subsp. *doylei*
>C. *jejuni* subsp. *jejuni*
>C. *lanienae*
>C. *lari*
>C. *mucosalis*
>C. *mustelae*
>C. *nitrofigilis*
>C. *pylori*
>C. *pylori* subsp. *mustelae*
>C. *rectus*
>C. *showae*
>C. *sputorum* subsp. *bubulus*
>C. *sputorum* subsp. *mucosalis*
>C. *sputorum* subsp. *sputorum*
>C. *upsaliensis*

Campylobacteraceae

campylobacteriosis

Campylobacter-like organism (CLO)

canadense
>Mycoplasma *c.*
>Simulium *c.*

canadensis
>Aedes *c.*
>Chromohalobacter *c.*
>Culicoides *c.*
>Echinococcus granulosus *c.*
>Flexibacter *c.*
>Halomonas *c.*
>Hansenula *c.*
>Onychocola *c.*
>Pichia *c.*
>Rickettsia *c.*

Canadian Infectious Disease Society

canal
>gynecophoric c.
>Laurer c.

canaliculata
>Ornithobilharzia *c.*

canaliculitis

Cananeia virus (CANV)

canariensis
>Pseudolynchia *c.*

canarius
>Streptomyces *c.*

canarypox virus

cancellatum
>Myxotrichum *c.*

C

NOTES

cancer
anal c.
cervical c.
European Organization for Research
and Treatment of C. (EORTC)
inflammatory breast c.
invasive cervical c. (ICC)
non-small cell lung c. (NSCLC)
Union Internationale Contre La C.
(UICC)
cancerogena
Erwinia c.
cancerogenus
Enterobacter c.
cancrum oris
Candida (f)
C. *aaseri*
C. *albicans*
C. *albicans* vaginitis
C. *albomarginata*
C. *amapae*
C. *anatomiae*
C. *ancudensis*
C. *antarctica*
C. *antillancae*
C. *apicola*
C. *apis*
C. arthritis
C. *atlantica*
C. *atmosphaerica*
C. *auringiensis*
C. *austromarina*
C. *azyma*
C. *bacarum*
C. balanitis
C. *beechii*
C. *bertae*
C. *berthetii*
C. *blankii*
C. blastoconidia
C. *bogoriensis*
C. *boidinii*
C. *boleticola*
C. *bombi*
C. *bombicola*
C. *bovina*
C. *brumptii*
C. *buinensis*
C. *butyri*
C. *cacaoi*
C. *cantarellii*
C. *cariosilignicola*
C. *caseinolytica*
C. *castellii*
C. *castrensis*
C. *catenulata*
C. *chalmersii*
C. *chilensis*

C. *chiropterorum*
C. *chodatii*
C. *ciferrii*
C. *coipomoensis*
C. *conglobata*
C. *cylindracea*
C. cystitis
C. *dendrica*
C. *dendronema*
C. *deserticola*
C. *diddensiae*
C. *diversa*
C. *drimydis*
C. *dubliniensis*
C. *edax*
C. endophthalmitis
C. *entomophila*
C. *ergastensis*
C. *ernobii*
C. esophagitis
C. *ethanolica*
C. *euphorbiae*
C. *euphorbiiphila*
C. *fabianii*
C. *famata*
C. *famata* var. *famata*
C. *famata* var. *flareri*
C. *fennica*
C. *fermenticarens*
C. *firmetaria*
C. *floricola*
C. *fluviatilis*
C. folliculitis
C. *freyschussii*
C. *friedrichii*
C. *fructus*
C. *galacta*
C. *geochares*
C. *glabrata*
C. *glabrata* endocarditis
C. *glaebosa*
C. glossitis
C. glossodynia
C. *glucosophila*
C. *gropengiesseri*
C. *guilliermondii*
C. *haemulonii*
C. *homilentoma*
C. *humicola*
C. *humilis*
C. *incommunis*
C. *inconspicua*
C. infection
C. *ingens*
C. *insectalens*
C. *insectamans*
C. *insectorum*
C. *intermedia*

C. ishiwadae
C. karawaiewii
C. kefyr
C. krissii
C. kruisii
C. krusei
C. lactiscondensi
C. lambica
C. laureliae
C. leukoplakia
C. lipolytica
C. llanquihuensis
C. lodderae
C. lusitaniae
C. lyxosophila
C. macedoniensis
C. magnoliae
C. maltosa
C. maris
C. maritima
C. melibiosica
C. membranifaciens
C. meningitis
C. mesenterica
C. methanosorbosa
C. milleri
C. mogii
C. montana
C. multigemmis
C. musae
C. mycoderma
C. naeodendra
C. natalensis
C. nemodendra
C. nitratophila
C. norvegensis
C. norvegica
C. odintsovae
C. oleophila
C. oregonensis
C. osteomyelitis
C. ovalis
C. palmioleophila
C. paludigena
C. parapsilosis
C. parapsilosis colonization
C. pararugosa
C. pelliculosa
C. peltata
C. peritonitis
C. petrohuensis
C. pignaliae

C. pini
C. pneumonia
C. populi
C. pseudointermedia
C. pseudolambica
C. pseudotropicalis
C. psychrophila
C. pulcherrima
C. punicea
C. pustula
C. quercitrusa
C. quercuum
C. railenensis
C. ravautii
C. reukaufii
C. rhagii
C. robusta
C. rugopelliculosa
C. rugosa
C. saitoana
C. sake
C. salida
C. salmanticensis
C. santamariae
C. santjacobensis
C. savonica
C. schatavii
C. septicemia
C. sequanensis
C. shehatae
C. shehatae var. *insectosa*
C. shehatae var. *lignosa*
C. shehatae var. *shehatae*
C. silvae
C. silvanorum
C. silvatica
C. silvicola
C. silvicultrix
C. skin test
C. solani
C. sonorensis
C. sophiae-reginae
C. sorbophila
C. sorbosa
C. sorboxylosa
C. spandovensis
C. stellata
C. succiphila
C. suecica
C. tanzawaensis
C. tapae
C. techellsii

C

NOTES

Candida (continued)
    C. tenuis
    C. torresii
    C. tropicalis
    C. tsuchiyae
    C. utilis
    C. vaccinii
    C. vaginitis
    C. valdiviana
    C. valida
    C. vanderwaltii
    C. vartiovaarae
    C. versatilis
    C. vini
    C. viswanathii
    C. vulvovaginitis
    C. wickerhamii
    C. xestobii
    C. zeylanoides
Candida-associated denture stomatitis
candidal
    c. arthritis
    c. esophagitis
    c. infection
    c. osteomyelitis
candidemia
    catheter-related c.
candidiasis
    acute atrophic oral c.
    atrophic c.
    chronic disseminated c.
    chronic hyperplastic c.
    chronic mucocutaneous c. (CMC)
    congenital c.
    cutaneous c.
    disseminated c.
    erythematous c.
    esophageal c.
    esophageal c.
    fluconazole-refractory oral c.
    follicular c.
    hematogenously disseminated c.
    hepatosplenic c.
    invasive c.
    mucocutaneous c.
    mucosal c.
    oral c.
    oropharyngeal c.
    osteoarticular c.
    pseudomembranous c.
    renal c.
    superficial c.
    systemic c.
    urinary tract c.
    urogenital c.
    vaginal c.
    vulvovaginal c.

candidosis
    esophageal c.
    oral c.
    vulvovaginal c.
candidum
    Cylindrocarpon c.
    Geotrichum c.
candiduria
candidus
    Aspergillus c.
    Streptomyces c.
    strophulus c.
    Thermoactinomyces c.
Candistatin
canefield fever
canescens
    Streptomyces c.
Canesten
cangingivalis
    Porphyromonas c.
canicola
    c. fever
    Leptospira interrogans serovar c.
canicruria
    Jensenia c.
canicularis
    Fannia c.
caniferus
    Streptomyces c.
canigenitalium
    Ureaplasma c.
canimorsus
    Capnocytophaga c.
Caninde virus (CNAV)
canine
    c. bite-associated septicemia
    minute virus of c. (MVC)
caninum
    Ancylostoma c.
    Dipylidium c.
    Episthmium c.
    Neospora c.
    Pneumonyssoides c.
    Pneumonyssus c.
caninus
    Centrocestus c.
canis
    Actinomyces c.
    Babesia c.
    Brucella c.
    Ctenocephalides c.
    Demodex c.
    Ehrlichia c.
    Giardia c.
    Haemobartonella c.
    Helicobacter c.
    Hepatozoon c.
    Isospora c.

Microsporum c.
Moraxella c.
Mycoplasma c.
Neisseria c.
Pasteurella c.
Streptococcus c.
Toxocara c.
Trichodectes c.
cannabina
   Pseudomonas c.
cannula
   indwelling c.
cannulation
canonicola
   Simulium c.
canorii
   Anopheles c.
canoris
   Porphyromonas c.
cansulci
   Porphyromonas c.
cantarellii
   Candida c.
cantator
   Aedes c.
Cantharellaceae
Cantharellales
cantharicola
   Spiroplasma c.
cantharidin
canthus, pl. **canthi**
   inner c.
Cantil
cantonensis
   Angiostrongylus c.
   Parastrongylus c.
canus
   Streptomyces c.
CANV
   Cananeia virus
Canyon
   Jamestown C.
CAP
   community-acquired bacterial pneumonia
cap
   Drixoral Cough & Congestion
     Liquid C.'s
   Drixoral Cough & Sore Throat
     Liquid C.'s
   ritonavir soft gel c.
   Sudafed Cold & Cough
     Liquid C.'s

cap1
   caprine adenovirus 1
capacity
   total iron-binding c. (TIBC)
Capastat Sulfate
CAPD
   continuous ambulatory peritoneal dialysis
CAPD-associated peritonitis
capensis
   Saccharomyces c.
Cape Wrath virus (CWV)
capillaceus
   Actinoplanes c.
Capillaria (p)
   C. aerophila
   C. granuloma
   C. hepatica
   C. philippinensis
   C. talpae
capillariasis
   intestinal c.
   Philippine c.
Capillariinae
capillaris
   Muellerius c.
capillary
   c. indirect hemagglutination test
   c. leak syndrome
   c. precipitin test
capillatus
   Cyclops c.
   Solenopotes c.
capillispiralis
   Streptomyces c.
capillosus
   Bacteroides c.
Capillovirus (v)
   C. group
capillus
   Bacteroides c.
Capim virus (CAPV)
capitatum
   Trichosporon c.
capitatus
   Blastoschizomyces c.
   Dipodascus c.
capitis
   inflammatory tinea c.
   pediculosis c.
   Pediculus humanus c.
   pityriasis c.
   pthiriasis c.

C

NOTES

capitis (continued)
    Staphylococcus capitis subsp. *c.*
    tinea c.
    trichophytosis c.
capitovis
    Corynebacterium c.
Capitrol
capitular
capitulum, pl. **capitula**
Caplets
    Advil Cold & Sinus C.
    Bayer Select Chest Cold C.
    Dimacol C.
    Dimetapp Sinus C.
    Dristan Sinus C.
Capnocytophaga (b)
    C. canimorsus
    C. cynodegmi
    C. gingivalis
    C. granulosa
    C. haemolytica
    C. ochracea
    C. sputigena
capnocytophagoides
    Dysgonomonas c.
Capnodiaceae
capoamus
    Streptomyces c.
caprae
    Bovicola c.
    Chorioptes c.
    Damalina c.
    Moraxella c.
    Mycobacterium tuberculosis subsp.
      c.
    Staphylococcus c.
Capravirine
capreolus
    Saccharothrix mutabilis subsp. *c.*
capreomycin
    c. sulfate
capri
    Mycoplasma mycoides subsp. *c.*
capricola
    Trichostrongylus c.
capricolum
    Mycoplasma capricolum subsp. *c.*
capricornii
    Haemagogus c.
caprine
    c. adenovirus 1 (cap1)
    c. arthritis encephalitis virus
    c. herpetovirus
caprinus
    Streptococcus c.
capripneumoniae
    Mycoplasma capricolum subsp. *c.*
Capripoxvirus (v)

caproate
    hydroxyprogesterone c.
caproni
    Echinostoma c.
Capronia puicherrima (f)
capsaicin
capsid
    phage with double c.
    virus c.
Capsin
capsomere
Capsularis zoogleiformans (b)
capsular K antigen
capsulata
    Friedmanniella c.
    Hansenula c.
    Methylopila c.
    Pichia c.
    Rhodopseudomonas c.
    Sphingomonas c.
capsulatum
    Acidobacterium c.
    Flavobacterium c.
    Histoplasma c.
    Histoplasma capsulatum var. *c.*
    Novosphingobium c.
capsulatus
    Actinobacillus c.
    Ajellomyces c.
    Blastobacter c.
    Cryptococcus c.
    Methylococcus c.
    Rhodobacter c.
capsule
    bacterial c.
    Banophen Decongestant C.
    brood c.
    Fortovase soft gel c.
    Glisson c.
    hard gel c. (HGC)
    Ordrine AT Extended Release C.
    polysaccharide c.
    Rescaps-D S.R. C.
    saquinavir hard gel c.
    saquinavir soft gelatin c.
    Tuss-Allergine Modified T.D. C.
    Tussogest Extended Release C.
Capsulets
    Sinumist-SR C.
capsuligenum
    Filobasidium c.
    Leucosporidium c.
Captia IgM assay
capture
    CMV DNA hybrid c.
    DNA hybrid c.
CAPV
    Capim virus

Capzasin-P
Carafate
Carajas virus
caramiphen and phenylpropanolamine
carampicillin hydrochloride
Caraparu virus (CARV)
carate
carbacephem class of drug
carbamazepine
carbamide peroxide
carbapenem
    c. class of drug
carbazochrome sodium sulfonate (AC-17)
carbenicillin
    c. indanyl sodium
    c. test
carbetapentane
    chlorpheniramine, ephedrine, phenylephrine, and c.
carbinolicum
    Acetobacterium c.
carbinolicus
    Desulfovibrio c.
    Pelobacter c.
carbinoxamine, pseudoephedrine, and dextromethorphan
Carbodec DM
carbohydrate
    c. antigen
    c. base test
carbol
    c. fuchsin stain
    c. xylene
carbolic acid
Carbomycetaceae
carbon
    c. dioxide laser
    source of c.
carbonacea
    Micromonospora c.
    Micromonospora carbonacea subsp. *c.*
carbonate
    lithium c.
carbonelli
    Crassicauda c.
carboniphilus
    Bacillus c.
Carbophilus carboxidus (b)
carboxidovorans
    Oligotropha c.

carboxidus
    Carbophilus c.
Carboxydibrachium pacificum (b)
carboxydohydrogena
    Pseudomonas c.
Carboxydothermus hydrogenoformans (b)
carboxymethylcellulose sodium
carboxypenicillin
carbuncle
carchariae
    Vibrio c.
carcinoembryonic antigen (CEA)
carcinogenic
carcinoma
    basal cell c.
    cervical c.
    condylomatous c.
    epidermoid c.
    gastric c.
    keratinizing squamoid c.
    lung c.
    nasopharyngeal c.
    oral squamous cell c.
    squamous cell c.
carcinomatosis
    disseminated c.
card
    c. agglutination trypanosomiasis test (CATT)
    GPI c.
    gram-positive Identification c.
    Vitek Anaerobe Identification (ANI) c.
    Vitek GPI c.
    Vitek *Neisseria-Haemophilus* Identification C.
    Vitek NHI C.
Cardec DM
cardiac
    c. abnormality
    c. infection
    c. rupture
    c. tamponade
Cardiobacteriaceae
Cardiobacterium (b)
    C. hominis
    C. hominis endocarditis
cardiolipin-cholesterol-lecithin antigen
cardiomegaly
cardiomyopathy
    alcohol-induced c.
    dilated c. (DCOM)

C

NOTES

cardiomyopathy *(continued)*
    drug-induced c.
    hypertrophic obstructive c.
    idiopathic dilated c.
    ischemic c.
cardiopulmonary
    c. phase
Cardioquin
cardiothoracic
cardiotoxic drug
cardiovascular
    c. brucellosis
    c. syphilis
Cardiovirus (v)
carditis
care
    meatal c.
    Tempra Cold C.
Carey-Coombs murmur
Carey Island virus (CIV)
cariaci
    Methanogenium c.
caribensis
    Burkholderia c.
caricae
    Laestadia c.
caricapapayae
    Pseudomonas c.
carindacillin
carinii
    Pneumocystis c.
cariosilignicola
    Candida c.
Carlavirus (v)
carlsbergensis
    Saccharomyces c. (*See*
      Saccharomyces cerevisiae)
carmelization
carminata
    Actinomadura c.
    Nonomuraea roseoviolacea subsp. *c.*
Carmol-HC Topical
Carmovirus (v)
carnaticus
    Staphylococcus sciuri subsp. *c.*
carnea
    Nocardia c.
carnegieana
    Erwinia c.
    Pectobacterium c.
carneum
    Streptosporangium c.
carneus
    Aspergillus c.
Carnimonas nigrificans (b)
carnis
    Clostridium c.
    Lactobacillus c.

carnitine
carnivorous
Carnobacterium (b)
    C. alterfunditum
    C. divergens
    C. funditum
    C. gallinarum
    C. inhibens
    C. mobile
    C. piscicola
carnosum
    Leuconostoc c.
carnosus
    Lactobacillus sakei subsp. *c.*
    Staphylococcus carnosus subsp. *c.*
carotene
    beta c.
carotenoid
carotid
carotinifaciens
    Paracoccus c.
carotovora
    Erwinia carotovora subsp. *c.*
carotovorum
    Pectobacterium carotovorum subsp.
      c.
carouselicus
    Macrococcus c.
carpaticus
    Streptomyces c.
carpinense
    Elytrosporangium c.
carpinensis
    Streptomyces c.
Carpoglyphidae
Carpoglyphus
    C. lactis
carrageenovora
    Alteromonas c.
    Pseudoalteromonas c.
carrier
    chronic HBsAg c.
    chronic hepatitis B surface
      antigen c.
    incubatory c.
    c. strain
Carrión disease
carrionii
    Cladophialophora c.
carsonii
    Pichia c.
cartae
    Cellulomonas c.
Carter black mycetoma (*See* Madura
foot)
carteri
    Leptoconops c.
    Volvox c.

cartilaginosus
CARV
    Caraparu virus
Caryophanales
Caryophanon (b)
    C. latum
    C. tenue
caryophila
    Holospora c.
caryophilus
    Caedibacter c.
caryophylli
    Burkholderia c.
    Pseudomonas c.
casamino acid
caseating granulomatous disease
case definition
casei
    Brevibacterium c.
    Corynebacterium c.
    Lactobacillus c.
    Piophila c.
caseilytica
    Bogoriella c.
casein
    c. hydrolysis test
    isoelectric c.
caseinolytica
    Candida c.
Caseobacter polymorphus (b)
caseolyticus
    Macrococcus o.
    Staphylococcus c.
caseous necrosis
Casoni antigen
cassavae
    Xanthomonas c.
casseliflavus
    Enterococcus c.
    Streptococcus c.
cassiicola
    Corynespora c.
cast
    broad waxy c.
    dirty brown granular c.
    epithelial c.
    fatty c.
    granular c.
    hemoglobin c.
    hyaline c.
    orange c.
    red cell c.

    renal tubular c.
    urine c.
    waxy c.
castaneus
    Catenuloplanes c.
castelarensis
    Streptomyces rutgersensis subsp. *c.*
castellanii
    Acanthamoeba c.
    Exophiala c.
castellii
    Candida c.
Castleman disease
castor oil
castration cell
castrensis
    Candida c.
cat
    c. bite
    c. scratch disease (CSD)
    c. scratch encephalitis
    c. scratch skin test
catalase
    c. test
catanella
    Gonyaulax c.
cataphylla
    Aedes c.
catarinense
    Simulium c.
catarrhal
    c. enteritis
    c. jaundice
    c. stage
catarrhalis
    Branhamella c.
    herpes c.
    Moraxella (Branhamella) c.
catecholicum
    Desulfobacterium c.
Catellatospora (b)
    C. citrea subsp. *citrea*
    C. citrea subsp. *methionotrophica*
    C. ferruginea
    C. koreensis
    C. matsumotoense
    C. tsunoense
catenaformis
    Lactobacillus c.
Catenariaceae
catenating

NOTES

catenatus
  Phaeococcomyces c.
Catenibacterium mitsuokai (b)
cateniformis
  Coprobacillus c.
Catenococcus thiocycli (b)
catenoid
catenulae
  Streptomyces c.
catenulata
  Candida c.
catenulate
catenulatum
  Bifidobacterium c.
catenulatus
  Chondromyces c.
Catenuloplanes (b)
  C. atrovinosus
  C. castaneus
  C. crispus
  C. indicus
  C. japonicus
  C. nepalensis
  C. niger
caterpillar
  buck moth c.
  c. dermatitis
  dermatitis-causing c.
  saddleback c.
  stinging c.
Cathaemasia (p)
  C. cabrerai
  C. hians
  C. nycticoracis
Cathaemasidae
cathartic
catheter
  Broviac c.
  Broviac-type c.
  central venous c. (CVC)
  condom c.
  CSF shunt c.
  Foley c.
  Hickman c.
  Hickman/Broviac c.
  hyperalimentation c.
  indwelling c.
  intraarterial c.
  intravascular c.
  intravascular c.-2 (IVc-2)
  Malecot-type c.
  Metras c.
  peripheral arterial c.
  peripheral intravenous c.
  peripherally inserted central c.
    (PICC)
  protected brush c. (PBC)
  Quinton and Groshong c.

  rifampin-impregnated c.
  silastic c.
  silicone-elastomer c.
  single-lumen c.
  subclavian c.
  Swan-Ganz c.
  swan-neck catheter Missouri c.
  Tenchoff c.
  c. tip culture
  triple-lumen central venous c.
  tunneled c.
  urethral c.
catheter-associated
  c.-a. bacteremia (CAB)
  c.-a. infection (CAI)
  c.-a. urinary tract infection
catheterization
  central venous c.
  suprapubic c.
catheterized urine
catheter-related
  c.-r. bacteremia
  c.-r. bacteremia/fungemia
  c.-r. bloodstream infection (CRBSI)
  c.-r. candidemia
  c.-r. sepsis (CRS)
  c.-r. septicemia (CRS)
  c.-r. urinary tract infection
cati
  Notoedres c.
  Toxocara c.
  Ureaplasma c.
cation-selective ion channel
Catonella morbi (b)
catoniae
  Oribaculum c.
  Porphyromonas c.
CATT
  card agglutination trypanosomiasis test
cattle
  infectious papilloma of c.
  malignant catarrh of c.
  winter dysentery of c.
cattleyae
  Acidovorax avenae subsp. *c.*
  Pseudomonas c.
catuli
  Actinomyces c.
catus
  Coprococcus c.
CATUV
  Catu virus
Catu virus (CATUV)
caucasica
  Borrelia c.
  Physaloptera c.
caucasicus
  Streptomyces globisporus subsp. *c.*

cauchense
   Simulium c.
caudatum
   Anaplasma c.
   Paramecium c.
caudatus
   Bodo c.
Caulimovirus (v)
caulinodans
   Azorhizobium c.
Caulobacter (b)
   C. *bacteroides*
   C. *crescentus*
   C. *fusiformis*
   C. *halobacteroides*
   C. *henricii*
   C. *intermedius*
   C. *leidyi*
   C. *maris*
   C. *segnis*
   C. *subvibrioides*
   C. *variabilis*
   C. *vibrioides*
Caulochora baumgartneri (f)
causative
caustic agent
cava
   Phoma c.
cavaticus
   Culicoides c.
cavernae
   Beutenbergia c.
Cavernicola pilosa (p)
cavernous sinus thrombosis
caviae
   Aeromonas c.
   Aeromonas punctata subsp. *c.*
   Chlamydophila c.
   Moraxella (Branhamella) c.
   Mycoplasma c.
   Neisseria c.
   Veillonella c.
cavigenitalium
   Acholeplasma c.
cavipharyngis
   Mycoplasma c.
caviscabies
   Streptomyces c.
cavitary
   c. lung
   c. lung lesion
   c. pulmonary disease

c. pulmonary histoplasmosis
c. tuberculosis
c. upper-lobe infiltrate
cavitating pulmonary nodule
cavitation
   pneumonia c.
Cavosteliaceae
cavourensis
   Streptomyces c.
   Streptomyces cavourensis subsp. *c.*
Cayenne
   mal de C.
cayetanensis
   Cyclospora c.
CbaAr 426 virus
CBC
   complete blood count
CCA
   circulating cathodic antigen
C-C chemokine receptor, CCR5
C-CHFV
   Crimean-Congo hemorrhagic fever
CCPD
   continuous cycling peritoneal dialysis
CD
   Ceclor CD
CD4
   C. depletion
   C. lymphocyte count
   C. T cell
   C. T lymphocyte
CD4+
   C. lymphocyte
   C. lymphocyte count
   C. receptor
   C. T-cell depletion
   C. T-cell homeostasis
   C. T lymphopenia
CD8
   C. T cell
   C. T lymphocyte
CD8+ cell subset
CD8+ T cell
CDAD
   Clostridium difficile-associated disease
CDC
   Centers for Disease Control
   CDC group DF-1, -3
   CDC NO-1 group
   CDC WO-1 group
CD4:CD8 ratio
CD4+:CD8+ ratio

NOTES

CDCP
  Centers for Disease Control and
    Prevention
CDDP
  cisplatin
CDE
  cyclophosphamide, doxorubicin, and
    etoposide
CD62L
  L-selectin molecule
CEA
  carcinoembryonic antigen
CEb virus
cecicola
    Roseburia c.
Ceclor
    C. CD
cecorum
    Enterococcus c.
    Streptococcus c.
cecum
Cedax
Cedecea (b)
    C. davisae
    C. lapagei
    C. neteri
CEE
  central European encephalitis
CeeNU
    C. Oral
CEEV
  central European encephalitis virus
cefaclor
cefadroxil
    c. monohydrate
Cefadyl
cefalexin
    c. monohydrate
cefamandole
    c. nafate
Cefanex
cefazolin
    c. sodium
cefdinir (CFDN)
cefepime
    c. hydrochloride
cefetamet
cefinase testing
cefixime
Cefizox
cefmenoxime
cefmetazole
    c. sodium
Cefobid
cefodizime
cefonicid
    c. sodium

cefoperazone
    c. sodium
    c. sulbactam
ceforanide
Cefotan
cefotaxime
    c. sodium
cefotetan
    c. disodium
cefoxitin
    c. sodium
cefpirome
cefpodoxime
    c. proxetil
cefprozil
cefsulodin
ceftazidime
ceftibuten
Ceftin
    C. Oral
ceftizoxime
    c. sodium
ceftriaxone
    c. sodium
cefuroxime
    c. axetil
    c. axetil suspension (CAE)
    c. sodium
Cefzil
celatum
    Clostridium c.
    Mycobacterium c.
celebensis
    Raillietina c.
celer
    Thermococcus c.
celere
    Thermobrachium c.
celerecrescens
    Clostridium c.
Celestoderm
Celestone
    C. Oral
    C. Phosphate Injection
    C. Soluspan
Celgene
cell
    antibody-secreting c. (ASC)
    antigen-presenting c. (APC)
    antigen-reactive T c.
    antigen-specific T c.
    c. association
    B c.
    B1 c.
    B7-positive tumor c.
    CaCo-2 c.
    castration c.
    CD4 T c.

CD8 T c.
CD8+ T c.
C. Cept
ciliated epithelial c.
Clara c.
clue c.
conidiogenous c.
c. count
crenated red blood c.
crypt c.
c. culture
cytolytic T helper c.
cytotoxic c.
Daudi c.
dendritic c. (DC)
Downey c.
dysmorphic red c.
encapsulated budding yeast c.
epithelial c.
epithelioid c.
erythroprogenitor c.
flame c.
ganglion c.
GHOST c.
giant c.
goblet c.
HeLa c.
helper c.
hematopoietic stem c. (HSC)
Hofbauer c.
Ia-expressing c.
immunoglobin-producing c.
inflammatory c.
Jurkat T c.
Kupffer c.
LAK c.
long-lived memory T c.
lymphokine-activated killer c.
M c.
McCoy c.
memory B, T c.
mesothelial c.
microfold c.
microglial rod c.
Mikulicz c.
monocyte-derived dendritic c.
 (MDDC)
multinucleated giant c.
natural killer c.
NK c.
nucleated red blood c.
c. organelle

palisading epithelioid c.
parenchymal c.
peptide-specific T c.
peripheral blood mononuclear c.
 (PBMC)
phagocytic c.
plasma c.
polymorphonuclear c.
precursor B c.
progenitor c.
pus c.
red blood c. (RBC)
Reed-Sternberg c.
Reed-Sternberg-like c.
satellite c.
sensitized c.
small noncleaved c.
smudge c.
somatic c.
c. sorting fluorescence activation
spindle c.
squamocolumnar epithelial c.
squamous c.
stem c.
stromal c.
suppressor T c.
T-helper c.
T-inducer c.
c. transfer
c. transformation
c. tropism
tubular c.
tumor-draining lymph node c.
 (TDLNC)
vacuolated prickle c.
virus-transformed c.
c. wall-defective bacteria
white blood c. (WBC)

cellasea
 Cellulomonas c.
cell-bound antibody
cellicolous
cell-mediated
 c.-m. immune (CMI)
 c.-m. immune response
 c.-m. immunity (CMI)
cellobioparum
 Clostridium c.
cellobiosa
 Pichia c.
cellobiose fermentation test

NOTES

C

cellobiosus
  Lactobacillus c.
cellophane
  c. tape swab
  c. thick smear technique
cellostaticus
  Streptomyces c.
cellulans
  Cellulomonas c.
  Cellulosimicrobium c.
  Nocardia c.
cellular
  c. adhesion molecule (CAM)
  c. atypia
  c. debris
  c. immune panel
  c. immune response
  c. immune theory
  c. immunity
  c. immunity deficiency syndrome
  c. transcription factor
  c. vaccine
cellularis
  balanitis circumscripta plasma c.
cellularity
  mixed c.
cellulitis
  acute scalp c.
  anaerobic c.
  crepitant c.
  demarcated c.
  dissecting c.
  eosinophilic c.
  epizootic c.
  erysipeloid c.
  fungal c.
  orbital c.
  pelvic c.
  perianal streptococcal c.
  periorbital c.
  phlegmonous c.
  posthysterectomy c.
  preseptal c.
  preseptal/orbital c.
  subacute c.
  synergistic c.
cellulofermentans
  Clostridium c.
celluloflavus
  Streptomyces c.
cellulolyticum
  Clostridium c.
cellulolyticus
  Acetivibrio c.
  Acidothermus c.
  Streptomyces c.
Cellulomonas (b)
  C. biazotea

C. cartae
C. cellasea
C. cellulans
C. fermentans
C. fimi
C. flavigena
C. gelida
C. hominis
C. humilata
C. iranensis
C. persica
C. turbata
C. uda
Cellulophaga (b)
  C. algicola
  C. baltica
  C. fucicola
  C. lytica
  C. uliginosa
cellulophilum
  Streptoverticillium olivoreticuli
   subsp. *c.*
cellulophilus
  Streptomyces olivoreticuli subsp. *c.*
cellulosae
  cysticercosis *c.*
  Cysticercus c.
  Streptomyces c.
cellulose
  c. acetate test
  c. tape
cellulosi
  Clostridium c.
cellulosilytica
  Halocella c
Cellulosimicrobium cellulans (b)
cellulosolvens
  Acetivibrio c.
  Bacteroides c.
  Eubacterium c.
cellulosum
  Polyangium c.
cellulovorans
  Clostridium c.
Cellumonadaceae
cellutitis
Cellvibrio (b)
  C. mixtus subsp. *dextranolyticus*
  C. mixtus subsp. *mixtus*
celom
CELO virus
celozoic
Celsus kerion
Cel-U-Jec Injection
CEM
  Center for Molecular Epidemiology
Cenafed
  C. Plus tablet

Cenestin
cenocyte
cenocytic
cenosite
centenaria
    Rhodocista c.
centenum
    Rhodospirillum c.
Center
    C. for Molecular Epidemiology
      (CEM)
    Veterans Administration Medical C.
      (VAMC)
Centers
    C. for Disease Control (CDC)
    C. for Disease Control and
      Prevention (CDCP)
    C. for Disease Control and
      Prevention anaerobe agar
    C. for Disease Control and
      Prevention M5 group
    C. for Disease Control and
      Prevention nonoxidizer-1 group
    C. for Disease Control and
      Prevention O-3 group
    C. for Disease Control and
      Prevention weak oxidizer-1 group
Centipeda (h)
    C. periodontii
centipede
central
    c. adiposity
    c. European encephalitis (CEE)
    c. European encephalitis virus
      (CEEV)
    c. European tick-borne fever
    c. line sepsis
    c. nervous system (CNS)
    c. nervous system infection
    c. nervous system lymphoma
    c. nervous system tuberculosis
    c. venous catheter (CVC)
    c. venous catheterization
centrale
    Anaplasma c.
Centratuss
    C. DM
    C. DM-D
    C. DM Expectorant
centrifugation
    high-speed c.

    lysis c.
    zinc sulfate flotation c.
centrifuge
centrifuged
centrilobular
Centrocestus (p)
    C. asadai
    C. caninus
Centrospora acerina (f)
centrosporus
    Bacillus c.
    Brevibacillus c.
Centruroides
    C. sculpturatus
centurionis
    Chrysops c.
cenuris
cenurosis
CEP
    chronic eosinophilic pneumonia
cepacia
    Burkholderia c.
    Pseudomonas c.
    c. syndrome
cephalad
cephalexin
    c. hydrochloride
    c. monohydrate
cephalgia
cephalhematoma
cephalic tetanus
Cephaliophora irregularis (f)
Cephalobaenida
Cephalobaenidae
Cephalobidae
Cephalomyia (p)
cephalont
cephaloridine
cephalosporin
    c. test
    third-generation c.
cephalosporinase production testing
Cephalosporium (f)
Cephalothecaceae
cephalothin
    c. sodium
Cephalotrichum (f)
cephamycin
Cephanol
cephapirin
    c. sodium
cephazolin

C

NOTES

cephradine
Ceporacin
Ceporex
Cept
    Cell C.
Ceptaz
Ceratobasidiaceae
Ceratocystis (f)
Ceratomycetaceae
Ceratophyllidae
Ceratophyllus (p)
    C. gallinae
    C. niger
Ceratopogonidae
cerbereus
    Meiothermus c.
cercaria, pl. **cercariae**
    schistosome c.
cercariae
cercarial
    c. agglutination test
    c. dermatitis
cerci (*pl. of* cercus)
cercocystis
cercomer
cercomonad
Cercomonas (p)
    C. hominis
    C. intestinalis
cercopithecine herpesvirus 1–2
Cercospora apii (f)
cercus, pl. **cerci**
cerealis
    Oidiodendron c.
cerebellar
    c. ataxia
    c. herniation
    c. hypoplasia
    c. syndrome
cerebellum, pl. **cerebella**
cerebral
    c. angiitis
    c. angiostrongyliasis
    c. cladosporiosis
    c. coenurosis
    c. cysticercosis
    c. lymphoma
    c. malaria
    c. paragonimiasis
    c. toxoplasmosis
    c. vasculitis
cerebralis
    coenurus c.
    mycetism c.
cerebri
    pseudotumor c.
cerebriforme
    Trichosporon c.

cerebritis
cerebrospinal
    c. fever
    c. fluid (CSF)
    c. fluid India ink preparation
    c. fluid pleocytosis
    c. fluid shunt
    c. meningitis
    c. nematodiasis
    c. rhinorrhea
    c. schistosomiasis
cerebrosus
    Morococcus c.
cereus
    Bacillus c.
cerevisiae
    Megasphaera c.
    Saccharomyces c.
cerevisiiphilus
    Pectinatus c.
Cerinosterus cyanescens (f)
cerinus
    Agromyces cerinus subsp. *c.*
    Gluconobacter c.
Cerithidea
cerivastatin
ceroid
cerophilum
    Ramichloridium c.
Cerose-DM
cerqueira
    Simulium c.
Certiomyxaceae
Certiomyxales
Certionyxomycetes
Certiva
cervi
    Lipotena c.
    Setaria c.
cervical
    c. adenitis
    c. adenopathy
    c. cancer
    c. carcinoma
    c. *Chlamydia* culture
    c. cytology
    c. dysplasia
    c. ectopy
    c. ectropion
    c. gonorrhea
    c. intraepithelial neoplasia (CIN)
    c. invasive neoplasia (CIN)
    c. lavage
    c. lymphadenitis
    c. mediastinoscopy
    c. motion tenderness
    c. mucopus

c. portio
c. *Trichomonas* smear
cervicalis
Onchocerca c.
Roseomonas c.
cervices (*pl. of* cervix)
cervicitis
chlamydial c.
cystitis c.
infectious c.
mucopurulent c. (MPC)
cervicofacial actinomycosis
cervicography
cervicovaginal
c. flora
c. mucosal swab
c. secretion
c. smear
cervicovaginitis
Cervigram
Cerviscope
cervix, pl. **cervices**
C.E.S.
cesarean
c. delivery
c. section (C-section)
Cestoda
Cestodaria
cestode
intestinal c.
tapeworm c.
cestodiases
cestodiasis
Cestoidea
Cestrum
Cetacaine
Cetacort Topical
Cetamide
Isopto C.
C. Ophthalmic
Cetapred Ophthalmic
ceti
Cetobacterium c.
Cetobacterium ceti (b)
cetonicum
Desulfobacterium c.
cetylpyridinium chloride
CEV
California encephalitis virus
ceylanicum
Ancylostoma c.

ceylonensis
Brugia c.
ceylonica
Haemadipsa c.
ceylonicum
Ancylostoma c.
CF
complement fixation
complement-fixing
cystic fibrosis
CF antibody
Guiatuss CF
Synacol CF
CF test
Cf1t virus
CFA
colonization factor antigen
CFDN
cefdinir
CfMNPV
Choristoneura fumiferana MNPV
CFS
chronic fatigue syndrome
CFU
colony forming unit
CFUV
Corfou virus
Cf virus
CGLV
Changuinola virus
cGMP
cyclic guanine monophosphate
CGV
Chobar Gorge virus
Chabertiidae
Chabertiinae
chacoense
Mesorhizobium c.
Chaco virus (CHOV)
Chadefaudiellaceae
Chaetomium (f)
C. atrobrunneum
C. funicola
C. globosum
C. strumarium
Chaetophoma dero-unguis (f)
Chaetosphaeronema (f)
chaffeensis
Ehrlichia c.
Chagas
C. disease
C. trypanosomiasis

C

NOTES

105

Chagas-Cruz disease
chagasi
    Leishmania c.
chagasic
    c. encephalopathy
    c. lesion
    c. megacolon
    c. megasyndrome
    c. meningoencephalitis
    c. thyroiditis
chagoma
Chagres virus (CHGV)
chain
    long c.
    respiratory c.
    short c.
Chainia (b)
    C. antibiotica
    C. flava
    C. fumigata
    C. kunmingensis
    C. minutisclerotica
    C. nigra
    C. ochracea
    C. olivacea
    C. poonensis
    C. purpurogena
    C. rosea
    C. rubra
    C. violens
chalazion
chalcea
    Micromonospora c.
chalcocoma
    Simulium c.
Chalder Fatigue Scale
challenge
    provocative c.
    tumor c.
chalmersii
    Candida c.
champavatii
    Streptomyces c.
chancre
    mixed c.
    mucous membrane c.
    soft c.
    sporotrichositic c.
    c. stage
    syphilis c.
    syphilitic c.
    trypanosomal c.
    tuberculous c.
chancriform
    c. pyoderma
    c. syndrome
chancroid
    c. chancroidal

    c. culture
    mucous membrane c.
    phagedenic c.
    c. ulcer
chancroidal
    c. bubo
    chancroid c.
    c. ulceration
chancrous
chandelier
    favic c.
    c. sign
Chandipura virus (CHPV)
change
    eczematous c.
Chang medium
Changuinola virus (CGLV)
channel
    c. catfish reovirus (CRV)
    cation-selective ion c.
chaotropic salt
chapellei
    Geobacter c.
charcoal agar
Charcot
    C. joint
    C. triad
Charcot-Leyden crystal
Charleville virus (CHVV)
Charlouis disease
chartarum
    Alternaria c.
    Myxotrichum c.
    Pithomyces c.
    Stachybotrys c.
    Ulocladium c.
chartatabidum
    Clostridium c.
chartreusis
    Streptomyces c.
Chasers
    Scot-Tussin DM Cough C.
chattanoogensis
    Streptomyces c.
chauliocola
    Mesoplasma c.
Chauveau bacterium
chauvoei
    Clostridium c.
CHC
    chronic hepatitis C
Chealamide
checkerboard assay
Chédiak-Higashi syndrome
cheek
    slapped c.
cheerisanensis
    Kitasatospora c.

cheese
    c. maggot
    c. worker's lung
CHEF
  contour-clamped homogeneous electric field
  contour-clamped homogenous fields electrophoresis
cheilitis
    angular c.
    erythematous c.
    pseudomembranous c.
Cheilospirura hamulosa (p)
chejuensis
    Hahella c.
Chelatobacter heintzii (b)
Chelatococcus asaccharovorans (b)
chelicera
Chelicerata
cheloid leishmaniasis
chelonae
    Dermatophilus c.
    Mycobacterium c.
    Mycobacterium chelonae subsp. c.
chemical meningitis
chemiluminescence assay
chemiluminescent DNA
chemoautotroph
chemoautotrophic
chemofluorescent optical brightening agent
chemoheterotroph
chemoheterotrophic
chemoimmunology
chemoimmunotherapy
chemokine receptor
chemolithotroph
chemolithotrophic
chemoluminescence
chemoorganotroph
chemoorganotrophic
chemoprophylaxis
chemoreceptor
chemosis
chemotactic
chemotaxis
    neutrophil c.
chemotherapeutic agent
chemotherapy
    ablative c.
    antineoplastic c.
    anti-RT c.

    antiviral c.
    combination c.
    cytotoxic c.
    EPOCH c.
    front-line c.
    high-dose c.
    c. induction
    induction c.
    intensive c.
    intralesional c.
    intralesional interferon c.
    PR c.
    prophylactic antianaerobe c.
    salvage c.
    single-agent c.
    systemic c.
    systemic cytotoxic c.
chemotherapy-induced neutropenia
Chenuda virus (CNUV)
cheopis
    Xenopsylla c.
Cheracol
    C. D
cherrii
    Legionella c.
cherry red epiglottis
chersina
    Micromonospora c.
chevalieri
    Aspergillus c.
    Eurotium c.
chewaclae
    Culicoides c.
Cheyletiella (p)
    C. blakei
    C. infestation
    C. parasitivorax
    C. yasguri
Cheyletiellidae
Cheyletoidea
CHF
  congestive heart failure
CHGV
  Chagres virus
chibaensis
    Streptomyces c.
chibensis
    Paenibacillus c.
Chibroxin Ophthalmic
chickenpox
    c. culture
    c. immune globulin

C

NOTES

chickenpox *(continued)*
   c. immunoglobulin
   c. titer
   c. vaccine
   c. virus
chiclero ulcer
chidesteri
   Culex c.
chief agglutinin
chigger
   c. mite
chigoe
chikungunya virus (CHIKV)
CHIKV
   chikungunya virus
childbed fever
children
   Cough Syrup DM Decongestant
     for C.
Children's
   C. Advil suspension
   C. Benylin DM-D
   C. Hold
   C. Motrin suspension
   C. Silfedrine
chileae
   Thioploca c.
chilensis
   Candida c.
   Thiomicrospira c.
chiliani
   Haemadipsa c.
Chilibre virus (CHIV)
chilomastigiasis
Chilomastigidae
Chilomastix mesnili (p)
chilomastosis
chilopodiasis
chimpanzee herpesvirus
CHIMV
   Chim virus
Chim virus (CHIMV)
chinatum
   Echinostoma c.
chinense
   Spiroplasma c.
Chinese letters
chiopterus
   Culicoides c.
chironomi
   Rickettsiella c.
Chironomus
   C. attenuatus
   C. plumosus
chiropterorum
   Candida c.
chitae
   Mycobacterium c.

chitinivorans
   Halanaerobacter c.
chitinolytica
   Telluria c.
chitinolyticus
   Bacillus c.
Chitinophaga pinensis (b)
chitonophagus
   Thermococcus c.
chitterlings
chitwoodi
   Meloidogyne c.
CHIV
   Chilibre virus
Chlamydia (b)
   C. culture
   C. disease
   LGV strain of C.
   C. muridarum
   C. pecorum
   C. pneumoniae
   C. pneumoniae serology
   C. pneumoniae sinusitis
   C. psittaci
   C. psittaci serology
   C. smear
   C. suis
   C. trachomatis (CT)
   C. trachomatis LCx
   C. trachomatis Probe Competition
     Assay
   C. TWAR
chlamydia
   genital c.
   c. probe
Chlamydiaceae
Chlamydiae
chlamydial
   c. antigen detection
   c. cervicitis
   c. conjunctivitis
   c. disease
   c. infection
   c. pneumonitis
   c. urethritis
Chlamydiales
Chlamydiamicrovirus (v)
Chlamydiazyme
chlamydiosis
Chlamydoabsidia padenii (f)
Chlamydophila (b)
   C. abortus
   C. caviae
   C. felis
   C. pecorum
   C. pneumoniae
   C. psittaci
Chlamydophrys

chlamydospora
    Alternaria c.
chlamydosporum
    Fusarium c.
chliarophilus
    Meiothermus c.
    Thermus c.
chloasma
Chlorafed Liquid
chloral hydrate
chlorambucil
chloramine-T
chloramphenicol
    c., polymyxin B, and
      hydrocortisone
    c. and prednisolone
    c. serum level
chlordiazepoxide
    clidinium and c.
chlorellavorus
    Vampirovibrio c.
chlorhexidine
    c. diacetate aqueous solution
    c. gluconate
Chlorhexseptic
chloride
    Adrenalin C.
    benzalkonium c. (BZK)
    benzethonium c.
    cetylpyridinium c.
    hydrocodone, phenylephrine,
      pyrilamine, phenindamine,
      chlorpheniramine, and
      ammonium c.
    mercuric c.
    methylbenzethonium c.
    methylrosaniline c.
    polyvinyl c. (PVC)
    saturated mercuric c.
    triphenyltetrazolium c. (TTC)
Chloridium (f)
chlorinated lime
Chloriridovirus (v)
chlorobenzoica
    Thauera c.
Chlorobiaceae
Chlorobium (b)
    C. chlorovibrioides
    C. limicola
    C. phaeobacteroides
    C. phaeovibrioides

C. tepidum
C. vibrioforme
chlorocephalum
    Haplographium c.
chlorocresol aqueous solution
chloroethenica
    Desulfuromonas c.
Chloroflexaceae
Chloroflexus (b)
    C. aggregans
    C. aurantiacus
Chloroherpeton thalassium (b)
chloromethanicum
    Hyphomicrobium c.
    Methylobacterium c.
Chloromycetin
    C. Injection
Chloronema giganteum (b)
chlorophenolica
    Sphingomonas c.
chlorophenolicum
    Mycobacterium c.
    Sphingobium c.
chlorophenolicus
    Arthrobacter c.
    Rhodococcus c.
Chlorophyllum molybdites (f)
Chloropidae
Chloroptic Ophthalmic
Chloroptic-P Ophthalmic
chloroquine
    c. phosphate
    c. PO$_4$
    primaquine and c.
    c. and primaquine
chloroquine-resistant
chlororaphis
    Pseudomonas c.
chlororespirans
    Desulfitobacterium c.
chlorotrianisene
chlorovibrioides
    Chlorobium c.
chloroxine
chloroxylenol
Chlorphed-LA Nasal solution
chlorphenesin
chlorpheniramine
    c., ephedrine, phenylephrine, and
      carbetapentane
    hydrocodone and c.
    c., phenylephrine, and codeine

C

NOTES

chlorpheniramine *(continued)*
    c., phenylephrine, and
       dextromethorphan
    c., phenylpropanolamine, and
       dextromethorphan
    c. and pseudoephedrine
    c., pseudoephedrine, and codeine
chlorpropamide
chlortetracycline
    c. hydrochloride
Chlor-Trimeton 4 Hour Relief tablet
Chlor-Tripolon Decongestant
chlorum
    Heliobacterium c.
Choanephoraceae
Choanotaenia filamentosa (p)
Chobar Gorge virus (CGV)
chocolate agar
chocolatum
    Microbacterium c.
chodatii
    Candida c.
    Endomycopsis c.
choerinum
    Bifidobacterium c.
cholangiocarcinoma
cholangiography
    endoscopic retrograde c.
    percutaneous c.
    percutaneous transhepatic c. (PTCA)
cholangiohepatitis
    oriental c.
cholangiopancreatography
    endoscopic retrograde c. (ERCP)
cholangiopathy
    AIDS c.
cholangitis
    acute obstructive c.
    acute suppurative c.
    fulminating acute suppurative c.
    pyogenic c.
    sclerosing c.
    septic c.
    toxic c.
cholecystectomy
cholecystitis
    acalculous c.
    acute c.
    emphysematous c.
cholecystoduodenal fistula
cholecystus
    Helicobacter c.
choledochal cyst
choledochocholedochostomy
choledochojejunostomy
choledocholithiasis
Choledyl
cholelithiasis

cholera
    c. agar
    Asiatic c.
    c. bacillus
    epidemic c.
    c. sicca
    c. toxin
    typhoid c.
    c. vaccine
cholerae
    Vibrio c.
choleraesuis
    Salmonella choleraesuis subsp. *c.*
choleragen
choleraic
choleraphage
cholera-red reaction
cholestasis
cholestatic liver disease
cholesteatoma
cholesterol
    HDL c.
       high-density lipoprotein cholesterol
       high-density lipoprotein c. (HDL
        cholesterol)
cholestyramine
    c. resin
choliformis
    mycetism c.
choline
    c. magnesium trisalicylate
    c. salicylate
choline-binding protein
cholinergic
cholodnii
    Leptothrix c.
chondroitin sulfatase
chondroitinus
    Bacillus c.
    Paenibacillus c.
Chondromyces (b)
    C. apiculatus
    C. catenulatus
    C. crocatus
    C. lanuginosus
    C. pediculatus
chondrophila
    Waddlia c.
CHOP
    cyclophosphamide, hydroxydaunomycin,
      Oncovin, and prednisone
chordatum
    Diphyllobothrium c.
Chordodes morgani (p)
Chordodidae
Chordodinae
Chordopoxvirinae

chorea
    Sydenham c.
choreoathetoid
choreoathetosis
chorioamnionitis
    maternal c.
choriomeningitis
    lymphocytic c. (LCM)
chorionic villus
Chorioptes (p)
    C. bovis
    C. caprae
    C. equi
    C. ovis
chorioretinal
chorioretinitis
    toxoplasmic c.
choriovillous
Choristoneura
    C. fumiferana MNPV (CfMNPV)
Chorizagrotis auxiliaris
choroid
    c. plexus
choroidal
    c. angiitis
choroiditis
    cryptococcal c.
    mycobacterial c.
    Pneumocystis carinii c.
choroidopathy
Chortoglyphus arcuatus (p)
CHORUS study
choshinensis
    Bacillus c.
    Brevibacillus c.
CHOV
    Chaco virus
CHPV
    Chandipura virus
chrestomyceticus
    Streptomyces c.
christensenii
    Aerococcus c.
Christian disease
Christie
    C., Atkins, and Munch-Petersen (CAMP)
    C., Atkins, and Munch-Petersen test
Chromatiaceae
chromatica
    trichomycosis c.

chromatin
    c. body
    marginated c.
Chromatium (b)
    C. buderi
    C. gracile
    C. minus
    C. minutissimum
    C. okenii
    C. purpuratum
    C. salexigens
    C. tepidum
    C. vinosum
    C. violascens
    C. warmingii
    C. weissei
chromatographic assay
chromatography
    affinity c.
    DEAE cellulose anion-exchange c.
    diethylaminoethyl cellulose anion-exchange c.
    gas c.
    gas-liquid c. (GLC)
    high-performance liquid c. (HPLC)
    liquid c.
    thin-layer c.
chromatoid
chromatoidal bar
chromatophore
chromatotropism
chromium-release assay
Chromobacterium (b)
    C. fluviatile
    C. violaceum
chromoblastomycosis
chromofuscus
    Streptomyces c.
chromogen
chromogena
    Thermomonospora c.
chromogenes
    Microbispora c.
    Staphylococcus c.
    Staphylococcus hyicus subsp. c.
chromogenesis
chromogenic
    c. cephalosporin test
    c. enzyme substrate test
Chromohalobacter (b)
    C. canadensis
    C. israelensis

C

NOTES

Chromohalobacter (continued)
  C. *marismortui*
  C. *salexigens*
chromomycosis
chromophoric
chromoplastid
chromosome
  giant c.
  lampbrush c.
  polytene c.
  ring c.
Chromotorula (f)
chromotrope-2R modified trichrome staining technique
chromotrope stain
chronic
  c. active gastritis
  c. active hepatitis (CAH)
  c. African sleeping sickness
  c. aggressive hepatitis
  c. appendiceal syndrome
  c. atrophic gastritis
  c. atrophic rhinitis
  c. bone marrow deficiency
  c. bronchitis
  c. coinfection
  c. conjunctivitis
  c. cryptosporidial diarrhea
  c. cutaneous leishmaniasis
  c. diffuse sclerosing osteomyelitis
  c. disseminated candidiasis
  c. EBV syndrome
  c. eosinophilic pneumonia (CEP)
  c. fatigue syndrome (CFS)
  c. fibrocavitary pneumonia
  c. granulomatous disease
  c. HBsAg carrier
  c. hematogenous tuberculosis
  c. hepatitis B surface antigen carrier
  c. hepatitis C (CHC)
  c. histiocytosis
  c. hyperplastic candidiasis
  c. ileitis
  c. inflammation
  c. inflammatory arthritis
  c. interstitial fibrosis
  c. interstitial pneumonitis
  c. intestinal cryptosporidiosis
  c. intestinal isosporiasis
  c. malaria
  c. monarticular arthritis
  c. mucocutaneous candidiasis (CMC)
  c. necrotizing aspergillosis
  c. obstructive pulmonary disease (COPD)
  c. otitis media

  c. paranasal sinusitis
  c. persistent hepatitis (CPH)
  c. pulmonary tuberculosis
  c. septicemia
  c. trypanosomiasis
  c. viral hepatitis
  c. viremia
chronica
  mycosis cutis c.
chroococcum
  Azotobacter c.
chroococcus
  Methylococcus c.
chrysanthemi
  Erwinia c.
  Pectobacterium c.
chrysea
  Oscillochloris c.
Chryseobacterium (b)
  C. *balustinum*
  C. *gleum*
  C. *indologenes*
  C. *indoltheticum*
  C. *meningosepticum*
  C. *scophthalmum*
Chryseomonas (b)
  C. *luteola*
  C. *polytricha*
chryseus
  Streptomyces c.
Chrysiogenes arsenatis (b)
chrysogenum
  Penicillium c.
chrysomallus
  Streptomyces c.
  Streptomyces chrysomallus subsp. c.
Chrysomyia
  C. *albiceps*
  C. *bezziana*
Chrysonilia sitophila (f)
chrysopicola
  Spiroplasma c.
Chrysops (p)
  C. *centurionis*
  C. *dimidiatus*
  C. *langi*
  C. *silaceus*
chrysorrhoea
  Euproctis c.
chrysospermus
  Hypomyces c.
Chrysosporium (f)
  C. *keratinophilum*
  C. *pannicola*
  C. *parvum*
  C. *parvum* var. *crescens*
  C. *tropicum*

chrysosporium
    Phanerochaete c.
Chrysovirus (v)
chub reovirus
chubuense
    Mycobacterium c.
chubuensis
    Rhodococcus c.
chungbukensis
    Sphingomonas c.
churchillensis
    Aedes c.
Churg-Strauss angiitis
CHVV
    Charleville virus
CHVX
chyluria
Chytridiaceae
Chytridiales
Chytridiomycctes
CI
    calcium ionophore
cicatricial lesion
cicatricosa
    Ambrosiozyma c.
cicatrization
ciceri
    Mesorhizobium c.
    Rhizobium c.
cichorii
    Pseudomonas c.
ciclopirox
    c. olamine
cidofovir
    c. gel
Cidomycin
cidovir
CIE, CIEP
    countercurrent immunoelectrophoresis
    counterimmunoelectrophoresis
ciferii
    Stephanoascus c.
ciferrii
    Candida c.
    Hansenula c.
    Pichia c.
cigar-shaped
ciguatera
    c. fish poisoning
ciguatoxin
CIK lymphocyte
Cilastatin

cilastatin
    imipenem and c.
cilia (*pl. of* cilium)
ciliary
    c. flush
    c. movement
Ciliata
ciliate
ciliated
    c. epithelial cell
ciliocytophthoria
Ciliophora
cilium, pl. **cilia**
Ciloxan Ophthalmic
cimetidine
Cimex (p)
    C. hemipterus
    C. lectularius
Cimicidae
cimicosis
CIN
    cervical intraepithelial neoplasia
    cervical invasive neoplasia
cinaedi
    Campylobacter c.
    Helicobacter c.
cincinnatiensis
    Legionella c.
    Vibrio c.
cinctum
    Myrothecium c.
cinerea
    Microellobosporia c.
    Neisseria c.
cinerella
cinereorectus
    Streptomyces c.
cinereoruber
    Streptomyces c.
    Streptomyces cinereoruber subsp. *c.*
cinereospinus
    Streptomyces c.
cinerescens
    Volutella c.
cinereus
    Aedes c.
    Coprinus c.
    Streptomyces c.
cinerochromogenes
    Streptomyces c.
cinetorchis
    Echinostoma c.

NOTES

cingulata
> Glomerella c.

cinnabarinus
> Streptomyces c.

cinnamivorans
> Papillibacter c.

cinnamonensis
> Streptomyces c.

cinnamoneum
> Streptoverticillium cinnamoneum
> subsp. c.

cinnamoneus
> Streptomyces cinnamoneus subsp. c.

cinnamopurpureum
> Eupenicillium c.

Cinobac Pulvules

Cinoxacin

cinoxacin

Cipro
> C. HC Otic
> C. injection
> C. I.V.
> C. Oral

ciprofloxacin
> c. hydrochloride
> c. and hydrocortisone

circinata
> tinea c.

circinate balanitis

circinelloides
> Mucor c.

circling disease of sheep

Circoviridae

Circovirus (v)

circovirus
> porcine c.

circulans
> Bacillus c.

circulating
> c. anodic antigen (CAA)
> c. cathodic antigen (CCA)
> c. immune complex

circulation
> total anomalous pulmonary c.
> (TAPC)

circulatory macrophage

circumcincta
> Ostertagia c.

circumcision wound abscess

circumdentaria
> Porphyromonas c.

circumoral paresthesia

circumoval precipitin test

circumscriptus
> Culicoides c.

circumsporozoite protein

cirratus
> Streptomyces c.

cirrhosis
> c. of the liver

cirrus, pl. **cirri**

cisapride

ciscaucasicus
> Streptomyces c.

cisplatin (CDDP)

cissicola
> Pseudomonas c.

citelli
> Mycoplasma c.

Citellus

Citeromyces matritensis (f)

citrate
> diethylcarbamazine c.
> magnesium c.
> piperazine c.
> ranitidine bismuth c.
> c. utilization test

citratiphilum
> Aquabacterium c.

citrea
> Actinomadura c.
> Alteromonas c.
> Catellatospora citrea subsp. c.
> Pantoea c.
> Promicromonospora c.
> Pseudoalteromonas c.

citreofluorescens
> Streptomyces c.

citreum
> Brevibacterium c.
> Curtobacterium c.
> Leuconostoc c.

citreus
> Agrococcus c.
> Arthrobacter c.
> Planococcus c.

citri
> Spiroplasma c.
> Xanthomonas c.

citric acid bladder mixture

citricus
> Formivibrio c.

citrinum
> Penicillium c.

Citrobacter (b)
> C. amalonaticus
> C. braakii
> C. diversus
> C. farmeri
> C. freundii
> C. gillenii
> C. koseri
> C. murliniae
> C. rodentium
> C. sedlakii

C. werkmanii
C. youngae
citronellolis
    Pseudomonas c.
citrulli
    Acidovorax avenae subsp. *c.*
    Pseudomonas avenae subsp. *c.*
    Pseudomonas pseudoalcaligenes
      subsp. *c.*
CIV
    Carey Island virus
CJD
    Creutzfeldt-Jacob disease
[14]C-labeled urea breath test
[13]C-labeled urea breath test
clade
Cladochytriaceae
Cladophialophora (f)
    C. arxii
    C. bantiana
    C. boppii
    C. carrionii
    C. devriesii
Cladorrhinum
    C. bulbillosum
cladosporioides
    Cludosporium c.
    Hormodendrum c.
cladosporiosis
    cerebral c.
Cladosporium (f)
    C. cladosporioides
    C. cucumerinum
    C. elatum
    C. herbarum
    C. oxysporum
    C. sphaerospermum
Claforan
clamp connection
Clara cell
clarithromycin
clarithromycin/ethambutol regimen
clarkei
    Simulium c.
clarkii
    Bacillus c.
    Spiroplasma c.
clarridgeiae
    Bartonella c.
class
classification
    ACTG c.

adansonian c.
Bethesda c.
Lancefield c.
Runyon c. of nontuberculous
    mycobacteria
UICC c.
Union Internationale Contre La
    Cancer c.
Clathraceae
clathratiforme
    Pelodictyon c.
clathrin-coated pit
claudication
clausii
    Bacillus c.
claussenii
    Brettanomyces c.
Claustulaceae
clava
    Leptoconops c.
Clavariaceae
clavata
    Curvularia c.
clavato-nanicus
    Aspergillus c.-n.
clavatum
    Geotrichum c.
clavatus
    Aspergillus c.
Clavibacter (b)
    C. iranicus
    C. michiganensis subsp. *insidiosus*
    C. michiganensis subsp.
     michiganensis
    C. michiganensis subsp. *nebraskensis*
    C. michiganensis subsp. *sepedonicus*
    C. michiganensis subsp. *tessellarius*
    C. rathayi
    C. toxicus
    C. tritici
    C. xyli subsp. *cynodontis*
    C. xyli subsp. *xyli*
clavibothrium
    Bothriocephalus c.
clavibranchium
    Simulium c.
claviceps
    Bothriocephalus c.
Claviceps purpurea (f)
Clavicipitaceae
Clavicipitales

C

NOTES

clavifer
  Streptomyces c.
claviforme
  Streptosporangium c.
Clavispora lusitaniae (f)
clavulanate
  ticarcillin c.
clavulanic acid
clavuligerus
  Streptomyces c.
Clavulin
clean
  c. catheter urine culture
  C. & Clear Deep Cleaning
    Astringent
  C. & Clear Invisible Clearasil
    Clearstick
clean-catch
  c.-c. midstream urine
  c.-c. urine specimen
Cleanser
  Perineal Skin C.
Cleansing
  Fostex Medicated C.
Clear
  C. Away Disc
  C. By Design Gel
  C. Pore Treatment
  Scot-Tussin Senior C.
  C. Tussin 30
clearance
  creatinine c. (CrCl)
  urea nitrogen c.
Clearasil
  C. B.P. Plus
  C. Maximum Strength
  C. Pads
Clearstick
  Clean & Clear Invisible
    Clearasil C.
Clearview *Chlamydia* test
cleavage
  progressive c.
cleft
  c. lip
  Maurer c.
clenched-fist injury
Cleocin
  C. HCl
  C. HCl Oral
  C. Pediatric
  C. Pediatric Oral
  C. Phosphate
  C. Phosphate Injection
  C. T
  C. T Topical
  C. Vaginal
cleptoparasite

Cleveland and Collier liver extract medium
Clevelandellida
clevelandensis
  Afipia c.
Clevelandina reticulitermitidis (b)
clidinium and chlordiazepoxide
cliftonensis
  Rubrimonas c.
c2-like viruses (v)
Climara Transdermal
clinafloxacin
  c. HCl
Clinda-Derm
  C.-D. Topical
  C.-D. Topical solution
clindamycin
  c. hydrochloride
  c. phosphate
clindamycin-primaquine
Clindex
clinical
  c. AIDS
  c. latency
clinicopathologic
clinicopathological
Clinostomatidae
Clinostomatoidea
Clinostomum marginatum (p)
clioquinol
  c. and hydrocortisone
Clitocybe dealbata (f)
CLO
  Campylobacter-like organism
  CLO test
Clo
  C. Mor virus (CMV)
cloacae
  Enterobacter c.
  Sphingomonas c.
cloacale
  Mycoplasma c.
clobetasol
Clocort Maximum Strength
clocortolone
Cloderm Topical
clofazimine
  c. palmitate
Clogmia
  C. albipunctata
clonal
  c. abortion
  c. aging
clonazepam
clone
  Iberian epidemic c.
clonogenic
clonorchiasis

clonorchiosis
Clonorchis sinensis (p)
Clonothrix (b)
clorazepate
closed
    c. drainage
    c. joint aspiration
    c. space infection
Closterovirus (v)
clostridial
    c. gas gangrene
    c. myonecrosis
    c. toxin
Clostridium (b)
    C. absonum
    C. aceticum
    C. acetireducens
    C. acetobutylicum
    C. acidisoli
    C. acidiurici
    C. aerotolerans
    C. akagii
    C. aldrichii
    C. algidicarnis
    C. algidixylanolyticum
    C. aminophilum
    C. aminovalericum
    C. arcticum
    C. argentinense
    C. aurantibutyricum
    C. barati
    C. barkeri
    C. beijerinckii
    C. bifermentans
    C. botulinum
    C. botulinum types A, B, C, D,
      E, F and G
    C. bryantii
    C. butyricum
    C. cadaveris
    C. carnis
    C. celatum
    C. celerecrescens
    C. cellobioparum
    C. cellulofermentans
    C. cellulolyticum
    C. cellulosi
    C. cellulovorans
    C. chartatabidum
    C. chauvoei
    C. coccoides
    C. cochlearium

C. cocleatum
C. colinum
C. collagenovorans
C. cylindrosporum
C. difficile
C. difficile-associated disease
  (CDAD)
C. difficile colitis
C. difficile sepsis syndrome
C. difficile test (CLOtest)
C. difficile toxin assay
C. difficile toxin B
C. disporicum
C. durum
C. estertheticum
C. fallax
C. felsineum
C. fervidum
C. fimetarium
C. formicoaceticum
C. frigidicarnis
C. gasigenes
C. ghoni
C. glycolicum
C. grantii
C. haemolyticum
C. halophilum
C. hastiforme
C. herbivorans
C. hiranonis
C. histolyticum
C. homopropionicum
C. hungatei
C. hydroxybenzoicum
C. hylemonae
C. indolis
C. innocuum
C. intestinale
C. irregularis
C. isatidis
C. josui
C. kluyveri
C. laramiense
C. lentocellum
C. lentoputrescens
C. leptum
C. limosum
C. litorale
C. lituseburense
C. ljungdahlii
C. lortetii
C. magnum

C

NOTES

Clostridium (continued)
C. malenominatum
C. mangenotii
C. mayombei
C. methoxybenzovorans
C. methylpentosum
C. neopropionicum
C. nexile
C. novyi
C. oceanicum
C. orbiscindens
C. oroticum
C. oxalicum
C. papyrosolvens
C. paradoxum
C. paraperfringens
C. paraputrificum
C. pascui
C. pasteurianum
C. peptidivorans
C. perenne
C. perfringens
C. perfringens enterotoxin (CPE)
C. perfringens type A
C. pfennigii
C. piliforme
C. polysaccharolyticum
C. populeti
C. propionicum
C. proteoclasticum
C. proteolyticum
C. puniceum
C. purinolyticum
C. putrefaciens
C. putrificum
C. quercicolum
C. quinii
C. ramosum
C. rectum
C. roseum
C. saccharolyticum
C. sardiniensis
C. sartgoformum
C. scatologenes
C. scindens
C. septicum
C. sordellii
C. sphenoides
C. spiroforme
C. sporogenes
C. sporosphaeroides
C. stercorarium subsp. *leptospartum*
C. stercorarium subsp. *stercorarium*
C. stercorarium subsp.
   thermolacticum
C. sticklandii
C. subterminale
C. symbiosum

C. termitidis
C. tertium
C. tetani
C. tetani, Harvard strain 401
C. tetanomorphum
C. thermoaceticum
C. thermoalcaliphilum
C. thermoautotrophicum
C. thermobutyricum
C. thermocellum
C. thermocopriae
C. thermohydrosulfuricum
C. thermolacticum
C. thermopalmarium
C. thermopapyrolyticum
C. thermosaccharolyticum
C. thermosuccinogenes
C. thermosulfurogenes
C. tyrobutyricum
C. uliginosum
C. ultunense
C. villosum
C. vincentii
C. viride
C. xylanolyticum
C. xylanovorans
CLOtest
   Clostridium difficile test
Clotrimaderm
clotrimazole
   betamethasone and c.
   c. troche
   c. vaginal tablet
cloudy vision
cloxacillin
   c. sodium
Cloxapen
clozapine
clubbing of fingers
clue
   c. cell
   c. cell test
clump
clumping
   c. factor
Clutton joints
CMC
   chronic mucocutaneous candidiasis
   complement-mediated cytotoxicity
CMG
   cystometrogram
CMI
   cell-mediated immune
   cell-mediated immunity
   CMI response
CMV
   Clo Mor virus
   Cytomegalovirus

CMV adrenalitis
CMV antigenemia
CMV antigen test
CMV culture
CMV DNA hybrid capture
CMV early antigen FA method
CMV end-organ disease
CMV esophagitis
CMV hyperimmune globulin
CMV mononucleosis syndrome
CMV pneumonia
CMV pneumonitis
CMV retinitis
CMV serology
CMV shell vial method
CMVIG
    cytomegalovirus immune globulin
CMVIg
    cytomegalovirus-specific intravenous
      immune globulin
CMV-IGIV
CM$_1$ virus
CMV-Vue assay
CNAV
    Caninde virus
Cnemidocoptes (p) (*var. of*
   Knemidocoptes)
Cnephia
    C. pecuarum
Cnidospora (p)
Cnidosporidia
CNNA
    culture-negative neutrocytic ascites
CNS
    central nervous system
    coagulase-negative staphylococcus
      CNS cryptococcosis
CNTV
    Connecticut virus
CNUV
    Chenuda virus
COA
    coagglutination
    staphylococcal protein A COA
CoActifed
Coactin
coagglutination (COA)
    staphylococcal c.
    staphylococcal protein A c.
    c. test
coagulans
    Bacillus c.

    Bacteroides c.
    Hyphomicrobium c.
    Staphylococcus schleiferi subsp. *c.*
coagulase
    bound c.
    c. test
coagulase-negative
    c.-n. staphylococcal
    c.-n. staphylococcal infection
    c.-n. staphylococcus (CNS, CONS)
    Staphylococcus species c.-n.
coagulase-reacting factor (CRF)
coagulation
    disseminated intravascular c. (DIC)
coagulopathy
coagulum
    necrobiotic c.
coal
    c. tar
    c. tar, lanolin, and mineral oil
    c. tar and salicylic acid
coalesce
coalescence
CoAr 1071 virus
CoAr 3624 virus
CoAr 3627 virus
coastal plains virus (CPV)
coat
    buffy c.
    quantitative buffy c. (QBC)
cobalamin
Cocadviroid (v)
cocaine
    aqueous c.
Cocal virus
Coccaceae
coccal
cocci (*pl. of* coccus)
coccidia (*pl. of* coccidium)
coccidial
    c. infection
coccidian
Coccidiasina
coccidioidal
    c. complement-fixation level
    c. spherule
Coccidioides (f)
    C. immitis
    C. immunodiffusion
coccidioidin skin test
coccidioidomas

NOTES

C

119

coccidioidomycosis
　disseminated c.
　c. immitis
　primary c.
　subclinical c.
coccidiosis
Coccidium
　C. bigeminum
　C. bigeminum var. *hominis*
coccidium, pl. **coccidia**
coccobacillary
coccobacilli
coccobacillus
coccodes
　Colletotrichum c.
coccoid
Coccoideaceae
coccoides
　Clostridium c.
　Eperythrozoon c.
coccus, pl. **cocci**
　gram-negative c.
　gram-positive c.
　gram-positive anaerobic c. (GPAC)
　Weichselbaum c. (*See Neisseria
　　meningitidis*)
cochisensis
　Culicoides c.
cochleae
　Kluyvera c.
cochlear
cochlearium
　Clostridium c.
cochleata
　Kitasatospora c.
cochleate
cochleatus
　Streptomyces c.
Cochliobolus (f)
　C. australiensis
　C. cynodontis
　C. geniculatus
　C. hawaiiensis
　C. lunatus
　C. pallescens
　C. spiciferus
　C. verruculosus
Cochliomyia (p)
　C. americana
　C. hominivorax
　C. macellaria
Cochlonemataceae
Cochlosoma anatis (p)
cockerellii
　Culicoides c.
cockle agent
cocleatum
　Clostridium c.

cocophilus
　Aphelenchoides c.
cocovenenans
　Burkholderia c.
　Pseudomonas c.
Codafed Expectorant
Codamine
　C. Pediatric
Codehist DH
codeine
　Benylin C.
　bromodiphenhydramine and c.
　brompheniramine,
　　phenylpropanolamine, and c.
　chlorpheniramine, phenylephrine,
　　and c.
　chlorpheniramine, pseudoephedrine,
　　and c.
　C. Contin
　Deproist Expectorant With C.
　guaifenesin, pseudoephedrine, and c.
　Guiatussin With C.
　NF Cough Syrup with C.
　Phenergan VC With C.
　Pherazine VC w/ C.
　Pherazine With C.
　promethazine and c.
　promethazine, phenylephrine, and c.
　Promethist With C.
　Prometh VC With C.
　terpin hydrate and c.
　triprolidine, pseudoephedrine, and c.
codiaei
　Xanthomonas c.
Codiclear DH
codiocampa
　Wyeomyia c.
codon
　transcription initiation c.
cod worm
Coelenterata
coelenterate
coelescens
　Streptomyces c.
coeliaca
　Nocardia c.
coelicoflavus
　Streptomyces c.
coelicolor
　Streptomyces c.
coelom
coelomyarian
Coelomycetaceae
Coelomycetes
coenocyte
coenocytic
Coenonia anatina (b)

coenurosis
  cerebral c.
coenurus
  c. cerebralis
  c. disease
  c. glomeratus
coenzyme
  c. I, II
  c. Q
coerulea
  Absidia c.
  Actinomadura c.
  Micromonospora c.
coeruleoflavus
  Streptomyces c.
coeruleofusca
  Actinomadura c.
  Nocardiopsis c.
  Saccharothrix c.
coeruleofuscus
  Streptomyces c.
coeruleoprunus
  Streptomyces c.
coeruleorubidus
  Streptomyces c.
coeruleoviolacea
  Actinomadura c.
  Saccharothrix c.
coerulescens
  Streptomyces c.
coexisting
cofactor
  Kaposi sarcoma c.
cohaerens
  Herpetosiphon c.
  Lewinella c.
Cohn-ethanol fractionation
cohnii
  Bacillus c.
  Staphylococcus cohnii subsp. *c.*
Cohnistreptothrix
cohort
  Aquitaine c.
  Omega c.
coho salmon reovirus
coinfected
coinfection
  chronic c.
coin lesion
coipomoensis
  Candida c.
coital exanthema virus

coitus
cokeri
  Septobasidium c.
Cokeromyces (f)
  C. recurvatus
ColAn 57389 virus
cold
  c. abscess
  c. agglutination
  c. agglutinin
  c. agglutinin titer
  c. antibody
  c. autoagglutinin
  c. autoantibody
  Benylin C.
  c. blade surgery
  common c.
  Histenol C.
  c. light
  C. Medication D
  C. Medication Daytime Relief
  Ornex C.
  c. panniculitis
  Robitussin Pediatric Cough & C.
  c. sore
  c. stain
  Sudafed Severe C.
cold-knife
  c.-k. cone biopsy
  c.-k. technique
Coldloc
Coldloc-LA
cold-reactive autoantibody titer
colectomy
coleocola
  Eremococcus c.
Coleoptera
  poxvirus of C.
coleopterae
  Mesoplasma c.
Coleviroid (v)
coli
  Balantidium c.
  Campylobacter c.
  diarrheagenic *Escherichia c.*
  diffusely adherent *Escherichia c.*
    (DAEC)
  Entamoeba c.
  enteroadherent *Escherichia c.*
    (EAEC)
  enteroaggregative *Escherichia c.*
    (EAggEC, EaggEC)

NOTES

C

coli (continued)
    enterohemorrhagic *Escherichia c.* (EHEC)
    enteroinvasive *Escherichia c.* (EIEC)
    enteropathogenic *Escherichia c.* (EPEC)
    enterotoxigenic *Escherichia c.* (ETEC)
    enterovirulent *Escherichia c.* (EEC)
    Escherichia c.
    Paramecium c.
    Shiga toxin-producing *Escherichia c.* (STEC)
    Streptococcus infantarius subsp. *c.*
    verocytotoxin-producing *Escherichia c.* (VTEC)
colic
    renal c.
colicin
colicinogeny
coliform
    c. bacillus
    c. bacteria
colinum
    Clostridium c.
coliphage
    c. fd group
    c. MS2
    c. MS2-GA group
    c. φx174
    c. Q-beta
    c. Q-beta-SP group
    c. T7H
colistimethate
colistin
    c., neomycin, and hydrocortisone
    c. susceptibility test
colitis
    amebic c.
    antibiotic-associated c. (AAC)
    antibiotic-related c.
    Clostridium difficile c.
    eosinophilic c.
    fulminant amebic c.
    hemorrhagic c.
    invasive c.
    pseudomembranous c. (PMC)
    recurrent c.
    tuberculous c.
    ulcerative c.
collagen
    c. cuff
    c. vascular disease
collagenovorans
    Clostridium c.
collare
    Hysterothylacium c.

collared flagellate
collarette
collection
    American Type Culture C. (ATCC)
    National Type Culture C. (NTCC)
Colletotrichum (f)
    C. coccodes
    C. dematium
    C. gloeosporioides
collinoides
    Lactobacillus c.
Collinsella (b)
    C. aerofaciens
    C. intestinalis
    C. stercoris
collinus
    Streptomyces c.
collis
    Mycoplasma c.
colloidal feces
collosoma
    Leptomonas c.
Colocort
colocutaneous fistula
colombiense
    Aminobacterium c.
colombiensis
    Streptomyces c.
colon
    c. bacillus
    sigmoid c.
colonial morphology test
colonic
    c. polyp
    c. polyposis
    c. pseudotumor
colonization
    atypical mycobacterial c.
    Candida parapsilosis c.
    c. factor antigen (CFA)
    intestinal c.
    perineal MRSA c.
    c. resistance
colonometer
colonoscopy
colony
    daughter c.
    filamentous c.
    c. forming unit (CFU)
    H c.
    lenticular c.
    mother c.
    mucoid c.
    O c.
    rough c.
    satellite c.

smooth c.
spheroid c.
colony-stimulating factor (CSF)
coloradensis
    Amycolatopsis c.
Colorado
    C. tick fever (CTF)
    C. tick fever virus (CTFV)
colorectal
colorimetric assay
Color Vue *Cryptosporidium* **assay**
colostrum
colposcope
colposcopy
Coltivirus (v)
colubriformis
    Trichostrongylus c.
columbae
    Enterococcus c.
columbianum
    Oesophagostomum c.
columbianus
    Spermospora c.
Columbia SK virus
columbina
    Riemerella c.
columbinasale
    Mycoplasma c.
columbinum
    Mycoplasma c.
columbinus
    Pleurotus c.
columborale
    Mycoplasma c.
columella, pl. **columellae**
columellifera
    Pilimelia columellifera subsp. *c.*
columnar
    c. epithelium
columnare
    Flavobacterium c.
columnaris
    Baylisascaris c.
    Cytophaga c.
    Flexibacter c.
Colwellia (b)
    C. demingiae
    C. hadaliensis
    C. hornerae
    C. maris
    C. psychroerythraea

C. psychrotropica
C. rossensis
colwelliana
    Alteromonas c.
    Shewanella c.
Coly-Mycin
    C.-M. M Parenteral
    C.-M. Otic
    C.-M. S Oral
    C.-M. S Otic Drops
Comamonadaceae
Comamonas (b)
    C. acidovorans
    C. denitrificans
    C. nitrativorans
    C. terrigena
    C. testosteroni
comandoni
    Acanthamoeba c.
comatosa
    malaria c.
comatose
Combantrin
combesii
    Eubacterium c.
combination
    beta-lactam-beta-lactamase c.
    binary c.
    c. chemotherapy
    new c.
    c. therapy
combined
    measles and rubella vaccines, c.
    penicillin G benzathine and
      procaine c.
Combivir
comes
    Coprococcus c.
comma bacillus
commensal
    c. parasite
commensalism
    epizoic c.
Committee
    Hospital Infection Control Practices
      Advisory C. (HICPAC)
    National Vaccine Advisory C.
      (NVAC)
common
    c. cold
    c. cold virus
    c. cold virus group

C

NOTES

common *(continued)*
    c. variable hypogammaglobulinemia
    c. variable immunodeficiency
    c. wart
commune
    Aquabacterium c.
    Oceanospirillum c.
    Penicillium c.
    Schizophyllum c.
    Thermodesulfobacterium c.
communicability
communicable
    c. disease
    C. Disease Surveillance and
      Response (CSR)
communis
    Aedes c.
    Alteromonas c.
    Azoarcus c.
    Marinomonas c.
community
    biotic c.
community-acquired
    c.-a. bacteremia
    c.-a. bacterial pneumonia (CAP)
    c.-a. organism
    c.-a. pneumonia
    c.-a. septicemia
    c.-a. sinusitis
comorbidity
Comovirus (v)
compacta
    Fonsecaea c.
    Pseudonocardia c.
compactum
companulata
    Haemaphysalis c.
compartment syndrome
compassionate release
compassionate-use basis
Compazine
competitive
    c. PCR (cPCR)
    c. RT-PCR (cRT-PCR)
competitor DNA
complement
    c. fixation (CF)
    c. fixation test
complement-fixing (CF)
    c.-f. antibody
    immunodiffusion c.-f. (IDCF)
complement-mediated cytotoxicity (CMC)
complete
    c. atrioventricular block
    c. blood count (CBC)
    c. heart block
    c. medium
    c. metamorphosis

complex
    Acinetobacter calcoaceticus-
      baumannii c.
    AIDS dementia c. (ADC)
    AIDS-related c. (ARC)
    amphotericin B cholesteryl
      sulfate c.
    antigen 85 c.
    apical c.
    circulating immune c.
    Ghon c.
    intrinsic factor c.
    MAI c.
    major histocompatibility c. (MHC
      molecule, MHC)
    major histocompatibility c. class I
      (MHC-I)
    major histocompatibility c. class II
      (MHC-II)
    c. multichannel cystometry
    Mycobacterium avium c. (MAC)
    Mycobacterium avium-
      intracellulare c.
    Mycobacterium fortuitum-chelonae c.
    Mycobacterium fortuitum third
      biovar c.
    Mycobacterium terrae-triviale c.
    ophthalmoganglionary c.
    periodic sharp wave c. (PSWC)
    Ranke c.
    c. ventricular shunt
complicating allergic conjunctivitis
complication
    HIV-associated c.
    noninfectious disease c.
Compositae
composite lymphoma
compound
    ampholytic c.
    Hycomine C.
    pentavalent antimony-containing c.
    quaternary ammonium c. (QAC)
    salicylic and benzoic acid c.
    c. S, W
    C. W Plus
compransoris
    Zavarzinia c.
compressipes
    Acanthocephala c.
compromised host
computed
    c. tomography (CT)
    c. tomography brain scan (CT)
    c. transaxial tomography
Comtrex Maximum Strength Non-Drowsy
Comvax

ConA
    concanavalin A
concanavalin A (ConA)
concatemer
concentrate
concentration
    absolute plasma c. (APC)
    bactericidal c. (MBC)
    Baermann c.
    buffy coat c.
    C peptide c.
    CSF neopterin c.
    E-test gradient minimal
      inhibitory c.
    fecal c.
    formalin-ether sedimentation c.
    formalin-ethyl acetate
      sedimentation c.
    fractional inhibitory c. (FIC)
    gravity c.
    hematocrit c.
    hemoglobin c.
    M c.
    microhematocrit c.
    minimal inhibitory c. (MIC)
    minimum bactericidal c. (MBC)
    minimum inhibitory c. (MIC)
    peak plasma c.
    plasma anti-SEA antibody c.
    plasma cortisol c.
    plasma HIV RNA c.
    plasma lipid c.
    serum creatinine c.
    serum neopterin c.
    serum prolactin c.
    serum T c.
    zinc sulfate flotation c.
concentrator
    darkfield c.
    Evergreen FPC fecal c.
conchicola
    Aspidogaster c.
concilii
    Methanosaeta c.
    Methanothrix c.
concinna
    Haemaphysalis c.
concisus
    Campylobacter c.
concomitant
concretivorus
    Thiobacillus c.

condimenti
    Staphylococcus c.
conditioning
    heating, ventilating, and air c.
      (HVAC)
condom catheter
conduction
    c. defect
    c. hearing loss
conductivity
    total body electrical c. (TOBEC)
condyle
    femoral c.
Condyline
condyloma, pl. **condylomata**
    c. acuminatum
    exophytic c.
    flat c.
    giant c.
    c. latum
    penile c.
    perianal condylomata
    spiked c.
condylomatous-appearing
condylomatous carcinoma
Condylox
Conex
confidentiality
configuration
    shephord crook c.
Confirmation
    AccuProbe *Gonorrhoeae* Culture C.
confluence
confluent
confluentis
    Mycobacterium c.
confraterna
    Acanthocephala c.
confusa
    Weissella c.
confusum
    Corynebacterium c.
confusus
    Lactobacillus c.
congener
congenital
    c. agammaglobulinemia
    c. anemia
    c. asplenia
    c. candidiasis
    c. CMV infection
    c. cytomegalic inclusion disease

NOTES

congenital *(continued)*
    c. cytomegalovirus
    c. HCMV infection
    c. hemoglobinopathy
    c. HIV infection
    c. immunodeficiency
    c. Lyme disease
    c. malformation
    c. ocular toxoplasmosis
    c. rubella
    c. rubella syndrome
    c. self-healing reticulohistiocytosis
    c. syphilis
    c. tuberculosis
    c. varicella
congeri
    Cristitectus c.
Congess
    C. Jr
    C. Sr
Congest
    C. Aid
Congestac
    C. ND
Congest-Eze
Congestion
    Contac Head & Chest C.
    Vicks 44D Cough & Head C.
congestive heart failure (CHF)
conglobata
    Candida c.
conglobate abscess
conglomeratum
    Brachybacterium c.
Conglomeromonas (b)
    C. largomobilis subsp. *largomobilis*
    C. largomobilis subsp. *parooensis*
congoense
    Cylindrocarpon c.
congolense
    Halanaerobium c.
    Methanobacterium c.
    Trypanosoma c.
congolensis
    Dermatophilus c.
    Thysanotaenia c.
Congolian red fever
Congo red stain
congreenarum
    Simulium c.
conica
    Pirenella c.
Conicera
conicus
    Aspergillus c.
conidia
    Aspergillus c.

conidiobolae
    entomophthoramycosis c.
Conidiobolus (f)
    C. coronatus
    C. incongruus
conidiogenous
    c. cell
conidiophore
    phialophore-type c.
conidium
Coniochaeta (f)
    C. ligniaria
    C. subcorticalis
Coniosporium (f)
    C. apollinis
    C. atrum
    C. olivaceum
    C. strobilinum
Coniosporium perforans
Coniothecium (f)
    C. austriacum
    C. epidermidis
    C. glumarum
Coniothyrium (f)
    C. fuckelii
coniothyrium
    Leptosphaeria c.
conjugant
conjugate
    diphtheria, tetanus toxoids, whole-cell pertussis, and *Haemophilus influenzae* type b c. (DtwP-HIB)
    c. division
    c. vaccine
conjugation
conjugative
    c. plasmid
    c. transposon
conjugatus
    Pseudocaedibacter c.
conjunctiva, pl. **conjunctivae**
    bulbar c.
conjunctivae
    Dirofilaria c.
    Mycoplasma c.
conjunctival
    c. hyperemia
    c. injection
    c. microangiopathy
    c. papilloma
    c. scraping
    c. smear
    c. swab
    c. tuberculosis
conjunctivitis
    acute contagious c.
    acute epidemic c.
    acute follicular c.

allergic c.
bacterial c.
chlamydial c.
chronic c.
complicating allergic c.
diphtheritic c.
follicular c.
gonococcal c.
granular c.
granulomatous c.
Haemophilus c.
herpes simplex c.
herpetic c.
inclusion c.
infantile purulent c.
lymphogranuloma venereum c.
membranous c.
meningococcal c.
nosocomial viral c.
primary meningococcal c.
purulent c.
squirrel plague c.
swimming pool c.
toxicogenic c.
trachoma inclusion c.
trachoma and inclusion c. (TRIC)
trachomatous c.
tularemic c.
vernal c.
viral c.
conjunctus
    Metorchis c.
Connecticut virus (CNTV)
connection
    clamp c.
connective tissue disorder
connori
    Brachiola c.
    Nosema c.
Conocybe cyanopus (f)
conoid
conoideum
    Hypoderaeum c.
conorii
    Rickettsia c.
CONS
    coagulase-negative staphylococcus
consensus
conservative surgery
conservator
    Culex c.

consettensis
    Actinoplanes c.
consolidation
    lobar c.
consortionis
    Cryptococcus c.
conspecific
Conspicuum (p)
conspicuum
    Mycobacterium c.
conspirator
    Culex c.
constellatus
    Streptococcus constellatus subsp. *c.*
constitutional
    c. homeopathy
    c. symptom
constitutive resistance
constricta
    Ochroconis c.
consulate disease
Contac
    C. Cold Non-Drowsy
    C. Coughcaps
    C. Cough Formula Liquid
    C. Head & Chest Congestion
contact
    c. dermatitis
    replicate organism direct agar c.
    (RODAC-TM)
contagiosa
    impetigo c.
    keratosis follicularis c.
contagiosum
    ecthyma c.
    epithelioma c.
    erythema c.
    giant disseminated molluscum c.
    molluscum c.
    pemphigus c.
contagious
    c. disease
    c. ecthyma
    c. pustular dermatitis (CPDV)
    c. pustular stomatitis virus
contagiousness
contagium
contamination
    bacterial c.
    fecal c.
    Salmonella c.

C

NOTES

contents
    aspiration of gastric c.
Contergan
contiguous
    c. suppuration
Contin
    Codeine C.
continua
    acrodermatitis c.
    acrodermatitis pustolosa c.
    epilepsia partialis c.
    Heterophyopsis c.
continuous
    c. ambulatory peritoneal dialysis
    (CAPD)
    c. cycling peritoneal dialysis
    (CCPD)
    c. focal epilepsy
    c. positive airway pressure (CPAP)
contortum
    Eubacterium c.
contortus
    Haemonchus c.
contour-clamped
    c.-c. gel electrophoresis
    c.-c. homogeneous electric field
    (CHEF)
    c.-c. homogenous fields
    electrophoresis (CHEF)
contracaeciasis
Contracaecinea
Contracaecum
    C. filiforme
    C. mulli
    C. osculatum
    C. papilligerum
    C. pedum
    C. rudolphii
    C. septentrionale
contraceptive
    barrier c.
    oral c. (OC)
    c. sponge
contractile vacuole
contractility
    bladder c.
contraindicated
contraindication
contralateral
contrast
    oral c.
control
    biologic c.
    Blemish C.
    Centers for Disease C. (CDC)
    infection c.
    Lander Dandruff C.
    Oxy C.

    Shaklee Dandruff C.
    Study on Efficacy of Nosocomial
    Infection C. (SENIC)
    c. test
Controller
    Maalox H2 Acid C.
    Pepcid AC Acid C.
controverting
Contuss
    C. XT
conus medullaris syndrome
convalescence
convalescent
    c. phase
    c. stage
conventional
    amphotericin B (conventional)
conventional-beam therapy
Convict
    C. Creek 104 virus
    C. Creek 74 virus
conviti
    Simulium c.
convulsion
    febrile c.
CONX virus
cookei
    Microsporum c.
Cookellaceae
cookiellum
    Arthroderma c.
cookii
    Lysobacter enzymogenes subsp. *c.*
    Mycobacterium c.
cooleyi
    Argas c.
coolhaasii
    Caloramator c.
coolie itch
cooling blanket
Coomassie blue stain
Coombs-negative hemolytic anemia
Coombs test
Cooperia curticei (p)
Cooperiinae
COPD
    chronic obstructive pulmonary disease
Copelandia (f)
copenhageni
    Leptospira interrogans serovar *c.*
copepod
Copepoda
Cophene XP
copiosus
    Culicoides c.
    Leptoconops c.
copious
Coplin jar

copper pennies
copra itch
Coprinaceae
coprine
Coprinus (f)
    C. cinereus
    C. micaceus
Coprobacillus cateniformis (b)
Coprococcus (b)
    C. catus
    C. comes
    C. eutactus
coprologic examination
coprophagous
coprophagy
coprophil
coprophile
coprophilus
    Rhodococcus c.
coprostanoligenes
    Eubacterium c.
Coprothermobacter (b)
    C. platensis
    C. proteolyticus
coprozoa
coprozoic
Coptin
copulation
Co-Pyronil 2 Pulvules
corallina
    Microbispora c.
corallinus
    Rhodococcus c.
Corallobothrium (p)
coralloides
    Myxococcus c.
corbis
    Simulium c.
corchorusii
    Streptomyces c.
cord
    c. blood
    c. compression syndrome
cordiformis
    Nyctotherus c.
Cordran
    C. SP
Cordylobia (p)
    C. anthropophaga
    C. rodhaini
cordylobiasis

core
    hepatitis B virus c.
    c. promoter
    c. of tissue
corea
    Euploea c.
co-receptor
coremiformis
    Trichosporon c.
Corfou virus (CFUV)
coriaceae
    Borrelia c.
coriense
    Halorubrobacterium c.
    Halorubrum c.
Coriobacterium glomerans (b)
Corium
corkscrew appearance
Cormax Ointment
cormonsi
    Simulium c.
corn
    c. ergot
    c. smut
cornea
    serpent ulcer of c.
corneae
    Vittaforma c.
corneal
    c. haze
    c. infection
    c. opacity
    c. scarring
    c. scraping
    c. smear
    c. trauma
    c. ulcer
corneum
    stratum c.
    Vittaforma c.
corniculatum
    Arthroderma c.
corniger
    Culex c.
cornigera
    Haemaphysalis c.
cornmeal agar
cornutum
    Hysterothylacium c.
corogypsi
    Mycoplasma c.
coronafaciens

C

NOTES

coronal sulcus
coronary arteriopathy
coronata
    Delacroixia c.
coronator
    Culex c.
coronatum
    Cyathostomum c.
coronatus
    Conidiobolus c.
    Diploscapter c.
Coronaviridae
Coronavirus (v)
    C. group
coronavirus
    bovine c.
    enteric c.
    human c.
    rabbit c.
    rat c.
    turkey c.
coronavirus-like
    c.-l. particle (CVLP)
Corophyllin
corporis
    Bacteroides c.
    pediculosis c.
    Pediculus humanus c.
    Prevotella c.
    pthiriasis c.
    tinea c.
    trichophytosis c.
cor pulmonale
corpuscle
    basal c.
    calcareous c.
    Rainey c.
Corque Topical
Corriparta virus (CORV)
corrodens
    Eikenella c.
corroding bacillus
corrugata
    Acrocarpospora c.
    Pseudomonas c.
corrugatum
    Hysterothylacium c.
    Streptosporangium c.
corruscae
    Mesoplasma c.
    Spiroplasma c.
Cortacet
CortaGel Topical
Cortaid
    C. Maximum Strength Topical
    C. with Aloe Topical
Cortate
Cortatrigen Otic

Cort-Dome Topical
Cortef
    C. Feminine Itch Topical
corti
    Mesocestoides c.
corticale
    Cryptostroma c.
cortical gyral malformation
Corticiaceae
corticola
    Griphosphaeria c.
corticosporin
corticosteroid
corticotropin
Corticoviridae
Corticovirus (v)
Cortimyxin
Cortinariaceae
Cortinarius orellanus (f)
cortisol
    c. excretion
    c. level
cortisone acetate
Cortisporin
    C. Ophthalmic Ointment
    C. Ophthalmic suspension
    C. Otic
    C. Topical Cream
    C. Topical Ointment
Cortisporin-TC
    C.-T. Otic
    C.-T. Otic suspension
Cortizone-5 Topical
Cortizone-10 Topical
Cortoderm
Cortone Acetate
Cortrosyn
    C. stimulation test
CORV
    Corriparta virus
corymbifera
    Absidia c.
    Lichtheimia c.
Coryneaceae
corynebacteria
Corynebacteriaceae
corynebacterioides
    Nocardia c.
corynebacteriophage
    beta c.
Corynebacterium (b)
    C. accolens
    C. afermentans subsp. *afermentans*
    C. afermentans subsp. *lipophilum*
    C. ammoniagenes
    C. amycolatum
    C. argentoratense
    C. auris

C. auriscanis
C. betae
C. beticola
C. bovis
C. callunae
C. camporealensis
C. capitovis
C. casei
C. confusum
C. coyleae
C. cystitidis
C. diphtheriae
C. durum
C. equi
C. falsenii
C. fascians
C. felinum
C. flaccumfaciens
C. flavescens
C. glucuronolyticum
C. glutamicum
C. hoagii
C. ilicis
C. imitans
C. insidiosum
C. iranicum
C. jeikeium
C. kroppenstedtii
C. kutscheri
C. lilium
lipophilic *C.*
C. lipophiloflavum
C. macginleyi
C. mastitidis
C. matruchotii
C. michiganense
C. michiganense subsp. *tessellarius*
C. minutissimum
C. mooreparkense
C. mucifaciens
C. mycetoides
C. nebraskense
nonlipophilic *C.*
C. oortii
C. paurometabolum
C. phocae
C. pilosum
C. poinsettiae
C. propinquum
C. pseudodiphtheriticum
C. pseudotuberculosis
C. pyogenes

C. rathayi
C. renale
C. riegelii
C. seminale
C. sepedonicum
C. simulans
C. singulare
C. striatum
C. sundsvallense
C. terpenotabidum
C. testudinoris
C. thomssenii
C. tritici
C. ulcerans
C. urealyticum
C. variabile
C. vitaeruminis
C. xerosis
coryneform
   c. bacterium
coryneforme
   Bifidobacterium c.
Coryneliaceae
Corynelialis
Corynespora cassiicola (f)
coryniformis
   Lactobacillus coryniformis subsp. *c.*
Corynosoma strumosum
Coryphen
coryza virus
Cosmegen
cosmesis
Cosmocephalus obvelatus (p)
Cosmocerella (p)
cosmopolitan
costa, pl. **costae**
costai
   Leptopsylla algira c.
costaricanus
   Streptomyces c.
costaricense
   Simulium c.
costaricensis
   Angiostrongylus c.
   Morerastrongylus c.
costicola
   Salinivibrio costicola subsp. *c.*
   Vibrio c.
costimulation
   T-cell c.
CoSudafed Expectorant
cosyntropin

C

NOTES

cothurnata
    Amanita c.
Cotia virus (CPV)
cotopaxi
    Simulium c.
Cotridin
Cotrifed
Cotrim
    C. DS
cotrimoxazole
cottewii
    Mycoplasma c.
cotton
    c. blue stain
    c. swab
cotton-wool spot
Cotylaspis (p)
Cotylogonimus
Cotylurus (p)
Couchioplanes (b)
    C. caeruleus subsp. *azureus*
    C. caeruleus subsp. *caeruleus*
Cough
    Diphen C.
    Sudafed Cold & C.
    C. Suppressant Syrup DM
    C. syrup
    C. Syrup DM-D-E
    C. Syrup DM Decongestant
    C. Syrup DM Decongestant for
      Children
    C. Syrup DM Decongestant
      Expectorant
    C. Syrup DM-E
    C. Syrup with Guaifenesin
    Tylenol C.
cough
    staccato c.
    whooping c.
Coughcaps
    Contac C.
Council
    National Research C.
Councilman body
counseling and testing (C&T)
count
    absolute CD4 cell c.
    absolute CD4 lymphocyte c.
    absolute neutrophil c. (ANC)
    blood c.
    CD4 lymphocyte c.
    CD4+ lymphocyte c.
    cell c.
    complete blood c. (CBC)
    dilution egg c.
    direct-smear egg c.
    joint-fluid leukocyte c.
    lymphocyte c.

    neutrophil leukocyte c.
    platelet c.
    total lymphocyte c.
countercurrent
    c. centrifugal elutriation
    c. immunoelectrophoresis (CIE,
      CIEP)
counterimmunoelectrophoresis (CIE,
    CIEP)
    c. technique
Cowbone Ridge virus (CRV)
Cowdria (b)
    C. ruminantium
cowpox virus
Coxiella (b)
    C. burnetii
    C. burnetii titer
Coxsackie
    C. B
    C. B_1 virus titer
    C. B_2 virus titer
    C. B_3 virus titer
    C. B_4 virus titer
    C. B_5 virus titer
    C. B_6 virus titer
    C. B virus serology
    C. encephalitis
    C. virus
    C. virus A1
    C. virus serology
coxsackievirus
    c. A, B
    human c. A1–A24
    human c. B1–B6
coyleae
    Corynebacterium c.
CP
    Vancocin CP
Cp-1 virus
CPAP
    continuous positive airway pressure
cPCR
    competitive PCR
CPCV
    Cacipacore virus
CPDV
    contagious pustular dermatitis
CPE
    Clostridium perfringens enterotoxin
CpGV
    Cydia pomonella granulovirus
CPH
    chronic persistent hepatitis
CPK
    creatine phosphokinase
CPS
    pneumococcal capsular polysaccharide
      CPS antigen

CPV
    coastal plains virus
    Cotia virus
    cytoplasmic polyhedrosis virus
CQIV
    Calchaqui virus
C-R
    Bicillin C.-R.
crab
    c. hand
    c. lice
crack cocaine
crackles
craigi
    Simulium c.
craniad
cranial
    c. nerve palsy
    c. neuritis
    c. neuropathy
craniotomy
crassa
    Neurospora c.
    Simonsiella c.
Crassicauda (p)
    C. anthonyi
    C. boopis
    C. carbonelli
    C. grampicola
crassiceps
    Taenia c.
crassipes
    Damalina c.
crassostreae
    Nocardia c.
crassum
    Cylindrocarpon destructans var. *c.*
    Cylindrocarpon olidum var. *c.*
crassus
Crataerina
    C. pallida
Craurococcus roseus (b)
craw-craw
CRBSI
    catheter-related bloodstream infection
CrCl
    creatinine clearance
C-reactive protein (CRP)
cream
    aclometasone dipropionate c.
    Acticin C.
    AVC C.

Benzashave C.
Cortisporin Topical C.
DV Vaginal C.
Elimite C.
Exact C.
fluocinonide c.
foscarnet c.
hydrocortisone c.
ketoconazole c.
Lamisil C.
Lotrimin AF C.
Maximum Strength Desenex
    Antifungal C.
miconazole c.
Mudd Acne C.
Neosporin C.
Noritate C.
Prevex Diaper Rash C.
silver sulfadiazine c.
SSD C.
Sween C.
Vaniqa C.
Zonalon Topical C.
creatine
    c. kinase
    c. phosphokinase (CPK)
creatinine
    c. clearance (CrCl)
    c. kinase BB
    serum c.
creatinini
    Tissierella c.
creatinolyticus
    Arthrobacter c.
creatinophila
    Tissierella c.
creeping
    c. eruption
    c. myiasis
creme
    Fungoid C.
    Pedi-Cort V C.
cremea
    Actinomadura cremea subsp. *c.*
cremeus
    Streptomyces c.
cremoris
    Lactococcus lactis subsp. *c.*
    Leuconostoc c.
    Leuconostoc mesenteroides subsp. *c.*
    Streptococcus c.
    Streptococcus lactis subsp. *c.*

C

NOTES

crenated red blood cell
Crenosoma vulpis (p)
Crenothrix polyspora (b)
Creo-Terpin
Crepidostomum (p)
Crepidotaceae
crepitant
    c. cellulitis
    c. myositis
crepitation
crepuscularis
    Culicoides c.
crescendo pain
crescens
    Chrysosporium parvum var. *c.*
crescent
    malarial c.
crescentus
    Caulobacter c.
crest
    iliac c.
cresta
Cresylate
Cresylecht violet stain
cretacea
    Herbidospora c.
cretosus
    Streptomyces griseus subsp. *c.*
Creutzfeldt-Jacob, Creutzfeldt-Jakob
Creutzfeldt-Jacob disease (CJD)
crevioricanis
    Porphyromonas c.
CRF
    coagulase-reacting factor
Cribbeaceae
criceti
    Streptococcus c.
    Veillonella c.
    Veillonella alcalescens subsp. *c.*
cricetuli
    Mycoplasma c.
Crimean-Congo
    C.-C. fever
    C.-C. hemorrhagic fever (C-CHFV)
    C.-C. hemorrhagic fever virus
Crinivirus (v)
crisis, pl. crises
    adrenal c.
    aplastic c.
    transient aplastic c. (TAC)
crispa
    Planopolyspora c.
crispatus
    Lactobacillus c.
crispus
    Catenuloplanes c.
cristatus
    Streptococcus c.

Cristispira pectinis (b)
Cristitectus congeri (p)
criterium, pl. criteria
    Amsel criteria
    Ranson criteria
crithidia
Crithidia fasciculata (p)
crithidial
crixbelly
Crixivan
crocatus
    Chondromyces c.
crocea
    Bullera c.
Crocicreas (f)
crocidurae
    Borrelia c.
crocodyli
    Mycoplasma c.
Crohn disease
cross
    c. agglutination
    c. infection
    maltese c.
    c. reaction
    c. sensitization
Crossiella cryophila (b)
crosslinking
    UV c.
crossotus
    Butyrivibrio c.
cross-perfusion
cross-react
cross-reacting
    c.-r. agglutinin
    c.-r. antibody
cross-reactive antigen
cross-reactivity
cross-strain infectivity
crotalariae
    Phaeotrichoconis c.
crotali
    Cryptosporidium c.
    Porocephalus c.
Crotalus antitoxin
crotamiton
croup
croup-associated virus
croxtoni
    Simulium c.
CRP
    C-reactive protein
^{51}Cr release assay
CRS
    catheter-related sepsis
    catheter-related septicemia
cRT-PCR
    competitive RT-PCR

crucians
    Anopheles c.
Cruex
crunogena
    Thiomicrospira c.
cruris
    tinea c.
    trichophytosis c.
cruris-hominis
    Phoma c.-h.
crush preparation
Crustacea
crustacean
crusted
    c. ringworm
    c. scabies
cruzi
    Trypanosoma c.
cruzii
    Anopheles c.
    Anopheles cruzii c.
CRV
    channel catfish reovirus
    Cowbone Ridge virus
cryaerophilus
    Arcobacter c.
    Campylobacter c.
crymophilic
crymophylactic
cryoablation
cryoapplication
Cryobacterium (b)
    C. psychrophilum
cryocautery
cryocrescens
    Kluyvera c.
cryoglobulin
cryoglobulinemia
    essential c.
    type II mixed c.
cryomicroscopy
    electron c.
cryopexy
cryophila
    Crossiella c.
cryophilic
cryophilis
    Saccharothrix c.
cryophylactic
cryoprecipitate transfusion
cryoprobe
cryosupernatant

cryosurgery
cryotherapy
Crypromycetaceae
crypt
    c. abscess
    anal c.
    c. cell
    c.'s of Lieberkühn
    tonsillar c.
cryptic
    c. miliary tuberculosis
    c. virus group
Cryptobacterium curtum (b)
Cryptobia salmostica (p)
Cryptoccus aquaticus
Cryptococcaceae
cryptococcal
    c. abscess
    c. antigen serology
    c. antigen testing
    c. choroiditis
    c. granuloma
    c. meningitis
Cryptococcales
cryptococcal lymphadenitis
cryptococcemia
cryptococcoma
cryptococcosis
    AIDS-related c.
    CNS c.
    extrapulmonary c.
    pulmonary c.
Cryptococcus (f)
    C. aerius
    C. albidosimilis
    C. albidus
    C. albidus var. *albidus*
    C. albidus var. *diffluens*
    C. amylolentus
    C. antarcticus
    C. ater
    C. bhutanensis
    C. capsulatus
    C. consortionis
    C. curvatus
    C. dimennae
    C. feraegula
    C. flavus
    C. friedmanni
    C. fuscescens
    C. gastricus
    C. gilvescens

C

NOTES

Cryptococcus (continued)
   C. heveanensis
   C. huempii
   C. humicolus
   C. hungaricus
   IFA *C.*
   C. kuetzingii
   C. latex antigen agglutination
   C. laurentii
   C. luteolus
   C. macerans
   C. magnus
   C. marinus
   C. neoformans
   C. neoformans var. *gattii*
   C. neoformans var. *grubii*
   C. neoformans var. *neoformans*
   C. podzolicus
   C. preparation
   C. serology
   C. skinneri
   C. stain
   C. terreus
   C. uniguttulatus
   C. vishniacii
   C. yarrowii
cryptogenic
   c. fibrosing alveolitis
   c. infection
   c. tetanus
Cryptomyces pleomorpha (f)
Cryptosporangium (b)
   C. arvum
   C. japonicum
cryptosporidia
cryptosporidial
   c. enteritis
Cryptosporidiidae
cryptosporidiosis
   biliary c.
   chronic intestinal c.
   gastric c.
   intestinal c.
   c. parvum
   pulmonary c.
   respiratory c.
   tracheal c.
Cryptosporidium (p)
   C. crotali
   C. meleagridis
   C. muris
   C. nasorum
   C. parvum
cryptosporidium
   stool for c.
Cryptostroma corticale (f)
cryptotrichotillomania

cryptoxanthin
   beta c.
cryptozoite
cryptum
   Acidiphilium c.
crystal
   calcium oxalate c.
   Charcot-Leyden c.
   cystine c.
   hippurate c.
   pyrophosphate dihydrate c.
   urate c.
   uric acid c.
   urine c.
   violet c.
   c. violet
crystalline
   c. nephropathy
   c. penicillin
crystallinus
   Streptomyces c.
crystallization
crystallography
   x-ray c.
crystallopoietes
   Arthrobacter c.
crystalluria
   acyclovir c.
Crysticillin A.S.
CS
   Pertussin C.
   Poly-Histine C.
CSD
   cat scratch disease
   CSD encephalopathy
C-section
   cesarean section
CSF
   cerebrospinal fluid
   colony-stimulating factor
      CSF cryptococcal antigen serology
      CSF glucose
      granulocyte-macrophage CSF (GM-CSF)
      CSF neopterin concentration
      CSF pleocytosis
      CSF protein
      CSF shunt catheter
      CSF tap
      CSF trypomastigote
      CSF VDRL
      CSF viral culture
      CSF viral load
CSIRO Village virus (CVGV)
CSR
   Communicable Disease Surveillance and Response

CT
   Chlamydia trachomatis
   computed tomography
   computed tomography brain scan
      CT guidance
C&T
   counseling and testing
CT4 virus
C/Taylor/1233/47
   influenzavirus C.
CTCL
   cutaneous T-cell lymphoma
Ctenocephalides (p)
     C. canis
     C. felis
CTF
   Colorado tick fever
CTFV
   Colorado tick fever virus
CTL
   cytotoxic T lymphocyte
C/T/S Topical solution
cubensis
     Psilocybe c.
cuboidea
     Arthrographis c.
cucumerina
     Plectosphaerella c.
     Trichosanthes c.
cucumerinum
     Cladosporium c.
     Tracheophilus c.
     Typhlocoelum c.
Cucumovirus (v)
cucurbitae
     Xanthomonas c.
Cucurbitariaceae
cuenoti
     Blattabacterium c.
cuff
   collagen c.
   vaginal c.
cuffing
   perivascular c.
culbertsoni
     Acanthamoeba c.
culdocentesis
culdoscopy
Culex
     C. abominator
     C. alpicalis
     C. anips

     C. apicalis
     C. arizonensis
     C. atratus
     C. bahamensis
     C. boharti
     C. chidesteri
     C. conservator
     C. conspirator
     C. corniger
     C. coronator
     C. declarator
     C. decorator
     C. erraticus
     C. erythrothorax
     C. idottus
     C. inflictus
     C. inimitabilis
     C. interrogator
     C. iolambdis
     C. lucifugus
     C. mollis
     C. mulrennani
     C. nigripalpus
     C. peccator
     C. peus
     C. pilosus
     C. pipiens
     C. pleuristriatus
     C. quinquefasciatus
     C. reevesi
     C. restuans
     C. salinarius
     C. similis
     C. taeniopus
     C. tarsalis
     C. territans
     C. thriambus
     C. toweri
culicicola
     Spiroplasma c.
Culicidae
culicis
Culicoides
     C. alachua
     C. alaskensis
     C. alexanderi
     C. amazonius
     C. arboricola
     C. arizonensis
     C. arubae
     C. atchleyi
     C. austini

C

NOTES

Culicoides (continued)
- C. barbosai
- C. baueri
- C. beckae
- C. belkini
- C. bergi
- C. bermudensis
- C. bickleyi
- C. biguttatus
- C. blantoni
- C. bottimeri
- C. brookmani
- C. butleri
- C. byersi
- C. cacticola
- C. calexicanus
- C. californiensis
- C. canadensis
- C. cavaticus
- C. chewaclae
- C. chiopterus
- C. circumscriptus
- C. cochisensis
- C. cockerellii
- C. copiosus
- C. crepuscularis
- C. daedalus
- C. davisi
- C. debilipalpis
- C. defoliarti
- C. denningi
- C. denticulatus
- C. doeringae
- C. downesi
- C. eadsi
- C. edeni
- C. erikae
- C. floridensis
- C. flukei
- C. footei
- C. franciemonti
- C. freeborni
- C. frohnei
- C. furens
- C. gregsoni
- C. guttipennis
- C. guyanensis
- C. haematopotus
- C. halophilus
- C. hawsi
- C. hieroglyphicus
- C. hinmani
- C. hirtulus
- C. hoguei
- C. hollensis
- C. husseyi
- C. insignis
- C. insolatus
- C. inyoensis
- C. jacksoni
- C. jamaicensis
- C. jamesi
- C. jamnbacki
- C. jonesi
- C. juddi
- C. kibunensis
- C. kirbyi
- C. knowltoni
- C. lahontan
- C. leechi
- C. loisae
- C. lophortygis
- C. loughnani
- C. luglani
- C. luteovenus
- C. machardyi
- C. maritimus
- C. marium
- C. melleus
- C. miharai
- C. mississippiensis
- C. mohave
- C. monoensis
- C. mortivallis
- C. mulrennani
- C. multidentatus
- C. multipunctatus
- C. nanellus
- C. nanus
- C. neofagineus
- C. neomontanus
- C. neopulicaris
- C. niger
- C. novamexicanus
- C. obscuripennis
- C. obsoletus
- C. oklahomensis
- C. oregonensis
- C. ousairani
- C. owyheensis
- C. palmerae
- C. pampoikilus
- C. paraensis
- C. parapiliferus
- C. pechumani
- C. pecosensis
- C. peliliouensis
- C. phlebotomus
- C. piliferus
- C. posoensis
- C. pusillus
- C. reevesi
- C. riggsi
- C. ryckmani
- C. salihi
- C. salinarius

C. saltonensis
C. sanguisuga
C. saundersi
C. scanloni
C. sierrensis
C. sitiens
C. snowi
C. sommermanae
C. sordidellus
C. sphagnumensis
C. spinosus
C. stellifer
C. stilobezzioides
C. stonei
C. subimmaculatus
C. sublettei
C. tenuistylus
C. testudinalis
C. tissoti
C. torreyae
C. torridus
C. travisi
C. tristriatulus
C. unicolor
C. usingeri
C. utahensis
C. utowana
C. variipennis
C. venustus
C. villosipennis
C. vistulensis
C. werneri
C. wirthi
C. wisconsinensis
C. yukonensis
culicosis
Culiseta
C. alaskensis
C. annulata
C. incidens
C. inornata
C. inpatiens
C. melanura
C. minnesotae
C. morsitans
C. particeps
C. subochrae
cultivation
culture
AccuProbe *Campylobacter* C.
Actinomyces c.
aerobic bone marrow c.

AFB c.
AIDS blood c.
anaerobic c.
appropriate c.
arterial line c.
BacT/Alert blood c.
BACTEC blood c.
bacterial corneal c.
beta hemolytic strep c.
biopsy c.
bone marrow c.
bone marrow fungus c.
bone marrow mycobacteria c.
brain viral c.
bronchoscopic *Legionella* c.
broth c.
buffy coat viral c.
catheter tip c.
cell c.
cervical *Chlamydia* c.
chancroid c.
chickenpox c.
Chlamydia c.
clean catheter urine c.
CMV c.
CSF viral c.
cyst c.
diarrheagenic stool c.
diphtheria c.
EBV virus c.
echovirus c.
elective c.
endocervical c.
endometrial c.
enterovirus c.
epithelial raft c.
eye swab *Chlamydia* c.
fungal corneal c.
fungus c.
genital c.
German measles c.
gonorrhea c. (GC)
hanging-block c.
Harada-Mori filter paper strip c.
Hemovac tip c.
herpes simplex c.
HSV virus c.
hyperalimentation line c.
influenza virus c.
intraluminal c.
intravenous catheter c.
intravenous device c.

C

NOTES

culture *(continued)*
    intravenous line c.
    IUD c.
    Legionella pneumophila c.
    lesion c.
    lymph node c.
    lymphocyte c.
    mammalian cell c.
    c. medium
    microslide c.
    monoxenic c.
    mumps virus c.
    mycobacteria c.
    mycobacterial c.
    Mycoplasma T-strain c.
    nasopharyngeal c.
    needle c.
    Neisseria gonorrhoeae c.
    neotype c.
    Nocardia c.
    organotypic c.
    Oxgall media c.
    parainfluenza virus c.
    Petri dish c.
    plastic envelope c.
    poliovirus c.
    pouch c.
    prostatic fluid c.
    pure c.
    c. of pus
    rabies viral c.
    rash viral c.
    roll tube c.
    RSV c.
    rubella virus c.
    screening c.
    semiquantitative c. (SQC)
    sensitized c.
    Septi-Chek blood c.
    shake c.
    shingles c.
    shunt c.
    skin viral c.
    slant c.
    slope c.
    smear c.
    spleen cell c.
    sputum fungus c.
    stab c.
    sterile urine c.
    stock c.
    stool adenovirus c.
    stool echovirus c.
    stool enterovirus c.
    stool poliovirus c.
    stool viral c.
    streak c.
    strep throat screening c.

    Swan-Ganz tip c.
    three-day measles c.
    throat viral c.
    TRIC agent c.
    Trichomonas c.
    Trichomonas vaginalis c.
    TV c.
    type c.
    Ureaplasma urealyticum c.
    urethral *Chlamydia* c.
    urine fungus c.
    vaginal c.
    varicella-zoster virus c.
    venous catheter c.
    viral c.
    wound c.
    xenic c.

culture-negative
    c.-n. endocarditis
    c.-n. neutrocytic ascites (CNNA)

Culturette
    Mini-Tip C.
    C. swab

cumminsii
    Arthrobacter c.

cuneata
    Gregarina c.

cuneatum
    Simulium c.

cuneatus
    Desulfovibrio c.

cuniculi
    Bifidobacterium c.
    Cuterebra c.
    Encephalitozoon c.
    Gemella c.
    Methanosphaera c.
    Moraxella (Branhamella) c.
    Neisseria c.
    Spilopsyllus c. (p)

Cunninghamella (f)
    C. bertholletiae
    C. blakesleeana
    C. echinulata
    C. elegans
    C. homothallica

Cunninghamellaceae

cupida
    Deleya c.
    Halomonas c.

cupidus
    Alcaligenes c.

cuprea
    Anomala c.

Cupriavidus necator (b)

cuprina
    Lucilia c.

Phaenicia c.
Thiomonas c.
cuprophane
curacoi
Streptomyces c.
curassoni
Schistosoma c.
curdlanolyticus
Bacillus c.
Paenibacillus c.
curettage
dilatation and c.
curl
currant jelly sputum
currens
larva c.
Curschmann spiral
curticei
Cooperia c.
curtisii
Mobiluncus curtisii subsp. c.
Curtobacterium (b)
C. albidum
C. citreum
C. flaccumfaciens
C. luteum
C. plantarum
C. pusillum
C. saperdae
C. testaceum
Curtovirus (v)
curtum
Cryptobacterium c.
curva
Wolinella c.
curvachelus
Leptoconops c.
Curvalaria
curvata
Thermomonospora c.
curvatum
Phialemonium c.
curvatus
Cryptococcus c.
Desulfobacter c.
Lactobacillus c.
Lactobacillus c. subsp. *curvatus*
Methanobrevibacter c.
curve
epidemic c.
saddleback fever c.

Curvularia (f)
C. brachyspora
C. clavata
C. geniculata
C. lunata
C. lunata var. aeria
C. pallescens
C. senegalensis
C. verruculosa
curvulum
Acremonium c.
curvus
Campylobacter c.
cushingoid appearance
Cushing syndrome
cuspidatus
Eratyrus c.
cuspidosporus
Streptomyces c.
custerianus
Brettanomyces c.
custersiana
Dekkera c.
custesii
Brettanomyces c.
cutaneous
c. abscess
c. amebiasis
c. ancylostomiasis
c. anthrax
c. aspergillosis
c. ATL
c. biopsy
c. blastomycosis
c. candidiasis
c. delayed-type hypersensitivity
c. diphtheria
c. eruption
c. gnathostomiasis
c. herpes
c. human papillomavirus infection
c. larva migrans
c. leishmaniasis
c. leishmaniasis granuloma
c. lesion
localized c.
c. lymphoma
c. manifestation
c. melanoma
c. plague
c. sporotrichosis
c. T-cell lymphoma (CTCL)

C

NOTES

cutaneous *(continued)*
    c. T-cell malignancy
    c. tuberculin test
    c. tuberculosis
    c. vasculitis
cutaneum
    Anatrichosoma c.
    Trichosporon c.
Cuterebra (p)
    C. americana
    C. angustifrons
    C. buccata
    C. cuniculi
    C. neomexicana
    C. tenebrosa
Cuterebridae
cuticle
cuticularis
    Methanobrevibacter c.
cutirubrum
    Halobacterium c.
cutis
    amebiasis c.
    ancylostomiasis c.
    tuberculosis c.
Cutivate
CV-AL1A virus
CV-AL2A virus
CV-AL2C virus
CVA 1 virus
CV-BJ2C virus
CVB 1 virus
CVC
    central venous catheter
CV-CA1A virus
CV-CA1D virus
CV-CA4A virus
CV-CA4B virus
CVGV
    CSIRO Village virus
CVG 1 virus
CV-IL2A virus
CV-IL2B virus
CV-IL3A virus
CV-IL3D virus
CV-IL5-2s1 virus
CVLP
    coronavirus-like particle
CV-MA1D virus
CV-MA1E virus
CVM 1 virus
CV-NC1A virus
CV-NC1B virus
CV-NC1C virus
CV-NC1D virus
CV-NE8A virus
CV-NE8D virus
CV-NY2A virus

CV-NY2B virus
CV-NY2C virus
CV-NY3F virus
CV-NYb1 virus
CV-NYs1 virus
CVR 1 virus
CV-SC1A virus
CV-SC1B virus
CV-SH6 virus
CVV
    Cache Valley virus
CV-XZ3A virus
CV-XZ4A virus
CV-XZ4C virus
CV-XZ5C virus
CV-XZ6E virus
CWV
    Cape Wrath virus
C-X-C chemokine receptor, CXCR4
cyanea
    Saccharomonospora c.
cyaneofuscatus
    Streptomyces c.
cyanescens
    Cerinosterus c.
    Cylindrocarpon c.
    Psorophora c.
    Sporothrix c.
cyaneus
    Actinoplanes c.
    Streptomyces c.
cyanide antidote kit
cyanoalbus
    Streptomyces c.
Cyanobacteria
cyanobacterium-like body
cyanogriseus
    Actinoalloteichus c.
cyanopus
    Conocybe c.
cyanosis
cyanotic congenital heart disease
Cyathostoma
Cyathostomum coronatum (p)
cyclase
    adenylate c.
    guanylate c.
cycle
    endogenous c.
    erythrocytic c.
    exoerythrocytic c.
    exogenous c.
    heterogonic life c.
    homogonic life c.
    infectious c.
    virus-cell infectious c.
cyclic
    c. adenosine monophosphate

c. guanine monophosphate (cGMP)
c. guanosine monophosphate
c. neutropenia
c. octapeptide
cyclitrophicus
    Vibrio c.
Cyclobacterium marinum (b)
Cycloclasticus pugetii (b)
Cyclocort Topical
Cyclodontostomum purvisi (p)
cycloheptanicus
    Alicyclobacillus c.
    Bacillus c.
cyclohexanicum
    Propionibacterium c.
cycloheximide
cyclophilin (CyP)
cyclophosphamide
    c., doxorubicin, and etoposide
      (CDE)
    c., hydroxydaunomycin, Oncovin,
      and prednisone (CHOP)
Cyclophyllidae
cyclopiroxolamine
cycloplegia
cycloplegic
cyclopropanone hydrate
Cyclops (p)
    C. bicuspidatus
    C. capillatus
    C. lubbocki
    C. scutifer
    C. vernalis
cyclopteri
    Hysterothylacium c.
Cyclorrhapha
cycloserine
Cyclosine
cyclosis
Cyclospora cayetanensis (p)
cyclosporiasis
cyclosporin A
cyclosporine
cyclosporine-prednisone
cyclozoonosis
Cycofed Pediatric
Cydia pomonella **granulovirus (CpGV)**
Cylex
cylindracea
    Candida c.
Cylindrium

Cylindrocarpon (f)
    C. album
    C. candidum
    C. congoense
    C. cyanescens
    C. cylindroides var. cylindroides
    C. cylindroides var. tenue
    C. destructans
    C. destructans var. crassum
    C. faginatum
    C. heteronema
    C. lichenicola
    C. magnusianum
    C. obtusisporum
    C. olidum
    C. olidum var. crassum
    C. radicicola
    C. tonkinense
    C. vaginae
cylindroides
    Cylindrocarpon cylindroides var. c.
    Eubacterium c.
cylindrospora
    Absidia c.
cylindrosporum
    Clostridium c.
cylindruria
cynarae
    Xanthomonas c.
cynodegmi
    Capnocytophaga c.
cynodontis
    Clavibacter xyli subsp. c.
    Cochliobolus c.
    Leifsonia c.
    Leifsonia xyli subsp. c.
cynomolgi
    Plasmodium c.
Cynomya
    C. cadaverina
    C. hirta
    C. mortuorum
cynos
    Mycoplasma c.
cynotes
    Otodectes c.
CyP
    cyclophilin
cypionate
    testosterone c.
Cypovirus (v)

NOTES

cypricasei
    Lactobacillus c.
cypripedii
    Erwinia c.
    Pectobacterium c.
cyriacigeorgici
    Nocardia c.
cyst
    alveolar hydatid c.
    choledochal c.
    c. culture
    daughter c.
    echinococcal c.
    echinococcus c.
    granddaughter c.
    hydatid c.
    mother c.
    multilocular hydatid c.
    osseous hydatid c.
    parasitic c.
    parent c.
    phaeohyphomycotic c.
    phaeomycotic c.
    protozoan c.
    racemose c.
    sterile c.
    synovial c.
    unilocular hydatid c.
cystacanth
cystarginea
    Kitasatospora c.
cystargineus
    Streptomyces c.
cystectomy
cystic
    c. calcification
    c. degeneration
    c. fibrosis (CF)
    c. hydatid disease
cysticerci (*pl. of* cysticercus)
cysticercoid
cysticercosis
    c. cellulosae
    cerebral c.
    ocular c.
    spinal intramedullary c.
    subcutaneous c.
Cysticercus
    C. bovis
    C. cellulosae
    C. fasciolaris
    C. longicollis
    C. ovis
    C. pisiformis
    C. racemosus
    C. tenuicollis
cysticercus, pl. **cysticerci**
    aberrant c.

cystine crystal
cystine-tellurite blood agar test
cystitidis
    Corynebacterium c.
cystitis
    alkaline-encrusted c.
    Candida c.
    c. cervicitis
    hemorrhagic c.
Cystobacter (b)
    C. ferrugineus
    C. fuscus
    C. minus
Cystobacteraceae
Cystobacterineae
cystocele
cystometrogram (CMG)
    filling c.
    simple c.
cystometry
    complex multichannel c.
Cystoopsis scomber (p)
cystoscopic
    c. biopsy
    c. prostatectomy
Cystospaz
Cystospaz-M
cystostomy
    trocar suprapubic c.
Cystoviridae
Cystovirus (v)
Cytauxcoon (p)
    C. felis
cytoadherent protein
cytobrush scraping
cytocentrifuge preparation
cytochrome
    c. oxidase test
    c. P-450
    c. P450-3A
    c. system
cytocyst
CytoGam
cytogenetic
cytogenetics study
cytohistopathology
cytokine
    angiogenic c.
    c. assay
    c. beta$_2$-microglobulin
    c. depot
    paracrine c.
    proinflammatory c.
    c. therapy
cytokine-induced killer lymphocyte
cytologic screening
cytology
    ascitic fluid c.

body cavity fluid c.
c. brush
cervical c.
effusion c.
fluid c.
herpes c.
ocular c.
paracentesis fluid c.
pericardial fluid c.
peritoneal fluid c.
pleural fluid c.
synovial fluid c.
thoracentesis fluid c.
cytolysin
cytolysis
hepatic c.
cytolytic
c. phenotype
c. T helper cell
c. virus
cytomegalic inclusion disease
Cytomegalovirus (v) **(CMV)**
cytomegalovirus
congenital c.
c. end-organ disease
c. group
human c. (HCMV)
c. immune globulin (CMVIG)
c. immune globulin intravenous,
human
mouse c.
rat c.
c. retinitis
**cytomegalovirus-specific intravenous
immune globulin (CMVIg)**
cytomere
cytometry
flow c.
cytopathic
cytopathicity
cytopenia
cytopenic
Cytophaga (b)
C. agarovorans
C. allerginae
C. aprica
C. aquatilis
C. arvensicola
C. aurantiaca
C. columnaris
C. diffluens
C. drobachiensis

C. fermentans
C. flevensis
C. heparina
C. hutchinsonii
C. johnsonae
C. latercula
C. lytica
C. marina
C. marinoflava
C. pectinovora
C. psychrophila
C. saccharophila
C. salmonicolor
C. succinicans
C. uliginosa
C. xylanolytica
Cytophagaceae
Cytophagales
cytophanere
cytopharynx
cytoplasmic
c. keratohyalin inclusion body
c. polyhedrosis virus (CPV)
c. polyhedrosis virus group
c. vacuolization
c. vesiculation
cytoplasmic granulation
cytopyge
Cytorhabdovirus (v)
Cyto Rich
cytostatic treatment
cytostome
Cytotec
cytotonic enterotoxin
cytotoxic
c. assay
c. cell
c. chemotherapy
c. drug
c. T lymphocyte (CTL)
c. T-lymphocyte activity
c. T lymphocyte-based
immunotherapy
cytotoxicity
antibody-dependent cell-mediated c.
antibody-dependent cellular c.
(ADCC)
antibody-directed cellular c.
(ADCC)
complement-mediated c. (CMC)
cytotoxic T lymphocyte (CTL)

C

NOTES

145

cytotoxin
    tracheal c. (TCT)
Cytovene
Cytovene-IV
Cytoxan
cytozoic

cytozoon
Cyttariaceae
Cyttariales
Czapek-Dox medium
Czapek solution agar

D3 virus
dφ3 virus
dφ4 virus
dφ5 virus
Dabakala virus
DAC
> Guiatuss D.
> Guiatussin D.
> Halotussin D.
> Mytussin D.

Dacampiaceae
dacarbazine
> Adriamycin, bleomycin,
> vinblastine, d. (ABVD)

Dacron swab
Dacrymycetaceae
Dacrymycetales
dacryoadenitis
dacryocystitis
dacryocystorhinostomy (DCR)
dactinomycin
Dactylaria gallopava (f)
dactylitis
> blistering distal d.
> multidigit d.
> septic d.
> syphilitic d.
> tuberculous d.

Dactylium dendroides (f)
Dactylogyrus (p)
> *D. anchoratus*
> *D. extensus*
> *D. magnus*
> *D. manicatus*
> *D. vastator*

Dactylosporangium (b)
> *D. aurantiacum*
> *D. fulvum*
> *D. matsuzakiense*
> *D. roseum*
> *D. thailandense*
> *D. vinaceum*

DAEC
> diffusely adherent *Escherichia coli*

daedalus
> *Culicoides* d.

DAF
> direct amplification fingerprinting

DAG
> diacylglycerol

daghestanicus
> *Streptomyces* d.

dagmatis
> *Pasteurella* d.

D'Aguilar virus (DAGV)

DAGV
> D'Aguilar virus

daily dose
daisy
Dakar bat virus (DBV)
DakArK 7292 virus
Dalacin
> D. C, T
> D. Vaginal

d-alanine
d-alanyl-d-alanine
dalfopristin
> quinupristin and d.

dalton
damage
> acoustic nerve d.

Damalina (p)
> *D. bovis*
> *D. caprae*
> *D. crassipes*
> *D. equi*
> *D. limbata*
> *D. ovis*

dammini
> *Ixodes* d.

damnosus
> *Pediococcus* d.

damsela
> *Listonella* d.
> *Vibrio* d.

damselae
> *Photobacterium damselae* subsp. d.

dandongensis
> *Lasiohelea* d.

Dandruff Treatment Shampoo
dandy fever
Dane particle
Dan-Gard
dankaliensis
> *Gymnoascus* d.

dantrolene sodium
Dapa
Dapacin
DAPD
Dapsone
dapsone
D-arabitol fermentation test
Daraprim
darkfield
> d. concentrator
> d. examination
> d. microscopy

Darling disease
darlingi
> *Anopheles* d.

Darna trima **virus**
Daskil
dassonvillei
    Nocardiopsis dassonvillei subsp. *d.*
Dasychira pudibunda
dasyorrhus
    Aedes d.
Dasyprocta
data
    VIRADAPT d.
date fever
Daudi cell
daughter
    d. colony
    d. cyst
daunorubicin
    liposomal d.
DaunoXome
daurensis
    Heliorestis d.
DAV
    Drosophila A virus
Davainea proglottina (p)
Davaineidae
Davidsohn differential
davisae
    Cedecea d.
davisi
    Anopheles d.
    Anopheles triannulatus d.
    Culicoides d.
davtiani
    Teladorsagia d.
Dawson encephalitis
5-day fever
40-day fever
Daycaps
    Neo Citran D.
Dayquil
    D. Sinus with Pain Relief
Daytime
    Triaminic DM D.
    Tylenol Cold Medication (D.)
DBV
    Dakar bat virus
DC
    dendritic cell
    Bromanate DC
    Myphetane DC
DC-based immunotherapy
DCOM
    dilated cardiomyopathy
DCR
    dacryocystorhinostomy
DCV
    Drosophila C virus
ddATP
    dideoxyadenosine triphosphate

ddC
    dideoxycytidine
    2′3′-dideoxycytidine
    zalcitabine
DDD
    defined daily dose
ddI
    didanosine
    dideoxyinosine
DDS
dDVI virus
DE
    Ru-Tuss DE
D-E
    Calmylin Codeine D-E
de
    de novo exposure
    de novo lipogenesis (DNL)
dead-end host
deadly agaric
DEAE
    diethylaminoethyl
    DEAE cellulose anion-exchange
      chromatography
deaerated
DEAFF
    detection of early antigen fluorescent
    focus
deafness
    sudden acquired d.
dealbata
    Clitocybe d.
deaminase
    adenosine d.
    ornithine d.
death
    activation-induced cell d.
    d. cap mushroom
Debaryomyces (f)
    D. hansenii
    D. hansonii var. *fabyrii*
debilipalpis
    Culicoides d.
debilitation
debontii
    Prosthecobacter d.
debridement
debris
    cellular d.
debulking
debut
    sexual d.
DEC
    diethylcarbamazine
Decadron
    D. Injection
    D. Oral
    D. Phosphate

Decadron-LA
Deca-Durabolin
Decaject
Decaject-LA
decanoate
    nandrolone d.
decant
decarboxylase
    d. enzyme
    lysine d.
    d. test
deccanensis
    Actinoplanes d.
decennium
decerebrate rigidity
dechloracetivorans
    Desulfovibrio d.
dechloratans
    Ideonella d.
Dechloromonas agitata (b)
Dechlorosoma suillum (b)
2D echocardiography
deciduitis
    plasma cell d.
decipiens
    Phocanema d.
    Pseudoterranova d.
    Terranova d.
declarator
    Culex d.
Declomycin
Decofed syrup
Decohistine
    D. DH
    D. Expectorant
decollectum
    Simulium d.
Deconamine
    D. SR
    D. syrup
    D. tablet
Decongestant
    Balminil D.
    Benylin D.
    Buckley's DM D.
    Chlor-Tripolon D.
    Cough Syrup DM D.
    DM Plus D.
    D. Tablets
    Tylenol Cough with D.

Deconsal
    D. II
    D. Sprinkle
decontamination
    selective digestive d. (SDD)
    selective intestinal d. (SID)
decorator
    Culex d.
decorticate posture
decorum
    Simulium d.
decoyicus
    Streptomyces hygroscopicus subsp.
    d.
decreased acuity
decticus
    Aedes d.
decubitus ulcer
decumbens
    Penicillium d.
deep
    d. dyspareunia
    d. neck infection
    d. pelvic inflammatory disease
    d. serious soft tissue infection
    d. tendon reflex (DTR)
    d. vein thrombosis (DVT)
deep-seated infection
deer
    d. fly
    d. fly disease
    d. fly fever
defect
    atrial septal d. (ASD)
    atrioventricular septal d.
    conduction d.
    host d.
    neural tube d. (NTD)
    opsonic d.
    visual field d.
defectiva
    Abiotrophia d.
defective
    d. bacteriophage
    d. phage
    d. probacteriophage
    d. prophage
defectivus
    Streptococcus d.
Defen-LA
defense mechanism
Deferribacter thermophilus (b)

D

NOTES

defibrillator
    implantable cardioverter d. (ICD)
deficiency
    alpha$_1$-antitrypsin d.
    B12 d.
    chronic bone marrow d.
    folate d.
    glucose-6-phosphatase d.
    glucose-6-phosphate
        dehydrogenase d. (G6PD)
    gonadotropin d.
    G6PD d.
    growth hormone d.
    lactose d.
    mammalian binding lectin d.
    primary growth hormone d.
    protein S d.
    pyruvate kinase d.
    selective IgG subclass d.
deficit
    ECF d.
defined daily dose (DDD)
definition
    case d.
definitive host
deflectus
    Aspergillus d.
deflexum
    Myxotrichum d.
Defluvibacter lusatiensis (b)
defluvii
    Acidovorax d.
    Aquamicrobium d.
    Methanobacterium d.
    Pseudaminobacter d.
    Thiothrix d.
defoliarti
    Culicoides d.
    Simulium d.
deformability
defragrans
    Alcaligenes d.
degeneration
    adenoid d. (AD)
    cystic d.
    fatty d.
    spongiform d.
    wallerian d.
degensii
    Ammonifex d.
degerming
    skin d.
deglycerolized
Dehalobacter restrictus (b)
Dehalococcoides ethenogenes (b)
dehalogenans
    Desulfitobacterium d.
Dehalospirillum multivorans (b)

dehemoglobinize
dehiscence
    wound d.
Dehydral
dehydration
2-dehydroemetine
dehydroepiandrosterone (DHEA)
    d. sulfate (DHEAS)
dehydrogenase
    glucose-6-phosphate d. (G6PD)
    inosine monophosphate d. (IMPDH)
    lactate d. (LDH)
Deinobacter (b)
    D. grandis
Deinococcaceae
Deinococcus (b)
    D. erythromyxa
    D. geothermalis
    D. grandis
    D. murrayi
    D. proteolyticus
    D. radiodurans
    D. radiophilus
    D. radiopugnans
deionized
    d. water
dejongeii
    Prosthecobacter d.
Dekkera
    D. anomala
    D. bruxellensis
    D. custersiana
    D. intermedia
    D. naardensis
Del
    D. Aqua-5, -10 Gel
Delacroixia coronata (f)
delafieldii
    Acidovorax d.
    Ilyobacter d.
    Pseudomonas d.
Delatestryl Injection
Delatretrovirus (v)
delavirdine (DLV)
    d. mesylate (DLV)
delayed-type hypersensitivity (DTH)
delbrueckii
    Lactobacillus delbrueckii subsp. *d.*
    Saccharomyces d.
Delcort Topical
Delestrogen
deletrix
    Halicephalobus d.
    Micronema d.
Deleya (b)
    D. aesta
    D. aquamarina
    D. cupida

D. *halophila*
D. *marina*
D. *pacifica*
D. *salina*
D. *venusta*
deleyianum
  Sulfurospirillum d.
Delftia acidovorans (b)
Delft School of Dutch Microbiologists
Delhi belly
delicatum
  Aquaspirillum d.
delicatus
  Thiobacillus d.
deliense
  Leptotrombidium d.
delineated
delirium
  d. tremens
delivery
  cesarean d.
  liposome drug d.
Del-Mycin Topical
delphini
  Staphylococcus d.
delphinicola
  Actinobacillus d.
Delsym
delta
  d. hepatitis
delta-aminolevulinic
  d.-a. acid (ALA)
  d.-a. acid porphyrin test
delta/antidelta
Delta-Cortef Oral
deltae
  Methanococcus d.
Deltasone
delta-toxin
Delta-Tritex Topical
Deltavirus (v)
delthoidea
  Anthopsis d.
delusional parasitosis
demarcate
demarcated cellulitis
Dematiaceae
dematiaceous
  d. fungus
dematioides
  Hormonema d.
  Phaeosclera d.

dematium
  Colletotrichum d.
dematoideum
  Helminthosporum d.
Demdec
demeclocycline
Demend
dementia
  d. complex of AIDS
  multiinfarct d.
  d. paralytica
Demetria terragena (b)
demilune
demineralization
  bone d.
demingiae
  Colwellia d.
deminutus
  Ternidens d.
demodectic
  d. acariasis
  d. mange
Demodema
  D. *boranensis*
  D. *entomopoxvirus*
Demodex (p)
  D. *bovis*
  D. *brevis*
  D. *canis*
  D. *equi*
  D. *folliculorum*
  D. *phylloides*
Demodicidae
Demodicoidea
demolitive surgery
Demser
demyelinating
  d. disease
demyclination
denaturation
Denavir
dendrica
  Candida d.
dendritic
  d. cell (DC)
dendriticum
  Dicrocoelium d.
  Diphyllobothrium d.
  Trichosporon d.
dendritiformis
  Paenibacillus d.
dendrogram

D

NOTES

dendronema
    Candida d.
dendrophila
    Bullera d.
Dendrosphaereaceae
Dendrosporobacter (b)
    D. quercicolus
Dendrostilbella byssina (f)
denervation
dengue
    d. facies
    d. fever
    hemorrhagic d.
    d. hemorrhagic fever (DHF)
    d. hemorrhagic fever/shock
      syndrome (DHF-DSS)
    d. immunochromatographic folder
    d. shock syndrome (DSS)
    d. virus 1–4 (DENV 1–4)
denguelike illness
denhamense
    Roseibium d.
denitration
denitrificans
    Achromobacter xylosoxidans subsp.
      d.
    Alcaligenes d.
    Alcaligenes xylosoxidans subsp. *d.*
    Alteromonas d.
    Blastobacter d.
    Brachymonas d.
    Comamonas d.
    Halobacterium d.
    Haloferax d.
    Hyphomicrobium d.
    Jonesia d.
    Kingella d.
    Listeria d.
    Neisseria d.
    Paracoccus d.
    Pseudoalteromonas d.
    Roseobacter d.
    Thialkalivibrio d.
    Thiobacillus d.
    Thiomicrospira d.
denitrification
denitrify
Denitrobacterium detoxificans (b)
Denitrovibrio acetiphilus (b)
denningi
    Culicoides d.
Denorex
de novo cellular infection
densa
    Isaria d.
densitometer
densitometry
Densovirus (v)

densovirus
    Acheta domestica d. (AdDNV)
densum
dental infection
dentalis
    Mitsuokella d.
    Prevotella d.
dentatum
    Oesophagostomum d.
dentatus
    Stephanurus d.
dentiae
    Neisseria d.
denticola
    Bacteroides d.
    Prevotella d.
    Treponema d.
denticolens
    Actinomyces d.
    Bifidobacterium d.
denticulatus
    Culicoides d.
dentipes
    Hydrotaea d.
dentition
dentium
    Bifidobacterium d.
dentocariosa
    Rothia d.
DENV 1–4
    dengue virus 1–4
deoxycholate
    d. agar
    amphotericin B d.
deoxycycline
3-deoxy-D-manno-octulosonic acid
    trisaccharide
deoxyguanosine triphosphate (dGTP)
deoxyribonuclease (DNase)
    d. test
deoxyribonucleic
    d. acid (DNA)
    d. acid probe hybridization
deoxyribovirus
    icosahedral cytoplasmic d.
deoxyspergualin
deoxyvirus
depAndro Injection
Dependovirus (v)
depGynogen Injection
depigmentation
depigmented spot
depletion
    CD4 d.
    CD4+ T-cell d.
    electrolyte d.
    lymphocyte d.
depMedalone Injection

Depo-Estradiol Injection
Depogen Injection
Depoject Injection
depolymerans
    Roseateles d.
Depo-Medrol Injection
depomedroxyprogesterone acetate
Depopred Injection
Depo-Provera
deposition
    immune complex d.
    iron d.
depot
    cytokine d.
    d. medroxyprogesterone acetate
    (DMPA)
Depotest Injection
Depo-Testosterone Injection
depressed cellular immunity
Deproist Expectorant With Codeine
depulization
Dequadin
dequalinium
Dera Ghazi Khan virus (DGKV)
derivative
    artemisinin d.
    diamidine d.
    ergot d.
    nitrofuran d.
    nitroimidazole d.
    purified protein d. (PPD)
    thiacytidine d.
    trimethylsilyl d.
    undecylenic acid and d.'s
Dermabacter hominus (b)
Dermacentor (p)
    D. albipictus
    D. marginatus
    D. parumapertus
    D. reticulatus
Dermacne
Dermacoccus (b)
    D. nishinomiyaensis
Dermacort Topical
Dermaflex HC
dermal
    d. leishmaniasis
    d. tuberculosis
Dermanyssidae
Dermanyssus gallinae (p)
Dermarest Dricort Topical
Derma-Smoothe/FS Topical

Dermasone
Dermateaceae
dermatitidis
    Ajellomyces d.
    Blastomyces d.
    Wangiella d.
dermatitis, pl. dermatitides
    ancylostoma d.
    atopic d.
    blastomycetic d.
    Calycophora d.
    caterpillar d.
    cercarial d.
    contact d.
    contagious pustular d. (CPDV)
    diaper d.
    eczematous d.
    exfoliative d.
    genital atopic d.
    d. herpetiformis
    d. herpetiformis antibody
    infectious eczematoid d.
    infective d.
    nonreactive d.
    Paederus d.
    d. pediculoides
    pellagra-associated d.
    pellagroid d.
    proliferative d.
    pustular d.
    rat mite d.
    reactive d.
    schistosomal d.
    seborrheic d. (SD)
    stasis d.
dermatitis-causing caterpillar
Dermatobia hominis (p)
dermatobiasis
Dermatocentor
    D. andersoni
    D. occidentalis
    D. variabilis
dermatologic infection
dermatome
    trigeminal d.
dermatomycosis
    d. pedis
dermatomyositis
Dermatop
dermatopathic
Dermatophagoides (p)
    D. farinae

D

NOTES

153

Dermatophagoides (continued)
   D. microceras
   D. pteronyssinus   •
   D. scheremetewskyi
Dermatophilaceae
Dermatophilus (b)
   D. chelonae
   D. congolensis
dermatophyte
   d. infection
   d. mycetoma
dermatophytic fungus
dermatophytid
Dermatophytin
Dermatophytin-O
dermatophytosis
dermatosis
   acarine d.
dermatozoiasis
dermatozoon
dermatozoonosis
Dermazin
dermis
dermofibroma
Dermolate Topical
Dermolepida albohirtum
dermonecrotic
   d. toxin (DNT)
dermo-unguis
   Chaetophoma d-u.
Dermovate
Dermoxyl
Dermtex HC with Aloe Topical
derwentensis
   Actinoplanes d.
Derxia gummosa (b)
derxii
   Beijerinckia derxii subsp. d.
descemetocele
descending infection
Desemzia incerta (b)
Desenex
   Prescription Strength D.
desensitized
desert
   d. fever
   D. Shield virus
deserta
   Loxosceles d.
deserticola
   Aedes d.
   Candida d.
desferrioxamine susceptibility test
desiccation
desiderata
   Halomonas d.
desipramine
Desitin

Desmodus rotundus
desmolans
   Eubacterium d.
desmopressin
Desocort
desonide
DesOwen Topical
desoximetasone
desoxycholate
despeciated antitoxin
desquamate
desquamation
   moist d.
Desquam-E Gel
Desquam-X
   D.-X. Gel
   D.-X. Wash
destain
   phosphotungstic acid d.
destroying angel mushroom
destructans
   Cylindrocarpon d.
destructiva
   Ramularia d.
destructive
   d. gonococcal arthritis
   d. tenosynovitis
destructor
   Ditylenchus d.
   Isaria d.
   Lepidoglyphus d.
Desulfacinum (b)
   D. hydrothermale
   D. infernum
Desulfitobacterium (b)
   D. chlororespirans
   D. dehalogenans
   D. frappieri
   D. hafniense
Desulfobacca acetoxidans (b)
Desulfobacter (b)
   D. curvatus
   D. halotolerans
   D. hydrogenophilus
   D. latus
   D. postgatei
   D. vibrioformis
Desulfobacterium (b)
   D. anilini
   D. autotrophicum
   D. catecholicum
   D. cetonicum
   D. indolicum
   D. macestii
   D. phenolicum
Desulfobacula (b)
   D. phenolica
   D. toluolica

Desulfobulbus (b)
   D. elongatus
   D. propionicus
   D. rhabdoformis
Desulfocapsa (b)
   D. sulfexigens
   D. thiozymogenes
Desulfocella halophila (b)
Desulfococcus (b)
   D. biacutus
   D. multivorans
Desulfofaba gelida (b)
Desulfofrigus (b)
   D. fragile
   D. oceanense
Desulfofustis glycolicus (b)
Desulfohalobium (b)
   D. retbaense
Desulfomicrobium (b)
   D. apsheronum
   D. baculatum
   D. escambiense
   D. norvegicum
   D. orale
Desulfomonas pigra (b)
Desulfomonile (b)
   D. limimaris
   D. tiedjei
Desulfonatronovibrio hydrogenovorans (b)
Desulfonatronum lacustre (b)
Desulfonema (b)
   D. ishimotonii
   D. limicola
   D. magnum
Desulfonispora thiosulfatigenes (b)
Desulforhabdus amnigena (b)
Desulforhopalus (b)
   D. singaporensis
   D. vacuolatus
Desulfosarcina variabilis (b)
Desulfospira joergensenii (b)
Desulfosporosinus (b)
   D. meridiei
   D. orientis
Desulfotalea (b)
   D. arctica
   D. psychrophila
Desulfotignum balticum (b)
Desulfotomaculum (b)
   D. acetoxidans
   D. aeronauticum
   D. alkaliphilum

D. antarcticum
D. auripigmentum
D. australicum
D. geothermicum
D. gibsoniae
D. guttoideum
D. halophilum
D. kuznetsovii
D. luciae
D. nigrificans
D. orientis
D. putei
D. ruminis
D. sapomandens
D. thermoacetoxidans
D. thermobenzoicum
D. thermocisternum
D. thermosapovorans
Desulfovibrio (b)
D. acrylicus
D. aespoeensis
D. africanus
D. alcoholivorans
D. aminophilus
D. baarsii
D. baculatus
D. burkinensis
D. carbinolicus
D. cuneatus
D. dechloracetivorans
D. desulfuricans subsp. *aestuarii*
D. desulfuricans subsp. *desulfuricans*
D. fructosivorans
D. furfuralis
D. gabonensis
D. giganteus
D. gigas
D. halophilus
D. indonesiensis
D. inopinatus
D. intestinalis
D. litoralis
D. longreachensis
D. longus
D. mexicanus
D. oxyclinae
D. profundus
D. salexigens
D. sapovorans
D. senezii
D. simplex
D. sulfodismutans

D

NOTES

155

Desulfovibrio (continued)
    D. termitidis
    D. thermophilus
    D. vulgaris subsp. *oxamicus*
    D. vulgaris subsp. *vulgaris*
    D. zosterae
Desulfovirga adipica (b)
Desulfurella (b)
    D. acetivorans
    D. kamchatkensis
    D. multipotens
    D. propionica
desulfuricans
    Desulfovibrio desulfuricans subsp. *d.*
    Gordonia d.
Desulfurobacterium thermolithotrophum
    (b)
Desulfurococcaceae
Desulfurococcus (b)
    D. mobilis
    D. mucosus
Desulfurolobus ambivalens (b)
Desulfuromonas (b)
    D. acetexigens
    D. acetoxidans
    D. chloroethenica
    D. palmitatis
    D. thiophila
Desulfuromusa (b)
    D. bakii
    D. kysingii
    D. succinoxidans
detachment
    retinal d.
detection
    antibody d.
    antigen d.
    Bartonella henselae d.
    chlamydial antigen d.
    C1q immune complex d.
    direct viral antigen d.
    d. of early antigen fluorescent
      focus (DEAFF)
    hepatitis B DNA d.
    hepatitis C RNA d.
    hepatitis C virus antibody d.
    Mycobacterium tuberculosis d.
    rabies d.
    rotavirus rapid d.
    virus d.
Detensol
determinant
    T-cell d.
Determine HIV 1/2 immunoassay kit
Dethiosulfovibrio (b)
    D. acidaminovorans
    D. marinus

    D. peptidovorans
    D. russensis
detoxificans
    Denitrobacterium d.
detoxification
detrusor hyperreflexia
Dettol antiseptic
Detussin
    D. Expectorant
    D. Liquid
deuterium dilution
deuteromycetes
Deuteromycota
Deuteromycotina
deutonymph
devascularization
deviation
    immune d.
device
    antimicrobial removal d. (ARD)
    home infusion d.
    intrauterine d. (IUD)
    left ventricular assist d. (LVAD)
    multipuncture d.
    Multitest CMI d.
device-specific
devitalized
devorans
    Flavobacterium d.
Devosia riboflavina (b)
devriesii
    Cladophialophora d.
Devrom
dew itch
DEXA
    dual-energy x-ray absorptiometer
    dual-energy x-ray absorptiometry
Dexacidin
Dexacort Phosphate in Respihaler
dexamethasone
    neomycin, polymyxin B, and d.
    d. oral inhalation
    d. suppression test
    d. (systemic)
    tobramycin and d.
    d. (topical)
dexamethasone elixir
Dexasone
    D. L.A.
Dexasporin
Dexone
    D. LA
dextran
dextran-70
dextranase
dextran-from-sucrose test

dextranicum
> Leuconostoc d.
> Leuconostoc mesenteroides subsp. d.

dextranolyticum
> Microbacterium d.

dextranolyticus
> Cellvibrio mixtus subsp. d.

dextrinicus
> Pediococcus d.

dextrinosolvens
> Succinivibrio d.

dextroamphetamine

dextromethorphan
> acetaminophen and d.
> carbinoxamine, pseudoephedrine, and d.
> chlorpheniramine, phenylephrine, and d.
> chlorpheniramine, phenylpropanolamine, and d.
> guaifenesin, phenylpropanolamine, and d.
> guaifenesin, pseudoephedrine, and d.
> Phenergan With D.
> promethazine and d.
> pseudoephedrine and d.

Dey-Dose Isoproterenol

Dey-Drop Ophthalmic solution

Dey-Lute Isoetharine

DF-2
> dysgonic fermenter 2

DFA
> direct fluorescence assay
> direct fluorescent antibody
> direct fluorescent antibody test
> direct fluorescent assay
> MicroTrak DFA
> DFA staining
> DFA tissue test for *Treponema pallidum* (DFAT-TP)

DFA-TP
> direct fluorescent antibody examination for *Treponema pallidum*

DFAT-TP
> DFA tissue test for *Treponema pallidum*

DGI
> disseminated gonococcal infection

DGKV
> Dera Ghazi Khan virus

dGTP
> deoxyguanosine triphosphate

DH
> Codehist DH
> Codiclear DH
> Decohistine DH
> Dihistine DH

DHBV
> duck hepatitis B virus

DHDA
> directed heteroduplex analysis

DHEA
> dehydroepiandrosterone

DHEAS
> dehydroepiandrosterone sulfate

DHF
> dengue hemorrhagic fever

DHF-DSS
> dengue hemorrhagic fever/shock syndrome

Dhori virus

DHPG sodium

DHS
> DHS Tar
> DHS Zinc

DI
> diabetes insipidus

diabetes
> d. insipidus (DI)
> d. mellitus

diabetes insipidus (DI)

Diabetic
> D. Tussin DM
> D. Tussin EX

diabetic
> d. ketoacidosis
> d. neuropathy
> d. osteopathy

diabetogenic

diabolicus
> Vibrio d.

diabroticae
> Spiroplasma d.

diacetate
> propylene glycol d.

diacetilactis
> Streptococcus lactis subsp. d.

diacylglycerol (DAG)

diagnosis, pl. **diagnoses**
> differential d.
> etiologic d.
> laboratory d.
> presumptive d.

diagnosis-related group (DRG)

D

NOTES

diagnostic
>d. bronchoscopy
>d. particle agglutination
>d. thoracentesis

Dialister pneumosintes (b)

dialysis, pl. **dialyses**
>continuous ambulatory peritoneal d. (CAPD)
>continuous cycling peritoneal d. (CCPD)
>high-flux d.
>peritoneal d. (PD)
>renal d.

Diamanus montanus (p)

diameter
>asymmetry, border, color, and d. (ABCD)

diamidine derivative

diamine
>dimethylparaphenylene d.
>tetramethylparaphenylene d.
>tetramethylphenylene d.

diaminodiphenylsulfone

Diamond-Blackfan anemia

Diamond TYM medium

Diamox
>D. Sequels

diana
>*Hypoderma d.*

dianae
>*Selenomonas d.*

diantaeus
>*Aedes d.*

dianthicola
>*Alternaria d.*

Dianthovirus (v)

Diaparene

diaper
>d. dermatitis
>D. Rash

Diaporthales

Diaptomus sanguineus (p)

diarizonae
>*Salmonella choleraesuis* subsp. *d.*

diarrhea
>antibiotic-associated d. (AAD)
>Brainerd d.
>chronic cryptosporidial d.
>endemic d.
>idiopathic d.
>infantile d.
>infectious d.
>inflammatory d.
>intractable d.
>malabsorptive d.
>mucoid d.
>mucous d.
>nonbacterial d.

>noninflammatory d.
>prolonged d.
>secretory d.
>*Shigella* d.
>toxin-induced d.
>traveler's d.
>watery d.
>weanling d.
>winter d.

diarrheagenic
>d. *Escherichia coli*
>d. stool culture

diarrheal
>d. enterotoxin
>d. toxin

diarrheic
>d. shellfish poisoning (DSP)
>d. stool

diarrheogenic

diarrhetic shellfish poisoning

diastatica
>*Microbispora d.*

diastaticus
>*Streptomyces d.*
>*Streptomyces diastaticus* subsp. *d.*

diastatochromogenes
>*Streptomyces d.*

diathermy
>d. snare

diathesis, pl. **diatheses**
>hemorrhagic d.

diatom

diatomaceous

diatoms
>Bacillariophyta d.

Diatrypaceae

Diatrypales

diazepam

diazotrophicus
>*Acetobacter d.*
>*Gluconacetobacter d.*
>*Vibrio d.*

Dibenzyline

Dibothriocephalus latus (p)

dibromopropamidine

DIC
>disseminated intravascular coagulation

dicarboxylicus
>*Propionivibrio d.*

Dichelobacter (b)
>*D. nodosus*

dichloroacetate

dichloroisocyanurate
>sodium d.

dichloromethanicum
>*Methylobacterium d.*

Dichotomicrobium (b)
>*D. thermohalophilum*

dichotomicus
    Thermoactinomyces d.
Dichotomophthora portulacae (f)
Dichotomophthoropsis nymphaerum (f)
dichotomous
diclazuril sodium
dicloxacillin
    d. sodium
dicroceliasis
Dicrocoeliidae
dicrocoeliosis
Dicrocoelium (p)
    D. dendriticum
    D. hospes
    D. lanceatum
Dictyocaulus (p)
    D. filaria
    D. viviparus
Dictyoglomus (b)
    D. thermophilum
    D. turgidum
Dictyonella (f)
Dictyosteliales
Dictyosteliomycetes
didanosine (ddI)
didanosine-associated pancreatitis
diddensiae
    Candida d.
didehydro-deoxythymidine (d4T)
Didelphis
didelphis
    Streptococcus d.
    Tetratrichomonas d.
didemni
    Prochloron d.
dideoxyadenosine triphosphate (ddATP)
dideoxycytidine (ddC)
2′3′-dideoxycytidine (ddC)
dideoxydidehydrothymidine triphosphate
dideoxyinosine (ddI)
2′3′-dideoxyinosine
dideoxynucleoside
    d. agent
2′,3′-dideoxy-3′thiacytidine (3TC)
Didymella phacidiomorpha (f)
Didymium nigripes
Didymosphaeriaceae
diecious
Diene stain
dienestrol

Dientamoeba fragilis (p)
diernhoferi
    Mycobacterium d.
diet
    BRAT d.
    semielemental d. (SED)
Dieterle stain
dietetic
diethylaminoethyl (DEAE)
    d. cellulose anion-exchange
      chromatography
diethylcarbamazine (DEC)
    d. citrate
diethylstilbestrol
diethyltetracycline
diethyltoluamide
Dietzia (b)
    D. maris
    D. natronolimnaea
dietzii
    Nonomuraea d.
Difco
    D. blood agar
    D. Extra Sensing Power (ESP)
      Blood Culture System
difference
    alveolar-to-arterial oxygen d. ($D_{A\text{-}a}O_2$)
differential
    Davidsohn d.
    d. diagnosis
differentiation
    biochemical d.
Differin
difficile
    Clostridium d.
difficilis
    Streptococcus d.
diffluens
    Cytophaga d.
    Persicobacter d.
Diff-Quik stain
diffusa
    leishmaniasis tegumentaria d.
diffuse
    d. cutaneous leishmaniasis
    d. infiltrative lymphocytosis
      syndrome (DILS)
    d. interstitial hemorrhage
    d. interstitial pneumonia (DIP)

D

NOTES

diffuse *(continued)*
    d. lepromatosis
    d. lymphadenitis
diffusely adherent *Escherichia coli* **(DAEC)**
diffusion
    agar gel d.
    bubble d.
    double d.
    d. method
    radial d.
    tube d.
diflorasone
Diflucan
difluens
    Cryptococcus albidus var. *d.*
Digenea
Digene CMV hybrid capture DNA
digenesis
digenetic
    d. trematode
digestion
    intercellular d.
    intracellular d.
Digibind
digitata
    Ampullariella d.
digitatis
    Actinoplanes d.
digitatus
    Mecistocirrus d.
digiti
    panaritium d.
digonicus
    Helicotylenchus d.
digoxin
    d. immune Fab
Digramma brauni (p)
Diheterospora (f)
Dihistine
    D. DH
    D. Expectorant
dihydrate
    azithromycin d.
dihydrochloride
    histamine d.
    quinine d.
dihydroergotamine
dihydromorphone
dihydropteroate synthase gene
diiodohydroxyquin
diiodohydroxyquine
Dilantin
dilatation and curettage
dilated cardiomyopathy (DCOM)
Dilepididae
Dilor
diloxanide furoate

DILS
    diffuse infiltrative lymphocytosis syndrome
diltiazem
dilute
    d. Russell viper venom (DRVV)
    d. Russell viper venom time (DRVVT)
dilution
    deuterium d.
    d. egg count
    macrobroth d.
    maximum bactericidal d. (MBD)
    microbroth d.
    microtube d. (MD)
    d. susceptibility test
Dimacol Caplets
Dimargaritaceae
Dimargaritales
dimennae
    Cryptococcus d.
dimercaprol
dimerum
    Fusarium d.
Dimetane-DC
Dimetapp Sinus Caplets
dimethylnitrosamine
dimethylparaphenylene diamine
dimidiatum
    Scytalidium d.
dimidiatus
    Chrysops d.
    Triatoma d.
diminazene aceturate
diminished libido
diminuta
    Brevundimonas d.
    Hymenolepis d.
    Pseudomonas d.
diminution
diminutum
    Spiroplasma d.
dimorpha
    Mycoplana d.
dimorphic
    d. fungus
dimorphous
    d. leprosy
dinellii
    Simulium d.
dinitrochlorobenzene (DNCB)
Dinobdella (p)
    D. ferox
Dinoflagellata
dinoflagellate
Dinophysis
    D. acuminata
    D. norvegicus

dinophysis toxin
dinucleotidase
    antinicotinamide adenine d.
dinucleotide
    nicotinamide adenine d.
Diochloram
Dioctophyma renale (p)
Dioctophymatidae
Dioctophymatoidea
dioctophymiasis
Diodoquin
Diogent
Diomycin
Diopred
Dioptimyd
Dioptrol
Diorchitrema formosanum
Diospor HC
Diosporin
diospyrosa
    Actinokineospora d.
Diosulf
Dioval Injection
DIP
    diffuse interstitial pneumonia
Dipetalogaster maximus
Dipetalonema (p)
    D. arbuta
    D. gracile
    D. interstitium
    D. perstans
    D. reconditum
    D. sprenti
    D. streptocerca
    D. viteae
diphasic milk fever
Diphen Cough
diphenhydramine
    d. and pseudoephedrine
diphenoxylate
    d. HCl
diphenoxylate/atropine
diphenoxylate with atropine
diphosphate
    guanosine d. (GDP)
diphtheria
    d. antitoxin
    avian d.
    d. culture
    cutaneous d.
    d., pertussis and tetanus (DPT)
    d. and tetanus (DT)

    tetanus and d. (tD)
    d., tetanus toxoids and acellular pertussis (DTaP)
    d., tetanus toxoids, whole-cell pertussis, and *Haemophilus influenzae* type b conjugate (DtwP-HIB)
    d., tetanus toxoids and whole-cell pertussis vaccine (DTP)
    d. toxin
    d. vaccine
diphtheriae
    Corynebacterium d.
diphtheria-pertussis-tetanus (DPT, DTaP)
diphtheria-tetanus-pertussis (DTP)
    d.-t.-p. vaccine
diphtheritic
    d. conjunctivitis
    d. ulcer
diphtheroid
    d. bacillus
Diphyllobothriidae
Diphyllobothrium (p)
    D. chordatum
    D. dendriticum
    D. erinacei
    D. grandis
    D. latum
    D. mansonoides
    D. pacificum
    D. ursi
diphyllobothrium
    d. anemia
dipivoxil
    adefovir d. (ADV)
diplobacillus
Diplocalyx (b)
    D. calotermitidis
Diplocarpon rosae **virus (DrV)**
diplococcemia
diplococci (*pl. of* diplococcus)
diplococcin
diplococcoid bacterium
diplococcus, pl. **diplococci**
    gram-negative intracellular diplococci (GNID)
Diplocystaceae
Diplodia (f)
Diplogonoporus grandis (p)
Diplomonadida
Diplomonadina
diplopia

D

NOTES

Diploscapter coronata (p)
diplospora
    Kitasatoa d.
Diplostephanus (f)
Diplostomatidae
Dipodascaceae
Dipodascus capitatus (f)
dipodomis
    Pterygodermatites d.
Diprolene
    D. AF Topical
    D. Glycol
Diprosone
    D. Topical
dipsaci
    Ditylenchus d.
dipsosauri
    Bacillus d.
    Gracilibacillus d.
dipstick
    d. immunoassay
    leukocyte esterase d.
    leukocyte esterase urine d. (LE
      urine dipstick)
    LE urine d.
        leukocyte esterase urine dipstick
    urine d.
Diptera
    poxvirus of Diptera
dipteran
dipterous
diptheria toxoid
Dipus sagitta
dipylidiasis
Dipylidiinae
Dipylidium caninum (p)
direct
    d. agglutination test
    d. amplification fingerprinting
      (DAF)
    d. antiglobulin test
    d. assay
    d. Coombs test
    d. detection of virus
    d. endoscopy
    d. fluorescence assay (DFA)
    d. fluorescent antibody (DFA)
    d. fluorescent antibody examination
      for *Treponema pallidum* (DFA-
      TP)
    d. fluorescent antibody staining
    d. fluorescent antibody test (DFA)
    d. fluorescent antibody test for
      virus
    d. fluorescent assay (DFA)
    d. *Helicobacter pylori* antigen
    d. immunofluorescence test
    d. laryngoscopy

    d. ophthalmoscopy
    d. saline mount
    d. shiga toxin test
    d. spot indole test
    d. viral antigen detection
    d. wet mount
    d. wet mount examination
    d. zoonosis
directed heteroduplex analysis (DHDA)
Directigen Meningitis Test
directive
    advance d.
directly observed therapy (DOT)
direct-smear egg count
dirithromycin
Dirofilaria (p)
    D. conjunctivae
    D. immitis
    D. magalhaesi
    D. repens
    D. striata
    D. subdermata
    D. tenuis
    D. uris
dirofilariasis
    pulmonary d.
Dirofilariinae
dirty brown granular cast
DIS
    disease intervention specialist
disaccharidase
disaccharide intolerance
Disalcid
disarticulation
    hip d.
disc
    Clear Away D.
    optic d.
Discellaceae
Discella effusa (f)
discharge
    adherent d.
    endocervical d.
    flocculent d.
    frothy d.
    homogenous d.
    malodorous d.
    mucopurulent d.
    purulent d.
    urethral d.
    vaginal d.
disciform
disciformis
    Angiococcus d.
    Myxococcus d.
Discomyces (See *Mycobacterium
    tuberculosis*)
Discomycetes

discophora
Leptothrix d.
disease
acute neurologic d.
acute respiratory d. (ARD)
acyclovir-resistant d.
advanced-stage d.
akamushi d.
Almeida d.
alveolar cyst d.
alveolar hydatid d.
Alzheimer d.
arthropod-borne viral d.
atherosclerotic cardiovascular d.
atherosclerotic heart d. (ASHD)
autoimmune d.
bacterial d.
Bang d.
Behçet d.
big spleen d.
blinding river d.
blue d.
border d.
Borna d.
Bornholm d.
Botkins d.
Bowen d.
Breda d.
Brill-Zinsser d.
bulging eye d.
bullous d.
Buschke d.
Carrión d.
caseating granulomatous d.
Castleman d.
cat scratch d. (CSD)
cavitary pulmonary d.
Chagas d.
Chagas-Cruz d.
Charlouis d.
Chlamydia d.
chlamydial d.
cholestatic liver d.
Christian d.
chronic granulomatous d.
chronic obstructive pulmonary d.
(COPD)
Clostridium difficile-associated d.
(CDAD)
CMV end-organ d.
Coenurus d.
collagen vascular d.

communicable d.
congenital cytomegalic inclusion d.
congenital Lyme d.
consulate d.
contagious d.
Creutzfeldt-Jacob d. (CJD)
Crohn d.
cyanotic congenital heart d.
cystic hydatid d.
cytomegalic inclusion d.
cytomegalovirus end-organ d.
Darling d.
deep pelvic inflammatory d.
deer fly d.
demyelinating d.
dog d.
Duke d.
Dutton d.
Eales d.
echinococcus d.
ectoparasitic d.
end-stage renal d. (ESRD)
English sweating d.
eosinophilic lung d.
fifth d.
focal airspace d.
foot-and-mouth d. (FMD)
fourth d.
gardener's d.
gastroesophageal reflux d. (GERD)
Gaucher d.
genital ulcer d. (GUD)
Gerstmann-Straüssler-Scheinker d.
(GSS)
Gilchrist d.
graft-versus-host d. (GVHD)
Greenhow d.
hand-foot-and-mouth d.
Hansen d.
hantavirus d. (HVD)
Hashimoto d.
Heck d.
hepatic d.
hepatobiliary d.
herring worm d.
His-Werner d.
HIV salivary gland d.
Hodgkin d.
hoof-and-mouth d.
hookworm d.
hydatid cyst d.
hydatid Pott d.

D

NOTES

disease *(continued)*
inclusion body d.
infectious d.
infiltrative liver d.
inflammatory d.
inflammatory bowel d. (IBD)
International Union Against
  Tuberculosis and Lung D.
d. intervention specialist (DIS)
invasive d.
island d.
Jakob-Creutzfeldt d.
Jewish housewife d.
Johne d.
Kashin-Bek d.
Katayama d.
Kawasaki mucocutaneous d.
Kyasanur Forest d. (KFDV)
Legg-Calve-Perthes d.
Legionnaires d.
Lemierre d.
LMN d.
Lobo d.
lower motor neuron d.
lumpy skin d.
Lutz-Splendore-Almeida d.
Lyme d. (LD)
lymphoproliferative d.
malignant catarrhal fever d.
malignant lymphocytic
  proliferation d. (MLPD)
Manson d.
maple bark d.
Marburg virus d.
Mayaro virus d.
Ménière d.
meningococcal d.
miner's d.
mixed cellular Hodgkin d.
multicentric Castleman d.
mycoplasma d.
mycotic corneal ulcer d.
myocardial d.
necrotizing bowel d. (NBD)
nodular d.
noncaseating granulomatous d.
nontreponemal genital ulcer d.
nosema d.
notifiable infectious d.
oculogenital d.
Paget d.
paper mill worker's d.
parasitic d.
parenchymatic liver d.
Parkinson d.
parrot d.
Paxton d.
pelvic inflammatory d. (PID)

peptic ulcer d. (PUD)
periodontal d.
Peyronie d.
polycystic hydatid d.
polycystic kidney d.
Posadas d.
Pott d.
primary progressive lung d.
prion d.
ragsorter's d.
Rasmussen d.
reactivated Chagas d.
Reiter d.
rickettsial d.
Ritter d.
rose handler's d.
salivary gland d.
Scandinavian housewife d.
Schenck d.
sexually transmitted d. (STD)
shimamushi d.
sickle cell d.
slapped-cheek d.
slim d.
slow virus d.
stage C HIV d.
swineherd's d.
swollen belly d.
systemic autoimmune d.
systemic febrile d.
tertiary d.
thromboembolic d.
toxin-mediated d.
transmissible neurodegenerative d.
tsutsugamushi d.
tunnel d.
ulcerative d.
ulceroglandular d.
UMN d.
upper motor neuron d.
Urov d.
usual d.
vagabond's d.
vagrant's d.
variant Creutzfeldt-Jakob d. (vCJD)
venoocclusive d.
Vincent d.
viral d.
virus X d.
visceral Hodgkin d.
von Willebrand d.
Wakana d.
wasting d.
Weil d.
Wernicke d.
Whipple d.
Wilson d.
wooden tongue d.

woolsorter's d.
X-linked lymphoproliferative d.
zoonotic d.
disfiguring lesion
dish
Petri d.
disiens
Bacteroides d.
Prevotella d.
disk
d. diffusion susceptibility test
MUG D.
diskitis
intervertebral d.
Kingella kingae intervertebral d.
Dismuke series
disodium
cefotetan d.
edetate d.
moxalactam d.
ticarcillin d.
disorder
autoimmune d.
connective tissue d.
HIV-associated motor cognitive d.
Kawasaki mucocutaneous d.
lymphoproliferative d.
MEG d.'s
metabolic, endocrine, and
gastrointestinal d.'s
posttransplantation
lymphoproliferative d. (PTLD)
posttransplant
lymphoproliferative d. (PTLD)
seizure d.
Disotate
dispar
Aquaspirillum d.
Entamoeba d.
Enterococcus d.
Lymantria d.
Mycoplasma d.
Veillonella d.
Veillonella alcalescens subsp. *d.*
dispersa
Pantoea d.
disperse
dispersion
amphotericin B colloid d. (ABCD)
amphotericin B colloidal d.
disporicum
Clostridium d.

disproportionate
dissecting
d. aortic aneurysm
d. cellulitis
d. fasciitis
d. microscope
disseminated
d. *Acanthamoeba*
d. anergic cutaneous leishmaniasis
d. candidiasis
d. carcinomatosis
d. coccidioidomycosis
d. cryptococcal infection
d. gonococcal infection (DGI)
d. herpes simplex virus type 2
d. histoplasmosis
d. intrauterine infection
d. intravascular coagulation (DIC)
d. lesion
d. *Mycobacterium avium* complex
infection
d. nocardial infection
d. nontuberculous mycobacterial
(DNTM)
d. nontuberculous mycobacterial
infection
d. penicilliosis
d. *Pneumocystis*
d. protothecosis
d. sporotrichosis
d. syphilis
dissemination
hematogenous d.
systemic d.
dissolvens
Enterobacter d.
Erwinia d.
Dissonus nudiventrus (p)
distallicum
Streptoverticillium d.
distallicus
Streptomyces d.
distasonis
Bacteroides d.
Distaval
distemper
d. virus
Distillate
Tar D.
distilled water

D

NOTES

distincta
    Alteromonas d.
    Pseudoalteromonas d.
Distoma (p)
distomiasis
    hemic d.
    pulmonary d.
Distomum (p)
    D. appendiculatum
    D. foecundum
distortum
    Microsporum canis var. *d.*
    Ophiostoma d.
distribution
    butterfly d.
    glove-and-stocking d.
distributum
    Halobacterium d.
    Halorubrobacterium d.
    Halorubrum d.
disturbance
    arteriovenous conduction d.
    motility d.
disulfidooxidans
    Sulfobacillus d.
disulfiram-like toxin
Ditchling agent
diterpene
dithiothreitol solution
Ditylenchus (p)
    D. destructor
    D. dipsaci
diuretic
    loop-acting d.
diurnal periodicity
divaricatum
    Brevibacterium d.
divergens
    Babesia d.
    Carnobacterium d.
    Lactobacillus d.
diversa
    Candida d.
diversibranchium
    Simulium d.
diversifurcatum
    Simulium d.
diversum
    Ureaplasma d.
diversus
    Citrobacter d.
diverticulitis
diverticulosis
division
    conjugate d.
    multiplicative d.
dixiense
    Simulium d.

dizziness
    orthostatic d.
djakartensis
    Streptomyces d.
DLT
    dose-limiting toxicity
DLV
    delavirdine
    delavirdine mesylate
DM
    Anatuss DM
    Balminil DM
    Benylin DM
    Bronchopan DM
    Buckley's DM
    Carbodec DM
    Cardec DM
    Centratuss DM
    Cough Suppressant Syrup DM
    DM Cough syrup
    Diabetic Tussin DM
    Dorcol DM
    DM E Suppressant Expectorant
    Fenesin DM
    Genatuss DM
    Guaifenex DM
    Halotussin DM
    Hold DM
    Humibid DM
    Iobid DM
    Koffex DM
    Maxifed DM
    Monafed DM
    Mytussin DM
    Novahistex DM
    Novahistine DM
    Personnelle DM
    Pharminil DM
    Pharmitussin DM
    Phenameth DM
    DM Plus Decongestant
    Profen II DM
    Pseudo-Car DM
    DM Sans Sucre
    Sedatuss DM
    Silphen DM
    Siltussin DM
    Sirop DM
    Sudafed DM
    Syrup DM
    Tolu-Sed DM
    Triaminic Long Lasting DM
    Tussodan DM
    Uni-tussin DM
D-mannitol fermentation test
D-mannose fermentation test
DM-D
    Benylin DM-D

Centratuss DM-D
Children's Benylin DM-D
Koffex DM-D
Syrup DM-D
Triaminic DM-D
DM-D-E
Cough Syrup DM-D-E
DM-E
Benylin DM-E
Cough Syrup DM-E
Syrup DM-E
D-Med Injection
DMFO
DMP-266, -450
DMPA
depot medroxyprogesterone acetate
DNA
deoxyribonucleic acid
B19 DNA
branched DNA (bDNA)
branched chain DNA (bDNA)
chemiluminescent DNA
competitor DNA
DNA detection test
Digene CMV hybrid capture DNA
DNA DipStick Kit
double-stranded DNA (dsDNA)
DNA extraction
DNA homology
DNA hybrid capture
DNA hybridization analysis
DNA hybridization test
parvovirus B19 DNA
DNA probe
DNA probe hybridization
DNA probe test
random amplified polymorphic DNA (RAPD)
recombinant DNA (rDNA)
DNA tumor virus
DNase
deoxyribonuclease
DNCB
dinitrochlorobenzene
DNL
de novo lipogenesis
DNR
do-not-resuscitate
DNT
dermonecrotic toxin

DNTM
disseminated nontuberculous mycobacterial
DNTM infection
D$_{A-a}$O$_2$
alveolar-to-arterial oxygen difference
Doak
Tar D.
Doak-Oil
Doan's
D. Backache Pills
Extra Strength D.
D., Original
Dobell and O'Connor solution
dobutamine
Dochmius
Döderlein bacillus (*See* ***Lactobacillus acidophilus***)
doebereinerae
Azospirillum d.
doenitzi
Haemaphysalis d.
doeringae
Culicoides d.
dog
d. bite sepsis
d. disease
dogma
Dohle body
dolii
Halomethanococcus d.
Dolichopsyllidae
dolichum
Eubacterium d.
dolichura
Caenorhabditis d.
dolor
Dolorac
doloresi
Gnathostoma d.
Dolosicoccus paucivorans (b)
Dolosigranulum pigrum (b)
Dolotic
Dolsed
domain
functional d.
immunodominant d.
dome
d. epithelium
transducer d.
Domeboro
Otic D.

NOTES

domestica
> *Musca d.*
> *Musca domestica d.*

domesticus
> *Anopheles albitarsis d.*
> *Glycophagus d.*

dome-transducer

domiciliated

domoic acid

donation
> autologous blood d. (ABD)

Donnamar

Donnatal

do-not-resuscitate (DNR)

Donovan body

donovani
> *Leishmania d.*
> *Piroplasma d.*

donovanosis
> oral d.

dopamine

Doppler echocardiography

Doratomyces stemonitis (f)

Dorcol
> D. DM

dorotheae
> *Flexithrix d.*

dorsalis
> *Aedes d.*
> *Hippelates d.*
> tabes d.

Dorset culture egg medium

dorsilinea
> *Muscina d.*

dorsocervical
> d. fat

dorsoventral

Doryx

dose
> d. adjustment
> daily d.
> defined daily d. (DDD)
> infecting d.
> infective d.
> d. interval

dose-limiting toxicity (DLT)

dose-related myelotoxicity

doshiae
> *Bartonella d.*

dosing regimen

DOT
> directly observed therapy

dot
> d. blot
> d. blot assay
> d. blot hybridization
> Maurer d.

> Schüffner d.'s
> Ziemann d.'s

Dothideaceae

Dothideales

Dothioraceae

Dothiorella mangiferae (f)

double
> d. antibody radioimmunoassay
> d. diffusion
> d. intensification
> d. quartan
> d. tertian malaria
> d. unicompartmental

double-edged sword

double-stranded DNA (dsDNA)

douche
> zinc sulfate d.

doudoroffii
> *Oceanimonas d.*
> *Pseudomonas d.*

doughnut lesion

Douglas virus (DOUV)

douthitti
> *Schistosomatium d.*

DOUV
> Douglas virus

downei
> *Streptococcus d.*

downesi
> *Culicoides d.*

Downey cell

downgrading reaction

downsi
> *Simulium d.*

Down syndrome

doxepin

doxorubicin
> liposomal encapsulated d.
> pegylated liposomal-encapsulated d.

Doxy

Doxy-200

Doxy-Caps

Doxychel

Doxycin

doxycycline
> d. hyclate
> d. monohydrate
> d. pleurodesis

Doxy-Tabs

Doxytec

doxytetracycline

doylei
> *Campylobacter jejuni* subsp. *d.*

DPOA
> durable power of attorney

DPT
> diphtheria-pertussis-tetanus
> diphtheria, pertussis and tetanus

DPV
Drosophila P virus
Dr
Dr Scholl's Athlete's Foot
Dr Scholl's Maximum Strength Tritin
dracontiasis
dracunculiasis
Dracunculidae
Dracunculoidea
dracunculosis
Dracunculus (p)
D. *insignis*
D. *lutrae*
D. *medinensis*
D. *persarum*
drain
Reliavac d.
drainage
closed d.
percutaneous d.
draining
d. fistula
d. lymph node
Draschia (p)
Drechslera
D. *avenae*
D. *biseptata*
D. *brizae*
D. *holmii*
D. *longirostrata*
D. *maydis*
D. *monoceras*
D. *pedicellata*
D. *pluriseptata*
D. *sorokiniana*
D. *teres*
D. *tetramera*
D. *turcica*
Drenison
drepanidium
Drepanidotaenia lanceolata (p)
dressing
Elastoplast wound d.
DRG
diagnosis-related group
Dri-Ear Otic
drift
antigenic d.
drimydis
Candida d.

Dristan
D. Long Lasting Nasal solution
D. Sinus Caplets
Drixoral
D. Cough & Congestion Liquid Caps
D. Cough & Sore Throat Liquid Caps
D. Non-Drowsy
drobachiensis
Cytophaga d.
dronabinol
drop
Afrin Children's Nose D.'s
Allergan Ear D.'s
Brolene D.
Coly-Mycin S Otic D.'s
Rondamine-DM d.'s
Tussafed D.'s
Drosophila
D. *ananassae*
D. A virus (DAV)
D. C virus (DCV)
D. *melanogaster*
D. P virus (DPV)
D. *repleta*
D. X virus (DXV)
Drosophilidae
Drotic Otic
Drowsiness
Tylenol Cold No D.
Droxia
drozanskii
Legionella d.
drug
d. addiction
d. allergy
antimalarial d.
antineoplastic d.
antiviral d.
azole d.
carbacephem class of d.
carbapenem class of d.
cardiotoxic d.
cytotoxic d.
d. fever
d. holiday
immunosuppressive d.
d. interaction
d. intolerance
investigational new d. (IND)
myelotoxic d.

NOTES

drug *(continued)*
    nonsteroidal antiinflammatory d.
    (NSAID)
    sedative-hypnotic d.
    d. susceptibility assay
drug-induced
    d.-i. cardiomyopathy
drug-induced bone marrow suppression
drug-induced uveitis
drug-maintenance program
drug-resistant
    d.-r. HIV
    multiple d.-r. (MDR)
    d.-r. *Streptococcus pneumoniae*
    d.-r. tuberculosis
drug-seeking behavior
drug-susceptible *Streptococcus pneumoniae*
DrV
    Diplocarpon rosae virus
DRVV
    dilute Russell viper venom
DRVVT
    dilute Russell viper venom time
dry
    d. cutaneous leishmaniasis
    d. tap
Dryox
    D. Gel
    D. Wash
DS
    Bactrim DS
    Cotrim DS
    Septra DS
    Sulfatrim DS
dsDNA
    double-stranded DNA
    dsDNA algal virus
    dsDNA phycovirus group
DSP
    diarrheic shellfish poisoning
DSS
    dengue shock syndrome
DT
    diphtheria and tetanus
d4T
    didehydro-deoxythymidine
    stavudine
ᴅ-tagatose fermentation test
DTaP
    diphtheria-pertussis-tetanus
    diphtheria, tetanus toxoids and acellular
    pertussis
DTH
    delayed-type hypersensitivity
    DTH testing
DTIC-Dome

DTP
    diphtheria-tetanus-pertussis
    diphtheria, tetanus toxoids and whole-cell
    pertussis vaccine
    DTP vaccine
DTR
    deep tendon reflex
DtwP-HIB
    diphtheria, tetanus toxoids, whole-cell
    pertussis, and *Haemophilus influenzae*
    type b conjugate
DU6859a
dual
    d. infection
    d. nucleoside therapy
dual-energy x-ray absorptiometer (DEXA)
dual-energy x-ray absorptiometry (DEXA)
dual-fluorescence analysis
dubliniensis
    Candida d.
duck
    d. embryo origin vaccine
    d. hepatitis B virus (DHBV)
    d. hepatitis group
    d. influenza virus
    d. plague
    d. plague virus
Ducrey bacillus
ducreyi
    Haemophilus d.
duct
    Skene d.
    Stensen d.
Duffy blood group
Duganella zoogloeoides (b)
Dugbe virus (DUGV)
dugesii
    Borrelia d.
DUGV
    Dugbe virus
Duke disease
Dukes C colorectal carcinoma stage
dulcitol fermentation test
dumdum
    d. fever
dumoffii
    Fluoribacter d.
    Legionella d.
d'Unna
    Pate d.
duodecadis
    Arthrobacter d.
duodenal
    d. string test
    d. ulcer

duodenale
>   Ancylostoma d.

duodenalis (p)
>   Giardia d.

DuoFilm
>   D. solution

Duoforte

duplex
>   Simulium d.

Duplex T

dupreei
>   Aedes d.

durable power of attorney (DPOA)

Durabolin

Durafedrin

Dura-Gest

Duralone Injection

Duramist Plus

durans
>   Enterococcus d.
>   Streptococcus d.

Dura-Tabs

Duratest Injection

Durathate Injection

duration

Duration Nasal solution

Duratuss-G

Dura-Vent

Durck granuloma

dureti
>   Simulium d.

durhamensis
>   Actinoplanes d.
>   Streptomyces d.

Duricef

durum
>   Clostridium d.
>   Corynebacterium d.

durus
>   Paenibacillus d.

dust
>   d. mite
>   d. phagocyte

Dutton
>   D. disease
>   D. relapsing fever

duttonii
>   Borrelia d.

duvalii
>   Mycobacterium d.

Duvenhage virus

DVT
>   deep vein thrombosis

DV Vaginal Cream

dwarfism
>   Nakalanga d.

DX
>   Naldecon Senior D.

DXV
>   *Drosophila* X virus

Dyadobacter (b)
>   D. fermentans

dyari
>   Mansonia d.

Dycill

dye
>   blue d.
>   Loeffler methylene blue d.

Dynabac

Dynacin Oral

Dyna-Hex
>   D.-H. Topical

Dynapen

dyphylline

dyschromic papulosquamous skin lesion

dysconjugate gaze

dyscrasia

dysenteriae
>   Shigella d.
>   Shigella d. serotype 1

dysenteric
>   d. illness
>   d. malaria

dysentery
>   acute amebic d.
>   amebic d.
>   d. antitoxin
>   bacillary d.
>   d. bacillus
>   balantidial d.
>   bilharzial d.
>   fulminant d.
>   helminthic d.

dysfunction
>   brainstem d.
>   left ventricular d.
>   mitochondrial d.
>   neurologic d.
>   prosthetic valve d.
>   renal d.

dysgalactiae
>   Streptococcus dysgalactiae subsp. d.

dysgammaglobulinemia

D

NOTES

dysgeusia
dysgonic
    d. fermenter 2 (DF-2)
    d. fermenter 3
Dysgonomonas (b)
    D. capnocytophagoides
    D. gadei
dyskaryosis
dyskeratosis
dyslipidemia
dysmenorrhea
dysmetria
dysmorphic red cell
Dysne-Inhal
dyspareunia
    deep d.

dyspepsia
dysphagia
dysplasia
    bronchopulmonary d. (BPD)
    cervical d.
    medial d.
dysplastic epithelial
dyspnea
    exertional d.
dysreflexia
dysregulation
    immune d.
dysrhythmia
dystrophic osteoarthritis
dysuria

E

E test
E virus

44E

Vicks Pediatric Formula 44E

EA

endotracheal aspiration

eadsi

Culicoides e.

EAEC

enteroadherent *Escherichia coli*

Eagan

Haemophilus influenzae strain E.

EAggEC, EaggEC

enteroaggregative *Escherichia coli*

Eagle phenomenon

Eales disease

ear

swimmer's e.
e. thermometry

Ear-Eze Otic

earlei

Anopheles e.

early

e. erythrocyte
e. false morel
e. latent (EL)
e. latent syphilis

early-stage disease

ear, nose, and throat (ENT)

Easprin

East

E. African sleeping sickness
E. African trypanosomiasis

eastern

e. equine encephalitis (EEE)
e. equine encephalitis virus (EEEV)
e. equine encephalomyelitis

Eaton agent (*See* **Mycoplasma pneumoniae**)

Eaton-Lambert myasthenic syndrome

EAV

equine abortion virus

EB

elementary body
Epstein-Barr
EB nuclear antigen

E-Base

Eberth bacillus (*See* **Salmonella typhi**)

EBMT

European bone marrow transplantation

EBNA

Epstein-Barr nuclear antigen

EBNA-1 protein

Ebola

E. virus (EBOV)
E. virus hemorrhagic fever

Ebola-like viruses

EBOV

Ebola virus

EB-PFA

EBV

Epstein-Barr virus
EBV capsid antigen
EBV early antigen
EBV mononucleosis
EBV titer
EBV virus culture
EBV virus serology

EBV-associated lymphoid neoplasia

EC

Videx EC

E-C

Apo-Erythro E.-C.

Ec9 virus

ECCE

extracapsular cataract extraction

ecchymosis

ecdysial gland

ecdysis

ECF

executive cognitive function
ECF deficit

ECG

electrocardiogram

Echidnophaga gallinacea (p)

Echinacea angustifolia

echinata

Stachybotrys e.

echinate

echinatus

Streptomyces e.

Echinobotryum (f)

Echinochasmus (p)

E. *japonica*
E. *perfoliatus*

echinococcal cyst

echinococcosis

polycystic e.

Echinococcus (p)

E. *felidis*
E. *granulosus*
E. *granulosus canadensis*
E. *granulosus equinus*
E. *intermedius*
E. *multilocularis*
E. *oligarthrus*
E. *vogeli*

E

173

echinococcus
    e. cyst
    e. disease
echinodiscus
    Gigantorhynchus e.
echinoides
    Methylocystis e.
    Pseudomonas e.
    Sphingomonas e.
Echinoparyphium recurvatum (p)
Echinorhynchidae
Echinorhynchus gadi (p)
echinoruber
    Streptomyces e.
echinospora
    Actinomadura e.
    Microbispora e.
    Micromonospora e.
    Micromonospora echinospora subsp.
       e.
Echinosteliales
Echinosteliopsidales
Echinostoma (p)
    E. caproni
    E. chinatum
    E. cinetorchis
    E. hortense
    E. ilocanum
    E. lindoense
    E. macrorchis
    E. melis
    E. paraensi
    E. revolutum
    E. trivolus
Echinostomatidae
Echinostomatoidea
echinostomatosis
echinostomiasis
Echinostomida
echinulata
    Cunninghamella e.
echinulate
ECHO
    echocardiogram
    enteric cytopathic human orphan
    enteric cytopathogenic human orphan
    ECHO virus
echocardiogram (ECHO)
    unidimensional e.
echocardiograph
    transesophageal e. (TEE)
echocardiography
    2D e.
    Doppler e.
    M-mode e.
    transesophageal e. (TEE)
    transthoracic e.

    two-dimensional transthoracic e.
       (TTE)
echogenic
echogram
echovirus
    e. culture
    human e. 1–34
    e. II
eclampsia
ECM
    erythema chronicum migrans
ecological system
econazole
    e. nitrate
ecospecies
Ecostatin
ecosystem
    parasite-host e.
Ecotrin
ecthyma
    e. contagiosum
    contagious e.
    e. gangrenosum
ectocyst
ectogenous
ectomerogony
ectoparasite
    e. identification
ectoparasitic disease
ectoparasiticide
ectoparasitism
ectophyte
ectopic
    e. parasitism
    e. pregnancy
    e. schistosomiasis
ectoplasm
ectopy
    cervical e.
ectosarc
Ectosone
Ectothiorhodospira (b)
    E. abdelmalekii
    E. haloalkaliphila
    E. halochloris
    E. halophila
    E. marina
    E. marismortui
    E. mobilis
    E. shaposhnikovii
    E. vacuolata
Ectothiorhodospiraceae
ectothrix
Ectotrichophyton (f)
ectozoon
Ectrogellaceae
ectromelia virus

ectropion
  cervical e.
ecuadoriense
  Simulium e.
ECW
  extracellular water
eczema
  e. marginatum
  e. parasiticum
  varicose e.
eczematous
  e. change
  e. dermatitis
edaphicus
  Bacillus e.
edax
  Candida e.
edema
  allergic laryngeal e.
  e. factor (EF)
  lid e.
  macular e.
  noncardiogenic pulmonary e.
  optic disk e.
  palpebral e.
  pedal e.
  periorbital e.
  peripheral e.
  e. toxin
  Yangtze river e.
edematous enteritis
edeni
  Culicoides e.
ederensis
  Streptomyces e.
edetate disodium
Edge Hill virus (EHV)
edrophonium
ED-SPAZ
educational program
edwardii
  Mycoplasma e.
Edwardsiella (b)
  E. anguillimortifera
  E. hoshinae
  E. ictaluri
  E. tarda
EEC
  enterovirulent *Escherichia coli*
  EEC group

EEE
  eastern equine encephalitis
    EEE virus
EEEV
  eastern equine encephalitis virus
EEG
  electroencephalogram
  electroencephalography
eel
  vinegar e.
E.E.S.
EF
  edema factor
EF-4
  eugonic fermenter 4
efavirenz
EFE
  endocardial fibroelastosis
effect
  graft-versus-leukemia e.
  inoculum e.
effector T lymphocyte
efficacy
efficiency
  respiratory isolation
    implementation e. (RIIE)
effusa
  Discella e.
effuse
effusion
  e. cytology
  e. lymphoma
  parapneumonic e.
  pericardial e.
  pleural e.
Efidac/24
eflornithine
EgAn 1825-61 virus
EGD
  esophagogastroduodenoscopy
EGF
  epidermal growth factor
egg
  operculate e.
Eggerthella lenta (b)
eggerthii
  Bacteroides e.
eglandulous
Egtved virus
Egyptian
  E. hematuria

E

NOTES

Egyptian *(continued)*
    E. ophthalmia
    E. splenomegaly
EHDV
    epizootic hemorrhagic disease virus 1–8
EHEC
    enterohemorrhagic *Escherichia coli*
    EHEC O157:H7 Sakai strain
ehimense
    Streptoverticillium e.
ehimensis
    Bacillus e.
    Streptomyces e.
Ehrlichia (b)
    E. canis
    E. chaffeensis
    E. equi
    E. ewingii
    E. muris
    E. phagocytophila
    E. risticii
    E. sennetsu
    E. serology
Ehrlichiaceae
Ehrlichieae
ehrlichiosis
    human e. (HE)
    human granulocytic e. (HGE)
    human monocytic e. (HME)
    monocytic e.
Ehrlich reagent
EHV
    Edge Hill virus
EI
    erythema infectiosum
EIA
    enzymatic immunoassay
    enzyme immunoassay
    S/LS EIA
EIA2
Eidamia viridescens (f)
EIEC
    enteroinvasive *Escherichia coli*
eikelboomii
    Thiothrix e.
Eikenella (b)
    E. corrodens
    E. corrodens and *Kingella kingii*
Eimeria (p)
    E. acervulina
    E. adenoeides
    E. alabamensis
    E. anatis
    E. auburnensis
    E. bovis
    E. meleagridis
    E. necatrix
    E. ovina

    E. porci
    E. stiedai
    E. tenella
    E. vermiformis
Eimeriida
Eimeriidae
Eimeriorina
eiseni
    Anopheles e.
    Anopheles e. eiseni
    Anopheles e. geometricus
EK
    electrophoretic karyotyping
ekimensis
    Streptomyces e.
EL
    early latent
    EL syphilis
El
    El Moro Canyon virus
    El Tor *Vibrio*
Elaeophora schneideri (p)
ELAM-1
    endothelial leukocyte adhesion molecule-
    1
Elaphomycetaceae
Elaphomycetales
Elasmomycetaceae
elastica
    Hellvella e.
elastin
    e. fiber
Elastoplast wound dressing
elastosis
    intimal e.
elatum
    Cladosporium e.
elbow arthrogram
ELBW
    extremely low birth weight
Eldecort Topical
elective culture
Electra 1000C coagulation analyzer
electrocardiogram (ECG)
electrocautery
electrocoagulating forceps
electrocoagulation
electrodessication
electrodiagnostic study
electroencephalogram (EEG)
electroencephalography (EEG)
electrokarotype
electrolyte
    e. depletion
    serum e.
electromyelography (EMG)
electromyographic (EMG)
electromyography (EMG)

electron
  e. beam therapy
  e. cryomicroscopy
  e. micrograph
  e. microscopic examination
  e. microscopy (EM)
  e. transport
  e. transport system
electron-dense excrescence
electropherotype
electrophoresis
  agarose gel e.
  contour-clamped gel e.
  contour-clamped homogenous
    fields e. (CHEF)
  field inversion gel e. (FIGE)
  multilocus enzyme e. (MEE,
    MLEE)
  polyacrylamide gel e. (PAGE)
  pulsed-field gel e. (PFGE)
  sodium dodecyl sulfate-
    polyacrylamide gel e. (SDS-
    PAGE)
  temporal temperature gradient
    gel e. (TTGE)
electrophoretic (EP)
  e. karyotyping (EK)
  e. mobility
  e. mobility shift analysis (EMSA)
  e. mobility shift assay (EMSA)
  e. protein typing
electroporation
electrosurgery
electrosurgical
elegans
  Abiotrophia e.
  Apophysomyces e.
  Caenorhabditis e.
  Cunninghamella e.
  Flexibacter e.
  Granulicatella e.
  Halobacteroides e.
  Holospora e.
  Phaeoannellomyces e.
  Prosthenorchis e.
  Rhodoplanes e.
  Thiodictyon e.
element
  transposable e.
elementary body (EB)

elephantiasis
  genital e.
  nonfilarial e.
elephantis
  Mycobacterium e.
  Mycoplasma e.
elephant leg
elevation
  bilirubin e.
  transaminase e.
elfii
  Thermotoga e.
elicitation
eligens
  Eubacterium e.
Elimite
  E. Cream
ELISA
  enzyme-linked immunosorbent assay
  IgM ELISA
  ELISA test
  ELISA unit
ELISPOT
  enzyme-linked immunospot assay
  ELISPOT assay
elixir
  Allergy E.
  zidovudine e.
Elixomin
Elixophyllin
elizabethae
  Bartonella e.
  Rochalimaea e.
elkanii
  Bradyrhizobium e.
**Ellinghausen-McCollough-Johnson-Harris
  medium**
ellipsoidea
  Pseudallescheria e.
ellipsoideus
  Saccharomyces cerevisiae var. *e.*
ellychniae
  Entomoplasma e.
  Mycoplasma e.
Elocom
Elocon
elongata
  Halomonas e.
  Hysterolecitha e.
  Nadsonia fulvescens var. *e.*
  Neisseria elongata subsp. *e.*
  Pseudomonas e.

E

NOTES

elongatus
  Desulfobulbus e.
  Fibrobacter succinogenes subsp. *e.*
elongisporus
  Lodderomyces e.
elsdenii
  Megasphaera e.
Elsinoaceae
elucidate
elucidation
elution
  agar disk e.
elutriation
  countercurrent centrifugal e.
elviae
  Sterigmatomyces e.
elyakovii
  Alteromonas e.
  Pseudoalteromonas e.
Elytrosporangium (b)
  E. carpinense
  E. spirale
EM
  electron microscopy
  erythema migrans
  EM examination
emaciated
emaciation
EMAP II
  endothelial-monocyte activating
  polypeptide II
emarginatum
  Simulium e.
Ematozoon
EMB
  eosin methylene blue
  ethambutol
  EMB agar
Embadomonas intestinalis (p)
Embellisia (f)
  E. allii
  E. hyacinthi
emboli (*pl. of* embolus)
embolic
  e. event
  e. pneumonia
embolism
  air e.
  systemic fat e.
embolization
  arterial e.
  septic e.
embolus, pl. **emboli**
  meningococcal e.
  pulmonary e.
embryo
  hexacanth e.
  oncosphere e.

embryogenesis
embryologic
embryonate
embryopathy
embryophore
Embu virus
EMC
  encephalomyocarditis
  EMC virus
  EMC virus group
EMCV
  encephalomyocarditis virus
emerging virus
Emericella nidulans (f)
emesis
emetica
  Russula e.
emetic toxin
emetine
  e. hydrochloride
  e. treatment
EMG
  electromyelography
  electromyographic
  electromyography
Emgel Topical
EMIT
  enzyme-multiplied immunoassay
  technique
Emivirine
Emmonsia (f)
  E. parva
  E. parva var. *parva*
Emo-Cort
Empedobacter brevis (b)
EM-PFA
emphysema
  gangrenous e.
  metapneumonic e.
  subcutaneous e.
emphysematous
  e. cholecystitis
  e. gangrene
  e. phlegmon
empiric
  e. antibiotic
  e. therapy
Empirin
emporiatrics
empyema
  extradural e.
  pleural e.
  sinus e.
  subdural e.
  tuberculous e.
  ventricular e.

EMRSA
> epidemic methicillin-resistant
> *Staphylococcus aureus*

EMSA
> electrophoretic mobility shift analysis
> electrophoretic mobility shift assay

emtricitabine

emulsification

E-Mycin

E-Mycin-E

en
> en grappe
> en thyrse

Enamovirus (v)

enanthate
> testosterone e.

enanthem

Enantiothamnus
> *E. braulti*

encainide

Encap
> Novo-Rythro E.

encapsidated

encapsulated
> e. budding yeast cell

encapsulated daunorubicin

encephalitis
> acute hemorrhagic e.
> acute necrotizing e.
> arthropod-borne viral e.
> bunyavirus e.
> California e.
> cat scratch e.
> central European e. (CEE)
> Coxsackie e.
> Dawson e.
> eastern equine e. (EEE)
> epidemic e.
> experimental autoimmune e.
> Far East Russian e.
> flaviviral e.
> granulomatous e.
> granulomatous amebic e. (GAE)
> herpes simplex e.
> herpesvirus e.
> HIV e.
> HIV-1 e.
> hyperergic e.
> Ilheus e.
> inclusion body e.
> Japanese e. (JE)
> Japanese B e.

> e. lethargica
> measles inclusion body e.
> Mengo e.
> mumps e.
> mycoplasmal e.
> Powassan virus e.
> rabies e.
> Rasmussen e.
> Russian spring-summer e. (RSSE)
> Russian tick-borne e.
> St. Louis e. (SLE)
> St. Louis equine e.
> tick-borne e. (TBE)
> e. titer
> toxoplasma e.
> *Toxoplasma gondii* e.
> toxoplasmic e.
> e. vaccine
> Venezuelan equine e. (VEE)
> vernal e.
> viral e.
> e. virus
> Von Economo e.
> western equine e.
> woodcutter's e.

Encephalitozoon cuniculi (p)

encephalomalasia

encephalomyelitis
> acute disseminated e.
> autoimmune e.
> avian infectious e.
> eastern equine e.
> enzootic e.
> herpes B e.
> infectious porcine e.
> postinfectious e.
> rabies vaccine-induced e.
> Vilyuisk e.
> viral e.
> virus e.

encephalomyocarditis (EMC)
> e. virus (EMCV)

encephalopathy
> bovine spongiform e.
> chagasic e.
> CSD e.
> HIV e.
> HIV-1 e.
> subacute spongiform e.
> toxic e.
> transmissible mink e.

NOTES

E

179

encheleia
: *Aeromonas* e.

encisoi
: *Simulium* e

encystment

Endal

Endantadine

endarteritis
: bacterial e.
: e. obliterans
: obliterative e.
: pulmonary e.
: syphilitic e.

endemic
: e. diarrhea
: e. funiculitis
: e. hematuria
: e. hemoptysis
: e. nonbacterial infantile gastroenteritis
: e. relapsing fever
: e. syphilis
: e. typhus

endemicity

End Lice Liquid

Endo
: E. agar
: E. medium

endobiotic

endobioticum
: *Synchytrium* e.

endobronchial
: e. biopsy
: e. tuberculosis

endocardial fibroelastosis (EFE)

endocarditis
: acute bacterial e. (ABE)
: artificial valve e.
: bacteria-free stage of bacterial e.
: bacterial e. (BE)
: brucellar e.
: *Candida glabrata* e.
: *Cardiobacterium hominis* e.
: culture-negative e.
: enterococcal e.
: *Haemophilus* e.
: infectious e.
: infective e. (IE)
: *Kingella kingae* e.
: MRSA e.
: native valve e.
: *Neisseria mucosa* e.
: nonbacterial thrombotic e. (NBTE)
: nosocomial infective e.
: pacemaker e.
: polymicrobial e.
: prosthetic valve e. (PVE)
: staphylococcal e.

streptococcal e.
: *Streptococcus bovis* e.
: subacute bacterial e.

endocardium
: e., vascular structures, interstitium of striated muscle (EVI)
: e., vascular structures, interstitium of striated muscle antibody

endocervical
: e. culture
: e. discharge
: e. enzyme immunoassay
: e. Gram stain
: e. specimen
: e. swab

endocrine
: e. gland failure

endocrinotoxin

endocyst

endocytic vesicle

endocytosis
: receptor-mediated e.

Endodermophyton (p) (*See* **Trichophyton**)

endodontalis
: *Bacteroides* e.
: *Porphyromonas* e.

endodyocyte

endodyogeny

end-of-treatment response

endogamy

endogenous
: e. cycle
: e. endophthalmitis
: e. infection
: e. latent virus
: e. pyrogen
: e. viral superantigen

Endogonaceae

Endogonales

endolaser photocoagulation

Endolimax nana (p)

endoluminal

endomerogony

endometrial
: e. culture
: e. tuberculosis

endometritis
: postabortal e.
: postpartum e. (PPE)
: puerperal e.

endometrium

Endomyces (f)
: *E. fibuliger*
: *E. krusei*

Endomycetaceae

Endomycetales

Endomycopsis (f)
: *E. burtonii*

E. *chodatii*
E. *fibuliger*
E. *lipolytica*
E. *ohmeri*
endomyometritis
endo/nasotracheal suctioning
endonuclease
endoparametritis
endoparasite
endophthalmitis
 Aspergillus e.
 bacterial e.
 Candida e.
 endogenous e.
 fungal e.
 parasitic e.
 viral e.
endophyte
endophytic
endoplast
endoplastic
endopolygeny
Endorimospora (p) (*See* **Sarcocystis**)
endosarc
endoscope
 flexible fiberoptic e. (FFE)
endoscopic
 e. retrograde cholangiography
 e. retrograde
  cholangiopancreatography (ERCP)
 e. sphincterotomy
endoscopic retrograde cholangiography
endoscopist
endoscopy
 direct e.
 flexible fibroptic e.
 gastrointestinal e.
 upper gastrointestinal e.
endosomal protease
endosome
endospore
endostatin
endostreptosin
endosymbiosus
 Methanoplanus e.
endoteric bacterium
endothelial
 e. leukocyte adhesion molecule-1
  (ELAM-1)
endothelial-monocyte activating
 polypeptide II (EMAP II)
endothelium

endothrix
endotoxemia
endotoxic
 e. shock
endotoxicosis
endotoxin
endotracheal
 e. aspiration (EA)
 e. intubation
endovascular
endpoint dilution assay
Endrate
end-stage renal disease (ESRD)
end-to-end anastomosis
endus
 Streptomyces e.
enflagellation
Engelmann basal knob
Engenix-B
Englerulaceae
English sweating disease
engraftment
Engyodontium album (f)
enhematospore
Enhydrobacter aerosaccus (b)
enhydrum
 Prosthecomicrobium e.
enissocaesilis
 Streptomyces e.
enlarging lymph node
Enlon
enoeca
 Prevotella e.
enolase
Enomine
Enoplida
enoxacin
enriettii
 Leishmania e.
ENS
 enteral nutrition solution
ensconced
Enseada virus (ENSV)
Enseals
 Potassium Iodide E.
Ensifer adhaerens (b)
Ensure
ENSV
 Enseada virus
ENT
 ear, nose, and throat

E

NOTES

EN-tabs
    Azulfidine E.-t.
entamebiasis
entamebic
Entamoeba (p)
    E. coli
    E. dispar
    E. gingivalis
    E. hartmanni
    E. histolytica
    E. histolytica serology
    E. invadens
    E. moshkovskii
    E. polecki
Entamoebidae
entanii
    Gluconacetobacter e.
Entebbe bat virus (ENTV)
Entemopoxvirus
enteral
    e. feeding
    e. nutrition solution (ENS)
enteric
    e. absorption
    e. adenovirus
    e. bacterium
    e. coated beadlet
    e. coronavirus
    e. cytopathic human orphan
        (ECHO)
    e. cytopathogenic human orphan
        (ECHO)
    e. fever
    e. gram-negative bacillus
    e. microsporidiosis
    e. pathogen
    e. virus
enterica
    Allomonas e.
enterically transmitted non-A non-B hepatitis (ET-NANBH)
entericoid fever
enteris
enteritidis
    Salmonella e.
enteritis
    acute e.
    e. anaphylactica
    bacterial e.
    Campylobacter e.
    catarrhal e.
    cryptosporidial e.
    edematous e.
    feline infectious e.
    hemorrhagic e.
    human eosinophilic e.
    e. necroticans

    tuberculous e.
    ulcerative e.
enteroadherent *Escherichia coli* **(EAEC)**
enteroaggregative *Escherichia coli* **(EAggEC, EaggEC)**
Enterobacter (b)
    E. aerogenes
    E. agglomerans
    E. amnigenus
    E. amnigenus biogroup 1. 2
    E. asburiae
    E. cancerogenus
    E. cloacae
    E. cloacae ribotyping
    E. cloacae septicemia
    E. dissolvens
    E. gergoviae
    E. hormaechei
    E. intermedius
    E. kobei
    E. nimipressuralis
    E. pyrinus
    E. sakazakii
    E. taylorae
Enterobacteriaceae
    extended-spectrum beta-lactamase-producing E. (ESBLPE)
enterobacteria phage fr
enterobacterium
enterobactin
enterobiasis
    e. test
Enterobius (p)
    E. granuloma
    E. vermicularis
    E. vermicularis preparation
enterococcal
    e. bacteremia
    e. endocarditis
    e. urinary tract infection
enterococcemia
Enterococcus (b)
    E. asini
    E. avium
    E. avium bacteremia
    E. casseliflavus
    E. cecorum
    E. columbae
    E. dispar
    E. durans
    E. faecalis
    E. faecalis bacteremia
    E. faecium
    E. flavescens
    E. gallinarum
    E. haemoperoxidus
    E. hirae
    E. malodoratus

E. *moraviensis*
E. *mundtii*
E. *pseudoavium*
E. *raffinosus*
E. *saccharolyticus*
E. *seriolicida*
E. *solitarius*
E. *sulfureus*
E. *villorum*
enterococcus, pl. **enterococci**
  group D e.
  vancomycin-resistant e. (VRE)
enterocolitica
  Yersinia enterocolitica subsp. *e.*
enterocolitis
  antibiotic e.
  necrotizing e. (NEC)
  necrotizing amebic e.
  neutropenic e.
  purulent e.
  e. syndrome
enterocyte
  villus-attached e.
Enterocytozoon bieneusi (p)
enteroendocrine cell granule
enterohemorrhagic
  e. *Escherichia coli* (EHEC)
enteroidea
enteroinvasive *Escherichia coli* **(EIEC)**
Enteromonadidae
Enteromonadina
Enteromonas (p)
  E. *hominis*
  E. *intestinalis*
enteropathica
  acrodermatitis e.
enteropathogen
enteropathogenic
  e. *Escherichia coli* (EPEC)
  e. virus
enteropathy
  HIV e.
  protein-losing e.
enteropelogenes
  Aeromonas e.
enterophila
  Promicromonospora e.
enterostomy
Entero-Test
Enterotest

enterotoxigenic
  e. *Escherichia coli* (ETEC)
  e. staphylococcus
enterotoxigenicity
enterotoxin
  accessory cholera e. (ace)
  Clostridium perfringens e. (CPE)
  cytotonic e.
  diarrheal e.
  Escherichia coli e.
  staphylococcal e.
Enterotube II
enteroviral
  e. exanthema
  e. infection
  e. myocarditis
enterovirulent
  e. *Escherichia coli* (EEC)
  e. *Escherichia coli* group
Enterovirus (v)
enterovirus
  bovine e. 1–2
  e. culture
  human e. 68–71
  myelitic e.
  nonpolio e.
  porcine e. 1–11
  simian e. 1–18
enterozoic
enterozoon
Entex
  E. LA
  E. PSE
entire
Entoloma
  E. *lividum*
  E. *sinuatum*
Entolomataceae
Entomobirnavirus (v)
entomology
entomophila
  Candida e.
  Serratia e.
entomophilum
  Acholeplasma e.
  Mesoplasma e.
Entomophthoraceae
Entomophthorales
Entomophthora muscae
entomophthoramycosis
  e. basidiobolae
  e. conidiobolae

E

NOTES

Entomoplasma (b)
    E. ellychniae
    E. freundtii
    E. lucivorax
    E. luminosum
    E. melaleucae
    E. somnilux
Entomopoxvirinae
entomopoxvirus
    Demodema e.
Entomopoxvirus A (v)
Entomopoxvirus B (v)
Entomopoxvirus C (v)
Entopolypoides macaci (p)
entosarc
entozoa
entozoal
entozoon
Entrophen
Entuss-D Liquid
ENTV
    Entebbe bat virus
enucleation
enuresis
envelope
envenomation
Env gene
environment
    intrauterine e.
Environmental Protection Agency (EPA)
enzootic
    e. bovine leukosis
    e. encephalomyelitis
enzymatic immunoassay (EIA)
enzyme
    decarboxylase e.
    hepatic e.
    e. immunoassay (EIA)
    liver e.
    $NADP^+$ dependent malic e.
    nicotinamide adenine dinucleotide
      phosphate positive dependent
      malic e.
    pancreatic e.
enzyme-linked
    e.-l. immunosorbent assay (ELISA)
    e.-l. immunospot assay (ELISPOT)
**enzyme-multiplied immunoassay
technique (EMIT)**
enzymogenes
    Lysobacter enzymogenes subsp. *e.*
enzymopathy
    red cell e.
Enzymun-Test DNA Detection Assay
Eoastrion (b)
EORTC
    European Organization for Research and
    Treatment of Cancer

eosin
    hematoxylin and e. (H&E)
    e. methylene blue (EMB)
    e. methylene blue agar
eosinopenia
eosinophil
eosinophilia
    familial e.
    peripheral e.
    postinfectious e.
    simple pulmonary e.
    tropical pulmonary e.
eosinophilic
    e. abscess
    e. abscess formation
    e. bronchopneumonia
    e. cellulitis
    e. colitis
    e. folliculitis
    e. gastroenteritis
    e. leukemia
    e. lung disease
    e. meningitis
    e. meningoencephalitis
    e. microabscess
    e. nuclear inclusion body
    e. pleocytosis
    e. pneumonitis
    e. pustular folliculitis
    e. vasculitis
eosinophiluria
EP
    electrophoretic
EPA
    Environmental Protection Agency
EPEC
    enteropathogenic *Escherichia coli*
ependymal glial granulation
ependymitis
    e. granulosis
Eperythrozoon (b)
    E. coccoides
    E. ovis
    E. parvum
    E. suis
    E. wenyonii
ephedrine
Ephemerovirus (v)
epicardium
Epicauta
    E. fabricii
    E. pestifera
Epicoccum purpurascens (f)
epicyte
epidemic
    e. cerebrospinal fever
    e. cerebrospinal meningitis
    e. cholera

e. curve
e. diaphragmatic pleurisy
e. encephalitis
e. exanthema
e. gastroenteritis virus
e. hemorrhagic fever
e. hepatitis
e. jaundice
e. keratoconjunctivitis
e. keratoconjunctivitis virus
e. methicillin-resistant
  Staphylococcus aureus (EMRSA)
e. myalgia
e. myalgia virus
c. myositis
e. nausea
e. nonbacterial gastroenteritis
e. parotiditis
e. parotitis virus
e. pleurodynia
e. pleurodynia virus
e. polyarthritis
e. relapsing fever
e. roseola
e. transient diaphragmatic spasm
e. tremor
e. typhus
e. vomiting

epidemica
nephropathia e.
neuropathia e.

epidemicum
erythema arthriticum e.

epidemiography
epidemiologic
e. typing
epidemiological
epidemiologist
epidemiology
Center for Molecular E. (CEM)
molecular e.

epidermal
e. growth factor (EGF)
e. hyperplasia

epidermidis
Brevibacterium e.
Coniothecium e.
Staphylococcus e.

epidermodysplasia verruciformis
epidermoid carcinoma
epidermolytic toxin A, B

Epidermophyton (f)
E. floccosum
E. stockdaleae

Epidermoptidae
epidermotropism
epididymal tuberculosis
epididymis
epididymitis
bacteremic e.

epididymoorchitis
epidural
e. abscess
e. anesthesia

epidural disease
Epi EZ
Epifrin
epigastric
epiglottis
cherry red e.

epiglottitis
epilepsia partialis continua
epilepsy
continuous focal e.
Jacksonian e.
Kozhevnikov e.

epilepticus
status e.

epimastical fever
epimastigote
epimerite
epinephrine
aqueous e.

EpiPen
E. Jr

epiphyseal
epiphysis
epipodophyllotoxin
episcleral
episcleritis
episialin tumor
episodic
episphaeria
Nectria e.

epistaxis
Episthmium caninum (p)
4-epitetrodotoxin
anhydrotetrodotoxin -e.

epithelial
e. cast
e. cell
dysplastic e.
e. hyperplasia

NOTES

E

epithelial *(continued)*
> e. keratitis
> e. raft culture

epithelialization
> squamous e.

epithelioid
> e. angiomatosis
> e. cell

epithelioma contagiosum

epithelium
> columnar e.
> dome e.
> follicular e.
> retinal pigment e. (RPE)
> squamous e.
> villus e.

epithet
> specific e.

epitope
> B cell e.
> serovar-specific e.

epitope-specific therapy

epitrochlea

epitrochlear

epituberculosis
> bronchial e.

Epivir-HBV

epizoic
> e. commensalism

epizoon

epizootic
> e. cellulitis
> e. hemorrhagic disease virus 1–8 (EHDV)

EPOCH chemotherapy

epoetin alfa

epoprostenol

EPP
> extrapulmonary pneumocystosis

epsilometer test (E-test)

Epsilonretrovirus (v)

Epstein-Barr (EB)
> E.-B. nuclear antigen (EBNA)
> E.-B. virus (EBV)

equator

equi
> *Bovicola e.*
> *Chorioptes e.*
> *Corynebacterium e.*
> *Damalina e.*
> *Demodex e.*
> *Ehrlichia e.*
> *Moraxella e.*
> *Papulaspora e.*
> *Streptococcus equi* subsp. *e.*

equifetale
> *Acholeplasma e.*

equigenitalis
> *Haemophilus e.*
> *Taylorella e.*

equigenitalium
> *Mycoplasma e.*

equina
> *Setaria e.*

equine
> e. abortion virus (EAV)
> e. antirabies serum
> antirabies serum (e.)

equinum
> *Microsporum e.*
> *Trypanosoma e.*

equinus
> *Echinococcus granulosus e.*
> *Haemagogus e.*
> *Streptococcus e.*

equipercicus
> *Macrococcus e.*

equiperdum
> *Trypanosoma e.*

equipment
> personal protective e. (PPE)

equirhinis
> *Mycoplasma e.*

equisimilis
> *Streptococcus dysgalactiae* subsp. *e.*

equorum
> *Parascaris e.*
> *Staphylococcus e.*

equuli
> *Actinobacillus e.*

era
> preantibiotic e.

Eramycin

Eratyrus
> *E. cuspidatus*

Erb point

ERCP
> endoscopic retrograde cholangiopancreatography

erecta
> *Stigmatella e.*

Eremococcus coleocola (b)

Eremomyces langeronii (f)

Eret-147 virus

ergastensis
> *Candida e.*

ergot
> corn e.
> e. derivative

ergotamine

ergotism

Ericaceae

erikae
> *Culicoides e.*

erinacei
  Diphyllobothrium e.
erinaceieuropaei
  Spirometra e.
Eristalis
  E. *tenax*
ernobii
  Candida e.
erose
erosio interdigitalis blastomycetica
erosive *Candida* **balanitis**
Errantivirus (v)
erraticus
  Culex e.
  Ornithodoros e.
erucism
erumpens
  Streptomyces e.
eruption
  creeping e.
  cutaneous c.
  morbilliform e.
  papular e.
  scarlatiniform e.
  seabather's e.
  vesicular e.
  zosteriform c.
eruptive fever
ERV
  Estero Real virus
Erve virus
Erwinia (b)
  E. *alni*
  E. *amylovora*
  E. *ananas*
  E. *aphidicola*
  E. *billingiae*
  E. *cacticida*
  E. *cancerogena*
  E. *carnegieana*
  E. *carotovora* subsp. *atroseptica*
  E. *carotovora* subsp. *betavasculorum*
  E. *carotovora* subsp. *carotovora*
  E. *carotovora* subsp. *odorifera*
  E. *carotovora* subsp. *wasabiae*
  E. *chrysanthemi*
  E. *cypripedii*
  E. *dissolvens*
  E. *herbicola*
  E. *mallotivora*
  E. *milletiae*
  E. *nigrifluens*

E. *nimipressuralis*
E. *paradisiaca*
E. *persicina*
E. *psidii*
E. *pyrifoliae*
E. *quercina*
E. *rhapontici*
E. *rubrifaciens*
E. *salicis*
E. *stewartii*
E. *tracheiphila*
E. *uredovora*
Erwinieae
Erybid
Eryc
Eryderm Topical
Erygel Topical
Erymax Topical
EryPed
erysipelas
  swine e.
erysipeloid
  e. cellulitis
  e. of Rosenbach
Erysipelothrix (b)
  E. *rhusiopathiae*
  E. *tonsillarum*
erysipelotoxin
Erysiphaceae
Erysiphales
Ery-Tab
erythema
  e. arthriticum
  e. arthriticum epidemicum
  e. chronicum migrans (ECM)
  e. contagiosum
  e. induratum of Bazin
  e. infectiosum (EI)
  e. marginatum
  e. migrans (EM)
  e. multiforme
  e. nodosum
  e. nodosum leprosum
Erythema-Tab
erythematosus
  lupus e.
  systemic lupus e. (SLE)
erythematous
  e. band
  e. candidiasis
  e. cheilitis
  e. hyperpigmented papule

NOTES

E

erythematous *(continued)*
   e. lesion
   e. maculopapular rash
   e. papule
   e. submucosal plaque
erythra
   Legionella e.
erythraea
   Saccharopolyspora e.
erythraeus
   Streptomyces e.
erythrasma
erythreum
   Aeromicrobium e.
erythrinae
   Samsonia e.
erythritol fermentation test
Erythrobacter (b)
   E. litoralis
   E. longus
Erythro-Base
erythroblast
erythroblastopenia
   transient e.
erythroblastosis fetalis
Erythrocin
erythrocyte
   early e.
   e. flux
   late e.
   leukocyte-free packed e.
   parasitized e.
   e. sedimentation rate (ESR)
   senescent e.
   e. stroma
erythrocytic
   e. cycle
erythroderma
erythrogenic toxin
erythrogriseus
   Streptomyces e.
erythroid
   e. hyperplasia
   e. hypoplasia
   e. progenitor
Erythromicrobium ramosum (b)
Erythromonas ursincola (b)
erythromycin
   e. base
   e. and benzoyl peroxide
   e. estolate
   e. ethylsuccinate
   e. gluceptate
   e. lactobionate
   e. (ophthalmic/topical)
   e. stearate
   e. and sulfisoxazole
   e. (systemic)

erythromycin ophthalmic ointment
erythromycin-sulfa
erythromyxa
   Deinococcus e.
   Kocuria e.
erythrophagocytosis
erythroplasia of Queyrat
erythropoiesis
erythropoietin
erythropolis
   Rhodococcus e.
erythroprogenitor cell
erythropyknosis
erythrothorax
   Culex e.
Erythrovirus (v)
erytremiasis
Eryzole
ES
   Pertussin ES
ESBLPE
   extended-spectrum beta-lactamase-
   producing Enterobacteriaceae
escambiense
   Desulfomicrobium e.
eschar
Escherichia (b)
   E. adecarboxylata
   E. blattae
   E. coli
   E. coli enterotoxin
   E. coli inactive
   E. coli K12
   E. coli 39R861
   E. coli shiga toxin
   E. coli strain V/517
   E. coli verocytotoxin
   E. fergusonii
   E. hermannii
   E. vulneris
Escherichia-**7-11 virus**
Escherichieae
Esclim Transdermal
escomeli
   Simulium e.
esculenta
   Gyromitra e.
   Helvella e.
esculentum
   Lycopersicon e.
esculin
   bile e.
   e. hydrolysis
   e. hydrolysis test
E-Solve-2 Topical
esophageal
   e. atresia
   e. candidiasis

e. candidosis
e. intramural pseudodiverticulosis
e. lesion
e. ulceration
esophagitis
Candida e.
candidal e.
CMV e.
herpes e.
reflux e.
Strongyloides e.
esophagogastroduodenoscopy (EGD)
esophagospasm
esophagostomiasis
esotropia
espanaensis
Saccharothrix e.
espanolae
Methanobacterium e.
espejiana
Alteromonas e.
Pseudoalteromonas e.
espundia
ESR
erythrocyte sedimentation rate
ESRD
end-stage renal disease
essential
e. cryoglobulinemia
e. thrombocythemia
Estar
estazolam
e. drug interaction
esteraromaticum
Aureobacterium e.
Flavobacterium e.
Microbacterium e.
esterase
leukocyte e. (LE)
urine leukocyte e.
Estero Real virus (ERV)
estertheticum
Clostridium e.
esthiomene
Estinyl
estolate
erythromycin e.
Estrace Oral
Estraderm Transdermal
estradiol
ethinyl e.
Estra-L Injection

estramustine
Estring
estrogen
PMS-Conjugated E.'s
estunensis
Acetobacter e.
Acetobacter pasteurianus subsp. *e.*
ETEC
enterotoxigenic *Escherichia coli*
E-test
epsilometer test
E-test gradient minimal inhibitory
concentration
ethambutol (EMB)
ethanol
ethanolgignens
Acetivibrio e.
ethanolica
Candida e.
ethanolicus
Thermoanaerobacter e.
ethelae
Simulium e.
ethenogenes
Dehalococcoides e.
ethidium bromide
ethinyl estradiol
ethionamide
ethyl
e. alcohol
e. chloride vinyl spray
e. hydrocupreine
ethylenediaminetetraacetic acid
ethylene oxide (ETO)
2-ethyl-phosphonoformate
ethylsuccinate
erythromycin e.
Etibi
etiologic
e. agent
e. diagnosis
etiology
etli
Rhizobium e.
ET-NANBH
enterically transmitted non-A non-B
hepatitis
ETO
ethylene oxide
etoposide
cyclophosphamide, doxorubicin,
and e. (CDE)

NOTES

E

etretinate
ETS-2% Topical
Euantennariaceae
eubacteria
Eubacteriales
Eubacterium (b)
    E. *acidaminophilum*
    E. *aerofaciens*
    E. *aggregans*
    E. *alactolyticum*
    E. *angustum*
    E. *barkeri*
    E. *biforme*
    E. *brachy*
    E. *budayi*
    E. *callanderi*
    E. *cellulosolvens*
    E. *combesii*
    E. *contortum*
    E. *coprostanoligenes*
    E. *cylindroides*
    E. *desmolans*
    E. *dolichum*
    E. *eligens*
    E. *exiguum*
    E. *fissicatena*
    E. *formicigenerans*
    E. *fossor*
    E. *hadrum*
    E. *hallii*
    E. *infirmum*
    E. *lentum*
    E. *limosum*
    E. *minutum*
    E. *moniliforme*
    E. *multiforme*
    E. *nitritogenes*
    E. *nodatum*
    E. *oxidoreducens*
    E. *plautii*
    E. *plexicaudatum*
    E. *ramulus*
    E. *rectale*
    E. *ruminantium*
    E. *saburreum*
    E. *saphenum*
    E. *siraeum*
    E. *suis*
    E. *sulci*
    E. *tarantellae*
    E. *tardum*
    E. *tenue*
    E. *timidum*
    E. *tortuosum*
    E. *uniforme*
    E. *ventriosum*
    E. *xylanophilum*
    E. *yurii* subsp. *margaretiae*

    E. *yurii* subsp. *schtitka*
    E. *yurii* subsp. *yurii*
Eubaculovirinae
Eubenangee virus (EUBV)
EUBV
    Eubenangee virus
eucalypti
eucaryote (*var. of* eukaryote)
eucaryotic (*var. of* eukaryotic)
Euceratomycetaceae
Eucestoda
Eucoccidiorida
Eucocytis meeki
Eucoleus
eucrenophila
    Aeromonas *e.*
Eudal-SR
euedes
    Aedes *e.*
Euflagellata
Euglena
    E. *gracilis*
    E. *viridis*
Euglenidae
euglycemia
eugonadal
eugonic
    e. fermenter 4 (EF-4)
Eugregarinida
Eukaryotae
eukaryote, eucaryote
eukaryotic, eucaryotic
    e. organism
eumorphum
    Graphium *e.*
eumycetes
eumycetoma
Eumycetozoea
Eumycota
eumycotic mycetoma
Euparyphium (p)
    E. *beaveri*
    E. *ilocanum*
    E. *melis*
Eupenicillium (f)
    E. *abidjanum*
    E. *baarnense*
    E. *cinnamopurpureum*
    E. *idahoense*
    E. *luzoniacum*
    E. *meridianum*
    E. *philippinese*
    E. *pinetorium*
    E. *terreneum*
euphorbiae
    Candida *e.*
euphorbiiphila
    Candida *e.*

euphoria
Euploea corea
Euproctis chrysorrhoea
eupyrena
    Phoma e.
Eurax Topical
eurihalina
    Halomonas e.
    Volcaniella e.
eurocidicum
    Streptoverticillium e.
eurocidicus
    Streptomyces e.
Euroglyphus maynei (p)
europaea
    Nitrosomonas e.
    Pelistega e.
europaeiscabiei
    Streptomyces e.
europaeus
    Acetobacter e.
    Actinomyces e.
    Gluconacetobacter e.
European
    E. bone marrow transplantation
      (EBMT)
    E. eel virus
    E. Organization for Research and
      Treatment of Cancer (EORTC)
    E. tarantula
Eurotiaceae
Eurotiales
Eurotium (f)
    E. amstelodami
    E. chevalieri
    E. herbariorum
    E. repens
euroxenous parasite
euryadminiculum
    Simulium e.
euryhalinum
    Rhodovulum e.
euryhalinus
    Rhodobacter e.
eurythermus
    Streptomyces e.
Eurytrema pancraticum (p)
eurytremiasis
Eusimulium (p)
eustachian
Eustrongylides (p)

Eustrongylinae
eustrongyloides
eustrongyloidiasis
Eustrongylus gigas (p)
eutactus
    Coprococcus e.
euthyroid syndrome
Eutrombicula (p)
    E. alfreddugesi
    E. splendens
eutropha
    Ralstonia e.
eutrophus
    Alcaligenes e.
Euxoa auxiliaris
EVA
    American eel virus
evandroi
    Anopheles e.
evanescent lesion
evansae
    Anopheles e.
    Anopheles e. evansae
evansi
    Trypanosoma e.
evansii
    Azoarcus e.
evasion
    immune e.
event
    embolic e.
Everglades virus (EVEV)
Evergreen FPC fecal concentrator
everninomicin
Everone Injection
evestigatum
    Methanohalobium e.
EVEV
    Everglades virus
EVI
    endocardium, vascular structures,
      interstitium of striated muscle
    EVI antibody
Ewingella americana (b)
ewingii
    Ehrlichia e.
EX
    Diabetic Tussin EX
    Naldecon Senior EX
Ex
    Touro Ex

E

NOTES

exacerbation
  acute e.
  acute bacterial e.
Exact Cream
examination
  bimanual e.
  coprologic e.
  darkfield e.
  direct wet mount e.
  electron microscopic e.
  EM e.
  fecal e.
  macroscopic e.
  morphologic e.
  ova and parasites e.
  permanent stained smear e.
  proctoscopic e.
exanthem
  petechial e.
  roseoliform e.
  e. subitum
  vesicular e.
exanthema
  enteroviral e.
  epidemic e.
  viral e.
exanthematous
exanthesis arthrosia
excavation
  archeologic e.
Excedrin IB
Excellospora viridilutea (b)
excentricus
  Asticcacaulis e.
exchange transfusion
Excipulaceae
excision
  marginal e.
  wide e.
excisional biopsy
excisum
  Simulium e.
excitability
excitation
  anomalous atrioventricular e.
exconjugant
excoriation
excrescence
  electron-dense e.
excretion
  cortisol e.
excrucians
  Aedes e.
excursion
  respiratory e.
excystation
excysted

excysting
executive cognitive function (ECF)
exedens
  Nannocystis e.
Exelderm
  E. Topical
exertional dyspnea
exflagellation
exfoliation
exfoliative
  e. dermatitis
  e. toxin
exfoliatus
  Streptomyces e.
Exidine Scrub
exigua
  Haematobia irritans e.
  Slackia e.
Exiguobacterium (b)
  E. acetylicum
  E. aurantiacum
exiguum
  Eubacterium e.
  Simulium e.
exit-site infection
exoantigen
  e. extraction test
  e. test
Exobasidiaceae
Exobasidiales
Exobasidium (f)
exocrine
exocytosis
exoenzyme S
exoerythrocytic
  e. cycle
  e. stage
exogamy
exogenetic
exogenous
  e. cycle
exogenously
Exophiala (f)
  E. castellanii
  E. jeanselmei
  E. jeanselmei var. *heteromorpha*
  E. jeanselmei var. *lecaniicorni*
  E. mansoni
  E. moniliae
  E. pisciphila
  E. salmonis
  E. spinifera
exophyte
exophytic
  e. condyloma
exophytic nodule
exoskeleton
exospore

Exosporina (f)
exosporium
exoteric bacterium
exotoxin
    e. A
    bacterial e.
    pertussis e.
    Pseudomonas e. (PE)
    streptococcal pyrogenic e.
exotropia
expanded
    e. access
    e. range HIV-1 RNA
expansum
    Penicillium e.
Expectorant
    Acet-Am E.
    Anti-Tuss E.
    Balminil E.
    Benylin E.
    Calmylin E.
    Centratuss DM E.
    Codafed E.
    CoSudafed E.
    Cough Syrup DM Decongestant E.
    Decohistine E.
    Detussin E.
    Dihistine E.
    DM E Suppressant E.
    Fedahist E.
    Genamin E.
    GuiaCough E.
    Isoclor E.
    Koffex E.
    Myminic E.
    Novahistex DM E.
    Novahistine DM E.
    Nucofed Pediatric E.
    Phenhist E.
    Ru-Tuss E.
    Silaminic E.
    Sirop E.
    SRC E.
    Sudafed E.
    Triaminic Decongestant & E.
    Tri-Clear E.
    Triphenyl E.
    Tussafin E.
expectorated sputum
expenditure
    resting energy e. (REE)
    total energy e. (TEE)

experience
    AIDS Link to Intravenous E.'s
    (ALIVE)
experimental
    e. allergic neuritis
    e. autoimmune encephalitis
exposure
    de novo e.
    limitation of e.
    potential e.
    repeated e.
expressed
    baculovirus e.
exsanguinating hemoptysis
exsanguination
Exsel
    E. Shampoo
Exserohilum (f)
    E. longirostratum
    E. mcginnisii
    E. rostratum
extended-spectrum
    e.-s. beta-lactamase-producing
    Enterobacteriaceae (ESBLPE)
extension
    reverse transcriptase primer e.
    (RTPE)
extensus
    Dactylogyrus e.
Extentabs
externa
    acute diffuse otitis e.
    gnathostomiasis e.
    malignant otitis e.
    otitis e.
external
    e. beam radiotherapy
    e. genital swab
externalization
extorquens
    Methylobacterium e.
    Protomonas e.
Extra
    E. Action Cough syrup
    E. Strength Doan's
extracapsular cataract extraction
    (ECCE)
extracellular
    e. water (ECW)
extracerebral *Toxoplasma gondii*
extrachromosomal
extrachromosomally

E

NOTES

extracorporeal
extract
    aqueous e.
extraction
    DNA e.
    extracapsular cataract e. (ECCE)
    intracapsular cataract e. (ICCE)
    phenol-chloroform e.
extracutaneous sporotrichosis
extracytoplasmic
extradural empyema
extragastrointestinal anisakidosis
extraglandular
extrahepatic
extraintestinal
    e. amebiasis
    e. infection
extraluminal
extramacular
extranodal disease
extranodal lymphoma
extraocularis
    Loa e.
extraocular motility
extrapolate
extrapolating
extrapulmonary
    e. cryptococcosis
    e. pneumocystosis (EPP)
    e. tuberculosis
extrapyramidal symptoms
extrarenal
extrasalivary mumps
extrasystole
extrauterine

extravasated
extravasation
extreme acanthosis
extremely low birth weight (ELBW)
extructa
    Bulleidia e. (b)
extubate
exudate
    fibrinopurulent e.
    mucopurulent endocervical e.
    purulent endocervical e.
    pyogenic e.
    seropurulent e.
    vitreous e.
    yellow e.
exudation
    retinal e.
exudative pharyngitis
Eyach virus (EYAV)
EYAV
    Eyach virus
eye
    e. infection
    red e.
    e. smear
    e. swab
    e. swab *Chlamydia* culture
    e. worm
eyelid
    e. infection
    tuberculosis of e.
eyespot
EZ
    Epi EZ

F

F agent
F pili
F plasmid
F116 virus
Fab

digoxin immune F.
Fabavirus (v)
fabianii

Candida f.
Fabospora
fabri

Hysterothylacium f.
fabricii

Epicauta f.
Fabry tinctura
fabyrii

Debaryomyces hansonii var. *f.*
Facey's Paddock virus (FPV)
facialis

Anthomyia f.
facial palsy
faciei

tinea f.
facies

dengue f.
moon f.
facile

Acidiphilium f.
Hyphomicrobium facile subsp. *f.*
facilis

Acidocella f.
Acidovorax f.
Pseudomonas f.
Facklamia (b)

F. *hominis*
F. *ignava*
F. *languida*
F. *miroungae*
F. *sourekii*
F. *tabacinasalis*
FACScan
factive
factor

anti-von Willebrand f. (anti-vWF)
bacteriocin f.
behavioral risk f.
bifidus f.
biotic f.
CAMP f.
cellular transcription f.
clumping f.
coagulase-reacting f. (CRF)
colony-stimulating f. (CSF)
edema f. (EF)

epidermal growth f. (EGF)
f. essential for resistance to
methicillin (*fem* factor)
fem f.
factor essential for resistance to
methicillin
fertility f.
granulocyte colony-stimulating f.
(G-CSF)
granulocyte/macrophage colony-
stimulating f. (GM-CSF, rGM-
CSF)
histamine-sensitizing f.
hyperglyccmic-glycogenolytic f.
(HGE)
islet-activating f.
lethal f. (LF)
lymphocytosis-promoting f.
macrophage colony-stimulating f.
(M-CSF)
mitogenic f.
neural growth f.
obstetric f.
platelet-activating f. (PAF)
recombinant f. VIII
rheumatoid f. (RF)
serum opacity f.
serum resistance f.
sex f.
SLR f.
tracheal colonization f.
tumor necrosis f. (TNF)
V f.
vascular endothelial growth
factor/vascular permeability f.
(VEGF/VPF)
X f.
factor-1
insulinlike growth f. (IGF-1)
factor-alpha
tumor necrosis f.-a. (TNF-a, TNF-
alpha)
factor H
facultative
f. anaerobe
f. bacteria
f. parasite
f. saprophyte
facultatively
faecale
Acetomicrobium f.
Trichosporon f.
faecalis
Alcaligenes faecalis subsp. *f.*

F

faecalis (*continued*)
> *Enterococcus f.*
> *Streptococcus f.*

faecitabidus
> *Rarobacter f.*

faecium
> *Brachybacterium f.*
> *Enterococcus f.*
> *Phascolarctobacterium f.*
> *Sphingobacterium f.*
> *Streptococcus f.*
> VanB *Enterococcus f.* (VBEF)
> vancomycin-resistant *Enterococcus f.* (VREF)

faeni
> *Frigoribacterium f.*
> *Micropolyspora f.*

Faenia rectivirgula (b)
Faget sign

faginatum
> *Cylindrocarpon f.*

failure
> congestive heart f. (CHF)
> endocrine gland f.
> fulminant hepatic f. (FHF)
> growth f.
> hepatic f.
> ovarian f.
> renal f.
> f. to thrive (FTT)
> virologic f.

fainei
> *Leptospira f.*

fairfieldensis
> *Legionella f.*

Fairley test

falcatus
> *Stellantchasmus f.*

falciforme
> *Acremonium f.*

falciparum
> f. fever
> *Laverania f.*
> f. malaria
> *Plasmodium f.*

Falcivibrio (b)
> *F. grandis*
> *F. vaginalis*

falconis
> *Mycoplasma f.*

fallax
> *Clostridium f.*
> *Leuconostoc f.*
> *Mycobacterium f.*

fallonii
> *Legionella f.*

fallopian
> f. tube
> f. tube tuberculosis

false
> f. agglutination
> f. branching
> f. labor
> f. morel

false-negative
> f.-n. patch test
> f.-n. reaction

falsenii
> *Corynebacterium f.*

falsus
> *Pseudocaedibacter f.*

famata
> *Candida f.*
> *Candida famata* var. *f.*

famciclovir
familial
> f. eosinophilia
> f. Mediterranean fever (FMF)

family
famotidine
Famvir
Fanconi-like syndrome
Fanconi syndrome
Fannia
> *F. benjamini*
> *F. canicularis*
> *F. incisurata*
> *F. leucosticta*
> *F. manicata*
> *F. pusio*
> *F. scalaris*

Fansidar
Fansimef
Farallon virus (FARV)
farauti
> *Anopheles f.*

Farazolidone
farciminis
> *Lactobacillus f.*

farciminosum
> *Histoplasma capsulatum* var. *f.*

farcinica
> *Nocardia f.*

farcinogenes
> *Mycobacterium f.*

Far East Russian encephalitis
farinae
> *Dermatophagoides f.*
> *Tyrophagus f.*

farinosa
> *Pichia f.*

farmeri
> *Citrobacter f.*

farmer's lung

FARV
> Farallon virus

FAS
> fluorescent actin staining
> FAS test

fascial plane

fascians
> *Corynebacterium f.*
> *Rhodococcus f.*

fasciatum
> *Heliophilum f.*

fasciatus
> *Nosopsyllus f.*

fasciculata
> *Crithidia f.*

fasciculation

fasciculus
> *Aquaspirillum f.*
> *Prolinoborus f.*

fasciitis
> dissecting f.
> necrotizing f.

fasciocutaneous flap

Fasciola (p)
> *F. gigantica*
> *F. hepatica*
> *F. jacksoni*
> *F. magna*

fasciolaris
> *Cysticercus f.*
> *Fimbriaria f.*

Fascioletta ilocana (p)

fascioliasis

fasciolid

Fasciolidae

Fascioloides magna (p)

fasciolopsiasis

Fasciolopsis

Fasciolopsis buski (p)

fasciotomy

fast

fastidiosa
> *Actinomadura f.*
> *Amycolatopsis f.*
> *Microtetraspora f.*
> *Nonomuraea f.*
> *Xylella f.*

fastidiosum
> *Aeromicrobium f.*
> *Mycoplasma f.*

fastidiosus
> *Bacillus f.*
> *Nocardioides f.*

fastidious
> f. anaerobe agar
> f. organism

fasting glucose

fastness
> acid f.

fastosum
> *Platynosomum f.*

fat
> dorsocervical f.
> fecal f.
> f. necrosis
> total abdominal f. (TAT)
> truncal f.
> visceral abdominal f. (VAT)
> f. wasting

fatal
> f. disseminated infection
> f. familial insomnia (FFI)

fatality rate

fat-free mass (FFM)

fatigability

fatty
> f. acid analysis
> f. cast
> f. degeneration
> f. infiltration of the liver
> f. liver

faucial

faucium
> *Mycoplasma f.*

fauriae
> *Roseomonas f.*

fausti
> *Anopheles f.*

favic chandelier

FA virus

favosa
> porrigo f.
> tinea f.

favus

FBL
> focal brain lesion

5-FC
> 5-flucytosine
> 5-fluorocytosine
> 5-FC level

5-Fc

FC3-9 virus

F

NOTES

FDA
Food and Drug Administration
Fdda
FDV
Fiji disease virus
feature
morphologic f.
febricitans
pes f.
febrile
f. agglutinin
f. convulsion
f. fasciolitic eosinophilic syndrome
fecal
f. alpha$_2$-antitrypsin
f. concentration
f. concentration test
f. contamination
f. examination
f. fat
f. leukocyte
f. leukocyte stain
f. smear
f. transmission
fecal-oral
f.-o. non-A non-B hepatitis
f.-o. route
f.-o. spread
feces
colloidal f.
fibrous f.
fecoculture technique
Fedahist
F. Expectorant
F. Expectorant Pediatric
F. tablet
feeding
enteral f.
tube f.
feeleii
Legionella f.
Feinberg-Whittington medium
Felicola subrostratus (p)
felid herpesvirus 1
felidis
Echinococcus f.
felifaucium
Mycoplasma f.
feliminutum
Mycoplasma f.
feline
f. calicivirus
f. herpesvirus
f. immunodeficiency virus (FIV)
f. infectious enteritis
f. infectious peritonitis virus
(FIPV)

f. panleukopenia virus (FPLV, FPV)
f. parvovirus
felineus
Opisthorchis f.
felinum
Corynebacterium f.
Ureaplasma f.
felis
Afipia f.
Chlamydophila f.
Ctenocephalides f.
Cytauxcoon f.
Haemobartonella f.
Haemophilus f.
Helicobacter f.
Isospora f.
Mycoplasma f.
Rickettsia f.
Staphylococcus f.
felleus
Streptomyces f.
felsineum
Clostridium f.
female
f. genital tract
f. genital tract infection
fem **factor**
Femguard
Femizole-7
Femizol-M
Femogen
F. Forte
Femogex
femoral
f. condyle
f. head
f. vein
Fenesin
F. DM
Fenestellaceae
fenestralis
Anisopus f.
fenestration
Fenicol
Fennellia (f)
F. flavipes
F. nivea
fennelliae
Campylobacter f.
Helicobacter f.
fennica
Candida f.
fentanyl patch
fenticonazole
feraegula
Cryptococcus f.
fer-de-lance virus

fergusonii
    Escherichia f.
Ferimmune
fermentans
    Acidaminococcus f.
    Brevibacterium f.
    Cellulomonas f.
    Cytophaga f.
    Dyadobacter f.
    Geothrix f.
    Halanaerobium f.
    Mycoplasma f.
    Pichia f.
    Rhodoferax f.
fermentati
    Saccharomyces f.
fermentation
    lactose f.
    mannitol f.
fermentative
fermentatus
    Saccharobacter f.
fermented
    f. beaver tail
    f. food
    f. food botulism
fermenter
    dysgonic f. 2 (DF-2)
    dysgonic f. 3
    eugonic f. 4 (EF-4)
    glucose f.
fermenticarens
    Candida f.
Fermentotrichon (f)
fermentum
    Lactobacillus f.
ferox
    Dinobdella f.
    Psorophora f.
ferragutiae
    Buttiauxella f.
Ferribacterium linneticum (b)
ferric ammonium sulfate
Ferrimonas balearica (b)
ferrireducens
    Geovibrio f.
    Thermoterrabacterium f.
Ferroglobus placidus (b)
ferrooxidans
    Acidimicrobium f.
    Acidithiobacillus f.

    Leptospirillum f.
    Thiobacillus f.
ferrophilus
    Palaeococcus f.
Ferroplasma acidiphilum (b)
ferruginea
    Actinomadura f.
    Catellatospora f.
    Gallionella f.
    Micromonospora echinospora subsp.
      f.
    Microtetraspora f.
    Nonomuraea f.
ferrugineum
    Agrobacterium f.
    Flavobacterium f.
    Microsporum f.
    Pedomicrobium f.
ferrugineus
    Actinoplanes f.
    Cystobacter f.
ferruginosa
    Tubifera f.
fertility
    f. agent
    f. factor
ferus
    Streptococcus f.
fervens
    Methanococcus f.
    Streptomyces f.
    Streptomyces fervens subsp. f.
    Streptoverticillium fervens subsp. f.
Fervidobacterium (b)
    F. gondwanense
    F. islandicum
    F. nodosum
    F. pennivorans
fervidum
    Clostridium f.
fervidus
    Caloramator f.
    Methanothermus f.
fessus
    Vagococcus f.
festoon
fetalis
    Alishewanella f.
    erythroblastosis f.
    hydrops f.
fetal resorption

F

NOTES

fetus

 Campylobacter fetus subsp. *f.*

fever

acute rheumatic f. (ARF)
Aden f.
aestivoautumnal f.
African hemorrhagic f.
Argentine hemorrhagic f.
arthropod-borne viral hemorrhagic f.
Assam f.
autumn f.
autumnal f.
benign tertian f.
black f.
blackwater f.
f. blister
blue f.
Bolivian hemorrhagic f.
bouquet f.
boutonneuse f.
bovine ephemeral f. (BEFV)
Brazilian hemorrhagic f.
Brazilian purpuric f. (BPF)
breakbone f.
Bunyamwera f.
Burdwan f.
cachectic f.
canefield f.
canicola f.
central European tick-borne f.
cerebrospinal f.
childbed f.
Colorado tick f. (CTF)
Congolian red f.
Crimean-Congo f.
Crimean-Congo hemorrhagic f. (C-CHFV)
dandy f.
date f.
5-day f.
40-day f.
deer fly f.
dengue f.
dengue hemorrhagic f. (DHF)
desert f.
diphasic milk f.
drug f.
dumdum f.
Dutton relapsing f.
Ebola virus hemorrhagic f.
endemic relapsing f.
enteric f.
entericoid f.
epidemic cerebrospinal f.
epidemic hemorrhagic f.
epidemic relapsing f.
epimastical f.
eruptive f.

falciparum f.
familial Mediterranean f. (FMF)
field f.
Filovirus hemorrhagic f.
flood f.
Fort Bragg f.
Gambian f.
glandular f.
grain f.
Haverhill f.
hematuric bilious f.
hemoglobinuric f.
hemorrhagic f.
herpetic f.
hospital f.
icterohemorrhagic f.
Ilheus f.
intermittent malarial f.
inundation f.
island f.
jail f.
Japanese river f.
jungle yellow f.
Katayama f.
kedani f.
Kew Gardens f.
Kinkiang f.
Korean hemorrhagic f. (KHF)
Lassa f.
laurel f.
lemming f.
louse-borne relapsing f.
low-grade f.
malarial f.
malignant catarrhal f.
malignant tertian f.
Malta f.
Manchurian f.
Marburg f.
Marseilles f.
marsh f.
Mediterranean erythematous f.
Mediterranean exanthematous f.
Mediterranean spotted f.
Meuse f.
Mexican spotted f.
miniature scarlet f.
monoleptic f.
Mossman f.
mud f.
nanukayami f.
neutropenic f.
nodal f.
North Queensland tick f.
Omsk hemorrhagic f.
O'nyong-nyong f.
Oroya f.
Pahvant Valley f.

paludal f.
pappataci f.
papular f.
paratyphoid f.
parenteric f.
parrot f.
Persian relapsing f.
pharyngoconjunctival f.
phlebotomus f.
f. phobia
polka f.
polyleptic f.
Pontiac f.
Potomac f.
pretibial f.
protein f.
puerperal f.
Pym f.
pyogenic f.
Q f.
quartan f.
query f.
quintan f.
quotidian f.
rabbit f.
rat bite f.
recrudescent typhus f.
recurrent f.
red f.
relapsing f.
remittent malarial f.
remitting f.
rheumatic f.
Rift Valley f.
Rocky Mountain spotless f.
Rocky Mountain spotted f. (RMSF)
Roman f.
rose f.
Ross River f.
sandfly f.
San Joaquin f.
São Paulo f.
scarlet f.
scarlet f. toxin A
Sennetsu f.
septic scarlet f.
seven-day f.
shank f.
shinbone f.
ship f.
shipping f.
Sindbis f.

slow f.
snail f.
solar f.
f. sore
South African tick-bite f.
f. spike
spirillum f.
spotted f.
staphylococcal scarlet f.
swamp f.
swine f.
swineherd f.
symptomatic f.
syphilitic f.
tertian f.
three-day f.
tick bite f.
tick-borne relapsing f.
Tobia f.
toxic scarlet f.
trench f.
Triaminic Cold & F.
tsutsugamushi f.
typhoid f.
undulant f.
f. of unknown origin (FUO)
urticarial f.
uveoparotid f.
Uzbekistan hemorrhagic f.
valley f.
Venezuelan hemorrhagic f.
viral hemorrhagic f.
vivax f.
Volhynia f.
Wesselsbron f.
West African f.
West Nile f.
wound f.
Yangtze Valley f.
yellow f. (YF)
Zika f.

Feverall
fexofenadine
FFA
    free fatty acid
FFE
    flexible fiberoptic endoscope
FFI
    fatal familial insomnia
FFM
    fat-free mass

F

NOTES

FFP
> fresh frozen plasma

FFPB
> flexible fiberoptic bronchoscopy with protected brush

F1, F2 virus

FH5 virus

FHA
> filamentous hemagglutinin

FHF
> fulminant hepatic failure

fiber
> elastin f.

fibergastroscopy

fiberoptic bronchoscopy (FOB)

fibrata
> *Methylosarcina f.*

Fibricola seoulensis (p)

fibril
> subpellicular f.

fibrin

fibrinflatum
> *Simulium f.*

fibrinogen

fibrinolysis test

fibrinopurulent
> f. exudate
> f. pneumonitis

fibrinous

fibrisolvens
> *Butyrivibrio f.*

Fibrobacter (b)
> *F. intestinalis*
> *F. succinogenes* subsp. *elongatus*
> *F. succinogenes* subsp. *succinogenes*

fibroblastic reaction

fibrocalcific arteriopathy

fibroelastosis
> endocardial f. (EFE)

fibroinflammatory
> immunoincompetent f.

fibronectin

fibrosa
> *Actinomadura f.*

fibrosing mediastinitis

fibrosis
> chronic interstitial f.
> cystic f. (CF)
> idiopathic pulmonary f.
> interstitial f.
> Jaccoud periarticular f.
> mediastinal f.
> periportal f.
> pipestem f.
> Symmers clay pipestem f.

fibrotic bladder

fibrous feces

fibuliger
> *Endomyces f.*
> *Endomycopsis f.*

FIC
> fractional inhibitory concentration
> FIC index

ficaria
> *Serratia f.*

fici
> *Geotrichum f.*

ficuserectae
> *Pseudomonas f.*

fiddleback spider

field
> contour-clamped homogeneous electric f. (CHEF)
> f. fever
> f. inversion gel electrophoresis (FIGE)
> f. trial
> f. vole

fiery serpent worm

fifth
> f. disease

FIGE
> field inversion gel electrophoresis

Figulus sublaevis

Fiji disease virus (FDV)

Fijivirus (v)

filaceous

filament
> axial f.
> parabasal f.

filamentary keratitis

filamentosa
> *Choanotaenia f.*

filamentosus
> *Streptomyces f.*

filamentous
> f. colony
> f. fungus
> f. hemagglutinin (FHA)
> f. phage virus

filamentus
> *Polaribacter f.*

filar

filaria
> *Dictyocaulus f.*

filarial
> f. funiculitis
> f. hydrocele
> f. infection
> f. parasite
> f. periodicity
> f. synovitis

filariasis
> bancroftian f.
> brugian f.

human lymphatic f.
lymphatic f.
Malayan f.
occult f.
periodic f.
f. peripheral blood preparation
filaricidal
filaricide
filariform
f. larva
Filariidae
Filaroidea
Filaroides hirthi (p)
Fildes medium
filgrastim
Filibacter limicola (b)
filicollis
Nematodirus f.
Filifactor (b)
F. alocis
F. villosus
filiform
f. wart
filiforme
Contracaecum f.
filiformis
Alysiella f.
Flexibacter f.
Holdemania f.
Methanobrevibacter f.
Thermus f.
Vitreoscilla f.
filing
iron f.
filipinensis
Streptomyces f.
Filisoma
filling cystometrogram
Filmtabs
Biaxin F.
Filobacillus milosensis (b)
Filobasidiaceae
Filobasidiales
Filobasidiella neoformans var. *neoformans*
(f)
Filobasidium (f)
F. capsuligenum
F. floriforme
F. uniguttulatum
Filomicrobium fusiforme (b)
Filoviridae

Filovirus (v)
F. hemorrhagic fever
filter
heat and moisture exchanging f.
(HMEF)
HEPA f.
high-efficiency particulate air f.
Millipore f.
Nucleopore f.
Nytrel f.
f. in situ hybridization test
filterable agent
Fimbriaria fasciolaris
Fimbriariinae
fimbriated
fimbriatus
Streptomyces f.
fimetarium
Acetobacterium f.
Clostridium f.
fimi
Cellulomonas f.
fimicarius
Streptomyces f.
fimicola
Sordaria f.
final host
finasteride
Finegoldia magna (b)
fine-needle
f.-n. aspirate
f.-n. aspiration
finger
clubbing of f.'s
fingerprinting
direct amplification f. (DAF)
finlandica
Pichia f.
finlayi
Streptomyces f.
finnii
Thermoanaerobacter f.
Thermoanaerobacter brockii subsp.
f.
FIPV
feline infectious peritonitis virus
fire ant
firmetaria
Candida f.
firmus
Bacillus f.
First aid Antibiotics + Moisturizer

NOTES

F

first-catch urine specimen
first-void
> f.-v. urine (FVU)
> f.-v. urine sample

fischeri
> Neosartorya f.
> Photobacterium f.
> Vibrio f.

fish
> f. poisoning
> f. tapeworm anemia

Fisher Guillain-Barré syndrome
fisherianus
> Aspergillus f.

fishtank granuloma
fissicatena
> Eubacterium f.

fission
> binary f.
> f. fungus
> multiple f.
> simple f.

fissiparity
fissiparous
fissure
> anal f.
> bowel f.

fissurella
> Phaeotheca f.

fistula
> arteriovenous f. (AVF)
> bronchohepatic f.
> bronchopleural f.
> cholecystoduodenal f.
> colocutaneous f.
> draining f.
> urethral f.

FITC
> fluorescein isothiocyanate

FITC-conjugated polyvalent antiserum
fitchii
> Aedes f.

Fitz-Hugh-Curtis syndrome
FIV
> feline immunodeficiency virus

fixation
> complement f. (CF)
> formalin f.

fixative
> AFA f.
> alcohol-glycerin f.
> PVA f.
> SAF f.
> single vial f.

flaccid paralysis
flaccumfaciens
> Corynebacterium f.
> Curtobacterium f.

flagella
flagellar
> f. agglutinin
> f. H antigen
> f. stain

Flagellata
flagellate
> collared f.

flagellated
flagellatum
> Lyticum f.

flagellatus
> Methylobacillus f.

flagellin
flagellosis
Flagyl
> F. Oral

Flamazine
flame cell
Flammeovirga aprica (b)
Flanders virus (FLAV)
flap
> fasciocutaneous f.

flareri
> Candida famata var. f.

FlashTrack DNA Probe assay
flask
> hatching f.
> volumetric f.

flat
> f. condyloma
> f. wart

flat-topped
flatulence
flatworm
> parasitic f.

FLAV
> Flanders virus

flava
> Actinomadura f.
> Chainia f.
> Haemaphysalis f.
> Hydrogenophaga f.
> Lechevalieria f.
> Neisseria f.
> Nocardiopsis f.
> Pseudomonas f.
> Saccharothrix f.

flavea
> Microellobosporia f.

flavefaciens
> Ruminococcus f.

flaveolus
> Streptomyces f.

flavescens
> Aedes f.
> Arthrobacter f.
> Arthroderma f.

Aureobacterium *f.*
Corynebacterium *f.*
Enterococcus *f.*
Microbacterium *f.*
Microsporum *f.*
Mycobacterium *f.*
Myxococcus *f.*
Neisseria *f.*
Pseudomonas *f.*

flaveus
Streptomyces *f.*

flavida
Kribbella *f.*
Nesotriatoma *f.*

flavidofuscus
Streptomyces *f.*

flavidovirens
Streptomyces *f.*

flavidum
Acetomicrobium *f.*

flavifemur
Simulium *f.*

flavigena
Cellulomonas *f.*

Flavimonas oryzihabitans (b)

flavipes
Aspergillus *f.*
Fennellia *f.*

flavipictum
Simulium *f.*

flaviscleroticus
Streptomyces *f.*

flaviscutellata
Lutzomyia *f.*

flavithermus
Anoxybacillus *f.*

flaviviral encephalitis
Flaviviridae
Flavivirus (v)
flavivirus
Flavobacteriaceae
Flavobacterium (b)
F. acidificum
F. acidurans
F. aquatile
F. balustinum
F. branchiophilum
F. breve
F. capsulatum
F. columnare
F. devorans
F. esteraromaticum

F. ferrugineum
F. flevense
F. frigidarium
F. gillisiae
F. gleum
F. gondwanense
F. halmephilum
F. heparinum
F. hibernum
F. hydatis
F. indologenes
F. indoltheticum
F. johnsoniae
F. marinotypicum
F. meningosepticum
F. mizutaii
F. multivorum
F. oceanosedimentum
F. odoratum
F. okeanokoites
F. pectinovorum
F. psychrophilum
F. resinovorum
F. saccharophilum
F. salegens
F. scophthalmum
F. spiritivorum
F. succinicans
F. tegetincola
F. thalpophilum
F. thermophilum
F. uliginosum
F. xanthum
F. yabuuchiae

flavochromogenes
flavofungini
Streptomyces *f.*

flavofuscus
Streptomyces *f.*
Streptomyces globisporus subsp. *f.*

flavogenita
Stemonitis *f.*

flavogriseus
Streptomyces *f.*

flavopersicum
Streptoverticillium *f.*

flavopersicus
Streptomyces *f.*

flavopubescens
Simulium *f.*

flavorosea
Nocardia *f.*

NOTES

flavotricini
    Streptomyces f.
flavovariabilis
    Streptomyces f.
flavovirens
    Streptomyces f.
flavoviridis
    Streptomyces f.
flavus
    Arthrobacter f.
    Aspergillus f.
    Cryptococcus f.
    Xanthobacter f.
flea
    sand f.
flea-borne typhus
flecainide
flectens
    Pseudomonas f.
Flectobacillus (b)
    F. glomeratus
    F. major
    F. marinus
fleroxacin
flesh fly
fletcheri
    Leptotrombidium f.
Fletcher medium
fleurettii
    Staphylococcus f.
FLEV
    Flexal virus
flevense
    Flavobacterium f.
flevensis
    Cytophaga f.
Flexal virus (FLEV)
Flexibacter (b)
    F. aggregans
    F. aurantiacus
    F. canadensis
    F. columnaris
    F. elegans
    F. filiformis
    F. flexilis
    F. japonensis
    F. litoralis
    F. maritimus
    F. ovolyticus
    F. polymorphus
    F. psychrophilus
    F. roseolus
    F. ruber
    F. sancti
    F. tractuosus
Flexibacteriae
flexibilis
    Serpens f.

flexible
    f. bronchoscopy
    f. fiberoptic bronchoscopy with protected brush (FFPB)
    f. fiberoptic endoscope (FFE)
    f. fiberoptic endoscopy
flexilis
    Flexibacter f.
Flexistipes sinusarabici (b)
Flexithrix dorotheae (b)
Flexner bacillus
flexneri
    Shigella f.
flexuosa
    Actinomadura f.
    Microtetraspora f.
    Nonomuraea f.
flexus
    Bacillus f.
FLN
    fluorescence-lactose-denitrification medium
floater
floccose
floccosum
    Epidermophyton f.
flocculare
    Mycoplasma f.
flocculation
    f. test
flocculent
    f. discharge
flocculiformis
    Trichococcus f.
flocculus
    Streptomyces f.
flock house virus
flood fever
flora
    aerobic microbial f.
    anaerobic microbial f.
    cervicovaginal f.
    infectious f.
    mixed aerobic and anaerobic f.
    normal gut f.
    vaginal f.
florentinus
    Saccharomyces f.
floricola
    Candida f.
    Spiroplasma f.
floridae
    Streptomyces f.
floridensis
    Culicoides f.
floriforme
    Filobasidium f.

Florone
  F. E
florum
  Acholeplasma f.
  Mesoplasma f.
flotation method
flow
  bone scan with f.
  f. cytometric analysis
  f. cytometry
  laminar air f. (LAF)
Floxin
  F. IV
flucloxacillin
fluconazole
fluconazole-refractory
  f.-r. oral candidiasis
fluconazole-refractory disease
fluctuant
fluctuating
flucytosine
  f. level
5-flucytosine (5-FC)
fludarabine
  f. monophosphate
fludrocortisone
flueggei
  Selenomonas f.
fluid
  ascitic f.
  bronchoalveolar lavage f.
  cerebrospinal f. (CSF)
  f. cytology
  peritoneal f.
  pleural f.
  f. replacement
  f. resuscitation
  synovial f.
  f. tetanus toxoid
  vesicular f.
  f. wave
Flu-Imune
fluke
  giant intestinal f.
  rat lung f.
flukei
  Culicoides f.
  Muscina f.
flu-like syndrome
Flumadine

fluminensis
  Anopheles f.
  Beijerinckia f.
fluocinolone
fluocinonide
  f. cream
Fluoderm
Fluogen
Fluonid Topical
fluorescein
  f. isothiocyanate (FITC)
fluorescein-conjugated polyclonal antibody
fluorescence
  f. microscopy
  f. polarization immunoassay (FPIA)
  f. spectroscopy
fluorescence-lactose-denitrification medium (FLN)
fluorescens
  Pseudomonas f.
  Streptomyces f.
fluorescent
  f. actin staining (FAS)
  f. actin staining test
  f. antibody kit
  f. treponemal antibody absorption (FTA-ABS, FTA-Abs)
  f. treponemal antibody absorption test (FTA-ABS, FTA-Abs)
  f. treponemal antibody adsorption (FTA-ABS, FTA-Abs)
  f. treponemal antigen-absorption
  f. treponemal antigen-absorption test
fluorescent-denitrification test
Fluoribacter (b)
  F. bozemanae
  F. dumoffii
  F. gormanii
fluoride
fluorochrome
  f. chitin staining
  f. stain
5-fluorocytosine (5-FC)
5-fluorocytozine
fluorodeoxyglucose
fluorogram
fluorometholone
  sulfacetamide sodium and f.
fluoronaphthyrodine antibiotic
fluoroquinolone
  f. monotherapy

F

NOTES

4-fluoroquinolone
fluoroquinolone(6)
fluoroquinolone-resistant
5-fluorouracil
fluoxetine
fluoxymesterone
flurandrenolide
flurazepam
Flurosyn Topical
flush
 ciliary f.
Flushield
flushing
Flutex Topical
fluticasone (topical)
Flutone
fluvialis
 Vagococcus f.
 Vibrio f.
fluviatile
 Chromobacterium f.
fluviatilis
 Candida f.
 Iodobacter f.
Fluviral
Fluvirin
flu virus vaccine
flux
 erythrocyte f.
fluximetry
 laser Doppler f.
Fluzone
fly
 f. agaric
 f. agaric mushroom
 f. blister
 flesh f.
 heel f.
 louse f.
 mangrove f.
 phlebotomus f.
 riverine tsetse f.
 savanna tsetse f.
 screwworm f.
 Spanish f.
 tabanid f.
 tsetse f.
 tumbu f.
 warble f.
FMD
 foot-and-mouth disease
FMF
 familial Mediterranean fever
FML-S Ophthalmic suspension
FMV
 Fort Morgan virus
foamy
 f. agent

 f. virus
 f. virus group
FOB
 fiberoptic bronchoscopy
focal
 f. airspace disease
 f. brain lesion (FBL)
 f. cellular infiltration
 f. epithelial hyperplasia of Heck
 f. histiocytosis
 f. infection
 f. inflammation
 f. mass lesion
 f. mycobacterial lymphadenitis
 f. pneumonia
 f. reaction
 f. sclerosis lesion
 f. segmental glomerulosclerosis
  (FSGS)
focus, pl. **foci**
 detection of early antigen
  fluorescent f. (DEAFF)
 Ghon f.
 Simon f.
 Weigart f.
focusing
 isoelectric f. (IEF)
fodinarum
 Methylomonas f.
foecundum
 Distomum f.
foenisicii
 Paneolus f.
foetida
 Holophaga f.
foetus
 Trichomonas f.
 Tritrichomonas f.
folate
 f. deficiency
 f. metabolism
fold
 Kerckring f.
folder
 dengue immunochromatographic f.
Foley catheter
folinic acid
foliorum
 Microbacterium f.
follicle
 hair f.
 f. mite
follicle-stimulating hormone (FSH)
follicular
 f. abscess
 f. candidiasis
 f. conjunctivitis
 f. epithelium

f. hyperplasia
f. invasion
f. mange
f. non-Hodgkin lymphoma
f. stimulating hormone (FSH)
f. trachoma
folliculitis
f. barbae
Candida f.
eosinophilic f.
eosinophilic pustular f.
hot tub f.
Malassezia f.
folliculorum
Demodex f.
pityriasis f.
Follman balanitis
Fomede virus (FOMV)
fomite
fomiversen
intravitreal f.
fomivirsen
FOMV
Fomede virus
Fonsecaea (f)
F. compacta
F. pedrosoi
fontanelle
full f.
fonticola
Serratia f.
fontium
Pragia f.
food
F. and Drug Administration (FDA)
fermented f.
f. poisoning
foodborne
f. botulism
f. intoxication
f. outbreaks
fools' mushroom
foot
Aftate for Athlete's F.
athlete's f.
Dr Scholl's Athlete's F.
fungous f.
Hong Kong f.
f. infection
Madura f.
puncture wound of f.
ringworm of f.

foot-and-mouth
f.-a.-m. disease (FMD)
f.-a.-m. disease virus
f.-a.-m. disease virus vaccine
football-shaped
footei
Culicoides f.
foramen
f. of Luschka
f. of Magendie
f. magnum
Foraminifera
foraminiferous
forceps
biopsy f.
electrocoagulating f.
Forcipomyia glauca (p)
Forecariah virus (FORV)
foreign-body sensation
foreshadow
forest yaw
form
accole f.
applique f.
bradyzoite f.
involution f.
L f.
sickle f.
tachyzoite f.
formaldehyde
aqueous f.
gaseous f.
formalin-ether
f.-e. sedimentation concentration
f.-e. sedimentation technique
formalin-ethyl
f.-e. acetate concentration technique
f.-e. acetate sedimentation
concentration
f.-e. acetate sedimentation technique
formalin fixation
formalin-fixed stool specimen
formalin-inactivated vaccine
formalin-killed
formation
calculus f.
eosinophilic abscess f.
formicicum
Methanobacterium f.
formicigenerans
Eubacterium f.

F

NOTES

formicilis
    Gemmiger f.
formicoaceticum
    Clostridium f.
formigenes
    Oxalobacter f.
Formivibrio (b)
    F. citricus
formol-gel test
formosa
    Amanita muscaria var. *f.*
formosanum
    Diorchitrema f.
formosensis
    Actinomadura f.
    Haemaphysalis f.
    Thermomonospora f.
formosus
    Bacillus f.
    Brevibacillus f.
Formula
    Anti-Acne Control F.
    F. Q
    Triaminic AM Decongestant F.
    Vicks Formula 44 Pediatric F.
formulation
    amphotericin B liposomal f.
fornicalis
    Lactobacillus f.
fornix, pl. **fornices**
    posterior f.
Forscheimer spot
Forssman antibody
forsythus
    Bacteroides f.
Fort
    F. Bragg fever
    F. Morgan virus (FMV)
    F. Sherman virus (FSV)
Fortaz
Forte
    Femogen F.
    Robinul F.
    Stieva-A F.
Fortovase
    F. soft gel capsule
fortuitum
    Mycobacterium fortuitum subsp. *f.*
FORV
    Forecariah virus
foscarnet (PFA)
    f. cream
    intravenous f.
foscarnet-induced nephrotoxicity
fosfomycin
    f. tromethamine
fossa, pl. **fossae**
    iliac f.

fossor
    Atopobium f.
    Eubacterium f.
fosteri
    Thermomicrobium f.
Fostex
    F. Bar
    F. 10% BPO Gel
    F. Medicated Cleansing
    F. 10% Wash
Fototar
foundation
fourchette
Fournier gangrene
fourth disease
fovea
foveal
Foveavirus (v)
fowl
    f. adenovirus 1
    f. typhoid
fowleri
    Naegleria f.
fowlpox
    f. virus
    f. virus subgroup
fozivudine tidoxil (FZD)
FPIA
    fluorescence polarization immunoassay
FPLV
    feline panleukopenia virus
FPV
    Facey's Paddock virus
    feline panleukopenia virus
fr
    enterobacteria phage f.
fractional
    f. inhibitory concentration (FIC)
    f. inhibitory concentration index
fractionation
    Cohn-ethanol f.
fracture
    basilar skull f.
    stress f.
fradiae
    Streptomyces f.
Fraenkel pneumococcus
fragariae
    Xanthomonas f.
fragi
    Pseudomonas f.
fragile
    Desulfofrigus f.
    Streptosporangium f.
fragilis
    Bacteroides f.
    Dientamoeba f.

Saccharomyces f.
Streptomyces f.
fragmentation
red cell f.
framboesioides
mycosis f.
frame
open reading f. (ORF)
franciemonti
Culicoides f.
franciscanus
Anopheles f.
Anopheles franciscanus f.
Francisella (b)
F. novicida
F. philomiragia
F. tularensis antibody
F. tularensis biogroup *holarctica*
F. tularensis biogroup *novicida*
F. tularensis biogroup *palearctica*
F. tularensis biogroup *tularensis*
F. tularensis subsp. *mediasiatica*
F. tularensis subsp. *tularensis*
Frankia ani (b)
frank pus
franzmannii
Polaribacter f.
Franz medium
frappieri
Desulfitobacterium f.
fraseri
Legionella pneumophila subsp. *f.*
Fraser Point virus
fraterna
Hymenolepis nana f.
Frateuria aurantia (b)
frateurii
Gluconobacter f.
fraudulenta
Pseudo-nitzschia f.
frederiksbergensis
Pseudomonas f.
frederiksenii
Yersinia f.
fredii
Rhizobium f.
Sinorhizobium f.
free
f. fatty acid (FFA)
Pain Aid F.
f. testosterone
f. thyroxine

freeborni
Anopheles f.
Culicoides f.
freelist
freelisting
Freezone solution
Frei test
frenum
fresh frozen plasma (FFP)
freudenreichii
Propionibacterium freudenreichii subsp. *f.*
freundii
Citrobacter f.
freundtii
Entomoplasma f.
freyschussii
Candida f.
friable
friedericiana
Providencia f.
Friedländer
F. bacillus
F. pneumonia
friedmanni
Cryptococcus f.
Friedmanniella (b)
F. antarctica
F. capsulata
F. lacustris
F. spumicola
friedrichii
Candida f.
frigidarium
Flavobacterium f.
frigidicarnis
Clostridium f.
frigidicola
Psychrobacter f.
frigidimarina
Shewanella f.
frigidum
Leucosporidium f.
Methanogenium f.
frigoramans
Subtercola f.
Frigoribacterium (b)
F. faeni
frigoritolerans
Brevibacterium f.
Frijoles virus (FRIV)

F

NOTES

211

frisia
　　Methanosarcina f.
　　Thiomicrospira f.
frisingense
　　Herbaspirillum f.
frisingensis
　　Pectinatus f.
frisius
　　Methanococcus f.
frittonii
　　Methanogenium f.
friuliensis
　　Actinoplanes f.
FRIV
　　Frijoles virus
fri virus
frog virus group
frohnei
　　Culicoides f.
frontal
front-line chemotherapy
frosted-branch angitis
frothy discharge
fructicola
　　Graphium f.
fructivorans
　　Lactobacillus f.
fructosivorans
　　Desulfovibrio f.
　　Thiothrix f.
fructosus
　　Lactobacillus f.
fructus
　　Candida f.
fruiting body
frumenti
　　Lactobacillus f.
FSGS
　　focal segmental glomerulosclerosis
FSH
　　follicle-stimulating hormone
　　follicular stimulating hormone
FS Shampoo Topical
FSV
　　Fort Sherman virus
F₃T

F$_3$T
FTA-ABS, FTA-Abs
　　fluorescent treponemal antibody
　　　absorption
　　fluorescent treponemal antibody
　　　absorption test
　　fluorescent treponemal antibody
　　　adsorption
　　　　serum FTA-ABS
　　　　FTA-ABS test
FTT
　　failure to thrive

fucicola
　　Cellulophaga f.
Fucidin
　　F. I.V.
　　F. Oral suspension
　　F. tablet
fuckelii
　　Coniothyrium f.
fucosus
　　Agromyces fucosus subsp. *f.*
fuelleborni
　　Strongyloides f.
Fuellebornius
　　F. medinensis
fugitive swelling
fugu poisoning
fujikori
　　Gibberella f.
fujisana
　　Haemaphysalis f.
fujisawaense
　　Methylobacterium f.
fukuiense
　　Streptosporangium amethystogenes
　　　subsp. *f.*
Fukuoka virus
fulgidus
　　Archaeoglobus f.
fuliginea
full-blown AIDS
full fontanelle
full-thickness retinal necrosis
fulminans
　　purpura f.
fulminant
　　f. amebic colitis
　　f. bronchiolitis
　　f. chorioretinitis
　　f. dysentery
　　f. hepatic failure (FHF)
　　f. hepatitis
　　f. sepsis
　　f. tracheitis
fulminating
　　f. acute suppurative cholangitis
fulva
　　Pseudomonas f.
fulvacrura
　　Muscina f.
fulvescens
　　Actinomadura f.
　　Aphanoascus f.
　　Nadsonia fulvescens var. *f.*
fulvibnotum
　　Simulium f.
Fulvicin
　　F. P/G
Fulvicin-U/F

fulvissimus
    Streptomyces f.
fulvius
    antivenin Micrurus f.
fulvorobeus
    Streptomyces f.
fulvum
    Arthroderma f.
    Dactylosporangium f.
    Microsporum f.
    Phaeospirillum f.
    Rhodospirillum f.
fulvus
    Aedes f.
    Aedes f. fulvus
fumagillin
fumanus
    Streptomyces f.
fumarii
    Pyrolobus f.
fumarioli
    Bacillus f.
fumaroxidans
    Syntrophobacter f.
fume hood
fumicolans
    Thermococcus f.
fumigata
    Chainia f.
fumigatiscleroticus
    Streptomyces f.
fumigatus
    Aspergillus f.
    Streptomyces chrysomallus subsp. f.
fumosum
    Polyangium f.
fumusoroseu
    Paecilomyces f.
function
    B-cell f.
    executive cognitive f. (ECF)
functional
    f. bladder outlet resistance
    f. domain
    f. proliferative assay
fundi (*pl. of* fundus)
Fundibacter jadensis (b)
funditum
    Carnobacterium f.
fundoscopic

funduliforme
    Fusobacterium necrophorum subsp.
        f.
fundus, pl. **fundi**
funduscopic
fungal
    f. cellulitis
    f. corneal culture
    f. endophthalmitis
    f. hypha
    f. immunodiffusion
    f. infection
    f. keratitis
    f. meningitis
    f. peritonitis
    f. precipitin test
    f. serology
    f. skin testing
fungate
fungemia
    Histoplasma capsulatum f.
fungi (*pl. of* fungus)
fungicidal
fungicide
Fungi-Fluor
Fungi Imperfecti
fungiphilus
    Azonexus f.
Fungiqual A
fungistatic
fungitoxic
fungitoxicity
Fungizone
Fungoid
    F. AF Topical solution
    F. Creme
    F. Tincture
fungoides
    mycosis f.
fungorum
    Burkholderia f.
fungous
    f. foot
fungus, pl. **fungi**
    f. ball
    f. call
    f. culture
    dematiaceous f.
    dermatophytic f.
    dimorphic f.
    filamentous f.
    fission f.

F

NOTES

fungus *(continued)*
    imperfect f.
    nondermatophyte f.
    perfect f.
    ray f.
    saprophytic f.
    f. smear
    sulfur shelf f.
    thrush f.
    yeast f.
    yeastlike f.
funicola
    Chaetomium f.
funiculitis
    endemic f.
    filarial f.
funiculosum
    Penicillium f.
funiculus
    Bothriocephalus f.
funisitis
funkei
    Actinomyces f.
FUO
    fever of unknown origin
Furacin topical
Furadantin
Furalan
Furamide
Furan
Furanite
Furatoin
furazolidone
    f. disk test
furcosa
    Anaerorhabdus f.
furcosus
    Bacteroides f.
furculatum
    Simulium f.
Furdantin
furens
    Culicoides f.
furfur
    Malassezia f.
furfuralis
    Desulfovibrio f.
furfurans
    porrigo f.
furiosus
    Pyrococcus f.
furnissii
    Vibrio f.
furoate
    diloxanide f.
    mometasone f.
furosemide
Furovirus (v)

Furoxone
furuncle
furunculoid
fusarioides
    Dactylium dendroides
    Pseudomicrodochium f.
fusariosis
    allergic bronchopulmonary f.
Fusarium (f)
    F. acuminatum
    F. aquaeductuum
    F. chlamydosporum
    F. dimerum
    F. graminearum
    F. lagenarium
    F. moniliforme
    F. neoceras
    F. nivale
    F. oxysporum
    F. phormii
    F. polymorphum
    F. proliferatum
    F. sacchari
    F. semitectum
    F. sporotrichioides
fusca
    Microtetraspora f.
    Mollisia f.
    Scopulariopsis f.
    Thermobifida f.
    Thermomonospora f.
fuscescens
    Cryptococcus f.
fuscidula
    Aposphaeria f.
fuscipes
    Glossina f.
fuscoatra
    Humicola fuscoatra var. *f.*
fuscovaginae
    Pseudomonas f.
fuscum
    Brevibacterium f.
fuscus
    Cystobacter f.
fuseau
Fusellovirus (v)
Fusibacter paucivorans (b)
Fusicoccum (f)
fusidic acid
fusiform
fusiforme
    Filomicrobium f.
    Fusobacterium nucleatum subsp. *f.*
fusiformis
    Bacillus f.
    Caulobacter f.
    Prosthecobacter f.

fusispora
  Acrophialophora f.
  Trichometasphaeria f.
Fusobacterium (b)
  F. alocis
  F. gonidiaformans
  F. mortiferum
  F. naviforme
  F. necrogenes
  F. necrophorum
  F. necrophorum subsp. funduliforme
  F. necrophorum subsp. necrophorum
  F. necrophorum subsp. necrophorum
   biovar C
  F. nucleatum subsp. animalis
  F. nucleatum subsp. fusiforme
  F. nucleatum subsp. nucleatum
  F. nucleatum subsp. polymorphum
  F. nucleatum subsp. vincentii
  F. perfoetens

  F. periodonticum
  F. plauti
  F. polysaccharolyticum
  F. prausnitzii
  F. pseudonecrophorum
  F. russii
  F. simiae
  F. sulci
  F. ulcerans
  F. varium
fusoidea
  Pseudallescheria f.
Fusoma
fusospirochetal
FVU
  first-void urine
    FVU sample
F-wave response
FZD
  fozivudine tidoxil

NOTES

F

215

G-1
    glycoprotein G.
G1
    aflatoxin G1
G2
    aflatoxin G2
G-2
    glycoprotein G.
G4 virus
G6 virus
G14 virus
g209-2M peptide vaccine
GA-1 virus
gabaldoni
    Anopheles g.
    Simulium g.
Gabek Forest virus (GFV)
GABHS
    GABHS pharyngitis
gabonensis
    Desulfovibrio g.
Gaboon ulcer
gadei
    Dysgonomonas g.
gadfly
Gadget's Gully virus (GGYV)
gadi
    Echinorhynchus g.
gadium
    Mycobacterium g.
gadolinium
GAE
    granulomatous amebic encephalitis
Gaeumannomyces (f)
    G. graminis
    G. graminis var. *tritici*
    G. graminis virus 019/6-A (GgV-019/6A)
    G. graminis virus 87-1-H (GgV-87-1-H)
    G. graminis virus T1-A (GgV-T1-A)
Gag
    G. gene
    G. polyprotein
Gag-Pol polyprotein
gag reflex
gaigeri
    Multiceps g.
gait
    slapping g.
gal 1–2
    Galius adenovirus 1–2
galacta
    Candida g.

galactanivorans
    Zobellia g.
Galactomyces geotrichum (f)
galactophilus
    Bacillus g.
galacturonicus
    Bacteroides g.
galbus
    Streptomyces g.
galegae
    Rhizobium g.
Galerina autumnalis (f)
galilaeus
    Streptomyces g.
Galius **adenovirus 1–2 (gal 1–2)**
gallaeciensis
    Roseobacter g.
gallbladder
galli
    Ascaridia g.
gallica
    Micromonospora g.
gallicida
    Pasteurella g.
    Pasteurella multicida subsp. g.
Gallicola barnesae (b)
gallicum
    Bifidobacterium g.
    Rhizobium g.
gallinacea
    Echidnophaga g.
gallinaceum
    Mycoplasma g.
gallinae
    Ceratophyllus g.
    Dermanyssus g.
    Knemidocoptes g.
    Microsporum g.
gallinarum
    Bifidobacterium g.
    Carnobacterium g.
    Enterococcus g.
    Heterakis g.
    Lactobacillus g.
    Mycoplasma g.
    Pasteurella g.
    Staphylococcus g.
    Streptococcus g.
Gallionellaceae
Gallionella ferruginea (b)
gallisepticum
    Mycoplasma g.
gallium
    g. abscess scan
    g. negative

G

gallium *(continued)*
    g. nitrate
    g. tumor scan
gallium-67
gallolyticus
    Streptococcus g.
gallop
    g. rhythm
gallopava
    Dactylaria g.
gallopavonis
    Mycoplasma g.
gallopavum
    Ochroconis g.
gallorale
    Ureaplasma g.
gallstone
GALT
    gut-associated lymphoid tissue
galvaoi
    Anopheles g.
GAL virus
gambiae
    Anopheles g.
Gambian
    G. fever
    G. sleeping sickness
    G. trypanosomiasis
gambiense
    Trypanosoma brucei g.
Gambierdiscus toxicus
Gamboa virus (GAMV)
gamete
gametic nucleus
gametocide
gametocyst
gametocyte
gametocyticides
gametogenesis
gametogonia
gametogony
gametoid
gametokinetic
gametophagia
Gamimune N
gamma
    g. benzene hexachloride
    g. benzene hexachloride shampoo
    g. gene
    g. globulin
    g. hemolysis
    g. hemolytic streptococcus
    g. herpesvirus
    interferon g.
    g. irradiation
    g. knife radiosurgery
    polymerase g.
gamma-2 herpesvirus

Gammabulin Immuno
gamma-Gandy body
Gammagard S/D
Gammagee
    Hep-B G.
gamma-glutamyl transpeptidase (gamma-GTP)
gamma-GTP
    gamma-glutamyl transpeptidase
Gammaherpesvirinae
gammaherpesvirus
gamma-interferon (IFN-gamma)
Gammaretrovirus (v)
Gammar-P I.V.
gamma-toxin
gammopathy
    monoclonal g.
gamogony
gamont
Gamsia (f)
Gamulin Rh
GAMV
    Gamboa virus
ganciclovir (GCV)
    g. intraocular implant
ganciclovir-resistant
gancidicus
    Streptomyces g.
Gan Gan virus (GGV)
ganglion, pl. **ganglia**
    basal g.
    g. cell
    sympathetic g.
gangosa
gangrene
    bacterial synergistic g.
    clostridial gas g.
    emphysematous g.
    Fournier g.
    gas g.
    infected vascular g.
    Meleney synergistic g.
    penile g.
    strep g.
    streptococcal g.
    symmetrical peripheral g.
    synergistic g.
    wet g.
gangrenosum
    ecthyma g.
    hemorrhagic pyoderma g.
    pyoderma g.
gangrenous
    g. emphysema
Gantanol
    Azo G.
Gantrisin
    Azo G.

Garamycin
Garatec
gardener's disease
Gardnerella (b)
    G. *vaginalis*
    G. vaginitis
gardneri
    Streptomyces g.
garinii
    Borrelia g.
garland chrysanthemum temperate virus
garlic
garrisoni
    Raillietina g.
garvieae
    Lactococcus g.
    Streptococcus g.
GAS
    group A *Streptococcus*
    GAS antigen
    GAS antigen test
    GAS infection
gas
    arterial blood g. (ABG)
    g. bacillus
    blood g.
    g. chromatography
    g. chromatography/mass
      spectrometry (GC/MS)
    g. from nitrate
    g. gangrene
    g. gangrene antitoxin
    g. isotope ratio mass spectrometry
      (GIRMS)
    nitrate to g.
    g. phlegmon
    g. plasma sterilization
gaseous formaldehyde
gasicomitatum
    Leuconostoc g.
gasigenes
    Clostridium g.
gas-liquid chromatography (GLC)
gasseri
    Lactobacillus g.
gaster
Gasterellaceae
Gasteromycetes
Gasterophilidae
Gasterophilus (p)
    G. *haemorrhoidalis*
    G. *intestinalis*

    G. *nasalis*
    G. *pecorum*
gastri
    Mycobacterium g.
gastric
    g. anisakidosis
    g. aspirate
    g. carcinoma
    g. cryptosporidiosis
    g. inflammation
    g. lymphoma
    g. metaplasia
    g. mucosal biopsy
gastricus
    Cryptococcus g.
gastritis
    atrophic g.
    chronic active g.
    chronic atrophic g.
    Helicobacter pylori g.
    Helicobacter pylori-associated g.
    Helicobacter pylori-related g.
Gastrodiscidae
Gastrodiscoides hominis
gastroenteritis
    acute infectious nonbacterial g.
    acute nonbacterial infectious g.
    acute viral g.
    bacterial g.
    Campylobacter g.
    endemic nonbacterial infantile g.
    eosinophilic g.
    epidemic nonbacterial g.
    infantile g.
    Norwalk g.
    nosocomial g.
    parasitic g.
    porcine transmissible g.
    rotavirus g.
    Vibrio cholerae g.
    Vibrio cholerae-induced g.
    Vibrio parahaemolyticus-
      associated g.
    viral g.
    g. virus type A, B
gastroesophageal
    g. reflux (GER)
    g. reflux disease (GERD)
gastroesophageal reflux (GER)
gastrointestinal (GI)
    g. anthrax
    g. endoscopy

G

NOTES

gastrointestinal *(continued)*
    g. infection
    g. irritant
    metabolic, endocrine, and g.
      (MEG)
    g. parasite
    g. tract
gastrointestinalis
    mycetism g.
Gastrophilidae
gastropod
Gastropoda
gastroscopy
Gastrosed
Gastrospirillum hominis
Gastrosporiaceae
gastrostomy
    percutaneous endoluminal g. (PEG)
    percutaneous endoscopic g. (PEG)
gateae
    Mycoplasma g.
gatifloxacin
gatifloxin
gattii
    Cryptococcus neoformans var. *g.*
Gaucher disease
gaudeatum
    Simulium g.
gaunt
gaurani
    Simulium g.
Gautieriaceae
Gautieriales
GAV
    Grand Arbaud virus
gaviniae
    Buttiauxella g.
GA virus
Gaviscon Prevent
gaze
    dysconjugate g.
gazogenes
    Beneckea g.
    Vibrio g.
GB
    GB virus (GBV)
    GB virus-A
    GB virus-B
    GB virus-C
GBS
    group B streptococcal sepsis
    group B streptococcus
GBV
    GB virus
GBV-C
    GB virus C
GB virus B
GB virus C (GBV-C)

GC
    gonococcus
    gonorrhea culture
GC/MS
    gas chromatography/mass spectrometry
G-CSF
    granulocyte colony-stimulating factor
GCU
    gonococcal urethritis
GCV
    ganciclovir
     GCV sodium
GDP
    guanosine diphosphate
Geastaceae
gedaensis
    Streptomyces g.
Gedoelstia (p)
gedoelstiosis
Gee
    Gee G.
geestiana
    Legionella g.
Gehan test
Gel
    Advanced Formula Oxy
     Sensitive G.
    Benzac AC G.
    Benzac W G.
    Brevoxyl G.
    Clear By Design G.
    Del Aqua-5, -10 G.
    Desquam-E G.
    Desquam-X G.
    Dryox G.
    Fostex 10% BPO G.
    H.P. Acthar G.
    Keralyt G.
    Perfectoderm G.
    Tisit Blue G.
    Vergogel G.
gel
    alitretinoin g.
    cidofovir g.
    Moist Again moisturizing g.
    N-9 g.
gelaticus
    Streptomyces g.
gelatin
    g. hydrolysis test
    g., pectin, and methylcellulose
gelatinase
    g. test
Gelatinodiscaceae
gelatinosa
    Rhodopseudomonas g.
    Thiocystis g.

gelatinosus
    Rhodocyclus g.
    Rubrivivax g.
gelatinovorans
    Ruegeria g.
gelatinovorum
    Agrobacterium g.
Gelfoam
gelida
    Cellulomonas g.
    Desulfofaba g.
Gelidibacter algens (b)
gelidicola
    Pseudomonas g.
gelidimarina
    Shewanella g.
gelidum
    Leuconostoc g.
    Leucosporidium g.
Gelopellidaceae
Gemella (b)
    G. *bergeri*
    G. *cuniculi*
    G. *haemolysans*
    G. *morbillorum*
    G. *sanguinis*
gemellus
    Paederus g.
gemfibrozil
gemifloxacin
geminata
    Solenopsis g.
gemistocytic astrocyte
Gemmata obscuriglobus (b)
Gemmiger formicilis (b)
Gemmobacter aquantilis (b)
Genac tablet
Genagesic
Genamin Expectorant
Gen-Amoxicillin
Genapap
Genapax
Genaspor
Genatuss
    G. DM
genavense
    Mycobacterium g.
gene
    alpha g.
    BCG host resistance g.
    beta g.
    dihydropteroate synthase g.

    Env g.
    Gag g.
    gamma g.
    JH g.
    mecA g.
    mini-exon-derived ribonucleic
      acid g.
    mini-exon-derived RNA g.
    nef g.
    resistance g.
    Rev g.
    Tat g.
    variant surface glycoprotein g.
    Vif g.
    vpu g.
    vpx-related g.
    VSG g.
Geneaceae
Genebs
generalisatus
    herpes zoster g.
generalized
    g. adenopathy
    g. lymphadenopathy
    g. tetanus
generation
    asexual g.
    nonsexual g.
    sexual g.
    virgin g
generator
    radiofrequency g.
genetic
    g. marker
    g. recombination
    g. transduction
genetically
geniculata
    Curvularia g.
    Pseudomonas g.
geniculatus
    Cochliobolus g.
GENIE HIV 1/2 assay
genital
    g. aphthous ulcer
    g. atopic dermatitis
    g. chlamydia
    g. chlamydial infection
    g. culture
    g. elephantiasis
    g. herpes
    g. herpes simplex

G

NOTES

genital *(continued)*
  g. herpes simplex virus
  g. lesion
  g. mutilation
  g. primordium
  g. ulceration
  g. ulcer disease (GUD)
  g. wart
genitalis
  herpes g.
genitalium
  Mycoplasma g.
genital wart
genitourinary
  g. infection
  g. prosthesis
  g. tract
  g. tuberculosis
genome
  minus sense-RNA g.
  plus sense-RNA g.
  RNA g.
  translation-competent g.
  viral g.
genomic
  g. repeat
Genoptic S.O.P. Ophthalmic
genospecies
genote
genotype
  anthroponotic g.
genotypic
  g. assay
  g. testing
  g. typing method
genotyping
  HCV g.
  hepatitis C viral RNA g.
  HIV g.
Genpril
Gen-Probe
  G.-P. PACE assay
  G.-P. Pace 2 *Chlamydia* test
Gentacidin
  G. Ophthalmic
Gentafair
Gent-AK
Gentak Ophthalmic
gentamicin
  g. level
  prednisolone and g.
gentianae
  Syntrophus g.
gentian violet
Gentrasul
Geobacillus (b)
  G. kaustophilus
  G. stearothermophilus

  G. subterraneus
  G. thermocatenulatus
  G. thermodenitrificans
  G. thermoglucosidasius
  G. thermoleovorans
  G. uzenensis
Geobacter (b)
  G. chapellei
  G. grbiciae
  G. hydrogenophilus
  G. metallireducens
  G. sulfurreducens
geochares
  Candida g.
Geocillin
Geodermatophilus obscurus (b)
Geoglossaceae
geolei
  Thermosipho g.
geometricus
Geomyces pannorus (f)
Geopen
geophilia
  Alternaria g.
geophilic
Geophilus
geophylla
  Inocybe g.
georgiae
  Actinomyces g.
georgiana
  Kluyvera g.
georgianus
  Anopheles g.
georgiense
  Marinobacterium g.
geothermalis
  Deinococcus g.
geothermicum
  Desulfotomaculum g.
Geothrix fermentans (b)
Geotoga (b)
  G. petraea
  G. subterranea
Geotrichoides (f)
Geotrichum (f)
  G. candidum
  G. clavatum
  G. fici
  G. klebhanii
geotrichum
  Galactomyces g.
Geovibrio ferrireducens (b)
gephyra
  Archangium g.
GER
  gastroesophageal reflux

GERD
    gastroesophageal reflux disease
gerencseriae
    Actinomyces g.
gergoviae
    Enterobacter g.
germ
    g. nucleus
    g. tube
    g. tube test
German
    G. measles
    G. measles culture
    G. measles vaccine
    G. measles virus
germanica
    Blattella g.
Germanin
germicidal preparation
germinal rod
Germiston virus (GERV)
gerontine
Gerstmann-Sträussler-Scheinker (GSS)
    G.-S.-S. disease (GSS)
    G.-S.-S. syndrome
gertleri
    Arthroderma g.
GERV
    Germiston virus
gessardii
    Pseudomonas g.
gestation
gestii
    Heliobacterium g.
Getah virus (GETV)
GETV
    Getah virus
geysericola
    Herpetosiphon g.
geysiriensis
    Streptomyces g.
GFR
    glomerular filtration rate
GFV
    Gabek Forest virus
GG
    Slo-Phyllin GG
gG1
    glycoprotein gG1
gG2
    glycoprotein gG2
gG-2 seropositive

GG/DM
    Kolephrin G.
GGV
    Gan Gan virus
GgV-019/6A
    Gaeumannomyces graminis virus 019/6-A
GgV-87-1-H
    Gaeumannomyces graminis virus 87-1-H
GgV-T1-A
    Gaeumannomyces graminis virus T1-A
GGYV
    Gadget's Gully virus
GH
    growth hormone
ghanaensis
    Streptomyces g.
Ghon
    G. complex
    G. focus
ghoni
    Clostridium g.
Ghon-Sachs bacillus (*See* **Clostridium septicum**)
GHOST
    G. cell
    G. cell assay
GI
    gastrointestinal
giant
    g. cell
    g. chromosome
    g. condyloma
    g. disseminated molluscum contagiosum
    g. intestinal fluke
    g. kidney worm
    g. pronormoblast
Giardia (p)
    G. agilis
    G. ardeae
    G. canis
    G. duodenalis
    G. intestinalis
    G. lamblia
    G. muris
    G. O-positive stool
    G. P-positive stool
    G. psittaci
    G.-specific antigen 65 (GSA65)
    G. trophozoite
giardiasis

NOTES

G

Giardiavirus (v)
giardinii
    Rhizobium g.
Gibberella (f)
    G. *fujikori*
    G. *monilformis*
    G. *zeae*
Gibbon ape leukemia virus
gibbonsii
    Haloferax g.
gibsoni
    Onchocerca g.
gibsoniae
    Desulfotomaculum g.
gibsonii
    Bacillus g.
    Kurthia g.
    Streptomyces g.
Giemsa-stained smear
Giemsa and Wilder reticulum stain
giesbergeri
    Aquaspirillum g.
gifhornensis
    Verrucosispora g.
gigantea
    Scolopendra g.
giganteum
    Chloronema g.
    Simulium g.
    Trichosporon g.
giganteus
    Desulfovibrio g.
gigantica
    Fasciola g.
Gigantobilharzia (p)
    G. *gyrauli*
    G. *huronensis*
    G. *sturniae*
Gigantorhynchus (p)
    G. *echinodiscus*
    G. *lopezneyrai*
    G. *lutzi*
    G. *oritzi*
    G. *pasteri*
    G. *ungiari*
gigas
    Desulfovibrio g.
    Eustrongylus g.
gilardii
    Ralstonia g.
    Roseomonas g.
Gilardi rod group 1
Gilbert syndrome
Gilchrist disease
gilesi
    Anopheles g.
gillenii
    Citrobacter g.

gillisiae
    Flavobacterium g.
gilvescens
    Cryptococcus g.
gilvum
    Mycobacterium g.
Gimenez stain
gingiva
    marginal g.
gingival
    g. swab
gingivalis
    Bacteroides g.
    Capnocytophaga g.
    Entamoeba g.
    Halicephalobus g.
    Porphyromonas g.
gingivicanis
    Porphyromonas g.
gingivitis
    acute necrotizing ulcerative g.
    HIV g.
    necrotizing ulcerative g.
    non-HIV chronic g.
    tuberculous g.
gingivostomatitis
    acute herpetic g.
    herpetic g.
    HSV-1 g.
    necrotizing g.
    ulcerative g.
Giopen
GIRMS
    gas isotope ratio mass spectrometry
GISA
    glycopeptide-intermediate *Staphylococcus aureus*
GIV
    Great Island virus
GJAV
    Guajara virus
glabrata
    Biomphalaria g.
    Candida g.
glabrosa
    tinea g.
glabrous
glabrum
glacial acetic acid
glacialis
    Leucorrhinia g.
Glaciecola (b)
    G. *pallidula*
    G. *punicea*
glacincola
    Psychrobacter g.
gladiatoris
    Spiroplasma g.

gladiatorum
　　herpes g.
gladioli
　　Burkholderia g.
　　Pseudomonas g.
glaebosa
　　Candida g.
gland
　　Bartholin g.
　　ecdysial g.
　　meibomian g.
　　g. of Moll
　　parotid g.
　　peritracheal g.
　　pituitary g.
　　prothoracic g.
　　Skene g.
　　surrenal g.
　　thoracic g.
　　ventral g.
　　g. of Zeiss
glanders
　　g. bacillus
glandis
　　papillae corona g.
glandular
　　g. fever
　　g. tularemia
glans
glasgowi
　　Androlaelaps g.
glathei
　　Burkholderia g.
　　Pseudomonas g.
glauca
　　Absidia g.
　　Forcipomyia g.
　　Microtetraspora g.
　　Saccharomonospora g.
glaucescens
　　Streptomyces g.
glaucoflava
　　Streptomycoides g.
glaucoma
　　acute angle-closure g.
　　secondary g.
Glaucon
glaucopis
　　Meniscus g.
glaucosporus
　　Streptomyces g.

glaucum
　　Trichoderma g.
glaucus
　　Aspergillus g.
　　Streptomyces g.
GLC
　　gas-liquid chromatography
glebosus
　　Streptomyces hygroscopicus subsp.
　　　g.
Glenospora graphii (f)
gleum
　　Chryseobacterium g.
　　Flavobacterium g.
glial proliferation
Gliocladium (f)
　　G. *penicilloides*
　　G. *virens*
gliocytosis
glioma
Gliomastix murorum (f)
gliosis
　　astrocytic g.
　　subependymal nodular g.
Glisson capsule
globactor
　　Volvox g.
global warming
globerula
　　Nocardia g.
globerulus
　　Rhodococcus g.
Globicatella sanguinis (b)
globicatena
　　Actinokineospora g.
globiformis
　　Arthrobacter g.
　　Rhodopila g.
　　Rhodopseudomonas g.
globispora
　　Bullera g.
　　Sporosarcina g.
globisporum
　　Amorphosporangium g.
globisporus
　　Actinoplanes g.
　　Bacillus g.
　　Streptomyces g.
　　Streptomyces globisporus subsp. g.
Globocephalus urosubulatus (p)
globoside

G

NOTES

globosum
 Bifidobacterium g.
 Bifidobacterium pseudolongum var. g.
 Chaetomium g.
globosus
 Bulinus g.
 Streptomyces g.
globulin
 antilymphocytic g. (ALG)
 anti-Rh(D) immune g.
 antithymocyte g. (ATG)
 chickenpox immune g.
 CMV hyperimmune g.
 cytomegalovirus immune g. (CMVIG)
 cytomegalovirus-specific intravenous immune g. (CMVIg)
 gamma g.
 hepatitis B immune g. (HBIG, H-BIG)
 human immune g.
 hyperimmune serum g. (HBIG, H-BIG)
 immune serum g. (ISG)
 intravenous immune g. (IVIG)
 respiratory syncytial virus immune g. (RSVIG, RSV-IGIV)
 Rh$_O$(D) immune g.
 serum g.
 serum hormone binding g. (SHBG)
 tetanus immune g. (TIG)
 varicella immune g. (VZIG)
 varicella-zoster immune g. (VZIG)
 zoster immune g.
gloeosporioides
 Colletotrichum g.
Gloeosporium (f)
glomerans
 Coriobacterium g.
glomerata
 Actinocorallia g.
 Actinomadura g.
 Phoma g.
glomeratus
 coenurus g.
 Flectobacillus g.
 Polaribacter g.
 Streptomyces g.
 Taenia g.
Glomerella (f)
 G. cingulata
 G. glycines
 G. phacidiomorpha
glomeroaurantiacus
 Streptomyces g.
glomerular
 g. filtration rate (GFR)

glomeruli (*pl. of* glomerulus)
glomerulitis
glomerulonephritis (GN)
 acute g. (AGN)
 acute hemorrhagic g.
 acute poststreptococcal g.
 antiglomerular basement membrane g.
 immune complex g.
 membranoproliferative g.
 membranous g.
 poststreptococcal acute g.
glomerulonephropathy
glomerulosclerosis
 focal segmental g. (FSGS)
glomerulus, pl. **glomeruli**
gloriae
 Arthroderma g.
 Trichophyton g.
Glossina (p)
 G. fuscipes
 G. morsitans
 G. pallidipes
 G. palpalis
 G. swynnertoni
 G. tabaniformis
 G. tachinoides
Glossinidae
glossinidia
 Wigglesworthia g.
glossinidius
 Sodalis g.
glossitis
 Candida g.
glossodynia
 Candida g.
glottis
GLOV
 Gray Lodge virus
glove-and-stocking
 g.-a.-s. distribution
 g.-a.-s. syndrome
GLSH
 glucose, lactalbumin, serum, and hemoglobin
 GLSH culture medium
glucagon
glucanolyticus
 Bacillus g.
 Paenibacillus g.
Glucantime
gluceptate
 erythromycin g.
glucocorticoid
Gluconacetobacter (b)
 G. azotocaptans
 G. diazotrophicus
 G. entanii

G. *europaeus*
G. *hansenii*
G. *intermedius*
G. *johannae*
G. *liquefaciens*
G. *oboediens*
G. *sacchari*
G. *xylinus* subsp. *sucrofermentans*
G. *xylinus* subsp. *xylinus*

gluconate
calcium g.
chlorhexidine g.
g. fermentation test
quinidine g.
topical chlorhexidine g.

Gluconobacter (b)
G. *asaii*
G. *cerinus*
G. *frateurii*
G. *oxydans* subsp. *industrius*
G. *oxydans* subsp. *melanogenes*
G. *oxydans* subsp. *oxydans*
G. *oxydans* subsp. *sphaericus*
G. *oxydans* subsp. *suboxydans*

glucose
CSF g.
fasting g.
g. fermentation test
g. fermenter
g. intolerance
isotonic g.
g., lactalbumin, serum, and
  hemoglobin (GLSH)
g., lactalbumin, serum, and
  hemoglobin culture medium
nonfasting g.
plasma g.
synovial g.
g. tolerance

glucose-6-phosphatase deficiency
glucose-6-phosphatase deoxyhydrogenase
glucose-6-phosphate
g.-p. dehydrogenase (G6PD)
g.-p. dehydrogenase deficiency
  (G6PD)

glucosida
Mannheimia g.
glucosophila
Candida g.
glucosotrophus
Methylovorus g.

glucozyma
Hansenula g.
Pichia g.
glucuronate
trimetrexate g.
glucuronolyticum
Corynebacterium g.
glucuronoxylomannan (GXM)
glucuronyltransferase
glumae
Burkholderia g.
Pseudomonas g.
glumarum
Coniothecium g.
glutamicum
Corynebacterium g.
glutaraldehyde
glutaraldehyde-based
glutarica
Pelospora g.
glutathione
glutathione-S-transferase (GST)
g.-t. pull-down assay (GST pull-
  down assay)
gluteal
glutinis
Rhodotorula g.
glutinosum
Metarhizium g.
GLV
Gumbo Limbo virus
Glyate
glyburide
glycerini
Anaerosinus g.
Anaerovibrio g.
Moorella g.
glycerol fermentation test
Glycerol-T
glycines
Glomerella g.
glycinophilus
Peptococcus g.
glycocalyx
glycocalyx-like
Glycofed
glycogen
g. fermentation test
g. hydrolysis test
g. vacuole
glycogenes
Methylobacillus g.

G

NOTES

glycogenica
  Micropruina g.
glycol
  Diprolene G.
  salicylic acid and propylene g.
glycolicum
  Clostridium g.
  Halochromatium g.
glycolicus
  Desulfofustis g.
  Syntrophobotulus g.
glycolytica
  Neisseria elongata subsp. *g.*
Glycomyces (b)
  G. *harbinensis*
  G. *rutgersensis*
  G. *tenuis*
glycopeptide
glycopeptide-intermediate *Staphylococcus*
  aureus (**GISA**)
glycopeptide-resistant *Staphylococcus*
  aureus (**GRSA**)
Glycophagus domesticus (p)
glycophilum
  Mycoplasma g.
glycoprotein
  g. 17-1A
  g. G-1
  g. G-2
  g. gG1
  g. gG2
  g. gp120
  variant surface g. (VSG)
glycoprotein-72
  tumor-associated g.
glycoprotein-based enzyme-linked
  immunosorbent assay (gpELISA)
glycopyrrolate
glycosaminoglycan
glycosuria
glycosylated
Glycotuss
Glycotuss-dM
glycovorans
  Pyrococcus g.
Glycyphagidae
Gly-Oxide Oral
glypizide
Glytuss
GM3
  typhimurium strain G.
GMAV
  Guama virus
GM-CSF
  granulocyte/macrophage colony-
    stimulating factor
  granulocyte-macrophage CSF

GMP
  good manufacturing practice
GMS
  Gomori methenamine silver
  Gomori methenamine silver stain
  methenamine silver stain
    GMS stain
G-myticin
  G.-m. Topical
GN
  glomerulonephritis
gnat
Gnathobdellida
Gnathostoma (p)
  G. *doloresi*
  G. *hispidum*
  G. *nipponicum*
  G. *procyonis*
  G. *spinigerum*
  G. *turgidum*
Gnathostomatidae
Gnathostomatinae
Gnathostomatoidea
gnathostomiasis
  cutaneous g.
  g. externa
  g. interna
  visceral g.
gnavus
  Ruminococcus g.
GNID
  gram-negative intracellular diplococci
Gnomoniaceae
Gnomoniopsis (f)
GnRH
  gonadotropin-releasing hormone
goatpox virus
gobitricini
  Streptomyces g.
goblet cell
goeidi
  Simulium g.
Goeldichironomus amazonicus
goetzii
  Trichophyton mentagrophytes var. *v.*
goiter
golden shiner virus (GSV)
gold sodium thiomalate
Golgi apparatus
gomezdelatorrei
  Anopheles g.
Gomoka virus (GOMV)
Gomori
  G. methenamine silver (GMS)
  G. methenamine silver stain (GMS
    stain, GMS)
  G. methenamine stain

gomorrense
  Halobaculum g.
Gomphidiaceae
Gomphrena **virus**
GOMV
  Gomoka virus
gonad
  g. nucleus
gonadotropin
  beta-human chorionic g. (beta-HCG)
  g. deficiency
  human chorionic g. (HCG)
gonadotropin-releasing hormone (GnRH)
gondii
  Toxoplasma g. (TG)
  Trypanosoma g.
gondwanense
  Fervidobacterium g.
  Flavobacterium g.
gondwanensis
  Psychroflexus g.
Gongylonema (p)
  G. neoplasticum
  G. orientale
  G. pulchrum
Gongylonematidae
gongylonemiasis
gonidiaformans
  Fusobacterium g.
Gonochek II
gonocide
gonococcal
  g. arthritis
  g. conjunctivitis
  g. infection
  g. meningitis
  g. ophthalmia neonatorium
  g. pharyngitis
  g. salpingitis
  g. scalp abscess
  g. septicemia
  g. stomatitis
  g. urethritis (GCU)
gonococci (*pl. of* gonococcus)
gonococcic
gonococcicide
gonococcus, pl. **gonococci (GC)**
  penicillinase-producing gonococci
    (PPNG)
  piliated g.

GonoGen
  G. II antigen detection system
  G. I test
gono-opsonin
gonorrhea
  anorectal g.
  cervical g.
  g. culture (GC)
  pharyngeal g.
gonorrheal
  g. arthritis
  g. urethritis
gonorrhoeae
  Neisseria g.
  penicillinase-producing *Neisseria* g.
    (PPNG)
  tetracycline-resistant *Neisseria* g.
    (TRNG)
gonotoxemia
gonotoxin
gonotyl
Gonyaulax catanella
goodii
  Mycobacterium g.
good manufacturing practice (GMP)
Goodpasture syndrome
goose parvovirus
Gordiacea oculata
Gordiidae
Gordil virus (GORV)
Gordioidea
Gordius (p)
  G. aquaticus
  G. medinensis
  G. robustus
Gordofilm Liquid
gordonae
  Bacillus g.
  Mycobacterium g.
  Paenibacillus g.
Gordonia (b)
  G. aichiensis
  G. alkanivorans
  G. amarae
  G. amicalis
  G. bronchialis
  G. desulfuricans
  G. hirsuta
  G. hydrophobica
  G. nitida
  G. polyisoprenivorans
  G. rhizosphera

G

NOTES

Gordonia (continued)
 G. *rubropertincta*
 G. *sputi*
 G. *terrae*
gordonii
 Streptococcus g.
gorgonarius
 Thermococcus g.
gormanii
 Fluoribacter g.
 Legionella g.
GORV
 Gordil virus
goshikiensis
 Streptomyces g.
Gossas virus (GOSV)
GOSV
 Gossas virus
gottschalkii
 Anaerobranca g.
gougerotii
 Streptomyces g.
gouldingi
 Simulium g.
goundou
gourvilii
 Trichophyton g.
gout
 tophaceous g.
gp120/160 viral protein
gp41 viral protein
GPAC
 gram-positive anaerobic coccus
G6PD
 glucose-6-phosphate dehydrogenase
 glucose-6-phosphate dehydrogenase
  deficiency
 G6PD deficiency
gpELISA
 glycoprotein-based enzyme-linked
  immunosorbent assay
gp120 envelope glycoprotein
gp41 glycoprotein
GPI
 gram-positive Identification
 GPI card
GP-ST
 Group A Streptococcus Direct Test
grabhami
 Anopheles g.
gracile
 Aquaspirillum g.
 Chromatium g.
 Dipetalonema g.
 Marichromatium g.
 Methylocaldum g.

Gracilibacillus (b)
 G. *dipsosauri*
 G. *halotolerans*
gracilis
 Bacteroides g.
 Campylobacter g.
 Euglena g.
 Nitrospina g.
grade 2 vomiting
gradient
 A-a g.
 alveolar-arterial oxygen g.
graevenitzii
 Actinomyces g.
graft
 g. suppression therapy
 g. versus host (GVH)
graft-versus-host disease (GVHD)
graft-versus-leukemia effect
Grahamella (b)
 G. *peromysci*
 G. *talpae*
grahamii
 Bartonella g.
grain
 g. fever
 g. itch
graingeri
 Borrelia g.
gralli
 Philophthalmus g.
Gram
 Spectro G.
gram
 G. iodine
 g. negative
 g. positive
 splenic g.
 G. stain
Gram-chromotrope stain
gramicidin
 neomycin, polymyxin B, and g.
graminearum
 Fusarium g.
graminearus
 Streptomyces g.
graminis
 Burkholderia g.
 Gaeumannomyces g.
 Lactobacillus g.
 Pseudomonas g.
graminofaciens
 Streptomyces g.
graminophila
 Heterodera g.
grammopterae
 Mesoplasma g.

gram-negative
- g.-n. aerobe
- g.-n. bacillus
- g.-n. bacteremia
- g.-n. coccus
- g.-n. intracellular diplococci (GNID)
- g.-n. organism
- g.-n. pneumonia
- g.-n. rod

gramnicola
- *Meloidogyne g.*

grampicola
- *Crassicauda g.*

gram-positive
- g.-p. aerobe
- g.-p. anaerobic coccus (GPAC)
- g.-p. bacillus
- g.-p. bacteremia
- g.-p. coccus
- g.-p. Identification (GPI)
- g.-p. Identification card
- g.-p. organism
- g.-p. rod

Gram-variable
- G.-v. bacteria

Gram-Weigert stain
Grand Arbaud virus (GAV)
granddaughter cyst
grandis
- *Demobacter g.*
- *Deinococcus g.*
- *Diphyllobothrium g.*
- *Diplogonoporus g.*
- *Falcivibrio g.*
- *Saprospira g.*

granivorans
- *Paenibacillus g.*

grantii
- *Clostridium g.*

granular
- g. cast
- g. conjunctivitis
- g. lid
- g. ophthalmia

granularity
granularum
- *Acholeplasma g.*

granulation
- ependymal glial g.
- toxic g.

granulatus
- *Ixodes g.*

granule
- basal g.
- enteroendocrine cell g.
- metachromatic g.
- Schüffner g.
- Snaplets-FR G.'s
- sulfur g.
- volutin g.

Granulicatella (b)
- *G. adiacens*
- *G. balaenopterae*
- *G. elegans*

granulocyte
- g. colony-stimulating factor (G-CSF)
- g. transfusion

granulocyte/macrophage colony-stimulating factor (GM-CSF, rGM-CSF)
granulocyte-macrophage CSF (GM-CSF)
granulocytic sarcoma
granulocytopenia
- transient grade 2 g.

granulocytopenic
granuloma, pl. granulomata
- g. annulare
- bilharzial g.
- *Capillaria* g.
- cryptococcal g.
- cutaneous leishmaniasis g.
- Durck g.
- *Enterobius* g.
- fishtank g.
- hepatic g.
- g. inguinale
- g. inguinale tropicum
- lymphatic filariasis g.
- Majocchi g.
- mediastinal g.
- noncaseating g.
- ocular larva migrans g.
- paracoccidioidal g.
- *Paragonimus* g.
- g. pudenda
- g. pudendi
- schistosome g.
- sterile g.
- swimming pool g.
- transmural eosinophilic g.
- trichinosis g.
- g. tropicum
- g. venereum

G

NOTES

granulomatis
  Calymmatobacterium g.
  Klebsiella g.
  Mannheimia g.
  Pasteurella g.
granulomatosa
  pneumocystosis g.
granulomatosis
  g. infantiseptica
  miliary g.
granulomatous
  g. amebic encephalitis (GAE)
  g. angiitis
  g. conjunctivitis
  g. encephalitis
  g. hepatitis
  g. infection
  g. inflammation
  g. lesion
  g. nodule
  g. pneumonitis
  g. reaction
  g. synovitis
  g. uveitis
granuloplasm
granulopoiesis
granulosa
  Capnocytophaga g.
  Limnatis g.
  Oospora g.
granulosis
  ependymitis g.
granulosum
  Propionibacterium g.
  Trichosporon g.
granulosus
  Aspergillus g.
  Echinococcus g.
Granulovirus (v)
granulovirus
  Cydia pomonella g. (CpGV)
granzyme B
grape cluster appearance
graphii (f)
  Glenospora g.
Graphiolaceae
Graphium (f)
  G. eumorphum
  G. fructicola
grappe
  en g.
grasserius
  Streptomyces lavendulae subsp. g.
grassi
  Monocercomonas g.
gratiana
  Legionella g.

gravis
  myasthenia g.
gravity concentration
gray
  G. Lodge virus (GLOV)
  g. pinkgill mushroom
grayanotoxin
  g. poisoning
gray-baby syndrome
grayi
  Listeria g.
grbiciae
  Geobacter g.
Great
  G. Island virus (GIV)
  G. Saltee virus
green
  brilliant g.
  g. gill mushroom
  g. nail syndrome
Greenhow disease
gregaloid
gregaria
  Schistocerca g.
Gregarina
  G. cuneata
  G. niphandrodes
  G. polymorpha
  G. steini
gregarine
Gregarinia
gregarinosis
gregarius
  Bothriocephalus g.
gregorii
  Saccharopolyspora g.
gregoryi
  Natronobacterium g.
gregsoni
  Culicoides g.
Grepafloxacin
grepafloxacin
grerreroi
  Simulium g.
Griesinger
  bilious typhoid of G.
griffini
  Acanthamoeba g.
Grifulvin V
grignonense
  Ochrobactrum g.
grimesii
  Serratia g.
grimontii
  Leminorella g.
Griphosphaeria corticola (f)
grippe

grippotyphosa
· *Leptospira interrogans* serovar *g.*
Grisactin
G. Ultra
Grisactin-500
grisea
Humicola grisea var. *g.*
Madurella g.
Microellobosporia g.
griseinus
Streptomyces g.
griseoaurantiacus
Streptomyces g.
griseobrunneus
Streptomyces g.
griseocarneum
Streptoverticillium g.
griseocarneus
Streptomyces g.
griseochromogenes
Streptomyces g.
griseoflavus
Streptomyces g.
griseofulvin
g. microsize
g. ultramicrosize
griseofulvum
Penicillium g.
griseofuscus
Streptomyces g
griseoincarnatus
Streptomyces g.
griseola
Kitasatospora g.
griseoloalbus
Streptomyces g.
griseolosporeus
Streptomyces g.
griseolus
Streptomyces g.
griseoluteus
Streptomyces g.
griseomycini
Streptomyces g.
griseoplanus
Streptomyces g.
griseorubens
Streptomyces g.
griseoruber
Streptomyces g.
griseorubiginosus
Streptomyces g.

griseosporeus
Streptomyces g.
griseostramineus
Streptomyces g.
griseoverticillatum
Streptoverticillium g.
griseoverticillatus
Streptomyces g.
griseoviridis
Streptomyces g.
griseum
Simulium g.
griseus
Streptomyces griseus subsp. *g.*
Grisonella
Grisovin-FP
Gris-PEG
grocer itch
Grocott
G. methenamine-silver stain
G. modified silver stain
groin
hanging g.
Groningen voice prosthesis
gropengiesseri
Candida g.
grossbecki
Aedes g.
ground
g. itch
g. itch anemia
ground-glass infiltrate
group
g. A, B, C, D, E, F virus
g. A beta-hemolytic streptococcal infection
g. A beta-hemolytic streptococcal pharyngitis
g. A beta-hemolytic streptococcus adenoassociated virus g.
g. agglutination
g. agglutinin
AIDS Clinical Trials G. (ACTG)
AIDS Vaccine Evaluation G. (AVEG)
g. A *Streptococcus* (GAS)
g. A *Streptococcus* antigen testing
G. A Streptococcus Direct Test (GP-ST)
g. A streptococcus infection
avian type C retrovirus g.
Bethesda-Ballerup G.

G

NOTES

group *(continued)*
   bipartite dsRNA mycovirus g.
   bisegmented dsRNA virus g.
   Brome mosaic virus g.
   g. B streptococcal sepsis (GBS)
   g. B streptococcus (GBS)
   g. B *Streptococcus* antigen test
   bullet-shaped virus g.
   Capillovirus g.
   CDC NO-1 g.
   CDC WO-1 g.
   Centers for Disease Control and
      Prevention M5 g.
   Centers for Disease Control and
      Prevention nonoxidizer-1 g.
   Centers for Disease Control and
      Prevention O-3 g.
   Centers for Disease Control and
      Prevention weak oxidizer-1 g.
   coliphage fd g.
   coliphage MS2-GA g.
   coliphage Q-beta-SP g.
   common cold virus g.
   Coronavirus g.
   g. C rotavirus
   cryptic virus g.
   cytomegalovirus g.
   cytoplasmic polyhedrosis virus g.
   g. D antigen test
   g. D enterococcus
   diagnosis-related g. (DRG)
   dsDNA phycovirus g.
   duck hepatitis g.
   Duffy blood g.
   EEC g.
   EMC virus g.
   enterovirulent *Escherichia coli* g.
   foamy virus g.
   frog virus g.
   HACEK g.
   Hantaan virus g.
   hepatitis A, B virus g.
   HIV-1 M g.
   HIV outlier g.
   HTLV-BLV g.
   human cytomegalovirus g.
   insect parvovirus g.
   International Antimicrobial
      Project G. (IAPG)
   lymphocytic choriomeningitis
      virus g.
   lymphoproliferative virus g.
   mammalian type B oncovirus g.
   mammalian type C retrovirus g.
   mammalian type D retrovirus g.
   Marburg virus g.
   measles-rinderpest-distemper virus g.
   monopartite dsRNA mycovirus g.

   mucosal disease virus g.
   Plasma Exchange/Sandoglobulin
      Guillain-Barré Syndrome Trial G.
   pseudomallei g.
   rabies virus g.
   respiratory syncytial virus g.
   sandfly fever and Uukuniemi
      virus g.
   TTV1 virus g.
   vesicular stomatitis virus g.
GROV
   Guaroa virus
growth
   g. failure
   g. hormone (GH)
   g. hormone deficiency
   g. hormone secretion
   g. inhibition test
GRSA
   glycopeptide-resistant *Staphylococcus
      aureus*
grub
grubii
      Cryptococcus neoformans var. *g.*
Grubyella (f)
grubyi
      Arthroderma g.
grubyii
      Procandida g.
grylli
      Rickettsiella g.
gryphiswaldense
      Magnetospirillum g.
GSA65
      Giardia-specific antigen 65
GSS
   Gerstmann-Straüssler-Scheinker
   Gerstmann-Straüssler-Scheinker disease
      GSS syndrome
GST
   glutathione-*S*-transferase
      GST pull-down assay
GSV
   golden shiner virus
GTP
   guanosine triphosphate
GU71U-344 virus
GU71U-350 virus
Guaifed
Guaifed-PD
guaifenesin
      Cough Syrup with G.
   hydrocodone and g.
   hydrocodone, pseudoephedrine,
      and g.
   g. and phenylpropanolamine
   g., phenylpropanolamine, and
      dextromethorphan

g., phenylpropanolamine, and phenylephrine
g. and pseudoephedrine
g., pseudoephedrine, and codeine
g., pseudoephedrine, and dextromethorphan
theophylline and g.
Guaifenex
G. DM
G. LA
G. PSE
Guaifenex PPA 75
GuaiMAX-D
Guaipax
Guaitab
Guaituss AC
Guaivent
Guai-Vent/PSE
Guajara virus (GJAV)
Guama virus (GMAV)
guamensis
Trabulsiella g.
Guanarito virus
guanidine
Guanieri body
guanosine
g. diphosphate (GDP)
g. triphosphatase
g. triphosphate (GTP)
guanylate cyclase
guurao
Anopheles g.
Guaratuba virus
Guard
Aspirin Plus Stomach G.
Guaroa virus (GROV)
guatemalensis
Anopheles parapunctipennis g.
guaymasensis
Thermococcus g.
GUD
genital ulcer disease
GuiaCough
G. Expectorant
guianense
Simulium g.
Guiatex
Guiatuss
G. CF
G. DAC
G. PE
Guiatuss-DM

Guiatussin
G. DAC
G. With Codeine
guidance
CT g.
ultrasound g.
Guignardia (f)
G. xanthosomae
Guillain-Barré syndrome
Guilliermondella (f)
guilliermondii
Candida g.
Oscillospira g.
Pichia g.
guinea
g. worm
g. worm infection
gulae
Porphyromonas g.
gull-winged
gulosa
Thelazia g.
Gumbo Limbo virus (GLV)
gumma
tuberculous g.
gummosa
Derxia g.
gummosus
Lysobacter g.
gunbarrel sight
Gurupi virus (GURV)
GURV
Gurupi virus
gut-associated lymphoid tissue (GALT)
guttaeformis
Planctomyces g.
guttatum
Simulium g.
guttiformus
Staleya g.
guttipennis
Culicoides g.
guttoideum
Desulfotomaculum g.
gutturosa
Onchocerca g.
guyanensis
Brugia g.
Culicoides g.
Leishmania g.
GVH
graft versus host

NOTES

G

GVHD
    graft-versus-host disease
G13 virus
G virus
G-well
GXM
    glucuronoxylomannan
Gymnamoebia
Gymnamoebida
Gymnoascaceae
Gymnoascales
Gymnoascus dankaliensis (f)
Gymnodia
      G. arcuata
      G. humilis
Gymnodinium breve
Gymnophalloides seoi (p)
gymnophalloidiasis
Gymnopilus spectabilis
gymnothecium
Gynazole*1
gynecomastia
gynecophoric canal

Gynecort Topical
Gynecure
Gyne-Lotrimin
Gyne-Lotrimin 3
Gyne-Sulf
Gynogen L.A. Injection
Gyno-Trosyd
gypis
      Mycoplasma g.
gypseum
      Arthroderma g.
      Microsporum g.
gypsy moth virus
gyrauli
      Gigantobilharzia g.
Gyrodactylus (p)
Gyrodontaceae
Gyromitra (f)
      G. ambigua
      G. esculenta
      G. infula
gyromitrin

H
Hauch
H agglutinin
H colony
H 2 Oxyl
87-1-H
Gaeumannomyces graminis virus -
H. (GgV-87-1-H)
h 1–47
human adenovirus 1–47
H-19J virus
H1N1 virus
H1-type plasmid-encoded resistance
H-1 virus
HA
hepatitis A
HA1 virus
HA2 virus
HAA
hepatitis A antigen
hepatitis-associated antigen
Ha-1A
HAAP
HTLV-1-associated arthropathy
HAART
highly active antiretroviral therapy
highly active antiretroviral treatment
habituation
Habronema (p)
H. megastoma
H. microstoma
H. muscae
H. zebrae
HACEK
Haemophilus aphrophilus, Actinobacillus
actinomycetemcomitans,
Cardiobacterium hominis, Eikenella
corrodens, and Kingella
HACEK group
hachijoense
Streptoverticillium h.
hachijoensis
Streptomyces h.
hackeliae
Legionella h.
hadaliensis
Colwellia h.
hadrum
Eubacterium h.
Hadrurus
HAD test
Haemadipsa
H. ceylonica
H. chiliani

H. japonica
H. zeylanica
Haemagogus
H. albomaculatus
H. capricornii
H. equinus
H. janthinomys
H. leucocelaenus
H. spegazzinii
Haemamoeba (p) (*See* **Plasmodium**)
Haemaphysalis (p)
H. companulata
H. concinna
H. cornigera
H. doenitzi
H. flava
H. formosensis
H. fujisana
H. humerosa
H. hystricis
H. japonica
H. kitaokai
H. leachi
H. leporispalustris
H. longicornis
H. megaspinosa
H. pentalagi
H. punctata
H. spinigera
H. wellingtoni
Haematobia (p)
H. irritans
H. irritans exigua
haematobium
Schistosoma h.
haematococcus
Hypomyces h.
Nectria h.
Haematopinidae
Haematopinus (p)
H. asini
H. quadripertusus
H. suis
H. tuberculatus
Haematopota (p)
H. americana
H. pluvialis
haematopotum
Simulium h.
haematopotus
Culicoides h.
Haemobartonella (b)
H. canis
H. felis
H. muris

H

Haemodipsus ventricosus (p)
haemoglobinophilus
 Haemophilus h.
Haemogregarinidae
haemolysans
 Gemella h.
haemolytica
 Capnocytophaga h.
 Mannheimia h.
 Pasteurella h.
haemolyticum
 Arcanobacterium h.
 Clostridium h.
haemolyticus
 Acinetobacter h.
 Haemophilus h.
 Staphylococcus h.
Haemonchinae
Haemonchus (p)
 H. contortus
 H. placei
haemoperoxidus
 Enterococcus h.
haemophilum
 Mycobacterium h.
Haemophilus (b)
 H. actinomycetemcomitans
 H. aegyptius
 H. aphrophilus
 *H. aphrophilus, Actinobacillus
  actinomycetemcomitans,
  Cardiobacterium hominis,
  Eikenella corrodens, and Kingella*
  (HACEK)
 H. avium
 H. b conjugate vaccine
 H. conjunctivitis
 H. ducreyi
 H. endocarditis
 H. equigenitalis
 H. felis
 H. haemoglobinophilus
 H. haemolyticus
 H. influenzae
 H. influenzae bacteremia
 H. influenzae biogroup *aegyptius*
 H. influenzae biotype III, IV
 H. influenzae otitis
 H. influenzae pneumonia
 H. influenzae sepsis
 H. influenzae serotype c strain
 H. influenzae strain Eagan
 H. influenzae susceptibility testing
 H. influenzae type b (HIB)
 H. influenzae type b meningitis
 H. influenzae type b vaccine
 H.-Neisseria
 H.-Neisseria identification (HNID)

H.-Neisseria identification panel
H. paracuniculus
H. paragallinarum
H. parahaemolyticus
H. parainfluenzae
H. parainfluenzae biotype II
H. paraphrohaemolyticus
H. paraphrophilus
H. parasuis
H. piscium
H. pleuropneumoniae
H. segnis
H. test medium (HTM)
H. vaginalis
Haemopis
Haemoproteus (p)
haemorrhoidalis
 Gasterophilus h.
Haemosol
Haemosporida
Haemosporidium
 H. undecimanae
 H. vigesim-tertanae
haemosporidium, pl. **haemosporidia**
Haemosporina
Haemospororina
haemulonii
 Candida h.
Haffkine vaccine
Hafnia alvei (b)
hafniense
 Desulfitobacterium h.
HAG
 Histoplasma capsulatum antigen
 HAG assay
Hahella chejuensis (b)
HAI
 hemagglutination inhibition
 HAI test
hainanense
 Rhizobium h.
hair
 h. follicle
 H. and Scalp
hair-baiting test
hairworm
hairy leukoplakia
hajdui
 Planctomyces h.
hakonensis
 Sulfolobus h.
Halanaerobacter (b)
 H. chitinivorans
 H. lacunarum
 H. salinarius
Halanaerobium (b)
 H. acetethylicum
 H. alcaliphilum

H. *congolense*
H. *fermentans*
H. *kushneri*
H. *lacusrosei*
H. *praevalens*
H. *saccharolyticum* subsp.
  saccharolyticum
H. *saccharolyticum* subsp.
  senegalense
H. *salsuginis*
halcinonide
Haldrone
Halfan
half-life
Halfprin
halicephalobiasis
Halicephalobus (p)
  H. *deletrix*
  H. *gingivalis*
  H. *(Micronema)*
halide
halioticoli
  Vibrio h.
Haliphthoraceae
Haliscomenobacter (b)
  H. *hydrossis*
Hallella seregans (b)
hallii
  Eubacterium h.
hallucination
halmapalus
  Bacillus h.
halmephilum
  Flavobacterium h.
halmophila
  Halomonas h.
halo
  perinuclear h.
haloalkaliphila
  Ectothiorhodospira h.
haloalkaliphilus
  Bacillus h.
Haloanaerobiaceae
Haloarcula (b)
  H. *argentinensis*
  H. *hispanica*
  H. *japonica*
  H. *marismortui*
  H. *mukohataei*
  H. *quadrata*
  H. *vallismortis*

Halobacillus (b)
  H. *halophilus*
  H. *litoralis*
  H. *trueperi*
Halobacterium (b)
  H. *cutirubrum*
  H. *denitrificans*
  H. *distributum*
  H. *halobium*
  H. *lacusprofundi*
  H. *mediterranei*
  H. *pharaonis*
  H. *saccharovorum*
  H. *salinarium*
  H. *sodomense*
  H. *trapanicum*
  H. *vallismortis*
  H. *volcanii*
Halobacteroides (b)
  H. *acetoethylicus*
  H. *elegans*
  H. *halobius*
  H. *lacunaris*
halobacteroides
  Caulobacter h.
Halobaculum gomorrense (b)
halobetasol
halobia
  Nesterenkonia h.
halobium
  Halobacterium h.
halobius
  Halobacteroides h.
  Micrococcus h.
Halocella cellulosilytica (b)
halochloris
  Ectothiorhodospira h.
  Halorhodospira h.
Halochromatium (b)
  H. *glycolicum*
  H. *salexigens*
Halococcus (b)
  H. *litoralis*
  H. *morrhuae*
  H. *saccharolyticus*
  H. *salifodinae*
  H. *turkmenicus*
halodenitrificans
  Bacillus h.
  Halomonas h.
  Paracoccus h.

NOTES

H

239

halodurans
    Bacillus h.
    Halomonas h.
    Roseivivax h.
Halofantrine
halofantrine
Haloferax (b)
    H. denitrificans
    H. gibbonsii
    H. mediterranei
    H. volcanii
Halog
Halog-E
halogenated
halogen-releasing
Halogeometricum borinquense (b)
Haloincola (b)
    H. saccharolyticus subsp.
     saccharolyticus
    H. saccharolyticus subsp.
     senegalensis
Halomethanococcus (b)
    H. doii
    H. mahii
Halomonadaceae
Halomonas (b)
    H. aquamarina
    H. campisalis
    H. canadensis
    H. cupida
    H. desiderata
    H. elongata
    H. eurihalina
    H. halmophila
    H. halodenitrificans
    H. halodurans
    H. halophila
    H. israelensis
    H. magadiensis
    H. marina
    H. meridiana
    H. pacifica
    H. pantelleriensis
    H. salina
    H. subglaciescola
    H. variabilis
    H. venusta
Halonatronum saccharophilum (b)
haloperidol
halophil
halophila
    Actinopolyspora h.
    Deleya h.
    Desulfocella h.
    Ectothiorhodospira h.
    Halomonas h.
    Halorhodospira h.
    Nocardiopsis h.

    Pseudomonas h.
    Spirochaeta h.
    Sporosarcina h.
    Thiocapsa h.
    Thiohalocapsa h.
halophilic
halophilum
    Clostridium h.
    Desulfotomaculum h.
    Microbacterium h.
halophilus
    Bacillus h.
    Culicoides h.
    Desulfovibrio h.
    Halobacillus h.
    Halothiobacillus h.
    Marinococcus h.
    Methanococcus h.
    Methanohalophilus h.
    Pediococcus h.
    Planococcus h.
    Tetragenococcus h.
    Thiobacillus h.
halophobica
    Pseudoamycolata h.
    Pseudonocardia h.
halophytica
    Micromonospora h.
    Micromonospora halophytica subsp.
     h.
haloplanktis
    Alteromonas h.
    Pseudoalteromonas h.
halopraeferens
    Azospirillum h.
haloprogin
Halorhabdus utahensis (b)
Halorhodospira (b)
    H. abdelmalekii
    H. halochloris
    H. halophila
Halorubrobacterium (b)
    H. coriense
    H. distributum
    H. lacusprofundi
    H. saccharovorum
    H. sodomense
Halorubrum (b)
    H. coriense
    H. distributum
    H. lacusprofundi
    H. saccharovorum
    H. sodomense
    H. trapanicum
    H. vacuolatum
Halosphaeriaceae
Halospirulina tapeticola (b)

Haloterrigena (b)
  H. thermotolerans
  H. turkmenica
Halotestin
Halotex
halothane
Halothermothrix orenii (b)
Halothiobacillus (b)
  H. halophilus
  H. hydrothermalis
  H. kellyi
  H. neapolitanus
halotolerans
  Brevibacterium h.
  Desulfobacter h.
  Gracilibacillus h.
  Lactobacillus h.
  Methanocalculus h.
  Roseivivax h.
  Weissella h.
Halotussin
  H. DAC
  H. DM
  H. PE
Halovibrio (b)
  H. variabilis
halstedii
  Streptomyces h.
Halteridium (p)
Haltran
halzoun
HAM
  HTLV-1-associated myelopathy
hamburgensis
  Nitrobacter h.
hamelinense
  Roseibium h.
hamsteri
  Lactobacillus h.
HAM/TSP
  HTLV-1-associated myelopathy/tropical
  spastic paraparesis
hamulosa
  Cheilospirura h.
Hancock porcine aortic valve
hand
  crab h.
hand-foot-and-mouth disease
hanedai
  Alteromonas h.
  Shewanella h.
hanging-block culture

hanging-drop
  h.-d. mount
  h.-d. procedure
hanging groin
Hannebertia (f)
Hansel stain
Hansen
  H. bacillus
  H. disease
hansenii
  Acetobacter h.
  Debaryomyces h.
  Gluconacetobacter h.
  Ruminococcus h.
  Streptococcus h.
  Torulaspora h.
Hansenula
  H. anomala
  H. californica
  H. canadensis
  H. capsulata
  H. ciferrii
  H. glucozyma
  H. henricii
  H. holstii
  H. minuta
  H. nonfermentans
  H. philodendri
  H. polymorpha
  H. saturnus
  H. subpelliculosa
  H. wickerhamii
  H. wingei
hansonii
  Methylosphaera h.
Hantaan
  H. virus (HTNV)
  H. virus group
Hantaan-like virus
H2 antagonist
Hantavirus (v)
  H. pulmonary syndrome
hantavirus
  h. disease (HVD)
  h. infection
  h. pulmonary syndrome (HPS)
  h. serology
HAP
  hyperthermic antiblastic perfusion
hapla
  Meloidogyne h.

NOTES

H

Haplographium (f)
   H. chlorocephalum
   H. pororicense
haplophila
   Pichia h.
Haplorchis (p)
   H. pumilio
   H. taichui
Haplosporangium parvum (f)
Haplosporidia
Harada-Mori filter paper strip culture
haranensis
   Biomphalaria h.
harbinensis
   Glycomyces h.
hard
   h. gel capsule (HGC)
   h. tick
hardjo
   Leptospira interrogans serovar *h.*
hare fibroma virus
harei
   Peptoniphilus h.
   Peptostreptococcus h.
Harpochytriaceae
Harpochytriales
hartmannellae
   Neochlamydia h.
Hartmannella veriformis (p)
Hartmannellidae
hartmanni
   Entamoeba h.
Hart Park virus (HPV)
harvest
   h. bug
   h. mite
harvester ant
harveyi
   Beneckea h.
   Borrelia h.
   Lucibacterium h.
   Vibrio h.
hasamiyami
Hashimoto
   H. disease
   H. thyroiditis
hassiacum
   Mycobacterium h.
hastiforme
   Clostridium h.
HAstV-1-7
   human astrovirus serotype 1-7
hatchetti
   Acanthamoeba h.
hatching flask
Hauch (H)
hauseri
   Proteus h.

HAV
   hepatitis A virus
Haverhill fever
Havrix
HAVRIX vaccine
Hawaii
   H. agent
   H. virus
hawaiiensis
   Cochliobolus h.
   Streptomyces h.
hawsi
   Culicoides h.
hay bacillus
Hayfebrol Liquid
haysi
   Simulium h.
Hazara virus (HAZV)
haze
   corneal h.
   vitreous h.
HAZV
   Hazara virus
HB
   Recombivax HB
   HB virus
HBAg
   hepatitis B antigen
HBeAg
   hepatitis B e antigen
HBIG, H-BIG
   hepatitis B immune globulin
   hepatitis B virus immunoglobulin
   hyperimmune serum globulin
HbOC vaccine
HBsAg
   hepatitis B surface antigen
   surface antigen of hepatitis B virus
HbsAg
   hepatitis B surface antigen
HbsAg-positive persistent hepatitis B virus infection
HBT
   human blood bilayer Tween
HBV
   hepatitis B virus
   HBV serology
HC
   Dermaflex HC
   Diospor HC
   Prevex HC
   Sarna HC
   HC testing
   Ti-U-Lac HC
HCG
   human chorionic gonadotropin
   HCG test

HCl
  amiodarone HCl
  Aralen HCl
  Cleocin HCl
  clinafloxacin HCl
  diphenoxylate HCl
  meperidine HCl
  proparacaine-HCl
  quinacrine HCl
  valacyclovir HCl
HCMV
  human cytomegalovirus
  human cytomegalovirus infection
HCV
  hepatitis C virus
    HCV genotyping
HCW
  health care worker
HD
  hemodialysis
HDCV
  human diploid cell culture rabies vaccine
  human diploid cell rabies vaccine
HDL cholesterol
HDoov
  Humpty Doo virus
HDS
  HIV Dementia Scale
HDV
  hepatitis delta virus
  hepatitis D virus
HE
  human ehrlichiosis
H&E
  hematoxylin and eosin
    H&E stain
head
  h. botfly
  femoral h.
  h. louse
  h. and neck tuberculosis
  H. & Shoulders
  H. & Shoulders Intensive
    Treatment
Headache Tablets
Headarest
healing
  ascended h.
health
  h. care worker (HCW)

National Institute for Occupational
  Safety and H. (NIOSH)
National Institutes of H. (NIH)
heart
  hypoplastic left h. (HLH)
  h. transplantation
  h. valve vegetation
heartworm
heat
  h. and moisture exchanging filter
    (HMEF)
  h. shock protein (HSP)
  h. shock protein antibody
  h. stroke
**heating, ventilating, and air
  conditioning (HVAC)**
heat-killed
heat-labile
  h.-l. toxin
heat-phenol inactivated vaccine
hebdomadis
  Leptospira interrogans serovar *h.*
Hebeloma mesophaeum (f)
hebraeum
  Amblyomma h.
Hecht pneumonia
Heck
  H. disease
  focal epithelial hyperplasia of H.
heckeshornense
  Mycobacterium h.
Hectopsyllidae
hectoris
  Anopheles h.
heel
  h. fly
  h. stick
hegeneri
  Philophthalmus h.
heidelbergense
  Mycobacterium h.
heimbachae
  Providencia h.
heintzii
  Chelatobacter h.
Hektoen agar
HeLa cell
Helcococcus (b)
  H. kunzii
  H. ovis
helcogenes
  Bacteroides h.

NOTES

H

243

Helenium
    H. S virus
    H. Y virus
helical
helicase
Helicobacter (b)
    H. acinonychis
    H. bilis
    H. bizzozeronii
    H. canis
    H. cholecystus
    H. cinaedi
    H. felis
    H. fennelliae
    H. hepaticus
    H. mesocricetorum
    H. muridarum
    H. mustelae
    H. nemestrinae
    H. pametensis
    H. pullorum
    H. pylori
    H. pylori-associated gastritis
    H. pylori culture and urease test
    H. pylori gastritis
    H. pylori-related gastritis
    H. pylori serology
    H. pylori urea breath test
    H. rodentium
    H. salomonis
    H. sp. strain Mainz
    H. trogontum
Helicocephalidaceae
helicoides
    Spiroplasma h.
Helicotylenchus (p)
    H. digonicus
    H. labiodiscinus
    H. leiocephalus
    H. platyurus
    H. pseudorobustus
Helidac
Heliobacillus mobilis (b)
Heliobacterium (b)
    H. chlorum
    H. gestii
    H. modesticaldum
    H. sulfidophilum
    H. undosum
heliomycini
    Streptomyces h.
Heliophilum fasciatum (b)
Heliorestis (b)
    H. baculata
    H. daurensis
heliothermus
    Antarctobacter h.
Heliothrix oregonensis (b)

heliotrinreducens
    Peptococcus h.
    Peptostreptococcus h.
    Slackia h.
Heliozoea
hellem
hellenica
    Weissella h.
hellenicus
    Staphylothermus h.
Hellvella elastica (f)
helminth
    h. infection
helminthagogue
helminthemesis
helminthiasis
helminthic, helmintic
    h. dysentery
    h. meningitis
    h. parasite
helminthism
helminthoeca
    Neorickettsia h.
helminthoid
helminthology
helminthoma
Helminthosporium (f)
Helminthosporum dematoideum (f)
helmintic (*var. of* helminthic)
Helophilus hybridus
Helotiaceae
Helotiales
helper
    h. cell
    h. cell/suppressor ratio
    h. virus
helvata
    Actinomadura h.
    Microtetraspora h.
    Nonomuraea h.
helvaticus
    Streptomyces h.
Helvellaceae
Helvella esculenta (f)
helvetianus
    Nematodirus h.
helvetica
    Methylopila h.
    Rickettsia h.
helveticus
    Campylobacter h.
    Lactobacillus h.
hemachromatosis
hemacytozoon
hemadsorbing virus
hemadsorption
    h. test (HAD test)

h. virus test
h. virus test type 1, 2
hemagglutinating unit
hemagglutination
h. inhibition (HAI)
h. inhibition test (HAI test)
reversed passive h. (RPHA)
Treponema pallidum h. (TPHA)
hemagglutination-inhibition (HI)
hemagglutinin
filamentous h. (FHA)
influenza virus h.
kidney bean h.
viral h.
hemagglutinin-neuraminidase (HN)
hemamebiasis
hematemesis
hematochezia
hematocrit
h. concentration
hematocytozoon
hematogenous
h. dissemination
h. pneumonia
h. spread
hematogenous dissemination
hematogenously
h. disseminated candidiasis
seed h.
hematologic
h. malignancy
h. toxicity
hematologist
hematoma
infected h.
subdural h.
hematopathologist
hematophagia
hematophagous
hematopoiesis
hematopoietic
h. progenitor
h. stem cell (HSC)
h. stem cell gene therapy
h. stem cell transplantation
hematopoietic cell
hematoxylin
h. and eosin (H&E)
h. and eosin stain
Mayer h.
hematoxylinophilic
hematozoic

hematozoon
hematuria
Egyptian h.
endemic h.
microscopic h.
terminal h.
hematuric bilious fever
hemianopia
Hemiascomycetes
hemic distomiasis
Hemichorda
Hemichordata
hemidiaphragm
hemihypesthesia
Hemiluca maia
hemimetabolous
hemin
hemiparesis
hemipelvectomy
Hemiphacidiaceae
hemiplegia
Hemiptera
hemipterus
Cimex h.
Hemispora stellata (f)
hemiteleus
Aedes h.
Hemiuridae
Hemivirus (v)
hemoagglutinin
hemocele
hemochromatosis
hemoconcentration
h. technique
hemocyanin
keyhole-limpet h. (KLH)
hemocytozoon
hemodialysis (HD)
hemodialyzer
hemodynamic
hemoflagellate
mitochondrion of h.
hemoglobin
h. A_{2C} value
h. cast
h. concentration
glucose, lactalbumin, serum, and h. (GLSH)
h. H
h. SC
hemoglobinemia

NOTES

H

hemoglobinopathy
    congenital h.
    iron-deficiency h.
hemoglobinophilic
hemoglobinuria
    malarial h.
    paroxysmal cold h.
hemoglobinuria and glomerular
   thrombosis (HUS/TTP)
hemoglobinuric
    h. fever
    h. nephrosis
hemogram
hemolymph
hemolymphatic stage
hemolysin
    alpha h.
    bacterial h.
    beta h.
    immune h.
    Kanagawa h.
    natural h.
    specific h.
    thermostable direct h. (TDH)
hemolysis
    alpha h.
    autoimmune h.
    beta h.
    biologic h.
    blood agar h.
    gamma h.
    immune h.
    h. inhibition
    viridans h.
hemolytic
    h. anemia
    beta h.
    h. streptococci
    h. uremic syndrome (HUS)
    h. uremic syndrome/thrombotic
      thrombocytopenia purpura
      (HUS/TTP)
hemoperitoneum
hemophagia
hemophagocytic syndrome
hemophagocytosis
hemophil
hemophilia
    h. A, B
hemophiliac
hemophilic
hemopoiesis
hemoptysis
    endemic h.
    exsanguinating h.
    parasitic h.
hemorrhage
    diffuse interstitial h.

    intracerebral h.
    intraretinal h.
    intraventricular h.
    petechial h.
    pulmonary h.
    splinter h.
    subarachnoid h. (SAH)
    subconjunctival h.
    subepithelial h.
    subungual splinter h.
    vitreous h.
hemorrhagic
    h. bulla
    h. colitis
    h. cystitis
    h. dengue
    h. diathesis
    h. enteritis
    h. fever
    h. fever renal syndrome
    h. fever with renal symptom
      (HFRS)
    h. fever with renal syndrome
      (HFRS)
    h. lesion
    h. leukoencephalopathy
    h. mediastinitis
    h. necrosis
    h. pain
    h. pancreatitis
    h. pneumonitis
    h. pyoderma gangrenosum
    h. rash
    h. septicemia
    h. smallpox
    h. telangiectasia
hemorrhoid
hemosiderin
hemosiderosis
hemosporidium
hemosporines
hemostasis
hemothorax
Hemovac tip culture
hemozoic
hemozoon
hendersoni
    Aedes h.
Hendersonula (f)
Hendra-like virus
Hendra virus
Henoch purpura
Henoch-Schönlein
    H.-S. purpura
    H.-S. syndrome
    H.-S. vasculitis
henrici
    Schizoblastosporion h.

henricii
  Blastobacter h.
  Caulobacter h.
  Hansenula h.
  Pichia h.
henselae
  Bartonella h.
  Rochalimaea h.
HEPA
  high-efficiency particulate air
  HEPA filter
Hepacivirus (v)
Hepadnaviridae
hepadnavirus
heparina
  Cytophaga h.
heparinized
heparinolytica
  Prevotella h.
heparinolyticus
  Bacteroides h.
heparinum
  Flavobacterium h.
  Sphingobacterium h.
heparinus
  Pedobacter h.
hepar lobatum
hepatic
  h. abscess
  h. amebiasis
  h. cytolysis
  h. disease
  h. enzyme
  h. failure
  h. granuloma
  h. transaminase
hepatica
  Capillaria h.
  Fasciola h.
Hepaticola (p) (*See Capillaria*)
hepaticus
  Helicobacter h.
hepatis
hepatitis, pl. **hepatitides**
  h. A (HA)
  h. A antigen (HAA)
  h. A, B virus group
  A-like non-A non-B h.
  anicteric virus h.
  autoimmune chronic h.
  h. A vaccine
  h. A virus (HAV)

h. B
h. B antigen (HBAg)
h. B core antibody
h. B core antigen
h. B, C seropositivity
h. B DNA detection
h. B e antigen (HBeAg)
h. B e antigen-positive
h. B immune globulin (HBIG, H-BIG)
B-like non-A non-B h.
h. B profile
h. B serology
h. B surface antibody (anti-HBs)
h. B surface antigen (HBsAg, HbsAg)
h. B surface antigen-positive persistent hepatitis B virus infection
h. B vaccine
h. B viral DNA assay
h. B virus (HBV)
h. B virus core
h. B virus immunoglobulin (HBIG, H-BIG)
chronic active h. (CAH)
chronic aggressive h.
chronic h. C (CHC)
chronic persistent h. (CPH)
chronic viral h.
h. C RNA detection
h. C serology
h. C viral RNA
h. C viral RNA genotyping
h. C virus (HCV)
h. C virus antibody detection
delta h.
h. delta virus (HDV)
h. D serology
h. D virus (HDV)
h. E
enterically transmitted non-A non-B h. (ET-NANBH)
epidemic h.
h. E serology
h. E virus (HEV)
fecal-oral non-A non-B h.
fulminant h.
granulomatous h.
h. G virus (HGV)
icteric h.
infectious canine h.

NOTES

H

hepatitis *(continued)*
> long incubation h.
> lupoid h.
> mouse h.
> NANB h.
> non-ABC h.
> non-A-E h.
> non-A-G h.
> non-A, non-B h.
> nonviral h.
> parenterally transmitted non-A non-B h. (PT-NANBH)
> posttransfusion h. (PTH)
> prolonged acute h.
> relapsing h. B
> serum h.
> short incubation h.
> transfusion h.
> type A viral h.
> viral h.
> h. virus

hepatitis-associated antigen (HAA)
hepatitis C
hepatobiliary
> h. disease
> h. tuberculosis

hepatocellular necrosis
Hepatocystis (p)
> *H. kochi* (*See Plasmodium kochi*)
> *H. simiae*

hepatocyte anisonucleosis
hepatoma
hepatomegaly
hepatopancreatic parvo-like virus
hepatosplenic
> h. candidiasis
> h. schistosomiasis

hepatosplenomegaly
hepatotoxic
hepatotoxicity
hepatotropic
Hepatovirus (v)
Hepatozoon (p)
> *H. canis*
> *H. muris*

Hep-B Gammagee
Heptavax immunization
Heptovir
HER
> HIV Epidemiology Research
> HER Study

herbal therapy
herbaricolor
> *Streptomyces h.*

herbariorum
> *Eurotium h.*
> *Muscor h.*

herbarum
> *Cladosporium h.*
> *Phoma h.*
> *Pleospora h.*

Herbaspirillum (b)
> *H. frisingense*
> *H. rubrisubalbicans*
> *H. seropedicae*

herbicidovorans
> *Sphingobium h.*
> *Sphingomonas h.*

herbicola
> *Erwinia h.*

herbicola-lathyri bacteria (*See Enterobacter agglomerans*)
herbida
> *Actinocorallia h.*

Herbidospora cretacea (b)
herbivorans
> *Clostridium h.*

herbivorous
Herbogesic
herd immunity
hereditary spherocytosis
Herisan
hermannii
> *Escherichia h.*

hermaphrodite
Hermetia
> *H. illucens*

hermsi
> *Ornithodoros h.*

hermsii
> *Borrelia h.*

hernia
> inguinal h.
> umbilical h.

herniation
> cerebellar h.
> intracranial h.
> uncal h.

herniorrhaphy
herpangina
HerpChek test
herpes
> acyclovir-resistant h.
> anogenital h.
> h. B encephalomyelitis
> h. catarrhalis
> h. circinatus bullosus
> cutaneous h.
> h. cytology
> h. esophagitis
> genital h.
> h. genitalis
> h. gladiatorum
> h. iris
> h. labialis

neonatal h.
h. neonatorium
h. progenitalis
h. simplex (HS)
h. simplex antibody
h. simplex conjunctivitis
h. simplex culture
h. simplex encephalitis
h. simplex infection
h. simplex keratitis
h. simplex recurrens
h. simplex viral shedding
h. simplex virus (HSV)
h. simplex virus 1 (HSV-1)
h. simplex virus 2 (HSV-2)
h. simplex virus arthritis
traumatic h.
h. whitlow
h. zoster
h. zoster generalisatus
h. zoster infection
h. zoster ophthalmicus
h. zoster oticus
h. zoster serology
h. zoster varicellosus
h. zoster virus
Herpesviridae
herpesvirus
h. ateles virus
bovine h. 1–5
cercopithecine h. 1–2
chimpanzee h.
h. encephalitis
felid h. 1
feline h.
gamma h.
gamma-2 h.
h. hominis
human h. (HHV)
human h. 1–8 (HHV 1–8)
human (alpha) h. 1
human herpesvirus 8/Kaposi
  sarcoma h. (HHV-8/KSHV)
human h. 6 variant A, B
Kaposi sarcoma h. (KSHV)
Kaposi sarcoma-associated h.
  (KSHV)
pongine h. 2
h. protein
h. saimiri (HVS)
saimiriine h. 1
suid h.

suid h. 2
h. type 1
Herpesvirus simiae
herpete
zoster sine h.
herpetic
h. angina
h. conjunctivitis
h. fever
h. gingivostomatitis
h. inclusion body
h. keratitis
h. keratoconjunctivitis
h. lesion
h. meningoencephalitis
h. paronychia
h. tracheobronchitis
h. ulcer
h. ulceration
h. vesicle
h. vulvovaginitis
h. whitlow
herpetiform
herpetiformis
dermatitis h.
impetigo h.
Herpetomonas (p)
Herpetosiphon (b)
  H. aurantiacus
  H. cohaerens
  H. geysericola
  H. nigricans
  H. persicus
Herpetoviridae
Herpetovirus
herpetovirus
caprine h.
Herpomycetaceae
Herpotrichia (f)
Herpotrichiellaceae
herreri
  Simulium h.
herring
h. worm
h. worm disease
hertigi
  Leishmania h.
Herxheimer
H. reaction
hesperidum
  Alicyclobacillus h.
Heterakidae

NOTES

H

Heterakis (p)
    H. gallinarum
    H. spumosa
Heterakoidea
heterecious
heterecism
Heterobasidiomyceter
Heterobilharzia americana (p)
heteroderae
    Torula h.
Heterodera graminophila (p)
Heteroderidae
Heterodoxus spiniger (p)
heteroduplex
    h. analysis
    h. mobility assay (HMA)
heterogamy
heterogeneity
heterogenetic parasite
heterogenic endobacterial antigen
heterogenicus
    Saccharomyces h.
heterogonic life cycle
heterograft
    bovine h.
heterohiochii
    Lactobacillus h.
heteromastigote
heterometabolous
heteromorpha
    Exophiala jeanselmei var. *h.*
heteronema
    Cylindrocarpon h.
heterophil
    h. antibody
    h. antibody test
heterophil-negative
    h.-n. mononucleosis
    h.-n. syndrome
Heterophyes (p)
    H. heterophyes
    H. katsuradai
heterophyes
    Heterophyes h.
heterophyiasis
heterophyid
    h. worm
Heterophyidae
heterophyidiasis
Heterophyopsis continua (p)
heteropolymer
Heteroptera
heterosexual
heterosporus
    Ophiobolus h.
heterothallic
heterothallica
    Thielavia h.

heterotopic ossification
heterotremus
    Paragonimus h.
Heterotrichia
heterotroph
heterotrophic
heterovaccine therapy
heteroxenous
    h. parasite
heterozygous
    h. thalassemia
Hetrazan
HEV
    hepatitis E virus
HEV1
    hibernal epidemic viral infection
heveanensis
    Cryptococcus h.
Hexa-Betalin
hexacanth
    h. embryo
hexachloride
    benzene h.
    gamma benzene h.
hexachlorocyclohexane
hexachlorophene
Hexadnovirus
Hexadrol
hexagonus
    Ixodes h.
hexamethylenetetramine
    methenamine h.
Hexamitidae
Hexapoda
Hexifoam
Hexit
hexodontus
    Aedes h.
hexon
HFA
    Proventil H.
H-F Antidote
HFRS
    hemorrhagic fever with renal symptom
    hemorrhagic fever with renal syndrome
HFR strain
HGC
    hard gel capsule
    saquinavir HGC
HGE
    human granulocytic ehrlichiosis
    hyperglycemic-glycogenolytic factor
hGH
    human growth hormone
HGV
    hepatitis G virus
HHAV
    human hepatitis A virus

HHV
   human herpesvirus
HHV 1–8
   human herpesvirus 1–8
HHV-8
    HHV-8 latent IgG antibody
    HHV-8 lytic IgG antibody
HHV-8/KSHV
   human herpesvirus 8/Kaposi sarcoma
     herpesvirus
HI
   hemagglutination-inhibition
hians
    Cathaemasia h.
HIB
    Haemophilus influenzae type b
hibernal epidemic viral infection
   (HEV1)
hiberniae
    Mycobacterium h.
hibernica
    Phoma h.
hibernum
    Flavobacterium h.
Hibiclens Topical
Hibidil
hibisca
    Actinomadura h.
hibiscicola
    Pseudomonas h.
Hibiscrub
Hibistat Topical
Hibitane
HibTITER
    H. vaccine
Hib-TT vaccine
HI-CAL VM bar
Hickman/Broviac catheter
Hickman catheter
Hi-Cor-1.0 Topical
Hi-Cor-2.5 Topical
HICPAC
   Hospital Infection Control Practices
    Advisory Committee
hidradenitis
    h. suppurativa (HS)
hidradenoma papilliferum
hiemalis
    acrodermatitis pustolosis h.
    Mucor h.
hienipiensis
    Saccharomyces h.

hieroglyphicus
    Culicoides h.
high
    h. affinity antigen receptor
    H. and Leifson test
    h. vaginal swab
high-density lipoprotein cholesterol
   (HDL cholesterol)
high-dose chemotherapy
high-efficiency
    h.-e. particulate air (HEPA)
    h.-e. particulate air filter
high-egg-passage vaccine
high-flux dialysis
high-frequency sensorineural
high-grade
    h.-g. extrahepatic biliary obstruction
    h.-g. squamous intraepithelial lesion
    (HSIL)
Highlands J virus (HJV)
highly active antiretroviral therapy
   (HAART)
highly active antiretroviral treatment
   (HAART)
high-performance
    h.-p. liquid chromatography (HPLC)
    h.-p. liquid chromatography assay
high-purity factor VIII
high-speed centrifugation
high-titer viremia
Hikojima
    Vibrio cholerae serotype 01 *H.*
hila (*pl. of* hilum)
hilar
    h. adenopathy
    h. lymphadenopathy
hilgardii
    Lactobacillus h.
hilli
    Anopheles amictus h.
HILP
   hyperthermic isolated limb perfusion
hilum, pl. hila
Himasthla (p)
hindustanus
    Streptoalloteichus h.
hinmani
    Culicoides h.
hinshawii
    Arizona h. (*See Salmonella*
    arizonae)

NOTES

H

251

hinzii
 Bordetella h.
hip
 h. arthrogram
 h. arthroplasty
 h. disarticulation
Hippea maritima (b)
Hippelates
 H. dorsalis
Hippel-Lindau
 von H.-L. (vHL)
hippikon
 Acholeplasma h.
Hippobosca (p)
 H. longipennis
Hippoboscidae
hippurate
 h. crystal
 h. hydrolysis
 methenamine h.
hippuratus
 Agromyces fucosus subsp. *h.*
Hip-Rex
Hiprex
hirae
 Enterococcus h.
hirame rhabdovirus
hiranonis
 Clostridium h.
hiroshimense
 Oceanospirillum h.
 Oceanospirillum maris subsp. *h.*
 Streptoverticillium h.
hiroshimensis
 Streptomyces h.
Hirsch charcoal agar modified medium
Hirschia baltica (b)
hirschiana
 Hyphomonas h.
hirschii
 Hydrogenophilus h.
 Prosthecomicrobium h.
hirsuta
 Gordonia h.
 Saccharopolyspora hirsuta subsp. *h.*
hirsutism
hirsutoid papillomatosis
hirsutus
 Streptomyces h.
hirta
 Cynomya h.
hirthi
 Filaroides h.
hirtipes
 Prosimulium h.
hirtipupa
 Simulium h.

hirtulus
 Culicoides h.
hirudinaceus
 Macracanthorhynchus h.
Hirudinea
hirudiniasis
Hirudo (p)
 H. medicinalis
 H. sjoestedi
Hismanal
Hispanic
hispanica
 Arthropsis h.
 Borrelia h.
 Haloarcula h.
hispanicus
 Marinococcus h.
 Salinicoccus h.
hispidum
 Gnathostoma h.
histamine
 h. dihydrochloride
 h. poisoning
histamine-2 receptor (H_2R)
 histamine-2-receptor antagonist
histamine-sensitizing factor
histaminum
 Photobacterium h.
Histenol Cold
Histerone Injection
histidine
histidine-rich protein-II (HRP-II)
histidinolovorans
 Arthrobacter h.
histidinovorans
 Natronincola h.
Histinex D Liquid
histiocyte
histiocytic
 h. hyperplasia
 h. lymphoma
histiocytoma
histiocytosis
 chronic h.
 focal h.
 malignant h.
 sinus h.
histocompatibility
histoid leprosy
Histolyn-CYL
histolytica
 Entamoeba h.
histolyticum
 Clostridium h.
Histomonas meleagridis (p)
histopathologic
histopathological
histopathologically

histopathology
Histoplasma (f)
    H. capsulatum
    H. capsulatum antibody and
      antigen
    H. capsulatum antigen (HAG)
    H. capsulatum var. *capsulatum*
    H. capsulatum var. *farciminosum*
    H. capsulatum fungemia
    H. capsulatum polysaccharide
      antigen (HPA)
histoplasma polysaccharide antigen
histoplasmin
    h. skin test
histoplasmoma
histoplasmosis
    acute pulmonary h.
    African h.
    cavitary pulmonary h.
    disseminated h.
    h. immunodiffusion
    mediastinal h.
    primary pulmonary h.
    progressive disseminated h. (PDH)
    pulmonary h.
    h. serology
history
    pathophysiology and natural h.
histotropic
histozoic
Histussin D Liquid
His-Werner disease
HIV
    human immunodeficiency virus
    HIV clade F
    HIV core antigen
    HIV Dementia Scale (HDS)
    HIV DNA amplication assay
    drug-resistant HIV
    HIV encephalitis
    HIV encephalopathy
    HIV enteropathy
    HIV Epidemiology Research (HER)
    HIV Epidemiology Research Study
    HIV genital ulcer
    HIV genotyping
    HIV gingivitis
    HIV group O
    HIV lipodystrophy
    HIV Network for Prevention Trials
      (HIVNET)
    HIV outlier group

    HIV p24 antigen
    HIV periodontitis
    HIV retinopathy
    HIV RNA level
    HIV salivary gland disease
    HIV shedding
    HIV subtype E
    HIV therapy
    HIV Vaccine Efficacy Trials
      Network (HIVNET)
    HIV Vaccine Efficacy Trials
      Network study
    HIV Vaccine Trials Network
      (HVTN)
    HIV viral load assay
    HIV viral protein
    HIV viremia
    HIV wasting syndrome
HIV-1
    human immunodeficiency virus 1, 2
    human immunodeficiency virus-type 1
    HIV-1 culture assay
    HIV-1 drug resistance testing
    HIV-1 encephalitis
    HIV-1 encephalopathy
    HIV-1 gene sequencing
    HIV-1 genome
    HIV-1 genomic sequence
    HIV-1 group O
    HIV-1 immunogen
    HIV-1 M group
    HIV-1 mutations testing
    HIV-1 RNA
    HIV-1 serology
    HIV-1 subtype C (HIV-1C)
HIV-2
    human immunodeficiency virus 1, 2
    human immunodeficiency virus-type 2
    HIV-2 proviral load
    HIV-2 viral load
HIV-1$_{IIIB}$ rgp160 polypeptide vaccine
HIV-1-specific reverse transcriptase
  inhibitor
Hivagen antibody test
HIV/AIDS
HIVAN
    HIV-associated nephropathy
HIV-associated
    H.-a. complication
    H.-a. lipodystrophy syndrome
    H.-a. motor cognitive disorder

NOTES

H

HIV-associated *(continued)*
    H.-a. nephropathy (HIVAN)
    H.-a. tuberculosis
HIV-1C
    HIV-1 subtype C
HIVCHEK-1/2 assay
HIVID
Hivid
HIV-induced microangiopathy
HIV-infected patient
HIV-negative
HIVNET
    HIV Network for Prevention Trials
    HIV Vaccine Efficacy Trials Network
    HIVNET study
HIV-positive
HIV-related thrombocytopenia
HIV-seronegative
HIV-seropositive
HIV-specific antibody
HJV
    Highlands J virus
HLA
    human leukocyte antigen
        HLA typing
HLA-A24
    human leukocyte antigen-A24
HLA-B27 histocompatibility antigen
HLH
    hypoplastic left heart
HLVd
HMA
    heteroduplex mobility assay
HME
    human monocytic ehrlichiosis
HMEF
    heat and moisture exchanging filter
HMG CoA reductase inhibitor
HMO
    hypothetical mean organism
HMS
    hypothetical mean strain
HN
    hemagglutinin-neuraminidase
HN131 virus
HN199 virus
HN295 virus
HN59 virus
HNID
    Haemophilus-Neisseria identification
        HNID panel
HOA
    hypertrophic osteoarthropathy
hoagii
    Corynebacterium h.
hobo spider

Hodgkin
    H. disease
    H. lymphoma
hodleri
    Mycobacterium h.
Hofbauer cell
hoffmanii
    Lecythophora h.
hoffmanni
    Simulium h.
Hofmann bacillus
hog cholera virus
hoguei
    Culicoides h.
höhn
    Physosporella h.
holarctica
    Francisella tularensis biogroup *h.*
Hold
    Children's H.
    H. DM
Holdemania filiformis (b)
holiday
    drug h.
hollandica
    Prochlorothrix h.
hollandicum
    Hyphomicrobium h.
hollandicus
    Aspergillus h.
Hollandina pterotermitidis (b)
hollensis
    Culicoides h.
hollisae
    Vibrio h.
holmesii
    Bordetella h.
    Mobiluncus curtisii subsp. *h.*
holmii
    Drechslera h.
    Setosphaeria h.
Holobasidiomycetidae
holocyclus
    Ixodes h.
holomastigote
holometabolous
    h. metamorphosis
holomyarian
Holophaga foetida (b)
holophytic
Holospora (b)
    H. caryophila
    H. elegans
    H. obtusa
    H. undulata
holotrichous
holozoic

holsaticus
    Sporobolomyces h.
holstii
    Hansenula h.
    Pichia h.
Homalomyia
homari
    Alcaligenes faecalis subsp. h.
homatropine
    hydrocodone and h.
home
    h. collection testing (HC testing)
    h. infusion device
    h. intravenous antibiotic
    nursing h. (NH)
homeless
homelessness
homeopathy
    constitutional h.
    patterned h.
homeostasis
    CD4+ T-cell h.
    T-cell h.
homilentoma
    Candida h.
hominis
    Actinobacillus h.
    Blastocystis h.
    Campylobacter h.
    Cardiobacterium h.
    Cellulomonas h.
    Cercomonas h.
    Coccidium bigeminum var. h.
    Dermatobia h.
    Enteromonas h.
    Facklamia h.
    Gastrodiscoides h.
    Gastrospirillum h.
    herpesvirus h.
    Microbacterium h.
    Mycoplasma h.
    Pentatrichomonas h.
    Pentratrichomonas h.
    poliovirus h.
    Polycytella h.
    Psilorchis h.
    Sarcocystis h.
    Sarcoptes h.
    Staphylococcus hominis subsp. h.
    Trachipleistophora h.

hominivorax
    Callitroga h.
    Cochliomyia h.
hominus
    Dermabacter h.
Homobasidiomycetes
homocysteine
homogeneous
homogenous discharge
homogonic life cycle
homograft
    saphenous h.
homohiochii
    Lactobacillus h.
homologous
homology
    DNA h.
homopolymer
homopropionicum
    Clostridium h.
homosexual
homothallic
homothallica
    Cunninghamella h.
homunculus
    Anopheles h.
honei
    Rickettsia h.
honeycomb ringworm
honey intoxication
Hong
    H. Kong foot
    H. Kong influenza
Hongia koreensis (b)
Honvol
hood
    fume h.
    laminar h.
hoof-and-mouth disease
hooklet
hookworm
    h. anemia
    h. disease
Hoplolaiminae
Hoplopsyllus anomalus (p)
hordei
    Saccharopolyspora h.
Hordeivirus (v)
hordeovulneris
    Actinomyces h.
Horder spot

NOTES

H

255

hordniae
    Lactococcus lactis subsp. *h.*
horikoshii
    Anaerobranca h.
    Bacillus h.
    Pyrococcus h.
horizontal spread
hormaechei
    Enterobacter h.
Hormodendron pedrosoi
Hormodendrum cladosporioides (f)
Hormographiella (f)
hormonal
    h. replacement therapy (HRT)
    h. therapy
hormone
    adrenocorticotrophin h.
    follicular stimulating h. (FSH)
    gonadotropin-releasing h. (GnRH)
    growth h. (GH)
    human growth h. (hGH)
    recombinant human growth h.
      (rhGH)
    syndrome of inappropriate secretion
      of antidiuretic h. (SIADH)
    thyroid-stimulating h. (TSH)
Hormonema dematioides (f)
hornerae
    Colwellia h.
horrida
    Psorophora h.
horse
    h. mushroom
    h. papilloma virus
horsefly
hortae
    Piedraia h.
Hortaea werneckii (f)
hortai
    Trichosporon h.
hortense
    Echinostoma h.
hortensis
    Ornithinicoccus h.
horti
    Bacillus h.
horton
    Streptomyces h.
hortorum
    Xanthomonas h.
hoshinae
    Edwardsiella h.
hospes
    Dicrocoelium h.
hospice care
hospital
    h. fever

H. Infection Control Practices
    Advisory Committee (HICPAC)
hospital-acquired
    h.-a. infection
host
    accidental h.
    amplifier h.
    compromised h.
    dead-end h.
    h. defect
    h. defense mechanism
    definitive h.
    final h.
    graft versus h. (GVH)
    h. immunity
    immunocompromised h.
    intermediate h.
    neutropenic h.
    paratenic h.
    reservoir h.
    h. response
    secondary h.
    transport h.
host-immune process
Hostuviroid (v)
hot
    h. flash
    h. stain
    h. tub folliculitis
hour
    Actifed 12 H.
    air changes per h. (ACH)
    Sudafed 12 H.
housefly
houtenae
    Salmonella choleraesuis subsp. *h.*
howellii
    Actinomyces h.
Howell-Jolly bodies
HPA
    Histoplasma capsulatum polysaccharide
    antigen
H.P. Acthar Gel
HPG
    hypothalamic-pituitary-gonadal
    HPG axis
HPLC
    high-performance liquid chromatography
    HPLC assay
HPMPC
HPS
    hantavirus pulmonary syndrome
HPV
    Hart Park virus
    human papillomavirus
    HPV viral subtyping
HPV-16
    human papillomavirus type 16

HPV-associated anogenital cancer
H₂R
   histamine-2 receptor
3H-radioimmunoassay (3H-RIA)
    3H-r. test kit
3H-RIA
   3H-radioimmunoassay
    3H-RIA test kit
HRP-II
   histidine-rich protein-II
HRSV
   human respiratory syncytial virus
HRT
   hormonal replacement therapy
HR virus
HS
   herpes simplex
   hidradenitis suppurativa
HSC
   hematopoietic stem cell
    HSC gene therapy
HSIL
   high-grade squamous intraepithelial
   lesion
HSP
   heat shock protein
H₂S test
HSV
   herpes simplex virus
    HSV antibody testing
    HSV shell vial method
    skin culture for HSV
    HSV virus culture
HSV-1
   herpes simplex virus 1
    HSV-1 gingivostomatitis
HSV-2
   herpes simplex virus 2
    HSV-2 antibody
HTIG
   human tetanus immunoglobulin
HTLV
   human T-cell lymphotropic virus
HTLV-1
   human T-lymphotropic virus
   human T-lymphotropic virus 1
    HTLV-1 myelitis
    HTLV-1 myelopathy
    HTLV-1 proviral load
    HTLV-1 provirus
    HTLV-1 uveitis

HTLV-2
   human T-lymphotropic virus 2
HTLV-1-associated
   H.-a. arthropathy (HAAP)
   H.-a. myelopathy (HAM)
   H.-a. myelopathy/tropical spastic
   paraparesis (HAM/TSP)
   H.-a. uveitis
HTLV-BLV group
HTLV-I
   human T-cell lymphotrophic virus type I
   human T-cell lymphotropic virus I
HTLV-I-Ab
HTLV-II
   human T-cell lymphotropic virus II
   human T-lymphotrophic virus type 2
HTLV-I/II antibody
HTLV-IIIB
HTLV-III/LAV
   human T-lymphotrophic
   virus/lymphadenopathy associated virus
HTM
   Haemophilus test medium
HTNV
   Hantaan virus
HU
   hydroxyurea
Huacho virus (HUAV)
huakuii
    Mesorhizobium h.
    Rhizobium h.
huautlense
    Rhizobium h.
HUAV
   Huacho virus
huempii
    Cryptococcus h.
Hughes virus (HUGV)
HUGV
   Hughes virus
humahuaquensis
    Trichosporon h.
(human)
    specific immune globulin (human)
    tetanus immune globulin (human)
human
   h. adenovirus 1–47 (h 1–47)
   h. (alpha) herpesvirus 1
   h. astrovirus serotype 1-7 (HAstV-
   1-7)
   h. babesiosis
   h. blood bilayer Tween (HBT)

NOTES

H

human *(continued)*
  h. botfly
  h. botfly myiasis
  h. botulism
  h. calcivirus
  h. chorionic gonadotropin (HCG)
  h. chorionic gonadotropin test
  h. coronavirus
  h. coxsackievirus A1–A24
  h. coxsackievirus B1–B6
  h. cytomegalovirus (HCMV)
  h. cytomegalovirus group
  cytomegalovirus immune globulin
    intravenous, h.
  h. cytomegalovirus infection
    (HCMV)
  h. diploid cell culture rabies
    vaccine (HDCV)
  h. diploid cell rabies vaccine
    (HDCV)
  h. echovirus 1–34
  h. ehrlichiosis (HE)
  h. enterovirus 68–71
  h. eosinophilic enteritis
  h. foamy virus
  h. granulocytic ehrlichiosis (HGE)
  h. growth hormone (hGH)
  h. hepatitis A virus (HHAV)
  h. herpesvirus (HHV)
  h. herpesvirus 1–8 (HHV 1–8)
  h. herpesvirus 8/Kaposi sarcoma
    herpesvirus (HHV-8/KSHV)
  h. herpesvirus 6 variant A, B
  h. immune globulin
  h. immunodeficiency virus (HIV)
  h. immunodeficiency virus 1, 2
    (HIV-1, HIV-2)
  h. immunodeficiency virus DNA
    antibody
  h. immunodeficiency virus-type 1
    (HIV-1)
  h. immunodeficiency virus-type 2
    (HIV-2)
  h. leukocyte antigen (HLA)
  h. leukocyte antigen-A24 (HLA-
    A24)
  h. lung fibroblast monolayer
  h. lymphatic filariasis
  h. measles immune serum
  h. monocytic ehrlichiosis (HME)
  h. orf virus
  h. papilloma virus
  h. papillomavirus (HPV)
  h. parvovirus
  h. pneumococcal meningitis
  h. poliovirus
  h. poliovirus 1, 2

  h. respiratory syncytial virus
    (HRSV)
  h. retrovirus
  h. rhinovirus 1–100
  h. rhinovirus 1A
  h. rotavirus
  h. scarlet fever immune serum
  h. spumavirus
  h. T-cell leukemia virus
  h. T-cell leukemia virus I
  h. T-cell leukemia virus II
  h. T cell lymphotrophic virus
  h. T cell lymphotrophic virus type
    II
  h. T-cell lymphotropic virus
    (HTLV)
  h. T-cell lymphotropic virus I
    (HTLV-I)
  h. T-cell lymphotropic virus II
    (HTLV-II)
  h. tetanus immunoglobulin (HTIG)
  h. T-lymphotrophic
    virus/lymphadenopathy associated
    virus (HTLV-III/LAV)
  h. T-lymphotrophic virus type 2
    (HTLV-II)
  h. T-lymphotropic virus (HTLV-1)
  h. T-lymphotropic virus 1 (HTLV-
    1)
  h. T-lymphotropic virus 2 (HTLV-
    2)
  h. T-lymphotropic virus type 3
human aminopeptidase N
human growth hormone (hGH)
humani
    Sarcoptes scabei var. *h.*
human leukocyte antigen (HLA)
human papillomavirus (HPV)
**human papillomavirus type 16 (HPV-
  16)**
human papillomavirus X
**human T-cell lymphotrophic virus type
  I (HTLV-I)**
humanus
    Pediculus h.
    Pediculus humanus h.
Humatin
humeral head
humerosa
    Haemaphysalis h.
humerus
Humibid
    H. DM
    H. L.A.
    H. Sprinkle
Humicola (f)
    H. fuscoatra var. *fuscoatra*

H. grisea var. *grisea*
H. insolens
humicola
    Candida h.
    Ochroconis h.
    Torula h.
    Vanrija h.
humicolus
    Cryptococcus h.
humidifier
    Puritan-Bennett Cascade h.
humidus
    Actinoplanes h.
    Streptomyces h.
humiferus
    Actinomyces h.
    Streptomyces h.
humilata
    Cellulomonas h.
humilis
    Candida h.
    Gymnodia h.
humiphilum
    Ornithinimicrobium h.
humor
    aqueous h.
humoral
    h. response
    h versus cellular immunity
humosa
    Stella h.
hump
    buffalo h.
Humpty Doo virus (HDoov)
hungaricus
    Cryptococcus h.
hungatei
    Clostridium h.
    Methanospirillum h.
Hung method
hunteri
    Simulium h.
Hurler syndrome
huronensis
    Gigantobilharzia h.
hurstbridge
    Leptospira fainei serovar H.
HUS
    hemolytic uremic syndrome
husseyi
    Culicoides h.

HUS/TTP
    hemoglobinuria and glomerular
      thrombosis
    hemolytic uremic syndrome/thrombotic
      thrombocytopenia purpura
Hutchinson
    H. incisor
    H. sign
hutchinsonii
    Cytophaga h.
huttiensis
    Pseudomonas h.
HVAC
    heating, ventilating, and air conditioning
HVD
    hantavirus disease
hveragerdense
    Thermodesulfobacterium h.
HVS
    herpesvirus saimiri
HVTN
    HIV Vaccine Trials Network
hv virus
hw virus
hyacinthi
    Embellisia h.
    Xanthomonas h.
hyalina
    Lampropedia h.
hyaline
    h. cast
    h. glomerular occlusion
    h. membrane
    h. pseudopodium
hyalinization
hyalinulum
    Acremonium h.
hyalinum
    Scytalidium h.
Hyalodendron lignicola (f)
hyalohyphomycosis
Hyalomma (p)
    H. anatolicum
    H. marginatum
    H. plumbeum
hyalophomycosis
Hyalopus nopporoensis (f)
Hyaloscyphaceae
hyaluronate
hyaluronidase
Hybolin Improved
Hybrid Capture assay

NOTES

H

hybridization
deoxyribonucleic acid probe h.
DNA probe h.
dot blot h.
nucleic acid h.
polymerase chain reaction in
situ h. (PCR-ISH)
in situ h. (ISH)
Southern blot h.
h. test
ultrasensitive fluorescence in situ h.
(UFISH)
hybridoma
B-cell h.
hybridus
Helophilus h.
hyclate
doxycycline h.
HycoClear Tuss
Hycodan
Hycomine
H. Compound
H. Pediatric
Hycort
H. Topical
Hycotuss Expectorant Liquid
Hydanangiaceae
hydatid
h. cyst
h. cyst disease
h. Pott disease
h. sand
h. thrill
hydatiduria
hydatigena
Taenia h.
hydatis
Flavobacterium h.
Hyderm
Hydnaceae
hydradenitis suppurativa
Hydramyn syrup
hydrate
chloral h.
cyclopropanone h.
terpin h.
hydrazide
isonicotinic acid h. (INH)
hydrazine
volatile h.
Hydrea
hydrocarbon
polyhydroxylated cyclic h.
hydrocarbon gel
hydrocarbonoclasticus
Marinobacter h.
hydrocarbonoxydans
Amycolata h.

Nocardia h.
Pseudonocardia h.
hydrocele
filarial h.
hydrocephalus
normal pressure h.
transient obstructive h.
hydrochloride
adamantanamine h.
amantadine h.
aminacrine h.
bacampicillin h.
butenafine h.
carampicillin h.
cefepime h.
cephalexin h.
chlortetracycline h.
ciprofloxacin h.
clindamycin h.
emetine h.
metformin h.
oxymetazoline h.
phenazopyridine h.
pseudoephedrine h.
ranitidine h.
tetracycline h.
hydrocodone
h. and chlorpheniramine
h., chlorpheniramine, phenylephrine,
acetaminophen, and caffeine
h. and guaifenesin
h. and homatropine
h. PA syrup
h., phenylephrine, pyrilamine,
phenindamine, chlorpheniramine,
and ammonium chloride
h. and phenylpropanolamine
h. and pseudoephedrine
h., pseudoephedrine, and
guaifenesin
hydrocortisone
acetic acid, propylene glycol
diacetate, and h.
bacitracin, neomycin, polymyxin B,
and h.
Bactine H.
benzoyl peroxide and h.
chloramphenicol, polymyxin B,
and h.
ciprofloxacin and h.
clioquinol and h.
colistin, neomycin, and h.
h. cream
lidocaine and h.
neomycin, polymyxin B, and h.
oxytetracycline and h.
polymyxin B and h.
h. (systemic)

h. (topical)
urea and h.
Hydrocortone Acetate
Hydrocort Topical
hydrocupreine
ethyl h.
hydroemetine
hydroextractor
hydrogen
h. peroxide
h. sulfide
h. sulfide production
h. sulfide triple sugar iron test
hydrogenalis
Anaerococcus h.
Peptostreptococcus h.
hydrogenans
Streptomyces h.
Hydrogenobacter (b)
H. acidophilus
H. subterraneus
H. thermophilus
hydrogenoformans
Acidaminobacter h.
Carboxydothermus h.
Hydrogenophaga (b)
H. flava
H. intermedia
H. palleronii
H. pseudoflava
H. taeniospiralis
hydrogenophila
Stetteria h.
hydrogenophilum
Calderobacterium h.
Hydrogenophilus (b)
H. hirschii
H. thermoluteolus
hydrogenophilus
Desulfobacter h.
Geobacter h.
hydrogenotrophicus
Ruminococcus h.
Hydrogenovibrio marinus (b)
hydrogenovorans
Desulfonatronovibrio h.
hydrolysate
hydrolysis
esculin h.
hippurate h.
sodium hippurate h.
urea h.

hydrolyticus
Microbulbifer h.
hydrolyze
Hydromet
hydromorphone
hydronephrosis
hydropelvis
Hydrophiinae
hydrophila
Aeromonas hydrophila subsp. *h.*
hydrophilic
hydrophobica
Gordonia h.
hydropneumothorax
hydrops
h. fetalis
nonimmune h.
Hydrosone
hydrossis
Haliscomenobacter h.
Hydrotaea
H. albipuncta
H. dentipes
H. irritans
H. meteorica
H. militaris
hydrotaxis
Hydro-Tex Topical
hydrotherapy
hydrothermale
Desulfacinum h.
hydrothermalis
Halothiobacillus h.
Thermococcus h.
Thiobacillus h.
hydrotropism
hydroureter
hydroxide
aluminum h.
potassium h. (KOH)
sodium h.
p-**hydroxyampicillin**
hydroxybenzoicum
Clostridium h.
Sporotomaculum h.
hydroxychloroquine
h. sulfate
hydroxyprogesterone caproate
5-hydroxytryptamine
hydroxyurea (HU)
h. salvage therapy
Hydrozoa

NOTES

H

261

Hygrophoraceae
hygroscope
hygroscopicus
    Streptomyces hygroscopicus subsp.
    h.
hyicus
    Staphylococcus h.
hylemonae
    Clostridium h.
Hylemya
Hylutin
Hymenobacter (b)
    H. actinosclerus
    H. roseosalivarius
Hymenogastraceae
Hymenogastrales
Hymenolepididae
Hymenolepidinae
Hymenolepis (p)
    H. diminuta
    H. microstoma
    H. nana
    H. nana fraterna
Hymenomyces
Hymenoptera
hyodysenteriae
    Brachyspira h.
    Serpulina h.
    Treponema h.
hyoilei
    Campylobacter h.
hyointestinalis
    Campylobacter hyointestinalis subsp.
    h.
    Streptococcus h.
hyopharyngis
    Mycoplasma h.
hyopneumoniae
    Mycoplasma h.
hyorhinis
    Mycoplasma h.
hyos
    Leptospira interrogans serovar *h.*
hyoscyamine
    h., atropine, scopolamine, and
      phenobarbital
Hyosophen
Hyostrongylus rubidus (p)
hyosynoviae
    Mycoplasma h.
hyovaginalis
    Actinomyces h.
    Streptococcus h.
hyperactivity
hyperalimentation
    h. catheter
    h. line culture
hyperbaric oxygen

hyperbilirubinemia
hypercalcemia
hypercapnia
hypercatabolism
hyperchlorination
hypercholesterolemia
hypercoagulability
hypercoagulable state
hypercortisolism
hyperemia
    conjunctival h.
    reactive h.
    rebound h.
hyperergic encephalitis
hyperesthesia
hyperesthetic
hypergammaglobulinemia
hypergic
hyperglucagonemia
hyperglycemia
hyperglycemic-glycogenolytic factor
    (HGE)
HyperHep
hyperhidrosis
hyperimmune
    h. group B-specific antiserum
    h. serum globulin (HBIG, H-BIG)
hyperimmunization
hyperimmunoglobulinemia D
hyperkeratosis
hyperkeratotic
hyperkinetic
hyperlactatemia
hyperlactemia
hyperleukocytosis
hyperlipidemia
    PI-induced h.
hypermagnesemia
hypermegale
    Megamonas h.
hypermegas
    Bacteroides h.
hypermetabolism
hyperosmolar
hyperparakeratosis
hyperparasite
hyperparasitemia
hyperparasitism
hyperpigmentation
hyperplasia
    adematous h.
    asymmetric nasopharyngeal
      lymphoid h.
    epidermal h.
    epithelial h.
    erythroid h.
    follicular h.
    histiocytic h.

lymphoid h.
nodular lymphoid h.
pseudoepitheliomatous h.
hyperplastic
hyperproliferative wart
hyperpyrexia
hyperreactive splenomegaly
hyperreflexia
detrusor h.
hyperreflexic bladder
hypersecretion
hypersensitivity
h. angiitis
Arthus h.
cutaneous delayed-type h.
delayed-type h. (DTH)
immediate-type h. (ITH)
h. pneumonitis
h. reaction
hypersplenism
hypertension
intracranial h.
portal h.
pregnancy-induced h. (PIH)
primary pulmonary h. (PPH)
hypertensive retinopathy
Hyper-Tet
hyperthermia
true h.
whole-body h. (WBH)
hyperthermic
h. antiblastic perfusion (HAP)
h. isolated limb perfusion (HILP)
Hyperthermus butylicus (b)
hyperthyroidism
hypertroph
hypertrophic
h. bladder
h. obstructive cardiomyopathy
h. osteoarthropathy (HOA)
hypertrophy
adenoidal h.
left ventricular h.
nonmalignant adenoidal h.
papillary h.
prostatic h.
right ventricular h. (RVH)
hyperuricemia
hypervascular appearance
hypha, pl. **hyphae**
fungal h.
racquet h.

saprophytic h.
spiral h.
true h.
Hyphelia
H. auriantica
H. nigrescens
H. rupestre
H. terrestris
H. umbrina
hyphema
hyphemia
intertropical h.
hyphessobryonchis
Pleistophora h.
Hyphochytriaceae
Hyphochytriales
Hyphochytriomycetes
Hyphomicrobiales
Hyphomicrobium (b)
H. aestuarii
H. chloromethanicum
H. coagulans
H. denitrificans
H. facile subsp. *facile*
H. facile subsp. *tolerans*
H. facile subsp. *ureaphilum*
H. hollandicum
H. indicum
H. methylovorum
H. neptunium
H. variabile
H. vulgare
H. zavarzinii
Hyphomonas (b)
H. adhaerans
H. hirschiana
H. jannaschiana
H. johnsonii
H. neptunium
H. oceanitis
H. polymorpha
H. rosenbergii
Hyphomycetales
hyphomycosis
Hyphozyma (f)
hypnocyst
hypnozoite
hypoactive bowel sounds
hypoadrenalism
hypoalbuminemia
hypoaldosteronism
hypocalcemia

NOTES

H

hypochlorhydria
hypochlorite
  sodium h.
hypochlorous acid
hypochondrial
hypochromic
  h. anemia
hypocomplementemia
Hypocrea (f)
Hypocreaceae
Hypocreales
Hypocrita jacobeae
hypodense
  h. lesion
  h. region
Hypoderaeum conoideum (p)
Hypoderma (p)
  H. bovis
  H. diana
  H. lineatum
Hypodermataceae
Hypodermatidae
hypodermatosis
hypoergic
hypogammaglobulinemia
  common variable h.
hypogea
  Thermotoga h.
hypoglycemia
hypoglycemic
hypoglycorrhachia
hypogonadism
  hypothalamic h.
hypogonadotropic hypogonadism
hypokalemia
hypolipidemic
hypomagnesemia
Hypomyces (f)
  H. aurantius
  H. broomeanus
  H. chrysospermus
  H. haematococcus
  H. mycophilus
  H. rosellus
  H. sepulcralis
  H. subiculosus
Hypomycetaceae
hyponatremia
  hypovolemic h.
hypopharynx
hypoplasia
  cerebellar h.
  erythroid h.
hypoplastic left heart (HLH)
hypoprothrombinemia

hypopyon
  h. ulcer
hypopyon uveitis
hyporeflexia
hyposegmentation
hyposplenia
hypostome
hypotension
hypothalamic hypogonadism
hypothalamic-pituitary-gonadal (HPG)
  h.-p.-g. axis
hypothalamus
hypothermia
hypothesis, pl. **hypotheses**
  null h.
hypothetical
  h. mean organism (HMO)
  h. mean strain (HMS)
hypothyroidism
hypotonia
hypotony
Hypovirus (v)
hypovolemia
hypovolemic
  h. hyponatremia
  h. shock
hypoxanthine
  arabinosyl h.
hypoxemia
hypoxia
hypoxic brain injury
Hypoxylon (f)
HypRho-D
  H.-D. Mini-Dose
Hyprogest 250
Hysterangiaceae
Hysterianceae
Hysterolecitha (p)
  H. elongata
  H. rosea
  H. trilocalis
Hysterothylacium
  H. aduncum
  H. arnoglossi
  H. auctum
  H. bifidalatum
  H. collare
  H. cornutum
  H. corrugatum
  H. cyclopteri
  H. fabri
  H. increscens
  H. incurvum
  H. legendrei

H. *reliquens*
H. *rhacodes*
H. *rigidum*
hystricis
  Haemaphysalis h.

Hytone Topical
Hytuss
Hytuss-2X

NOTES

I_2-2 virus
I3 virus
IA
invasive aspergillosis
IACOV
Iaco virus
Iaco virus (IACOV)
Ia-expressing cell
IAI
intraamniotic infection
IAIS
intraamniotic infection syndrome
iakyrus
Streptomyces i.
I-alpha virus
IAPG
International Antimicrobial Project Group
iatrogenic
i. immunosuppression
iatrogenically
IB
Excedrin IB
Midol IB
Motrin IB
Pamprin IB
Sine Aid IB
Ibaraki virus (IBAV)
IBAV
Ibaraki virus
IBD
inflammatory bowel disease
IBDV
infectious bursal disease virus
Iberian epidemic clone
IBL
immunoblastic lymphoma
ibotenic acid
IBRV
Ibuprin
ibuprofen
pseudoephedrine and i.
Ibuprohm
Ibu-Tab
IBV
avian infectious bronchitis virus
ICAM-1
intercellular adhesion molecule-1
ICAM-2
intercellular adhesion molecule-2
ICAM-3
intercellular adhesion molecule-3
ICC
invasive cervical cancer
ICCE
intracapsular cataract extraction

ICD
implantable cardioverter defibrillator
ICD p24
immune complex-dissociated p24 antigen
ice-water bath
Ichnovirus (v)
ichthiosmia
Aeromonas i.
ichthyoenteri
Vibrio i.
Ichthyophthirius multifiliis (p)
Icoaraci virus (ICOV)
ICON
I. Strep A test
I. Strep A test kit
I. Strep B enzyme immunoassay
icosahedral
i. cytoplasmic deoxyribovirus
i. virus
ICOV
Icoaraci virus
ICP
infection control practitioner
infection control professional
ictaluri
Edwardsiella i.
Ictalurid herpes-like viruses
icteric hepatitis
icterohaemorrhagiae
Leptospira interrogans serovar *i.*
icterohemorrhagic fever
icterus
infectious i.
scleral i.
ICU
intensive care unit
ICW
intracellular water
ID
immunodiffusion
ID32 Staph strip test
Idaeovirus (v)
idahoense
Eupenicillium i.
IDCF
immunodiffusion complement-fixing
IDCF test
identification
arthropod i.
ectoparasite i.
gram-positive I. (GPI)
Haemophilus-Neisseria i. (HNID)
insect i.
Neisseria-Haemophilus I. (NHI)

Ideonella (b)
    I. dechloratans
Idiomarina (b)
    I. abyssalis
    I. zobellii
idiopathic
    i. diarrhea
    i. dilated cardiomyopathy
    i. HIV-related disease
    i. nephrotic syndrome
    i. oral aphthous ulcer
    i. polymyositis
    i. pulmonary fibrosis
    i. thrombocytopenic purpura (ITP, ITTP)
idiosyncratic
idottus
    Culex i.
Idoxuridine
id reaction
IDTP
    immunodiffusion tube precipitin
        IDTP test
IDU
    injecting drug use
    injecting drug user
    injection drug user
IDV
    indinavir
IE
    infective endocarditis
IEF
    isoelectric focusing
IEM
    immune electron microscopy
IERIV
    Ieri virus
Ieri virus (IERIV)
IF
    immunofluorescent
        IF stain
IFA
    immune fluorescent antibody
    immunofluorescence antibody
    immunofluorescence assay
    immunofluorescent antibody
    immunofluorescent antibody assay
    indirect fluorescent antibody
    indirect immunofluorescent antibody
        IFA *Cryptococcus*
        LANA IFA
        IFA titer
IFAT
    indirect fluorescent antibody test
IFA test
IFEV
    Ife virus
Ife virus (IFEV)

IFI
    indirect immunofluorescence
If1, If2 virus
IFLrA
IFN-alpha
    IFN-alpha 2-alpha
IFN-gamma
    gamma-interferon
Ig
    immunoglobulin
IgA
    immunoglobulin A
        IgA antibody
        IgA anti-*Toxoplasma*
        IgA immunofluorescent antibody (IgA-IFA)
IgA-IFA
    IgA immunofluorescent antibody
IgE
    immunoglobulin E
        IgE antibody
        Aspergillus-specific IgE
        blood IgE
IgE-mediated
    I.-m. reaction
I-Gent
IGF-1
    insulinlike growth factor-1
IGFBP-1
    insulinlike growth factor binding protein-1
IgG
    immunoglobulin G
        IgG antibody to rubella
        IgG antibody titer
        anti-tat IgG
        IgG hepatitis E antibody
        IgG HEV antibody
        IgG nuclear antibody
        IgG response
        IgG serology
IgG-RF-complement aggregate
IgM
    immunoglobulin M
        IgM antibody to rubella
        IgM antibody titer
        anti-*Giardia* IgM
        IgM anti-GM1 antibody
        antiparvovirus B19-specific IgM
        IgM ELISA
        IgM enzyme-linked immunosorbent assay
        IgM immunofluorescent antibody (IgM-IFA)
        IgM response
        IgM test
IgM-IFA
    IgM immunofluorescent antibody

I

ignacioi
> *Simulium i.*
> *Simulium ignescens*

ignava
> *Facklamia i.*
> *Johnsonella i.*
> *Tepidimonas i.*

Ignavigranum ruoffiae (b)

ignescens
> *Simulium i.*

igneus
> *Methanococcus i.*

Ignicoccus (b)
> *I. islandicus*
> *I. pacificus*

igniterrae
> *Thermus i.*

iguanae
> *Neisseria i.*

IHA
> indirect hemagglutination assay
> indirect hemagglutinin assay
> IHA test

IHNV
> infectious hematopoietic necrosis virus

IIIB-Mel-J allogeneic tumor cell vaccine

Ikari syndrome

IL-1
> interleukin-1

IL-2
> interleukin-2
> IL-2 infusion
> liposome-encapsulated IL-2

IL-6
> interleukin 6

IL-8
> interleukin-8

IL-13
> interleukin-13

IL-2-based biotherapy

Ilarvirus (v)

ileal

ileitis
> chronic i.
> terminal i.

ileocecal tuberculosis

Ilesha virus (ILEV)

ileum

ileus
> paralytic i.

ILEV
> Ilesha virus

Ilheus
> I. encephalitis
> I. fever
> I. virus (ILHV)

ILHV
> Ilheus virus

iliac
> i. crest
> i. fossa

ilicis
> *Arthrobacter i.*
> *Corynebacterium i.*

iliopiscarium
> *Photobacterium i.*

iliopiscarius
> *Vibrio i.*

illini
> *Leptonema i.*

illinoisensis
> *Paenibacillus i.*

illness
> AIDS-defining i.
> denguelike i.
> dysenteric i.
> staphylococcal foodborne i.
> terminal i.

illucens
> *Hermetia i.*

illudens
> *Omphalotus i.*

illustris
> *Lucilia i.*

ilocana
> *Fascioletta i.*

ilocanum
> *Echinostoma i.*
> *Euparyphium i.*

Ilosone
> I. Pulvules

Ilotycin
> I. Ophthalmic

Ilyobacter (b)
> *I. delafieldii*
> *I. polytropus*
> *I. tartaricus*

IM
> infectious mononucleosis

IMA
> internal mammary artery

imaging
> magnetic resonance i. (MRI)

imago

NOTES

imbricata
     tinea i.
imidazole
     topical i.
imidazoquinolineamine
imipemide
imipenem
     i. and cilastatin
imipenem/meropenem
imipenem-resistant *Acinetobacter*
  baumannii
imipramine
imiquimod
imitans
     Corynebacterium i.
     Mycoplasma i.
immediate-type hypersensitivity (ITH)
immitis
     Coccidioides i.
     coccidioidomycosis i.
     Dirofilaria i.
immobile
     Phenylobacterium i.
immobilis
     Psychrobacter i.
immobilization
     Treponema pallidum i. (TPI)
ImmuCyst
immune
     i. agglutination
     i. agglutinin
     cell-mediated i. (CMI)
     i. complex assay
     i. complex deposition
     i. complex-dissociated p24 antigen
       (ICD p24)
     i. complex glomerulonephritis
     i. deviation
     i. dysregulation
     i. electron microscopy (IEM)
     i. evasion
     i. globulin (intramuscular)
     i. globulin (intravenous)
     i. hemolysin
     i. hemolysis
     i. hemolytic anemia
     i. inflammation
     i. interferon
     i. memory
     i. modulation
     i. opsonin
     i. paralysis
     i. precipitation
     i. protein
     i. reactivity
     i. response
     i. serum
     i. serum globulin (ISG)

     i. status testing
     i. surveillance
     i. system
     i. theory
     i. thrombocytopenia
     i. thrombocytopenic purpura (ITP)
immune-electrophoresis assay
immune-mediated
     i.-m. toxicity
immune-modulating
     i.-m. therapy
immunity
     acquired i.
     active i.
     antibody-mediated i. (AMI)
     anti-TB cellular i.
     antiviral i.
     cell-mediated i. (CMI)
     cellular i.
     depressed cellular i.
     herd i.
     host i.
     humoral versus cellular i.
     infection i.
     innate i.
     local i.
     maternal i.
     mucosal i.
     natural i.
     passive i.
     relative i.
     specific active i.
     specific passive i.
immunization
     active i.
     antiinterferon-alpha i.
     Heptavax i.
     passive i.
     i. requirement
     Standards for Pediatric I.
     viral i.
immunize
Immuno
     Gammabulin I.
immunoadsorption
immunoagglutination
immunoassay
     antibody capture i.
     dipstick i.
     endocervical enzyme i.
     enzymatic i. (EIA)
     enzyme i. (EIA)
     fluorescence polarization i. (FPIA)
     ICON Strep B enzyme i.
     microparticle enzyme i. (MEIA)
     microparticulate enzyme i. (MEIA)
     optimal i. (OIA)
     PCR i.

PCR-enzyme i.
Prima Toxin A enzyme i.
reactive enzyme i.
sensitive/less sensitive enzyme i.
serologic enzyme i.
Toxin CD enzyme i.
urethral enzyme i.
immunoblastic lymphoma (IBL)
immunoblot
    i. assay
    Lyme disease i.
immunoblotting
    SPN i.
immunochemotherapy
immunochromatographic assay
immunocompetent
immunocompromised
    i. host
    i. individual
immunocytochemical stain
immunocytochemistry
immunodeficiency
    bovine i.
    common variable i.
    congenital i.
immunodeficient
immunodiffusion (ID)
    Aspergillus i.
    blastomycosis i.
    Coccidioides i.
    i. complement-fixing (IDCF)
    i. complement-fixing test
    fungal i.
    histoplasmosis i.
    radial i. (RID)
    i. tube precipitin (IDTP)
    i. tube precipitin test
immunodominant domain
immunodysfunction
immunoelectron microscopy
immunoelectroosmophoresis
immunoelectrophoresis
    countercurrent i. (CIE, CIEP)
immunoelectrotransfer blot technique
immunoenzymatic assay
immunofluorescence
    i. analysis
    i. antibody (IFA)
    i. antibody test
    i. assay (IFA)
    indirect i. (IFI)

    i. skin biopsy
    i. stain
immunofluorescence antibody (IFA)
immunofluorescent (IF)
    i. antibody (IFA)
    i. antibody assay (IFA)
    i. study
immunogen
    HIV-1 i.
immunogenic
immunogenicity
immunoglobin-producing cell
immunoglobulin (Ig)
    i. A (IgA)
    i. A nephropathy
    anticytomegalovirus i.
    chickenpox i.
    i. E (IgE)
    hepatitis B virus i. (HBIG, H-BIG)
    human tetanus i. (HTIG)
    intravenous i. (IVIG, IVIg)
    rabies i. (RIG)
    serum i.
    tetanus i. (TIG)
    varicella-zoster i. (VZIG)
immunoglobulin G (IgG)
    antiparvovirus B19 i. G.
immunoglobulin M (IgM)
    antiparvovirus B19 i. M.
immunohistochemical
    i. probe technique
    i. staining
immunoincompetent fibroinflammatory
immunologic
immunomodulating
    i. therapy
immunomodulator
    i. therapy with interferon-gamma
immunomodulatory
immunomonitoring
immunopathy
    virus-induced i.
immunoperoxidase
    i. stain
    i. study
    i. technique
immunopotentiator
immunoprophylaxis
    active i.
    passive i.

NOTES

immunosenescence
immunosorbent agglutination assay (ISAGA)
immunostaining
immunosuppressant
immunosuppressed
    i. protocol (ISP)
immunosuppression
    iatrogenic i.
immunosuppressive
    i. drug
    i. therapy
immunosurveillance
immunotherapy
    active specific i. (ASI)
    adoptive i. (AIT)
    adoptive cellular i.
    cytotoxic T lymphocyte-based i.
    DC-based i.
    specific i.
    targeted i.
immunotoxin therapy (IT)
Imodium
Imovax Rabies I.D. Vaccine
impar
    Simulium i.
IMPDH
    inosine monophosphate dehydrogenase
impedance
    bioelectric i. (BIA)
Impenem/Meropenem
imperfect
    i. fungus
    i. stage
    i. state
Imperfecti
    Fungi I.
imperiale
    Brevibacterium i.
    Microbacterium i.
impetiginization
impetigo
    bullous i.
    i. contagiosa
    i. contagiosa bullosa
    i. herpetiformis
    i. neonatorum
    nonbullous i.
    streptococcal i.
    i. vulgaris
impiger
    Aedes i.
impingement
implant
    intravitreal i.
    progestin i.

implantable
    i. cardioverter defibrillator (ICD)
    i. cardioverter defibrillator infection
implant-associated
implicatus
    Aedes i.
importance
    Surveillance and Control of Pathogens of Epidemiologic I. (SCOPE)
impotence
imprint
    tissue i.
Improved
    Hybolin I.
Imuran
IMViC
in
    in situ
    in situ hybridization (ISH)
    in situ hybridization technique
    in situ polymerase chain reaction (IS-PCR)
    in utero
    in vitro pull-down assay
    in vivo
    in vivo confocal microscopy
    in vivo expression technology (IVET)
Inaba
    Vibrio cholerae serotype 01 I.
inactivated
    i. Japanese encephalitis virus vaccine
    Japanese encephalitis virus vaccine, i.
    i. poliomyelitis virus vaccine
    i. poliovirus
    i. whole virus vaccine
inactive
    i. brucellosis
    Escherichia coli i.
inadai
    Leptospira i.
inaequale
    Simulium i.
inagensis
    Actinokineospora i.
inanimate
incanus
    Rarobacter i.
incerta
    Desemzia i.
incertae sedis
incertum
    Brevibacterium i.
    Simulium i.

inchonensis
    Tsukamurella i.
incidence
incidens
    Culiseta i.
incidental parasite
incilis
    Laelaps i. (*See Plasmodium kochi*)
incisional biopsy
incisor
    Hutchinson i.
incisurata
    Fannia i.
inclusion
    i. blennorrhea
    i. body
    i. body disease
    i. body encephalitis
    i. body stain
    i. conjunctivitis
    i. conjunctivitis virus
    intracytoplasmic i.
    owl's eye i.
    viral i.
incognita
    Meloidogyne i.
    Oxyuris i.
incognito
    tinea i.
incognitum
    Schistosoma i.
incognitus
    Mycoplasma i.
incommunis
    Candida i.
incomplete
    i. agglutinin
    i. intestinal metaplasia
    i. metamorphosis
incongruus
    Conidiobolus i.
inconspicua
    Candida i.
inconstans
    Proteus i.
increpitus
    Aedes i.
increscens
    Hysterothylacium i.
incrustatum
    Simulium i.
incubating syphilis

incubation
    i. period
incubative stage
incubator
incubatory carrier
inculcated
incurvata
incurvatum
    Arthroderma i.
incurvum
    Hysterothylacium i.
IND
    investigational new drug
indanyl sodium
Inderal
    I. LA
indeterminate
    i. leprosy
indeterminate test
index, pl. indices
    body mass i. (BMI)
    FIC i.
    fractional inhibitory concentration i.
    intrathecal *Treponema pallidum*
        antibody i.
    ITPA i.
    i. lesion
    RBC i.
India
    I. ink
    I. ink preparation
    I. ink stain
indiaensis
    Streptomyces i.
indianense
    Streptosporangium i.
indianensis
indica
    Beijerinckia indica subsp. *i.*
    Microbispora i.
    Salmonella choleraesuis subsp. *i.*
indicator cell assay
indices (*pl. of* index)
indicum
    Arthrinium phaeospermum var. *i.*
    Bifidobacterium i.
    Hyphomicrobium i.
    Schistosoma i.
indicus
    Caloramator i.
    Catenuloplanes i.
    Muscor i.

NOTES

indiense
 Mycoplasma i.
indigens
 Azoarcus i.
indigofera
 Pseudomonas i.
 Vogesella i.
indigoferus
 Streptomyces i.
indinavir (IDV)
indirect
 i. agglutination
 i. calorimetry
 i. Coombs test
 i. fluorescent antibody (IFA)
 i. fluorescent antibody test (IFAT)
 i. hemagglutination assay (IHA)
 i. hemagglutination serologic assay
 i. hemagglutinin assay (IHA)
 i. immunofluorescence (IFI)
 i. immunofluorescence technique
 i. immunofluorescent antibody
  (IFA)
 i. laryngoscopy
 i. ophthalmoscopy
indium-III
indium-labeled white blood cell scan
indium leukocyte scan
individual
 immunocompromised i.
indol
indole
 i. positive
 i. production test
indolent respiratory infection
indolicum
 Desulfobacterium i.
indolicus
 Actinobacillus i.
 Peptococcus i.
 Peptoniphilus i.
 Peptostreptococcus i.
indolis
 Clostridium i.
indologenes
 Chryseobacterium i.
 Flavobacterium i.
 Kingella i.
 Pantoea stewartii subsp. *i.*
 Suttonella i.
indoltheticum
 Chryseobacterium i.
 Flavobacterium i.
indomethacin
indonesiensis
 Acetobacter i.
 Desulfovibrio i.
indoxyl acetate hydrolysis test

induced
 i. malaria
 i. sputum technique
induction
 chemotherapy i.
 i. chemotherapy
 lysogenic i.
induration
industrius
 Gluconobacter oxydans subsp. *i.*
indwelling
 i. cannula
 i. catheter
 i. voice prosthesis
Inermicapsiferinae
Inermicapsifer madagascariensis (p)
inermis
 Rhabditoides i.
iners
 Lactobacillus i.
 Mycoplasma i.
 Pseudomonas i.
inexorabile
 Simulium i.
INF-alpha
 interferon-alpha
Infanrix
infant
 i. botulism
 I. Formula Act
infantarius
 Streptococcus infantarius subsp. *i.*
infantile
 i. diarrhea
 i. gastroenteritis
 i. leishmaniasis
 i. papular acrodermatitis
 i. periarteritis nodosa
 i. purulent conjunctivitis
infantis
 Bifidobacterium i.
 Streptococcus i.
infantiseptica
 granulomatosis i.
infantum
 acrodermatitis papulosa i.
 Leishmania i.
 roseola i.
infarction
 myocardial i. (MI)
Infazinc
infect
infected
 i. ascites
 i. hematoma
 i. vascular gangrene
infecting dose

infection

abdominal i.
acute HIV-1 i. (AHI)
amniotic fluid i.
anaerobic i.
anal HPV i.
anal human papilloma virus i.
arboviral i.
arteriovenous shunt i.
ascending gonococcal i.
bacterial i.
balantidium i.
beta hemolytic streptococci i.
biliary tract i.
bloodstream i. (BSI)
bone i.
borrelial i.
breast i.
Candida i.
candidal i.
cardiac i.
catheter-associated i. (CAI)
catheter-associated urinary tract i.
catheter-related bloodstream i.
  (CRBSI)
catheter-related urinary tract i.
central nervous system i.
chlamydial i.
closed space i.
coagulase-negative staphylococcal i.
coccidial i.
congenital CMV i.
congenital HCMV i.
congenital HIV i.
i. control
i. control practitioner (ICP)
i. control professional (ICP)
corneal i.
cross i.
cryptogenic i.
cutaneous human papillomavirus i.
deep neck i.
deep-seated i.
deep serious soft tissue i.
dental i.
dermatologic i.
dermatophyte i.
descending i.
disseminated cryptococcal i.
disseminated gonococcal i. (DGI)
disseminated intrauterine i.

disseminated *Mycobacterium avium*
  complex i.
disseminated nocardial i.
disseminated nontuberculous
  mycobacterial i.
DNTM i.
dual i.
endogenous i.
enterococcal urinary tract i.
enteroviral i.
exit-site i.
extraintestinal i.
eye i.
eyelid i.
fatal disseminated i.
female genital tract i.
filarial i.
focal i.
foot i.
fungal i.
GAS i.
gastrointestinal i.
genital chlamydial i.
genitourinary i.
gonococcal i.
granulomatous i.
group A beta-hemolytic
  streptococcal i.
group A streptococcus i.
guinea worm i.
hantavirus i.
HbsAg-positive persistent hepatitis
  B virus i.
helminth i.
hepatitis B surface antigen-positive
  persistent hepatitis B virus i.
herpes simplex i.
herpes zoster i.
hibernal epidemic viral i. (HEV1)
hospital-acquired i.
human cytomegalovirus i. (HCMV)
i. immunity
implantable cardioverter
  defibrillator i.
insertion site i.
intervertebral disc space i. (IVDSI)
intraabdominal i.
intraamniotic i. (IAI)
intraocular i.
intrauterine i.
joint i.
laboratory-acquired i. (LAI)

NOTES

infection *(continued)*
    lacrimal apparatus i.
    laryngeal i.
    late i.
    latent i.
    leptospiral i.
    lower genital tract i.
    lower respiratory tract i.
    luminal i.
    lytic i.
    MAI i.
    mass i.
    metastatic i.
    microsporidial i.
    middle ear i.
    mixed nail i.
    musculoskeletal i.
    mycobacterial i.
    Mycoplasma i.
    natural focus of i.
    necrotizing i.
    necrotizing soft-tissue i. (NSTI)
    nonbacterial i.
    nontyphoidal salmonella i.
    nosocomial eye i.
    nosocomial rotavirus i.
    nosocomial urinary tract i.
    nosocominal i.
    ocular i.
    odontogenic i.
    opportunistic systemic fungal i.
    oral i.
    orbital i.
    orofacial odontogenic i.
    papillomavirus i.
    parasitic i.
    paravaccinia virus i.
    periocular i.
    permanent cardiac pacemaker i.
    pneumococcal i.
    polymicrobial i.
    postabortal i.
    primary i.
    protozoal i.
    protozoan i.
    pulmonary i.
    pyodermatous i.
    pyogenic i.
    recrudescent i.
    recurrent i.
    repeated respiratory i.
    reservoir of i.
    respiratory tract i.
    rhinocerebral i.
    Rickettsia i.
    rickettsial i.
    scalp i.
    secondary bacterial i.

    self-limited HBsAg-positive i.
    self-limited hepatitis B surface
        antigen-positive i.
    Seoul virus i.
    sexually transmitted i. (STI)
    Shigella i.
    skin i.
    smoldering i.
    soft tissue i.
    spirochetal i.
    spirochete i.
    spurious i.
    staphylococcal i.
    Streptococcus i.
    subclinical i.
    subcutaneous fungal i.
    subcutaneous necrotizing i.
    superficial i.
    suppurative oral i.
    surgical site i. (SSI)
    surgical wound i. (SWI)
    sycosiform fungous i.
    symptomatic urinary tract i.
    systemic CMV i.
    systemic fungal i.
    toxigenic bacterial i.
    trichomonal i.
    tunnel i.
    unusual opportunistic i.
    upper respiratory i. (URI)
    upper respiratory tract i.
    ureaplasmal i.
    urethral chlamydial i.
    urinary tract i. (UTI)
    vaccine strain i.
    vaccinia i.
    varicella-zoster i.
    ventriculoatrial shunt i.
    vesicular viral i.
    Vincent i.
    viral respiratory i.
    viscerotropic *Leishmania tropica* i.
    Western blot i.
    white piedra i.
    wound i.
    yeast i.
    zoonotic listerial i.
infectiosum
    erythema i. (EI)
infectious
    i. arthritis
    i. avian bronchitis
    i. bovine rhinotracheitis
    i. bursal disease virus (IBDV)
    i. bursitis
    i. canine hepatitis
    i. cervicitis
    i. crystalline keratopathy

i. cycle
i. diarrhea
i. disease
i. disease therapy
i. eczematoid dermatitis
i. endocarditis
i. flora
i. hematopoietic necrosis virus (IHNV)
i. icterus
i. jaundice
i. keratitis
i. lymphocytosis
i. mononucleosis (IM)
i. mononucleosis-like syndrome
i. mononucleosis serology
i. pancreatic necrosis virus (IPNV)
i. papilloma of cattle
i. plasmid
i. porcine encephalomyelitis
i. units per million (IUPM)
i. vaginitis
i. virion
infectiousness
infectiva
polioencephalitis i.
infective
i. dermatitis
i. dose
i. endocarditis (IE)
i. jaundice
infectivity
cross-strain i.
infectoria
Alternaria i.
Lewia i.
infelix
Selenomonas i.
Infergen
inferior
infernum
Desulfacinum i.
infernus
Acidianus i.
Bacillus i.
Methanococcus i.
infertility
postsalpingitis i.
tubal factor i.
infest
infestans
Scytalidium i.

Triatoma i.
Trichosporon i.
infestation
Cheyletiella i.
infiltrate
airspace ground-glass i.
cavitary upper-lobe i.
ground-glass i.
interstitial i.
mononuclear cell i.
nodular i.
plasma cell i.
pneumonic i.
T-cell i.
infiltration
focal cellular i.
myeloid cell i.
neutrophilic i.
perivascular i.
polymorphic i.
infiltrative liver disease
infirmatus
Aedes i.
infirmum
Eubacterium i.
Inflamase
inflammation
acute i. (AI)
chronic i.
focal i.
gastric i.
granulomatous i.
immune i.
lobular i.
meningeal i.
necrotizing granulomatous i.
vaginal i.
inflammatory
i. bowel disease (IBD)
i. breast cancer
i. cell
i. diarrhea
i. disease
i. tinea capitis
inflatum
Tolypocladium i.
inflatus
Wardomyces i.
inflictus
Culex i.
influenza
i. A, B serology

NOTES

influenza *(continued)*
    avian i.
    i. A virus
    i. bacillus
    i. B virus
    i. C virus influenzavirus
    Hong Kong i.
    i. pneumonia
    sequela of i.
    Spanish i.
    swine i.
    i. virus
    i. virus culture
    i. virus hemagglutinin
    i. virus type A, B
    i. virus vaccine
influenzae
    Haemophilus i.
    nontypeable *Haemophilus i.*
influenzavirus
    influenza C virus i.
Influenzavirus A (v)
Influenzavirus B (v)
Influenzavirus C (v)
influenzavirus C/Taylor/1233/47
infrastructure
infrasubspecific
infula
    Gyromitra i.
Infus-a-port
infusion
    brain-heart i. (BHI)
    IL-2 i.
    peripheral blood stem cell i.
    i. pyelogram
    i. therapy
infusion-related reaction
Infusoria
infusorian
ingens
    Candida i.
ingenuity
ingrica
    Thioploca i.
inguinal
    i. adenopathy
    i. bubo
    i. hernia
    i. lymphadenopathy
    i. lymph node
inguinale
    granuloma i.
inguinalis
    tinea i.
INGV
    Ingwavuma virus
Ingwavuma virus (INGV)

INH
    isoniazid
    isonicotinic acid hydrazide
inhalation
    i. anthrax
    dexamethasone oral i.
    NebuPent I.
Inhaler
    Azmacort Oral I.
inhibens
    Carnobacterium i.
inhibition
    hemagglutination i. (HAI)
    hemolysis i.
inhibitor
    alpha 1-proteinase i.
    angiotensin-converting enzyme i.
    beta-lactamase i.
    beta-lactam-beta-lactamase i.
    HIV-1-specific reverse
      transcriptase i.
    HMG CoA reductase i.
    nonnucleoside reverse
      transcriptase i. (NNRTI, NRTI)
    nonnucleoside RT i.
    nucleoside analog reverse
      transcriptase i. (NRTI)
    nucleoside reverse transcriptase i.
      (NRTI)
    piston-pump i.
    potent protease i.
    PR i.
    protease i. (PI)
    proton pump i. (PPI)
    reverse transcriptase i. (RTI)
    RT i.
    serotonin-reuptake i.
    topoisomerase II i.
iniae
    Streptococcus i.
inimitabilis
    Culex i.
ininii
    Anopheles i.
Inini virus (INIV)
INIV
    Inini virus
injecting drug use (IDU)
injecting drug user (IDU)
Injection
    Adlone I.
    Amcort I.
    A-methaPred I.
    Amikin I.
    Andro-L.A. I.
    Andropository I.
    Aristocort Forte I.
    Aristocort Intralesional I.

Aristospan Intra-articular I.
Aristospan Intralesional I.
Baci-IM I.
Celestone Phosphate I.
Cel-U-Jec I.
Chloromycetin I.
Cleocin Phosphate I.
Decadron I.
Delatestryl I.
depAndro I.
depGynogen I.
depMedalone I.
Depo-Estradiol I.
Depogen I.
Depoject I.
Depo-Medrol I.
Depopred I.
Depotest I.
Depo-Testosterone I.
Dioval I.
D-Med I.
Duralone I.
Duratest I.
Durathate I.
Estra-L I.
Everone I.
Gynogen L.A. I.
Histerone I.
Jenamicin I.
Kefurox I.
Kenaject I.
Kenalog I.
Key-Pred I.
Key-Pred-SP I.
Lyphocin I.
Medralone I.
Metro I.V. I.
Minocin IV I.
Monistat i.v. I.
M-Prednisol I.
Nafcil I.
Nallpen I.
Nebcin I.
Neupogen I.
Neutrexin I.
Ornidyl I.
Pentacarinat I.
Pentam-300 I.
Prednisol TBA I.
Rifadin I.
Serostim I.
Solu-Medrol I.

Tac-3 I.
Tac-40 I.
Terramycin I.M. I.
Tesamone I.
Triam-A I.
Triam Forte I.
Triamonide I.
Tri-Kort I.
Trilog I.
Trilone I.
Trisoject I.
Unipen I.
Vancocin I.
Vancoled I.
Zinacef I.

injection
amphotericin B lipid complex i.
Bicillin C-R 900/300 i.
Bicillin L-A i.
Cipro i.
conjunctival i.
i. drug user (IDU)
intradermal i.
intratumoral i.

injury
clenched-fist i.
hypoxic brain i.

ink
India i.

inkin
Sarcinosporon i.
Trichosporon i.

Inkoo virus (INKV)
INKV
Inkoo virus
inky cap mushroom
innate immunity
inner canthus
innidiation
innocens
Brachyspira i.
Serpulina i.
Simulium i.
Treponema i.
innocua
Listeria i.
Propioniferax i.
innocuum
Clostridium i.
Propionibacterium i.
inocula (*pl. of* inoculum)
inoculate

NOTES

279

inoculation
  intraperitoneal i.
inoculum, pl. **inocula**
  i. effect
Inocybe geophylla (f)
inopinatum
  Bifidobacterium i.
inopinatus
  Desulfovibrio i.
  Pediococcus i.
inornata
  Culiseta i.
inosine
  i. monophosphate dehydrogenase (IMPDH)
  i. pranobex
inositola
  Micromonospora i.
inositol fermentation test
Inoviridae
Inovirus (v)
inpatiens
  Culiseta i.
InPouch system
inquiline
  i. parasite
inquirenda
  Loa i.
INR
  international normalized ratio
insect
  i. identification
  i. parvovirus group
  i. vector
Insecta
insectalens
  Candida i.
insectorum
  Candida i.
insectosa
  Candida shehatae var. *i.*
Insert
  Lubrin I.
insertion
  i. sequence
  i. site infection
  tympanostomy tube i.
insidiosum
  Corynebacterium i.
  Pythium i.
insidiosus
  Clavibacter michiganensis subsp. *i.*
insignis
  Azomonas i.
  Culicoides i.
  Dracunculus i.
insingulare
  Arthroderma i.

insipidus
  diabetes i. (DI)
insolatus
  Culicoides i.
insolens
  Humicola i.
insolitum
  Spiroplasma i.
insolitus
  Bacillus i.
insolutum
  Polypaecilum i.
insomnia
  fatal familial i. (FFI)
inspiratory stridor
instar
insufficiency
  adrenal i.
  i. murmur
insulinlike
  i. growth factor-1 (IGF-1)
  i. growth factor binding protein-1 (IGFBP-1)
insulin resistance
integrase
integrase enzyme
integrin
integron
integrum
  Aquaspirillum peregrinum subsp. *i.*
integument
intensification
  double i.
intensive
  i. care unit (ICU)
  i. chemotherapy
interactance
  near-infrared i. (NIR)
interaction
  drug i.
  estazolam drug i.
  organism-host i.
  virus-host i.
intercalary
intercalatum
  Schistosoma i.
intercellular
  i. adhesion molecule-1 (ICAM-1)
  i. adhesion molecule-2 (ICAM-2)
  i. adhesion molecule-3 (ICAM-3)
  i. antibody basement membrane antibody
  i. digestion
intercostal
  i. artery
  i. retraction
interdigitale

interference
    bacterial i.
interferon
    i. alfa-2a
    i. alfa-2b
    i. alfa-2b and ribavirin combination
      pack
    i. alfacon-1
    i. alfa-n3
    i. alpha
    i. gamma
    immune i.
    lymphoblastoid i.
    pegylated i.
    recombinant consensus i.
    i. therapy
interferon-alfa-2B-n1
interferon-alpha (INF-alpha)
    i.-a. 2-alpha (IFN-alpha 2-alpha)
    i.-a. 2b
interferon-beta
interferon-gamma
    aerosolized i.-g.
    immunomodulator therapy with i.-g.
    systemic i.-g.
interferon-inducible protein 10 (IP-10)
interjectum
    Mycobacterium i.
interleukin
    systemic i.
interleukin-1 (IL-1)
interleukin-2 (IL-2)
    intravenous bolus i.
    subcutaneous i.
interleukin-3
    recombinant human i. (rhIL-3)
interleukin-4
interleukin-6 (IL-6)
interleukin-8 (IL-8)
interleukin-10
interleukin-12
interleukin-13 (IL-13)
intermedia
    Brevundimonas i.
    Candida i.
    Dekkera i.
    Hydrogenophaga i.
    Ornithobilharzia i.
    Prevotella i.
    Serpulina i.
    Thiomonas i.
    Yersinia i.

intermediate
    i. host
    i. wart
intermedilysin
intermedium
    Anaeroplasma i.
    Mycobacterium i.
    Ochrobactrum i.
intermedius
    Acetobacter i.
    Anopheles i.
    Bacteroides i.
    Bacteroides melaninogenicus subsp.
      i.
    Brettanomyces i.
    Caulobacter i.
    Echinococcus i.
    Enterobacter i.
    Gluconacetobacter i.
    Staphylococcus i.
    Streptococcus i.
    Streptomyces i.
    Thermoactinomyces i.
    Thiobacillus i.
Intermenstrual bleeding
intermittent
    i. malaria
    i. malarial fever
    i. positive-pressure breathing (IPPB)
interna
    gnathostomiasis i.
internal
    i. carotid artery thrombosis
    i. jugular vein
    i. mammary artery (IMA)
International
    I. Antimicrobial Project Group
      (IAPG)
    I. Union Against Tuberculosis and
      Lung Disease
international normalized ratio (INR)
internatus
    Micropolyspora i.
interpalpebral cornea
inter-repeat PCR (IR-PCR)
interrogans
    Leptospira i.
interrogator
    Culex i.
intersonii
interstice

NOTES

interstitial
    i. bronchopneumonia
    i. fibrosis
    i. infiltrate
    i. keratitis
    i. myocarditis
    i. nephritis
    i. plasma cell pneumonia
    i. pneumonitis
interstitium
    Dipetalonema i.
intertriginous
intertrigo
intertropical hyphemia
intertypic recombinant
interval
    dose i.
intervertebral
    i. disc space infection (IVDSI)
    i. diskitis
intervillitis
intervillositis
intestinal
    i. anisakidosis
    i. capillariasis
    i. cestode
    i. colonization
    i. cryptosporidiosis
    i. metaplasia
    i. myiasis
    i. schistosomiasis
    i. spirochetosis
    i. toxemia botulism
    i. tuberculosis
intestinale
    Clostridium i.
intestinalis
    Cercomonas i.
    Collinsella i.
    Desulfovibrio i.
    Embadomonas i.
    Enteromonas i.
    Fibrobacter i.
    Gasterophilus i.
    Giardia i.
    Lactobacillus i.
    Ligula i.
    mycosis i.
    Octomitus i.
    Retortamonas i.
    Septata i.
    Streptococcus i.
    Tricercomonas i.
intimal elastosis
intolerance
    disaccharide i.
    drug i.

    glucose i.
    lactose i.
intoxication
    foodborne i.
    honey i.
    mad honey i.
    pyrrolizidine alkaloid i.
    staphylococcal i.
intraabdominal
    i. abscess
    i. infection
    i. sepsis
intraamniotic
    i. infection (IAI)
    i. infection syndrome (IAIS)
intraaortic balloon pump
intraarterial catheter
intraassay
intrabladder balloon
intracapsular cataract extraction (ICCE)
intracardiac
intracavitary
intracellular
    i. digestion
    i. HIV RNA level
    i. parasite
    i. toxin
    i. water (ICW)
intracellulare
    Mycobacterium i.
intracellularis
    Lawsonia i.
intracerebral
    i. hemorrhage
intracranial
    i. bleeding
    i. herniation
    i. hypertension
    i. lesion
    i. pressure
intractable diarrhea
intracutaneous
    i. tuberculin skin testing
intracytoplasmic
    i. inclusion
intradermal
    i. injection
    i. method
    i. skin testing
    i. test
intraepidermal
    i. abscess
    i. microabscess
intraepithelial neoplasia
intraerythrocytic
intrafamilial
intrahepatic
intralaboratory

intralesion
intralesional
  i. chemotherapy
  i. injection
  i. interferon chemotherapy
  i. therapy
intralesional injection
intralumbar
intraluminal
  i. culture
intramedullary fixation nail
intramural
intramuscular
  i. antibiotic
  immune globulin (i.)
intranuclear
intraocular
  i. infection
  i. lymphoma
intraoperative
intraoral
  i. herpes simplex
  i. ulcer
intrapatient
intraperitoneal
  i. anisakidosis
  i. inoculation
intraprostatic
intrarenal abscess
intraretinal
  i. hemorrhage
intraretinal lesion
Intrasporangium (b)
  I. calvum
intrathecal
  i. *Treponema pallidum* antibody
  (ITPA)
  i. *Treponema pallidum* antibody
  index
intrathecal cytosine arabinoside
intratubular
intratumoral injection
intraurethral
intrauterine
  i. device (IUD)
  i. environment
  i. infection
intravaginal insemination
intravascular
  i. catheter
  i. catheter-2 (IVc-2)
  i. catheter-acquired sepsis

intravenous
  i. bolus interleukin-2
  i. catheter culture
  i. device culture
  i. drug user (IVDU)
  i. foscarnet
  i. immune globulin (IVIG)
  immune globulin (i.)
  i. immunoglobulin (IVIG, IVIg)
  i. line culture
  i. line sepsis
  i. pyelogram (IVP)
(intravenous-human)
intraventricular
  i. hemorrhage
intravesical
  i. BCG monotherapy
  i. polymorphonuclear leukocyte
intravirion gene therapy
intravitreal
  i. fomiversen
  i. implant
intrinsic
  i. factor complex
  i. muscular atrophy
introitus
Intron A
intrudens
  Aedes i.
intubate
intubation
  endotracheal i.
intussusception
inulin test
inulinus
  Sanguibacter i.
  Sporolactobacillus i.
inundation fever
inusitatus
  Saccharomyces i.
  Streptomyces i.
invadens
  Entamoeba i.
  Naegleria i.
  Trichomaris i.
invasive
  i. amebiasis
  i. aspergillosis (IA)
  i. candidiasis
  i. cervical cancer (ICC)
  i. colitis
  i. disease

NOTES

inventory
    Beck Depression I. (BDI)
invermination
investigational new drug (IND)
invicta
    Solenopsis i.
Invirase
involucrum
involution form
involutus
    Paxillus i.
involvement
    meningovascular i.
    node i.
    parenchymatous i.
inyoensis
    Culicoides i.
Iobid DM
Iodamoeba
    I. buetschlii
    I. suis
iodate
    sodium i.
iodide
    potassium i.
    saturated solution of potassium i. (SSKI)
    supersaturated potassium i. (SSKI)
iodine
    Gram i.
    i. mordant
    i. mount
    i. stain
iodinum
    Brevibacterium i.
***Iodobacter fluviatilis* (b)**
iodochlorhydroxyquin
iododeoxyuridine
iodophor
iodophore
iodoquinol
iodosum
    Rhodovulum i.
iolambdis
    Culex i.
Ionil
Ionil-T
    I.-T. Plus
ionized hypocalcemia
ionophore
    calcium i. (CI)
ions
    silver i.
iowae
    Mycoplasma i.
IP-10
    interferon-inducible protein 10

IPNV
    infectious pancreatic necrosis virus
IPOL
ipomoeae
    Streptomyces i.
***Ipomovirus* (v)**
IPPB
    intermittent positive-pressure breathing
IPPYV
    Ippy virus
Ippy virus (IPPYV)
ipratropium
ipsefact
IPV
    polio vaccine
IPy-1 virus
iracouboense
    Simulium i.
irakense
    Azospirillum i.
iranensis
    Cellulomonas i.
iranicum
    Corynebacterium i.
iranicus
    Clavibacter i.
    Rathayibacter i.
iraqiensis
    Actinopolyspora i.
irgensii
    Polaribacter i.
iridocyclitis
Iridoviridae
***Iridovirus* (v)**
iris
    i. atrophy
    herpes i.
iris-nodule
iritis
    tuberculous i.
Irituia virus (IRIV)
IRIV
    Irituia virus
iron
    i. deposition
    i. filing
    i. overload syndrome
    i. stain
    triple sugar i. (TSI)
    i. uptake
    i. uptake test
iron-alum mordant
iron-deficiency
    i.-d. anemia
    i.-d. hemoglobinopathy
iron-deficiency anemia
iron-hematoxylin-phosphotungstic acid technique

iron-hematoxylin stain
IR-PCR
 inter-repeat PCR
irradiation
 gamma i.
 total body i. (TBI)
 ultraviolet i.
 ultraviolet germicidal i. (UVGI)
irrational
irregularis
 Cephaliophora i.
 Clostridium i.
Irrigant
 Neosporin G.U. I.
irritability
irritans
 Haematobia i.
 Hydrotaea i.
 Leptoconops i.
 Siphona i.
irritant
 gastrointestinal i.
ISAGA
 immunosorbent agglutination assay
Isaria (f)
 I. densa
 I. destructor
 I. shiotae
 I. tenella
 I. vexans
isatidis
 Clostridium i.
ischemia
 mesenteric i.
 villus i.
ischemic
 i. cardiomyopathy
ischial tuberosity
ischiorectal abscess
Ischnocera
isethionate
 pentamidine i.
Isfahan virus (ISFV)
ISFV
 Isfahan virus
ISG
 immune serum globulin
ISH
 in situ hybridization
ishimotonii
 Desulfonema i.

ishiwadae
 Candida i.
ISKV
 Issyk-Kul virus
island
 i. disease
 i. fever
islandicum
 Fervidobacterium i.
 Pyrobaculum i.
islandicus
 Ignicoccus i.
 Thermodesulfovibrio i.
Isla Vista virus
islet-activating factor
isoagglutinin
isobetadine
Isochromatium (b)
 I. buderi
Isoclor Expectorant
isoconazole
isoelectric
 i. casein
 i. focusing (IEF)
 i. focusing technique
isoenzyme
 i. analysis
 i. technique
Isoetharine
 Arm-a-Med I.
 Dey-Lute I.
isoctharine
isoform
 prion protein normal i. (PrP^c)
 prion protein scrapie i. (PrP^{Sc})
isohemagglutinin
 anti-A i.
 anti-B i.
isolate
isolation
 rapid CMV i.
 rapid HSV i.
 viral i.
isolator
Isolator system
isolette
isomastigote
isomer
isometric phage with ssDNA
Isoniazid
isoniazid (INH)
 rifampin and i.

NOTES

isoniazid-resistant MTB
isoniazid+rifampin+pyrinamide
isonicotinic acid hydrazide (INH)
isoosmolar
Isoparorchiidae
isopropanol
isopropyl alcohol
Isoproterenol
    Arm-a-Med I.
    Dey-Dose I.
Isopto
    I. Cetamide
    I. Cetamide Ophthalmic
    I. Cetapred Ophthalmic
Isosphaera pallida (b)
Isospora (p)
    I. belli
    I. canis
    I. felis
    I. ohioensis
    I. rivolta
isosporiasis
    chronic intestinal i.
Isotamine
isothiocyanate
    fluorescein i. (FITC)
isothionate
    propamidine i.
    tetramethylrhodamine i. (TMRI)
isotonic
    i. glucose
    i. saline
    i. solution
isotonic saline
isotope
isotretinoin
Isotrex
isovalerica
    Spirochaeta i.
isoxazolyl penicillin
ISP
    immunosuppressed protocol
IS-PCR
    in situ polymerase chain reaction
israelensis
    Chromohalobacter i.
    Halomonas i.
    Legionella i.
israelii
    Actinomyces i.
Issatchenkia orientalis (f)
Issyk-Kul virus (ISKV)
I-Sulfacet
Isuprel
IT
    immunotoxin therapy
Itaituba virus (ITAV)

italicus
    Actinoplanes i.
    Saccharomyces i.
    Thermoanaerobacter i.
Itaporanga virus (ITPV)
Itaqui virus (ITQV)
itaunense
    Simulium i.
ITAV
    Itaituba virus
itch
    Absorbine Jock I.
    Aftate for Jock I.
    barber's i.
    coolie i.
    copra i.
    dew i.
    grain i.
    grocer i.
    ground i.
    kabure i.
    Malabar i.
    i. mite
    Norway i.
    poultryman's i.
    prairie i.
    rice i.
    straw i.
    swamp i.
    swimmer's i.
    Tinactin for Jock I.
    toe i.
    water i.
itching
    vulvovaginal i.
Iteravirus (v)
itersonii
    Aquaspirillum itersonii subsp. *i.*
ITH
    immediate-type hypersensitivity
Itimirim virus (ITIV)
ITIV
    Itimirim virus
ITP
    idiopathic thrombocytopenic purpura
    immune thrombocytopenic purpura
ITPA
    intrathecal *Treponema pallidum* antibody
        ITPA index
ITPV
    Itaporanga virus
ITQB
    Molecular Genetics Unit of the Institute
        of Biotechnology
ITQV
    Itaqui virus

itraconazole
    IV i.
    i. level
ITTP
    idiopathic thrombocytopenic purpura
Itupiranga virus (ITUV)
ITUV
    Itupiranga virus
IUD
    intrauterine device
    IUD culture
IUPM
    infectious units per million
IV
    Vibramycin IV
    IV virus
I.V.
    Cipro I.V.
    Fucidin I.V.
    Gammar-P I.V.
    Merrem I.V.
ivanovii
    Listeria i.
    Listeria i. subsp. *ivanovii*
    Listeria i. subsp. *londoniensis*
    Methanobacterium i.
IVc-2
    intravascular catheter-2
IVDSI
    intervertebral disc space infection
IVDU
    intravenous drug user
Ivecgam
ivermectin
IVET
    in vivo expression technology
IV ganciclovir
IVIG
    intravenous immune globulin
    intravenous immunoglobulin

IVIg
    intravenous immunoglobulin
I virus
ivoii
    Peptoniphilus i.
ivorii
    Peptostreptococcus i.
IVP
    intravenous pyelogram
IVP-Salk vaccine
IvyBlock
Ixodes (p)
    I. affinis
    I. apronophorus
    I. dammini
    I. granulatus
    I. hexagonus
    I. holocyclus
    I. japonensis
    I. lividus
    I. marxi
    I. muris
    I. nipponensis
    I. pacificus
    I. pavlovskyi
    I. persulcatus
    I. ricinus
    I. scapularis
    I. spinipalpis
ixodetis
    Spiroplasma i.
ixodic
ixodid
    i. tick
Ixodida
Ixodidae
Ixodinae
Ixodoidea
izardii
    Buttiauxella i.

NOTES

Jaa
    J. Amp
    J. Amp Trihydrate
    J. Pyral
Jaa-Prednisone
Jacareacanga virus (JACV)
Jaccoud periarticular fibrosis
jack o'lantern mushroom
jacksoni
    Culicoides j.
    Fasciola j.
Jacksonian epilepsy
jacobeae
    Hypocrita j.
jacumbae
    Simulium j.
JACV
    Jacareacanga virus
jadensis
    Fundibacter j.
jadinii
    Pichia j.
jail fever
jaimoramirezi
    Simulium j.
JAK
    Janus kinase
Jakob-Creutzfeldt disease
jamaicensis
    Culicoides j.
    Knemidocoptes j.
Jamanxi virus (JAMV)
jamesi
    Culicoides j.
Jamestown
    J. Canyon
    J. Canyon virus (JCV)
jamestowniensis
    Legionella j.
jamnbacki
    Culicoides j.
Jamshidi needle
JAMV
    Jamanxi virus
jandaei
    Aeromonas j.
Janeway lesion
Janibacter (b)
    J. brevis
    J. limosus
    J. terrae
jannaschiana
    Hyphomonas j.

jannaschii
    Methanococcus j.
    Oceanospirillum j.
janthinellum
    Penicillium j.
Janthinobacterium (b)
    J. agaricidamnosum
    J. lividum
janthinomys
    Haemagogus j.
janthinus
    Streptomyces j.
janus
    Aspergillus j.
Janus kinase (JAK)
Japanaut virus (JAPV)
Japanese
    J. B encephalitis
    J. B encephalitis vaccine
    J. B encephalitis virus
    J. encephalitis (JE)
    J. encephalitis virus (JEV)
    J. encephalitis virus vaccine, inactivated
    J. river fever
japonensis
    Flexibacter j.
    Ixodes j.
japonica
    Amycolatopsis j.
    Borrelia j.
    Echinochasmus j.
    Haemadipsa j.
    Haemaphysalis j.
    Haloarcula j.
    Limnatis j.
    Moritella j.
    Rickettsia j.
    Shewanella j.
    Tetrasphaera j.
    Xenorhabdus j.
japonicum
    Bradyrhizobium j.
    Cryptosporangium j.
    Microsporum j.
    Oceanospirillum j.
    Rhizobium j.
    Schistosoma j.
    Scytalidium j.
japonicus
    Aspergillus j.
    Catenuloplanes j.
    Luteococcus j.
    Thermosipho j.

J

JAPV
 Japanaut virus
jar
 Coplin j.
Jarisch-Herxheimer (JH) (*See*
 Herxheimer)
JARIV
 Jari virus
Jari virus (JARIV)
jaundice
 catarrhal j.
 epidemic j.
 infectious j.
 infective j.
 leptospiral j.
javanica
 Meloidogyne j.
javanicus
 Mucor j.
 Paecilomyces j.
jaw
 lumpy j.
JC
 JC polyomavirus
JCAHO
 Joint Commission on Accreditation of
 Healthcare Organizations
JCV
 Jamestown Canyon virus
JDV
 Juan Diaz virus
JE
 Japanese encephalitis
jeanselmei
 Exophiala j.
 Pullularia j.
jeikeium
 Corynebacterium j.
jejuni
 Campylobacter j.
 Campylobacter jejuni subsp. *j.*
jejunitis
jejunoileal
jejunostomy
 percutaneous endoscopic j. (PEJ)
jejunum
 tuberculosis of j.
jelly
 Xylocaine j.
Jenamicin
 J. Injection
jenense
 Thiospirillum j.
jenensis
 Agrococcus j.
 Streptomyces pentaticus subsp. *j.*
Jennerian approach

jenningsi
 Simulium j.
Jensenia canicruria (b) (*See*
 Rhodococcus)
jensenii
 Lactobacillus j.
 Nocardioides j.
 Pimelobacter j.
 Propionibacterium j.
jeotgali
 Bacillus j.
Jersey virus
jessenii
 Pseudomonas j.
jet-impeller nebulizer
jetmari
 Laelaps j. (*See Plasmodium kochi*)
JEV
 Japanese encephalitis virus
JE-VAX
Jewish housewife disease
JH
 Jarisch-Herxheimer
 JH gene
 JH reaction
 JH virus
jigger
jiroveci
 Pneumocystis j.
jirovecii
 Trichosporon j.
JKT-6423 virus
JKT-6969 virus
JKT-7041 virus
JKT-7075 virus
Joa virus
Job syndrome
joergensenii
 Desulfospira j.
johannae
 Gluconacetobacter j.
johannseni
 Simulium j.
Johne
 J. bacillus
 J. disease
johnsonae
 Cytophaga j.
Johnsonella ignava (b)
johnsoniae
 Flavobacterium j.
johnsonii
 Acinetobacter j.
 Hyphomonas j.
 Lactobacillus j.
johnsonli
 Sporidiobolus j.

Johnson-Trussel medium
Joinjakaka virus (JOIV)
joint
j. aspirate
j. aspiration
Charcot j.
Clutton j.'s
J. Commission on Accreditation of Healthcare Organizations (JCAHO)
j. infection
seeding of j.
sternoclavicular j.
j. study
j. tap
joint-fluid leukocyte count
JOIV
Joinjakaka virus
jonesi
Culicoides j.
Simulium j.
Jonesia denitrificans (b)
jonesii
Synergistes j.
jordanis
Legionella j.
Jordan tartrate test
josui
Clostridium j.
Jr
Congess Jr
EpiPen Jr
Juan Diaz virus (JDV)
juccuya
juddi
Culicoides j.
judithae
Anopheles j.
Jugra virus (JUGV)

jugular venous pressure
JUGV
Jugra virus
jujuyense
Simulium j.
julia
Rhodopseudomonas j.
juncopox virus
junction
anorectal j.
neosquamocolumnar j.
oronasal j.
squamocolumnar j.
jundiaiense
Simulium j.
jungle yellow fever
junii
Acinetobacter j.
Junin virus (JUNV)
Junior Strength Motrin
JUNV
Junin virus
Jurkat T cell
Jurona virus (JURV)
JURV
Jurona virus
Jutiapa virus (JUTV)
JUTV
Jutiapa virus
juvenile
j. chronic myelogenous leukemia
j. rheumatoid arthritis
j. wart

J

NOTES

K12
> *Escherichia coli* K12

K19 virus
kabanayense
> *Simulium* k.

kabure
> k. itch

Kachemak Bay virus
Kadam virus (KADV)
KADV
> Kadam virus

Kaeng Khoi virus (KKV)
Kahn test
Kaikalur virus (KAIV)
Kairi virus (KRIV)
Kaisodi virus (KSOV)
KAIV
> Kaikalur virus

kala azar
Kalcinate
Kaletra
kalimantani
> *Wuchereria* k.

kalrae
> *Arthrographis* k.

kamchatkensis
> *Desulfurella* k.

Kamese virus (KAMV)
Kammavanpettai virus (KMPV)
KAMV
> Kamese virus

Kanagawa hemolysin
kanamyceticus
> *Streptomyces* k.

kanamycin
> k. level
> k. susceptibility test

kanamycin-resistant
kanamycin-vancomycin
> k.-v. laked blood (KVLB)
> k.-v. laked blood agar

kandleri
> *Lactobacillus* k.
> *Methanopyrus* k.
> *Weissella* k.

kanei
> *Trichophyton* k.

Kannamangalam virus (KANV)
Kantrex
> K. level

KANV
> Kannamangalam virus

kaolin
Kao Shuan virus (KSV)

kaplicensis
> *Amaricoccus* k.

Kaposi
> K. sarcoma (KS)
> K. sarcoma-associated herpesvirus (KSHV)
> K. sarcoma cofactor
> K. sarcoma herpesvirus (KSHV)

kappa particle
karawaiewii
> *Candida* k.

Karimabad virus
karnatakensis
> *Microbispora* k.

Karnofsky
> K. Performance Scale
> K. Performance Score

Karshi virus (KSIV)
karyogonad
karyophage
karyosome
karyotype
karyotyping
> electrophoretic k. (EK)

karyozoic
Kasba virus (KASV)
Kashin-Bek disease
kashmirense
> *Streptoverticillium* k.

kashmirensis
> *Streptomyces* k.

Kasokero virus
kasugaensis
> *Streptomyces* k.

KASV
> Kasba virus

Katayama
> K. disease
> K. fever
> K. syndrome

Kato-Katz thick smear technique
Kato thick smear technique
katrae
> *Streptomyces* k.

katsuradai
> *Heterophyes* k.

kauaiensis
> *Kitasatoa* k.

kaustophilus
> *Bacillus* k.
> *Geobacillus* k.

Kawasaki
> K. mucocutaneous disease
> K. mucocutaneous disorder
> K. syndrome

K

KCV
    Kern Canyon virus
kedani fever
keddieii
    Sanguibacter k.
Keep Clear Anti-Dandruff Shampoo
kefiranofaciens
    Lactobacillus k.
kefirgranum
    Lactobacillus k.
kefiri
    Lactobacillus k.
Keflex
Keflin
Keftab
Kefurox
    K. Injection
kefyr
    Candida k.
Kefzol
Keissleriella (f)
kellicotti
    Paragonimus k.
kellyi
    Halothiobacillus k.
keloidal blastomycosis
Kemerovo virus (KEMV)
KEMV
    Kemerovo virus
Kenacort Oral
Kenaject Injection
Kenalog
    K. Injection
    K. in Orabase
    K. Topical
Kenonel Topical
kentuckense
    Streptoverticillium k.
kentuckensis
    Streptomyces k.
Keralyt
    K. Gel
Kerandel sign
keratanolyticum
    Aureobacterium k.
    Microbacterium k.
keratic precipitate
keratinized
keratinizing squamoid carcinoma
Keratinomyces
    K. ajelloi
keratinophilic
keratinophilum
    Chrysosporium k.
keratitis
    acanthamebic k.
    Acanthamoeba k.
    amebic k. (AK)

bacterial k.
epithelial k.
fungal k.
herpes simplex k.
herpetic k.
infectious k.
interstitial k.
microbial k.
mycotic k.
nosocomial k.
ocular amoebic k.
parasitic k.
punctate k.
sclerosing k.
serpiginous k.
keratoconjunctivitis
    epidemic k.
    herpetic k.
    microsporidian k.
keratoderma
keratomycosis
keratopathy
    infectious crystalline k.
    punctate k.
keratoplasty
    penetrating k.
keratosis, pl. **keratoses**
    k. follicularis contagiosa
    seborrheic k.
keratotomy
Kerckring fold
kerion
    Celsus k.
    tinea k.
Kern Canyon virus (KCV)
Kernia (f)
Kernig sign
kerteszi
    Leptoconops k.
Kestrone
Ketapang virus (KETV)
Ketek
ketoacidosis
    diabetic k.
ketoconazole
    k. cream
    k. level
Ketogulonicigenium (b)
    K. robustum
    K. vulgare
ketolide
ketone
ketosireducens
    Microbacterium k.
KETV
    Ketapang virus
Keuraliba virus (KEUV)

KEUV
  Keuraliba virus
Kevadon
Kew Gardens fever
keyhole-limpet hemocyanin (KLH)
Key-Pred Injection
Key-Pred-SP Injection
Keystone virus (KEYV)
KEYV
  Keystone virus
Kf1 virus
KFDV
  Kyasanur Forest disease
Khasan virus
KHF
  Korean hemorrhagic fever
Khuskia (f)
Ki67 antigen
Kibdelosporangium (b)
  K. albatum
  K. aridum subsp. *aridum*
  K. aridum subsp. *largum*
  K. philippinense
kibunensis
  Culicoides k.
Kickxellaceae
Kickxellales
kidney
  k. bean hemagglutinin
  k. bean lectin
  k. bean-shaped
  k. ultrasound
  k.'s, ureters and bladder (KUB)
kielensis
  Ahrensia k.
kifunensis
  Streptomyces k.
kijaniata
  Actinomadura k.
Kikuchi syndrome
kiliense
  Acremonium k.
killed vaccine (KV)
killer
  lymphokine-activated k. (LAK)
  natural k. (NK)
kilocalorie
kilonensis
  Pseudomonas k.
Kimberley virus (KIMV)

kimchii
  Lactobacillus k.
  Leuconostoc k.
KIMV
  Kimberley virus
kinase
  Janus k. (JAK)
  receptor protein tyrosine k. (RPTK)
  threonine k.
  thymidine k.
Kineococcus aurantiacus (b)
Kineosporia (b)
  K. aurantiaca
  K. mikuniensis
  K. rhamnosa
  K. rhizophila
  K. succinea
kinetics
kinetoplast
Kinctoplastida
kinetosome
kingae
  Kingella k.
Kingella (b)
  K. denitrificans
  Haemophilus aphrophilus,
    Actinobacillus
    actinomycetemcomitans,
    Cardiobacterium hominis,
    Eikenella corrodens, and K.
    (HACEK)
  K. indologenes
  K. kingae
  K. kingae endocarditis
  K. kingae intervertebral diskitis
  K. kingae osteomyelitis
  K. oralis
kingii
  Eikenella corrodens and
    Kingella k.
kinin
Kinkiang fever
kinkoti bean poisoning
Kinyoun
  K. acid-fast stain
  K. carbol-fuchsin stain
Kirby-Bauer
  K.-B. agar
  K.-B. disc diffusion test
  K.-B. susceptibility test
  K.-B. type assay

K

NOTES

kirbyi
    Culicoides k.
Kiricephalus (p)
kirishiense
    Thermohydrogenium k.
kirschneri
    Leptospira k.
kishiwadense
    Streptoverticillium k.
kishiwadensis
    Streptomyces k.
Kismayo virus (KISV)
kissing
    k. bug
    k. bug lesion
KISV
    Kismayo virus
kit
    Amplicor HCV Detection K.
    cyanide antidote k.
    Determine HIV 1/2
      immunoassay k.
    DNA DipStick K.
    fluorescent antibody k.
    3H-radioimmunoassay test k.
    3H-RIA test k.
    ICON Strep A test k.
    latex agglutination k.
    Meridian Merifluor k.
    MY-PAP cervicovaginal lavage k.
    Para-pak fecal collection k.
    TPHA Test K.
kitamiense
    Microbacterium k.
kitaokai
    Haemaphysalis k.
Kitasatoa (b)
    K. diplospora
    K. kauaiensis
    K. nagasakiensis
    K. purpurea
Kitasatospora (b)
    K. azatica
    K. cheerisanensis
    K. cochleata
    K. cystarginea
    K. griseola
    K. mediocidica
    K. paracochleata
    K. phosalacinea
    K. setae
kivui
    Acetogenium k.
    Thermoanaerobacter k.
KKV
    Kaeng Khoi virus
Klamath virus (KLAV)
Klaron Lotion

KLAV
    Klamath virus
klebahnii
    Trichosporon k.
klebhanii
    Geotrichum k.
Klebsiella (b)
    K. granulomatis
    K. mobilis
    K. ornithinolytica
    K. oxytoca
    K. ozaenae
    K. planticola
    K. pneumonia
    K. pneumoniae
    K. pneumoniae subsp. *ozaenae*
    K. pneumoniae subsp. *pneumoniae*
    K. pneumoniae subsp.
      rhinoscleromatis
    K. rhinoscleromatis
    K. trevisanii
Klebs-Loeffler bacillus (*See***
  *Corynebacterium***)**
Klerist-D tablet
KLH
    keyhole-limpet hemocyanin
Kline test
kloosii
    Staphylococcus k.
Kluveromyces (f)
Kluyvera (b)
    K. ascorbata
    K. cochleae
    K. cryocrescens
    K. georgiana
kluyveri
    Clostridium k.
    Saccharomyces k.
Kluyveromyces
    K. bulgaricus
    K. marxianus
    K. thermotolerans
    K. veronae
    K. wikenii
KMPV
    Kammavanpettai virus
knee
    k. arthrogram
    Nantucket k.
Knemidocoptes, Cnemidocoptes
    K. gallinae
    K. jamaicensis
    K. mutans
    K. pilae
knob
    Engelmann basal k.
    malarial k.
Knodell score

Knott technique
knowlesi
    Plasmodium k.
knowltoni
    Culicoides k.
koalarum
    Lonepinella k.
kobei
    Enterobacter k.
kobensis
    Bacillus k.
    Paenibacillus k.
    Saccharopolyspora hirsuta subsp. *k.*
Koch
    K. bacillus (*See Mycobacterium*
      tuberculosis)
    K. postulate
    K. tuberculin
kochi
    Hepatocystis k. (*See Plasmodium*
      kochi)
    Laelaps k. (*See Plasmodium kochi*)
    Plasmodium k.
Koch-Weeks bacillus (*See **Haemophilus***
aegyptius)
Kocuria (b)
    K. erythromyxa
    K. kristinae
    K. palustris
    K. rhizophila
    K. rosea
    K. varians
kocurii
    Paracoccus k.
    Planococcus k.
Kodachrome slide
koebnerization
Koebner phenomenon
koehlerae
    Bartonella k.
Koffex
    K. DM
    K. DM-D
    K. Expectorant
kofuense
    Streptosporangium viridogriseum
      subsp. *k.*
kofuensis
    Kutzneria k.
    Sporolactobacillus k.
KOH
    potassium hydroxide

KOH microscopy
KOH mount
KOH prep
KOH preparation
KOH solution
KOH stain
KOH testing
koilocyte
koilocytosis
koilocytotic atypica
Kokobera virus (KOKV)
Kokoskin stain
KOKV
    Kokobera virus
Kolephrin GG/DM
Kolongo virus (KOLV)
KOLV
    Kolongo virus
komogatae
    Leucobacter k.
komossense
    Mycobacterium k.
kompi
    Anopheles k.
konaensis
    Meloidogyne k.
Kondon's Nasal
koningii
    Scopulariopsis k.
konjaci
    Acidovorax k.
    Pseudomonas avenae subsp. *k.*
    Pseudomonas pseudoalcaligenes
      subsp. *k.*
Koongol virus (KOOV)
KOOV
    Koongol virus
Kopeloff modification
Koplik spot
Korean
    K. hemorrhagic fever (KHF)
    K. hemorrhagic fever virus
koreense
    Planomicrobium k.
koreensis
    Catellatospora k.
    Hongia k.
    Paenibacillus k.
    Rhodococcus k.
    Sphingomonas k.
Koserella trabulsii (b)

K

NOTES

koseri
    Citrobacter k.
kostiense
    Sinorhizobium k.
Kotonkan virus (KOTV)
KOTV
    Kotonkan virus
Koutango virus (KOUV)
KOUV
    Koutango virus
Kowanyama virus (KOWV)
KOWV
    Kowanyama virus
Kozhevnikov epilepsy
KPG
    potassium penicillin G
    KPG skin test
kra-kra
Kribbella (b)
    K. flavida
    K. sandramycini
kriegii
    Oceanospirillum k.
krissii
    Candida k.
kristensenii
    Yersinia k.
kristinae
    Kocuria k.
    Micrococcus k.
kristjanssonii
    Caldicellulosiruptor k.
KRIV
    Kairi virus
KRM-1648
kroppenstedtii
    Corynebacterium k.
kruisii
    Candida k.
Kruse brush
krusei
    Candida k.
    Endomyces k.
    Saccharomyces k. (*See Candida krusei*)
    Trichosporon k.
Kruskal-Wallis test
KS
    Kaposi sarcoma
KSHV
    Kaposi sarcoma-associated herpesvirus
    Kaposi sarcoma herpesvirus
        KSHV latent IgG antibody
        KSHV lytic IgG antibody
KSIV
    Karshi virus
KSOV
    Kaisodi virus

KSV
    Kao Shuan virus
KSY1 virus
KUB
    kidneys, ureters and bladder
kubicae
    Mycobacterium k.
kuenenii
    Thiomicrospira k.
kuetzingii
    Cryptococcus k.
Kunjin virus (KUNV)
kunkeei
    Lactobacillus k.
kunkelii
    Spiroplasma k.
kunmingensis
    Chainia k.
    Streptomyces k.
kunsanensis
    Nocardiopsis k.
KUNV
    Kunjin virus
kunzii
    Helcococcus k.
Kupffer cell
kurssanovii
    Streptomyces k.
Kurthia (b)
    K. gibsonii
    K. sibirica
    K. zopfii
kuru
kururiensis
    Burkholderia k.
kushneri
    Halanaerobium k.
kutscheri
    Corynebacterium k.
Kutzneria (b)
    K. albida
    K. kofuensis
    K. viridogrisea
kuznetsovii
    Desulfotomaculum k.
KV
    killed vaccine
K virus
KVLB
    kanamycin-vancomycin laked blood
        KVLB agar
Kwatta virus (KWAV)
KWAV
    Kwatta virus
Kwelcof
Kwell
Kwellada

Kyasanur
K. Forest disease (KFDV)
K. Forest disease virus
kysingii
Desulfuromusa k.
Kytococcus sedentarius (b)

KYZV
Kyzylagach virus
Kyzylagach
Sindbis virus subtype K.
K. virus (KYZV)

NOTES

K

L
L AmB
L form
L-756,423
L3 virus
L-929 bioassay
LA
latex agglutination
Ami-Tex LA
Apo-Theo LA
Dexone LA
Entex LA
Guaifenex LA
Inderal LA
Nolex LA
Partuss LA
Profen LA
LA test
Touro LA
Zephrex LA
L-A
Bicillin L.-A.
L.A.
Dexasone L.A.
Humibid L.A.
Phenylfenesin L.A.
Solurex L.A.
Theoclear L.A.
La
La Crosse virus (LACV)
La Joya virus (LJV)
labedae
Streptomyces l.
labetalol
labialis
herpes l.
recurrent HSV l.
labilomyceticus
Streptomyces albosporeus subsp. l.
labiodiscinus
Helicotylenchus l.
labor
false l.
prodromal l.
laboratory
l. diagnosis
Venereal Disease Research L.
(VDRL)
l. worker (LW)
laboratory-acquired infection (LAI)
labor-intensive
Laboulbeniaceae
Laboulbeniales
Laboulbeniomycetes

labreanum
Methanocorpusculum l.
Labrys monachus (b)
labyrinthitis
Labyrinthulales
Labyrinthulomycetes
Lacazia loboi (f)
Lachnospira (b)
L. multipara
L. pectinoschiza
lacrimal
l. abscess
l. apparatus infection
l. sac
lacrimalis
Peptoniphilus l.
Peptostreptococcus l.
lacrimation
lacrymalis
Thelazia l.
lactamica
Neisseria l.
lactaris
Ruminococcus l.
lactate
l. dehydrogenase (LDH)
l. dehydrogenase elevating virus
(LDV)
plasma l.
lacteus
Mycetocola l.
lactic
l. acid bacillus
l. acidosis
l. dehydrogenase virus (LDHV)
LactiCare-HC Topical
lacticifex
Selenomonas l.
lacticogenes
Beijerinckia indica subsp. l.
lacticola
Mycobacterium phage l.
lacticum
Microbacterium l.
lactiethylicus
Thermoanaerobacter brockii subsp.
l.
lactilytica
Selenomonas ruminantium subsp. l.
lactis
Bifidobacterium l.
Carpoglyphus l.
Lactobacillus l.
Lactobacillus delbrueckii subsp. l.
Lactococcus lactis subsp. l.

lactis (continued)
    Leuconostoc l.
    Saccharomyces l.
    Streptococcus l.
lactiscondensi
    Candida l.
lactoaceticus
    Caldicellulosiruptor l.
Lactobacillaceae
Lactobacillus (b)
    L. *acetotolerans*
    L. *acidipiscis*
    L. *acidophilus*
    L. *agilis*
    L. *algidus*
    L. *alimentarius*
    L. *amylolyticus*
    L. *amylophilus*
    L. *amylovorus*
    L. *animalis*
    L. *arizonensis*
    L. *aviarius* subsp. *araffinosus*
    L. *aviarius* subsp. *aviarius*
    L. *bavaricus*
    L. *bifermentans*
    L. *brevis*
    L. *buchneri*
    L. *bulgaricus*
    L. *carnis*
    L. *casei*
    L. *casei* subsp. *alactosus*
    L. *casei* subsp. *pseudoplantarum*
    L. *casei* subsp. *rhamnosus*
    L. *casei* subsp. *tolerans*
    L. *catenaformis*
    L. *cellobiosus*
    L. *collinoides*
    L. *confusus*
    L. *coryniformis* subsp. *coryniformis*
    L. *coryniformis* subsp. *torquens*
    L. *crispatus*
    L. *curvatus*
    L. *curvatus* subsp. *curvatus*
    L. *curvatus* subsp. *melibiosus*
    L. *cypricasei*
    L. *delbrueckii* subsp. *bulgaricus*
    L. *delbrueckii* subsp. *delbrueckii*
    L. *delbrueckii* subsp. *lactis*
    L. *divergens*
    L. *farciminis*
    L. *fermentum*
    L. *fornicalis*
    L. *fructivorans*
    L. *fructosus*
    L. *frumenti*
    L. *gallinarum*
    L. *gasseri*
    L. *graminis*

L. *halotolerans*
L. *hamsteri*
L. *helveticus*
L. *heterohiochii*
L. *hilgardii*
L. *homohiochii*
L. *iners*
L. *intestinalis*
L. *jensenii*
L. *johnsonii*
L. *kandleri*
L. *kefiranofaciens*
L. *kefirgranum*
L. *kefiri*
L. *kimchii*
L. *kunkeei*
L. *lactis*
L. *leichmannii*
L. *lindneri*
L. *malefermentans*
L. *mali*
L. *maltaromicus*
L. *manihotivorans*
L. *minor*
L. *minutus*
L. *mucosae*
L. *murinus*
L. *nagelii*
L. *oris*
L. *panis*
L. *parabuchneri*
L. *paracasei* subsp. *paracasei*
L. *paracasei* subsp. *tolerans*
L. *parakefiri*
L. *paralimentarius*
L. *paraplantarum*
L. *pentosus*
L. *perolens*
L. *piscicola*
L. *plantarum*
L. *pontis*
L. *psittaci*
L. *reuteri*
L. *rhamnosus*
L. *rimae*
L. *rogosae*
L. *ruminis*
L. *sakei*
L. *sakei* subsp. *carnosus*
L. *sakei* subsp. *sakei*
L. *salivarius* subsp. *salicinius*
L. *salivarius* subsp. *salivarius*
L. *sanfranciscensis*
L. *sharpeae*
L. *suebicus*
L. *trichodes*
L. *uli*
L. *vaccinostercus*

L. *vaginalis*
L. *viridescens*
L. *vitulinus*
L. *xylosus*
L. *yamanashiensis*
L. *zeae*
lactobacillus, pl. **lactobacilli**
lactobionate
    erythromycin l.
Lactococcus (b)
    L. *garvieae*
    L. *lactis* subsp. *cremoris*
    L. *lactis* subsp. *hordniae*
    L. *lactis* subsp. *lactis*
    L. *piscium*
    L. *plantarum*
    L. *raffinolactis*
**lactoferrin latex bead agglutination
    (LFLA)**
lactolyticus
    Anaerococcus l.
    Peptostreptococcus l.
lactophenol
    l. aniline blue stain
    l. cotton blue (LPCB)
    l. cotton blue mount
lactose
    l. deficiency
    l. fermentation
    l. fermentation test
    l. intolerance
Lactosphaera pasteurii (b)
lactosus
    Sporolactobacillus l.
lactucae
    Mesoplasma l.
    Mycoplasma l.
lactulose
lacunaris
    Halobacteroides l.
lacunar stroke
lacunarum
    Halanaerobacter l.
lacunata
    Moraxella (Moraxella) l.
lacuscaerulensis
    Silicibacter l.
lacusprofundi
    Halobacterium l.
    Halorubrobacterium l.
    Halorubrum l.

lacusrosei
    Halanaerobium l.
lacustre
    Desulfonatronum l.
lacustris
    Friedmanniella l.
LACV
    La Crosse virus
ladakanum
    Streptomyces l.
    Streptoverticillium l.
laden
    amastigote l.
Laelaps (p)
    L. *incilis* (See *Plasmodium kochi*)
    L. *jetmari* (See *Plasmodium kochi*)
    L. *kochi* (See *Plasmodium kochi*)
    L. *multispinosus* (See *Plasmodium
        kochi*)
Laelaptidae
Laestadia
    L. *caricae*
    L. *lonchocarpi*
    L. *musae*
laeta
    Loxosceles l.
Laetiporus sulphureus (f)
laevaniformans
    Microbacterium l.
laevolacticus
    Bacillus l.
LAF
    laminar air flow
lagena
    Torulomyces l.
lagenarium
    Fusarium l.
Lagenidiaceae
Lagenidiales
Lagochilascaris (p)
    L. *minor*
    L. *sprenti*
    L. *turgida*
lagogenitalium
    Mycoplasma l.
lagophilus
    Otobius l.
lagophthalmos
Lagos bat virus (LBV)
Lagovirus (v)
lag phase

L

NOTES

303

lahillei
> *Simulium l.*

lahontan
> *Culicoides l.*

LAI
> laboratory-acquired infection

lai
> *Leptospira interrogans* serovar *l.*

laidlawii
> *Acholeplasma l.*

LAK
> lymphokine-activated killer
> LAK cell

Lake Clarendon virus (LCV)

lakei
> *Simulium l.*

lambica
> *Candida l.*

lambicus
> *Brettanomyces l.*

lamblia
> *Giardia l.*

lambliasis

lambo
> lambo l.

lamina propria

laminar
> l. air flow (LAF)
> l. hood

laminectomy

laminin

laminosum
> *Phormidium l.*

Lamisil
> L. Cream
> L. Oral

lamivudine (3TC)
> l. triphosphate (3TC)
> zidovudine and l.

lamp
> slit l.
> Wood l.

lampbrush chromosome

Lamprene

Lamprobacter modestohalophilus (b)

Lamprocystis roseopersicina (b)

Lampropedia hyalina (b)

lampyridicola
> *Spiroplasma l.*

LANA
> latency-associated nuclear antigen
> LANA antibody assay
> LANA IFA
> LANA seropositivity

Lanabiotic

Lanacillin VK

Lanacort Topical

lanatus
> *Streptomyces l.*

lanceatum
> *Dicrocoelium l.*

Lancefield
> L. capillary precipitin method
> L. classification
> L. classification system
> L. group D streptococci
> L. grouping antiserum
> L. group-specific antiserum

lanceolata
> *Drepanidotaenia l.*
> *Pseudomonas l.*

lancet-shaped

Lander Dandruff Control

Landjia virus (LJAV)

Landry-Guillain-Barré syndrome

laneanus
> *Anopheles cruzii l.*

lanei
> *Anopheles l.*

laneportoi
> *Simulium l.*

langaaensis
> *Pasteurella l.*

Langat virus (LGTV)

Langer line

langeronii
> *Eremomyces l.*
> *Microsporum audouinii* var. *l.*
> *Pithoascus l.*
> *Procandida l.*

langi
> *Chrysops l.*

languida
> *Facklamia l.*

Langur virus

Laniazid
> L. syrup

lanienae
> *Campylobacter l.*

Lanjan virus

Lanosa nivalis (f)

lanosum
> *Streptoverticillium cinnamoneum* subsp. *l.*

lanosus
> *Streptomyces cinnamoneus* subsp. *l.*

lansingensis
> *Legionella l.*

lansoprazole

lantha
> *Atherix l.*

lanuginosus
> *Chondromyces l.*
> *Thermomyces l.*

LAP
leucine aminopeptidase
LAP test
lapagei
Cedecea *l.*
laparoscopic
laparoscopy
laparotomy
La-Piedad-Michoacan-Mexico virus
lapine parvovirus
lapsum
Thermonema *l.*
laramiense
Clostridium *l.*
larbish
larense
Pseudochaetosphaeronema *l.*
large
l. cell anaplastic lymphoma
l. cell lymphoma (LCL)
l. roundworm
large-bowel perforation
largimobile
Azospirillum *l.*
largomobilis
Conglomeromonas largomobilis
subsp. *l.*
largum
Kibdelosporangium aridum subsp. *l.*
lari
Campylobacter *l.*
Lariam
larrymoorei
Agrobacterium *l.*
larva, pl. **larvae**
anisakine l.
l. currens
filariform l.
l. migrans
plerocercoid l.
rhabditiform l.
sonicated l.
larvae
Bacillus *l.*
Paenibacillus *l.*
Paenibacillus larvae subsp. *l.*
Schineria *l.*
larval
larvatum
larvicidal
larvicide
larviparous

larviphagic
laryngeal
l. infection
l. tuberculosis
laryngectomy
total l.
larynges (*pl. of* larynx)
laryngeus
Mammomonogamus *l.*
laryngitis
viral l.
laryngoepiglottitis
laryngoscopy
direct l.
indirect l.
laryngospasm
laryngotracheitis
avian infectious l.
laryngotracheobronchitis
acute l.
larynx, pl. **larynges**
laser
carbon dioxide l.
l. Doppler fluximetry
l. photocoagulation
Lash casein hydrolysate-serum medium
Lasiodiplodia (f)
L. *theobromae*
L. *triflorae*
L. *tubericola*
Lasiohelea (p)
L. *dandongensis*
L. *lushana*
L. *mujiangensis*
L. *wuyiensis*
Lasiosphaeriaceae
Las Maloyas virus
Lassa
L. fever
L. virus (LASV)
lassitude
lassmanni
Simulium *l.*
LASV
Lassa virus
LAT
latency-associated transcript
lata
late
l. benign syphilis
l. erythrocyte
l. infection

NOTES

L

305

late *(continued)*
l. latent (LL)
l. latent syphilis
l. phase response
l. PVE
latency
clinical l.
latency-associated
l.-a. nuclear antigen (LANA)
l.-a. transcript (LAT)
latent
early l. (EL)
l. infection
late l. (LL)
l. microbism
l. nuclear antigen (LNA)
l. period
l. stage
l. syphilis
lateral
l. fixation of penis
l. pharyngeal space (LPS)
latercula
Cytophaga l.
lateritius
Streptomyces l.
laterosporus
Bacillus l.
Brevibacillus l.
latex
l. agglutination (LA)
l. agglutination kit
l. agglutination test
l. particle agglutination (LPA)
laticalx
Simulium l.
latidigitus
Simulium l.
latina
Actinomadura l.
Latino virus (LATV)
latipes
Simulium l.
lato
Borrelia burgdorferi sensu l.
sensu l.
Lato river virus
Latrodectus
L. mactans
latum
Caryophanon l.
condyloma l.
Diphyllobothrium l.
latus
Alcaligenes l.
Desulfobacter l.
Dibothriocephalus l.

LATV
Latino virus
latyschewii
Borrelia l.
laumondii
Photorhabdus luminescens subsp. *l.*
laurel fever
laureliae
Candida l.
laurentii
Cryptococcus l.
Streptomyces l.
Laurer canal
Lautropia mirabilis (b)
lautus
Bacillus l.
Paenibacillus l.
LAV
lymphadenopathy-associated virus
lavage
bronchoalveolar l. (BAL)
bronchopulmonary l.
cervical l.
lavendofoliae
Streptomyces l.
lavendulae
Streptomyces lavendulae subsp. *l.*
lavenduligriseum
Streptoverticillium l.
lavenduligriseus
Streptomyces l.
lavendulocolor
Streptomyces l.
Laverania falciparum (p)
law of priority
Lawsonia intracellularis (b)
lawsonii
Campylobacter hyointestinalis subsp. *l.*
lazaretto
lazarine leprosy
Lazaro
mal de San L.
LazerSporin-C Otic
LBM
lean body mass
little brown mushroom
LBV
Lagos bat virus
LCL
large cell lymphoma
LCM
lymphocytic choriomeningitis
LCM virus
LCMV
lymphocytic choriomeningitis virus
LCR
ligase chain reaction

Abbott LCx LCR
LCR assay
LCT
long-chain triglyceride
LCV
Lake Clarendon virus
LCx
Chlamydia trachomatis L.
L. *Chlamydia trachomatis* LCR
assay
L-D
Leishman-Donovan
L-D body
LD
Lyme disease
LDH
lactate dehydrogenase
LDHV
lactic dehydrogenase virus
LDL
low density lipoprotein
LDMA
lymphocyte detected membrane antigen
LDV
lactate dehydrogenase elevating virus
Le Dantec virus
LE
leukocyte esterase
LE antibody
LE urine dipstick
Le
Le Dantec virus (LDV)
leachi
Haemaphysalis l.
lean
l. body mass (LBM)
l. body muscle mass
Leanyer virus
Lebombo virus (LEBV)
LEBV
Lebombo virus
lecaniicorni
Exophiala jeanselmei var. l.
Lechevalieria (b)
L. *aerocolonigenes* subsp.
aerocolonigenes
L. *flava*
lecithinase
lecithinolyticum
Treponema l.
Lecithodendriidae
Leclercia adecarboxylata (b)

lectin
kidney bean l.
mitogenic adherence l.
lectularius
Cimex l.
Symbiotes l.
Lecythophora (f)
L. *hoffmanii*
L. *lignicola*
L. *mutabilis*
Lednice virus (LEDV)
LEDV
Lednice virus
leech
leechi
Culicoides l.
LEEP
loop electrosurgical excisional procedure
left
l. anterior mediastinoscopy
l. atrial myxoma
l. ventricle (LV)
l. ventricular assist device (LVAD)
l. ventricular dysfunction
l. ventricular hypertrophy
left-sided endocarditis
leg
Barbados l.
elephant l.
legendrei
Hysterothylacium l.
Legg-Calve-Perthes disease
Legionella (b)
L. *adelaidensis*
L. *anisa*
L. antigen test
L. antigenuria
L. assay
L. *birminghamensis*
L. *bozemaii*
L. *bozemanii*
L. *brunensis*
L. *cherrii*
L. *cincinnatiensis*
L. DFA stain
L. DNA probe
L. *drozanskii*
L. *dumoffii*
L. *erythra*
L. *fairfieldensis*
L. *fallonii*
L. *feeleii*

L

NOTES

307

Legionella (continued)
    L. *geestiana*
    L. *gormanii*
    L. *gratiana*
    L. *hackeliae*
    L. *israelensis*
    L. *jamestowniensis*
    L. *jordanis*
    L. *lansingensis*
    L. *londiniensis*
    L. *longbeachae*
    L. *lytica*
    L. *maceachernii*
    L. *micdadei*
    L. *moravica*
    L. *nautarum*
    L. *oakridgensis*
    L. *parisiensis*
    L. *pittsburghensis*
    L. *pneumophila* antibody
    L. *pneumophila* culture
    L. *pneumophila* subsp. *fraseri*
    L. *pneumophila* subsp. *pascullei*
    L. *pneumophila* subsp. *pneumophila*
    L. *pneumophila* serogroup Lansing 3
    L. *pneumophila* smear
    L. *quateirensis*
    L. *quinlivanii*
    L. *rowbothamii*
    L. *rubrilucens*
    L. *sainthelensi*
    L. *santicrucis*
    L. *serology*
    L. *shakespearei*
    L. *spiritensis*
    L. *steigerwaltii*
    L. *taurinensis*
    L. *tucsonensis*
    L. *wadsworthii*
    L. *waltersii*
    L. *worsleiensis*
Legionellaceae
Legionella-like amebal pathogen
Legionnaires
    L. disease
    L. disease antibody
leguminosarum
    Rhizobium l.
leichmannii
    Lactobacillus l.
leidyi
    Caulobacter l.
Leifson flagellar stain
Leifsonia (b)
    L. *aquatica*
    L. *cynodontis*
    L. *naganoensis*
    L. *poae*

    L. *shinshuensis*
    L. *xyli* subsp. *cynodontis*
    L. *xyli* subsp. *xyli*
leiocephalus
    Helicotylenchus l.
leiognathi
    Photobacterium l.
leiomyosarcoma
Leishman-Donovan (L-D)
    L.-D. body
Leishmania (p)
    L. *aethiopica*
    L. *amazonensis*
    L. *braziliensis*
    L. *chagasi*
    L. *donovani*
    L. *enriettii*
    L. *guyanensis*
    L. *hertigi*
    L. *infantum*
    L. *major*
    L. *mexicana*
    L. *panamensis*
    L. *peruviana*
    L. *tropica*
    L. *venezuelensis*
leishmaniae
leishmanial
leishmaniasis
    acute cutaneous l.
    American l.
    anergic l.
    anthroponotic cutaneous l.
    cheloid l.
    chronic cutaneous l.
    cutaneous l.
    dermal l.
    diffuse cutaneous l.
    disseminated anergic cutaneous l.
    dry cutaneous l.
    infantile l.
    leproid l.
    lupoid l.
    mucocutaneous l.
    mucosal l.
    nasopharyngeal l.
    New World l.
    nondisseminated cutaneous l.
    Old World l.
    post-kala azar dermal l.
    pseudolepromatous l.
    l. recidivans
    rural cutaneous l.
    sporotrichoid l.
    l. tegumentaria
    l. tegumentaria diffusa
    urban cutaneous l.

visceral l.
wet cutaneous l.
zoonotic cutaneous l.
Leishmaniavirus (v)
leishmanin skin test
leishmaniosis
leishmanoid
Leishman stain
leisingeri
    Methylophilus l.
lemic
Lemierre
    L. disease
    L. syndrome
Leminorella (b)
    L. grimontii
    L. richardii
lemming fever
lemoignei
    Paucimonas l.
    Pseudomonas l.
length of stay (LOS)
lens
    Medallion suture l.
    phase-contrast l.
lenta
    Eggerthella l.
lenticular colony
lenticularum
    Arthroderma l.
lenticulata
    Acanthamoeba l.
lentiflavum
    Mycobacterium l.
lentimorbus
    Bacillus l.
    Paenibacillus l.
Lentivirinae
Lentivirus (v)
lentocellum
    Clostridium l.
lentoputrescens
    Clostridium l.
lentum
    Eubacterium l.
lentus
    Bacillus l.
    Staphylococcus l.
    Staphylococcus sciuri subsp. *l.*
    Vibrio l.
Lentzea (b)
    L. albida

    L. albidocapillata
    L. californiensis
    L. violacea
    L. waywayandensis
Leo
    Mycobacterium phage L.
leonicaptivi
    Mycoplasma l.
leonina
    Toxascaris l.
leopard skin
leopharyngis
    Mycoplasma l.
Lepidoglyphus destructor (p)
Lepidoptera
Lepidoptera and Orthoptera
    poxvirus of a.
lepidopterism
lepidum
    Methylocaldum l.
lepori
    Brugia l.
leporina
    Podospora l.
leporinum
    Arnium l.
Leporipoxvirus (v)
leporispalustris
    Haemaphysalis l.
leprae
    Mycobacterium l.
lepraemurium
    Mycobacterium l.
lepra type-1, -2 reaction
leproid leishmaniasis
leprologist
leprology
leproma
lepromatosis
    diffuse l.
lepromatous
    borderline l. (BL)
    l. leprosy
lepromin skin test
leprosarium
leprostatic
leprosum
    erythema nodosum l.
leprosy
    articular l.
    l. bacillus (*See Mycobacterium leprae*)

L

NOTES

leprosy *(continued)*
    borderline l.
    dimorphous l.
    histoid l.
    indeterminate l.
    lazarine l.
    lepromatous l.
    Lucio l.
    macular l.
    Malabar l.
    multibacillary l.
    mutilating l.
    neural l.
    nodular l.
    paucibacillary l.
    smooth l.
    tuberculoid l.
leprotic
leprous
leptinotarsae
    Spiroplasma l.
Leptocimex boueti
Leptoconops (p)
    L. carteri
    L. clava
    L. copiosus
    L. curvachelus
    L. irritans
    L. kerteszi
    L. primaevus
    L. torrens
Leptolegniellaceae
leptomeningeal malignancy
leptomeninges
leptomeningitis
Leptomitaceae
Leptomitales
leptomonad
Leptomonas (p)
    L. collosoma
    L. seymouri
Leptonema illini (b)
Leptopeltidaceae
Leptopsylla (p)
    L. aethiopica
    L. aethiopica nakuruensis
    L. algira costai
    L. algira tuggertensis
    L. sciurobia
    L. segnis
Leptopsyllidae
leptospartum
    Clostridium stercorarium subsp. l.
    Thermobacteroides l.
Leptosphaeria (f)
    L. coniothyrium
    L. senegalensis
    L. tompkinsii

Leptospira (b)
    L. alexanderi
    L. biflexa
    L. borgpetersenii
    L. fainei
    L. fainei serovar hurstbridge
    L. inadai
    L. inadai serovar lyme
    L. interrogans
    L. interrogans sensu stricto
    L. interrogans serovar australis
    L. interrogans serovar autumnalis
    L. interrogans serovar ballum
    L. interrogans serovar bataviae
    L. interrogans serovar canicola
    L. interrogans serovar copenhageni
    L. interrogans serovar grippotyphosa
    L. interrogans serovar hardjo
    L. interrogans serovar hebdomadis
    L. interrogans serovar hyos
    L. interrogans serovar
      icterohaemorrhagiae
    L. interrogans serovar lai
    L. interrogans serovar pomona
    L. interrogans serovar pyrogenes
    L. interrogans serovar tarassovi
    L. kirschneri
    L. meyeri
    L. noguchii
    L. parva
    L. santarosai
    L. serology
    L. weilii
    L. wolbachii
Leptospiraceae
leptospiral
    l. infection
    l. jaundice
leptospire
Leptospirillum (b)
    L. ferrooxidans
    L. thermoferrooxidans
leptospirosis
    anicteric l.
    subclinical l.
Leptostromataceae
leptothricosis
Leptothrix (b)
    L. cholodnii
    L. discophora
    L. lopholea
    L. mobilis
    L. ochracea
Leptotrichia buccalis (b)
Leptotrombidium (p)
    L. arenicola

L. *deliense*
L. *fletcheri*
leptum
Clostridium l.
lesion
achromic macular skin l.
actinomycotic l.
anal squamous intraepithelial l.
anular l.
bulbous skin l.
cavitary lung l.
chagasic l.
cicatricial l.
coin l.
l. culture
cutaneous l.
disfiguring l.
disseminated l.
doughnut l.
dyschromic papulosquamous skin l.
erythematous l.
esophageal l.
evanescent l.
focal brain l. (FBL)
focal mass l.
focal sclerosis l.
genital l.
granulomatous l.
hemorrhagic l.
herpetic l.
high-grade squamous
  intraepithelial l. (HSIL)
hypodense l.
index l.
intracranial l.
intraretinal l.
Janeway l.
kissing bug l.
lichenoid l.
low-grade squamous
  intraepithelial l. (LSIL)
lymphoproliferative skin l.
lytic l.
macroscopic l.
maculopapular skin l.
Margarinos-Torres l.
marker l.
miliary l.
mucocutaneous HSV l.
mulaire l.
neoplastic l.
nickel and dime l.

nodular l.
oral l.
oropharyngeal l.
papillomatous skin l.
papular l.
papulosquamous skin l.
pedunculated l.
perineal l.
peripheral coin l.
pseudomembranous l.
pustular l.
ring-enhancing l.
satellite l.
signal l.
space-occupying l.
spinal compressive l.
squamous intraepithelial l. (SIL)
syphilitic l.
target l.
tubulointerstitial l.
varicelliform l.
violaceous papule verrucous l.
LET
leukocyte esterase test
lethal
l. factor (LF)
l. toxin
lethargic
lethargica
encephalitis l.
Von Economo encephalitis l.
lethargy
letrazuril
letter
Chinese l.'s
leucine
l. aminopeptidase (LAP)
l. aminopeptidase test (LAP test)
Leucobacter komogatae (b)
leucocelaenus
Haemagogus l.
Leucocytozoon (p)
L. *simondi*
L. *smithi*
Leuconostoc (b)
L. *amelibiosum*
L. *argentinum*
L. *carnosum*
L. *citreum*
L. *cremoris*
L. *dextranicum*
L. *fallax*

L

NOTES

Leuconostoc (continued)
.L. gasicomitatum
L. gelidum
L. kimchii
L. lactis
L. mesenteroides subsp. cremoris
L. mesenteroides subsp. dextranicum
L. mesenteroides subsp.
  mesenteroides
L. oenos
L. paramesenteroides
L. pseudomesenteroides
leucopoiesis
Leucorrhinia glacialis
Leucosporidium (f)
L. capsuligenum
L. frigidum
L. gelidum
L. nivale
L. scotti
L. stokesii
leucosticta
Fannia l.
Leucothrix mucor (b)
Leucotrichales
leucotrichum
Myrothecium l.
leucovorin
leukapheresis
leukemia
acute promyelocytic l.
adult T-cell l. (ATL)
B-cell chronic lymphocytic l.
B-chronic lymphocyte l. (B-CLL)
bovine l. (BLV)
eosinophilic l.
juvenile chronic myelogenous l.
lymphoblastic l.
myeloid l.
T-prolymphocytic l.
leukemia/lymphoma
adult T-cell l. (ATLL)
leukemic burden
leukoagglutinin
leukocidin
leukocoria
leukocyte
l. esterase (LE)
l. esterase dipstick
l. esterase test (LET)
l. esterase urine dipstick (LE urine
  dipstick)
fecal l.
intravesical polymorphonuclear l.
polymorphonuclear l. (PMN,
  PMNL)
tenesmus l.
tumor-infiltrating l.

leukocyte/epithelial cell ratio
leukocyte-free packed erythrocyte
leukocytoclastic
leukocytoclastic vasculitis
leukocytosis
perinephrial l.
peripheral l.
leukocyturia
leukoencephalitis
acute epidemic l.
acute hemorrhagic l.
postinfectious l.
leukoencephalopathy
hemorrhagic l.
multifocal l.
progressive multifocal l. (PML)
leukopenia
leukoplakia
Candida l.
hairy l.
oral hairy l. (OHL)
leukorrhea
leukosis
enzootic bovine l.
leukotriene
Leukovirus
Levaquin
Levbid
level
alanine aminotransferase l.
amikacin l.
amphotericin B l.
Ancobon l.
antimicrobial l.
aspartate aminotransferase l.
basal cortisol l.
biosafety l. (BSL)
blood Amikin l.
blood Fungizone l.
blood Sporanox l.
blood Vancocin l.
blood Vancoled l.
chloramphenicol serum l.
coccidioidal complement-fixation l.
cortisol l.
5-FC l.
flucytosine l.
gentamicin l.
HIV RNA l.
intracellular HIV RNA l.
itraconazole l.
kanamycin l.
Kantrex l.
ketoconazole l.
peak blood l.
plasma HIV RNA l.
plasma retinol l.
plasma selenium l.

plasma viral l.
pleural pH l.
proviral HIV RNA l.
rebound of plasma HIV RNA l.
ritonavir plasma l.
serum bacterial inhibitory l.
serum beta-carotene l.
serum endostatin l.
serum erythropoietin l.
serum retinol l.
serum testosterone l.
serum total bilirubin l.
spontaneous growth hormone l.
subnanogram l.
tobramycin l.
trough blood l.
vancomycin l.

levicastilloi
   Anopheles franciscanus l.

levida
   Muscina l.

levii
   Bacteroides l.
   Porphyromonas l.

Levinea (b)
   L. amalonatica
   L. malonatica

levis
   Streptomyces l.

Leviviridae
Levivirus (v)
levofloxacin
levonorgestrel
levothyroxine
Levsin
Levsinex
Levsin/SL
Lewia infectoria (f)
Lewinella (b)
   L. cohaerens
   L. nigricans
   L. persica

lewisi
   Simulium l.
   Trypanosoma l.

LF
   lethal factor
LFLA
   lactoferrin latex bead agglutination
L-form
   Lister-form

LGTV
   Langat virus
LGV
   lymphogranuloma venereum
      LGV strain of *Chlamydia*
LH
   luteinizing hormone
liaoningense
   Bradyrhizobium l.
libanensis
   Pseudomonas l.
libani
   Streptomyces libani subsp. *l.*
libanotica
   Actinocorallia l.
   Actinomadura l.
libido
   diminished l.
Liborius method
Librax
lice
   crab l.
   pubic l.
Liceales
Lice-Enz Shampoo
lichen
   l. albus
   l. nitidus
   l. planus
   l. sclerosus et atrophicus
lichenicola
   Cylindrocarpon l.
   Melittangium l.
licheniformis
   Bacillus l.
lichenoid lesion
lichen planus
Lichtheimia curymbifera (f)
lid
   l. edema
   granular l.
   l. lag
Lida-Mantle HC Topical
Lidemol
Lidex
Lidex-E
lidocaine
   bacitracin, neomycin, polymixin B,
      and l.
   l. and hydrocortisone
Lieberkühn
   crypts of L.

L

NOTES

lienomycini
  Streptomyces l.
Liesegang ring
life-long
life-threatening
ligase chain reaction (LCR)
ligation
  tubal l.
light
  cold l.
  l. microscopy
lignan
ligniaria
  Coniochaeta l.
lignicola
  Hyalodendron l.
  Lecythophora l.
  Scytalidium l.
lignieresii
  Actinobacillus l.
lignorum
  Trichoderma l.
lignosa
  Candida shehatae var. *l.*
Ligula intestinalis (p)
λ-like viruses (v)
lilacinum
  Streptoverticillium l.
lilacinus
  Paecilomyces l.
  Streptomyces l.
lilium
  Corynebacterium l.
limbata
  Damalina l.
limbatum
  Simulium l.
Lim Benyesh-Melnick intersecting antiserum pool
limbus
lime
  chlorinated l.
limicola
  Chlorobium l.
  Desulfonema l.
  Filibacter l.
  Methanoplanus l.
limimaris
  Desulfomonile l.
liminatans
  Methanofollis l.
  Methanogenium l.
limitation of exposure
limnaeus
  Thialkalicoccus l.
Limnatis (p)
  L. africana
  L. granulosa

L. japonica
L. nilotica
limnemia
limnemic
limneticum
  Ferribacterium l.
Limnobacter thiooxidans (b)
limnology
limnophilus
  Planctomyces l.
limosum
  Clostridium l.
  Eubacterium l.
limosus
  Janibacter l.
  Streptomyces l.
limulus amoebocyte lysate assay
linaloolentis
  Thauera l.
lincolnensis
  Streptomyces l.
lincolnii
  Moraxella l.
lincomycin
lincosamide
Linctus Codeine Blac
lindane
lindane-resistant
lindaniclasticus
  Rhodanobacter l.
lindneri
  Lactobacillus l.
lindnerii
  Pichia l.
lindoense
  Echinostoma l.
line
  Langer l.
  Pastia l.
  percutaneously placed l.
  l. probe assay (LIPA, LiPA)
  l. sepsis
linear gingival erythema
linear opacity
lineata
  Monocelis l.
  Phytobdella l.
lineatum
  Hypoderma l.
linens
  Brevibacterium l.
lineolae
  Spiroplasma l.
linezolid
linguale
  Spirosoma l.
lingual ulcer

Linguatula (p)
    L. rhinaria
    L. serrata
linguatuliasis
Linguatulida
Linguatulidae
linnaean system of nomenclature
Linognathus (p)
    L. africanus
    L. pedalis
    L. setosus
    L. vituli
linum
    Oceanospirillum l.
Liopygia argyrostoma
LIP
    lymphoid interstitial pneumonia
    lymphoid interstitial pneumonitis
lip
    cleft l.
LIPA
    line probe assay
LiPA
    line probe assay
    LiPA strip assay
lipase
lipemia
lipid-associated amphotericin B
lipid-lowering agent
lipmanii
    Streptomyces l.
lipoatrophy
    peripheral l.
lipocalidus
    Syntrophothermus l.
lipochrome
lipodystrophy
    HIV l.
    peripheral l.
    l. syndrome
lipofaciens
    Mycoplasma l.
lipofer
    Lipomyces l.
lipoferum
    Azospirillum l.
lipogenesis
    de novo l. (DNL)
lipohypertrophy
lipolytic
lipolytica
    Candida l.

Endomycopsis l.
Selenomonas l.
Thermosyntropha l.
Yarrowia l.
lipolyticus
    Anaerovibrio l.
lipomastia
lipomatosis
Lipomyces (f)
    L. lipofer
    L. starkeyi
    L. tetrasporus
Liponyssoides (p)
Liponyssus
    L. bacoti
    L. bursa
    L. sylviarum
lipophilic
    l. *Corynebacterium*
lipophiloflavum
    Corynebacterium l.
lipophilum
    Corynebacterium afermentans subsp. *l.*
    Mycoplasma l.
lipopolysaccharide (LPS)
lipoprotein
    low density l. (LDL)
liposomal
    amphotericin B l.
    l. amphotericin B (L AmB)
    l. daunorubicin
    l. encapsulated anthracycline
    l. encapsulated doxorubicin
liposome drug delivery
liposome-encapsulated
    l.-e. gentamicin
    l.-e. IL-2
liposuction
lipoteichoic acid
Lipotena cervi (p)
Lipothrixviridae
Lipothrixvirus (v)
lipotrophy
Lipovnik virus (LIPV)
lipoxenous
lipoxeny
LIPV
    Lipovnik virus
liquefaciens
    Acetobacter aceti subsp. *l.*
    Aureobacterium l.

L

NOTES

liquefaciens (continued)
      Brevibacterium l.
      Gluconacetobacter l.
      Microbacterium l.
      Serratia l.
liquefaction necrosis
liquefied carbolic acid
Liquibid
Liqui-Caps
      Vicks 44 Non-Drowsy Cold &
        Cough L.-C.
Liquid
      Anaplex L.
      Baby L.
      Barc L.
      Brontex L.
      Chlorafed L.
      Contac Cough Formula L.
      Detussin L.
      End Lice L.
      Gordofilm L.
      Hayfebrol L.
      Histinex D L.
      Histussin D L.
      Hycotuss Expectorant L.
      Lotrimin AF Spray L.
      Naldecon DX Adult L.
      Occlusal-HP L.
      L. Pred
      Pyrinyl II L.
      Rhinosyn L.
      Rhinosyn-PD L.
      Rhinosyn-X L.
      Ryna L.
      Ryna-C L.
      Tisit L.
      Triple X L.
      Tyrodone L.
liquid
      l. chromatography
      Entuss-D L.
      l. nitrogen
Liqui-Gels
      Alka-Seltzer Plus Flu & Body
        Aches Non-Drowsy L.-G.
      Robitussin Severe Congestion L.-G.
Liquiprin
Listerella paradoxus (f)
listeremia
      typhoidal l.
Lister-form (L-form)
listeri
      Nocardiopsis l.
Listeria (b)
      L. denitrificans
      L. grayi
      L. innocua
      L. ivanovii

      L. ivanovii subsp. *ivanovii*
      L. ivanovii subsp. *londoniensis*
      L. meningitis
      L. monocytogenes
      L. murrayi
      L. seeligeri
      L. welshimeri
listeria
listerial meningitis
listeriolysin O
listeriosis
Listonella (b)
      L. anguillarum
      L. damsela
      L. pelagia
lithiasis
lithium carbonate
Lithobius
lithogenes
      Paracoccidioides l.
      Trichosporon l.
lithoptysis
Lithostat
lithotroph
litmocidini
      Streptomyces l.
litorale
      Clostridium l.
      Spiroplasma l.
litoralis
      Desulfovibrio l.
      Erythrobacter l.
      Flexibacter l.
      Halobacillus l.
      Halococcus l.
      Roseobacter l.
      Spirochaeta l.
      Thiocapsa l.
litoralum
      Prosthecomicrobium l.
Litostomatea
little brown mushroom (LBM)
liturata
      Anthomyia l.
lituricollis
      Blattella l.
lituseburense
      Clostridium l.
LIV
      louping ill virus
live
      l. attenuated virus vaccine
      l. measles virus vaccine
      measles virus vaccine, l.
      l. mumps virus vaccine
      l. oral polio vaccine
      l. oral poliovirus vaccine
      l. rubella virus vaccine

rubella virus vaccine, l.
l. vaccine strain (LVS)
varicella virus vaccine, l.

liver
l. abscess
l. biopsy
cirrhosis of the l.
l. enzyme
l. enzyme test
fatty infiltration of the l.
l. function test
l. toxicity
transjugular needle biopsy of the l.
liver/kidney microsomal antibody
livida
Actinomadura l.
lividans
Streptomyces l.
lividum
Entoloma l.
Janthinobacterium l.
lividus
Ixodes l.
living will
lizard skin
LJAV
Landjia virus
LJP
localized juvenile periodontitis
ljungdahlii
Clostridium l.
LJV
La Joya virus
LL
late latent
LL syphilis
Llano Seco virus (LLSV)
llanquihuensis
Candida l.
lloydi
Anopheles evansae l.
LLSV
Llano Seco virus
LMN
lower motor neuron
LMN disease
LNA
latent nuclear antigen
Loa (p)
L. extraocularis
L. inquirenda
L. loa

loa
Loa l.
load
antigen l.
blood viral l.
body plasma viral l.
CSF viral l.
HIV-2 proviral l.
HIV-2 viral l.
HTLV-1 proviral l.
plasma HIV l.
plasma viral l. (PVL, pVL)
proviral l.
RNA viral l.
semen viral l.
viral l. (VL)
lobar
l. consolidation
l. pneumonia
lobata
Ampullariella l.
lobate
lobatum
hepar l.
lobatus
Actinoplanes l.
Loboa loboi (f)
Lobo disease
loboi
Lacazia l.
Loboa l.
Lobomyces (f)
lobomycosis
lobopodium
lobose
Lobosea
lobular inflammation
local immunity
localized
l. adenopathy
l. cutaneous
l. juvenile periodontitis (LJP)
l. tetanus
lockjaw
Lock solution
Locoid Topical
loculated abscess
Locusta migratoria
lodderae
Candida l.
Lodderomyces elongisporus (f)
Lodenosine

L

NOTES

Iodoxamide tromethamine
Loeffler
>L. bacillus
>L. blood culture medium
>L. methylene blue dye
>L. methylene blue stain

loescheii
>*Bacteroides l.*
>*Prevotella l.*

Löffler, Loeffler
>L. syndrome

logarithmic phase
1-log decrease
2-log decrease
logei
>*Photobacterium l.*
>*Vibrio l.*

loiasis
loisae
>*Culicoides l.*

Lokern virus (LOKV)
LOKV
>Lokern virus

lomefloxacin
Lomentospora (f)
Lomidine
lomondensis
>*Streptomyces l.*

Lomotil
lomustine
lonchocarpi
>*Laestadia l.*

londiniensis
>*Legionella l.*

subsp. *londoniensis*
Lone
>L. Star tick
>L. Star virus (LSV)

Lonepinella koalarum (b)
long
>l. chain
>l. incubation hepatitis
>l. thoracic nerve

Long-Acting
>Sinex L.-A.

long-acting sulfonamide
longbeachae
>*Legionella l.*

long-chain triglyceride (LCT)
longibrachiatrum
>*Trichoderma l.*

longicatena
>*Actinocorallia l.*
>*Actinomadura l.*
>*Nonomuraea l.*

longiceps
>*Monocelis l.*

longicollis
>*Cysticercus l.*

longicornis
>*Haemaphysalis l.*

longilobus
>*Senecio l.*

longior
>*Tyroglyphus l.*

longipalpis
>*Lutzomyia l.*

longipennis
>*Hippobosca l.*

longipes
>*Alternaria l.*

longirostrata
>*Drechslera l.*

longirostratum
>*Exserohilum l.*

longispora
>*Actinomadura l.*
>*Nocardiopsis l.*
>*Planobispora l.*
>*Saccharothrix l.*

longisporoflavus
>*Streptomyces l.*

longispororuber
>*Streptomyces l.*

longisporum
>*Streptosporangium l.*

longisporus
>*Streptomyces l.*

longissimespiculata
>*Nematodirella l.*

longistylatum
>*Simulium l.*

long-lived memory T cell
longreachensis
>*Desulfovibrio l.*

long-term nonprogressive disease
longum
>*Acetonema l.*
>*Bifidobacterium l.*

longus
>*Desulfovibrio l.*
>*Erythrobacter l.*

longwoodensis
>*Streptomyces l.*

Loniten Oral
loop
>autocrine-paracrine growth l.
>l. electrosurgical excisional
> procedure (LEEP)

loop-acting diuretic
Loossia
loperamide
lopezneyrai
>*Gigantorhynchus l.*

lophii
> *Nosema l.*

Lophiostomataceae

lopholea
> *Leptothrix l.*

lophortygis
> *Culicoides l.*

lophotrichate

lophotrichous

lopinavir
> l. and ritonavir

Loprox

Lorabid

loracarbef

loratadine

lorazepam

Lordsdale virus

Loridine

Loroxide

lortetii
> *Clostridium l.*
> *Sporohalobacter l.*

LOS
> length of stay

Losec

loss
> conduction hearing l.
> peripheral visual field l.

loti
> *Mesorhizobium l.*
> *Rhizobium l.*

lotion
> BlemErasc L.
> Klaron L.
> Lotrimin AF L.
> Neutrogena On-The-Spot Acne L.
> Nova Perfecting L.
> Panscol L.
> Sebizon Topical L.

Lotriderm

Lotrimin
> L. AF Cream
> L. AF Lotion
> L. AF solution
> L. AF Spray Liquid
> L. AF Spray Powder

Lotrisone

loughnani
> *Culicoides l.*

Louis Pasteur

louping ill virus (LIV)

louse
> biting l.
> body l.
> l. fly
> head l.
> pubic l.
> sea l.
> sucking l.

louse-borne
> l.-b. relapsing fever
> l.-b. typhus

lousiness

lousy

lovaniensis
> *Acetobacter pasteurianus* subsp. *l.*

lovastatin

Loviride

loviride

low
> l. affinity antigen receptor
> l. density lipoprotein (LDL)

low-dose VV therapy

low-egg-passage vaccine

Lowenstein-Jensen, Löwenstein-Jensen
> L.-J. agar
> L.-J. culture medium

lower
> l. genital tract infection
> l. motor neuron (LMN)
> l. motor neuron disease
> l. respiratory tract infection

low-grade
> l.-g. fever
> l.-g. squamous intraepithelial lesion (LSIL)

low-titer viremia

Loxosceles
> *L. deserta*
> *L. laeta*
> *L. reclusa*

lozenge
> amphotericin B l.

LP
> lumbar puncture

LPA
> latex particle agglutination
> lymphocyte proliferation assay
> lymphocytic proliferation assay

LPCB
> lactophenol cotton blue

L-phase variant

LPP-1 virus

L

NOTES

LPS
lateral pharyngeal space
lipopolysaccharide
L-pyrrolidonyl-beta-naphthylamide (PyR)
L-rhamnose fermentation test
L-selectin molecule (CD62L)
LSIL
low-grade squamous intraepithelial lesion
LSV
Lone Star virus
LT virus
Lu-III virus
lubbocki
Cyclops l.
lubricus
Agitococcus l.
Lubrin Insert
lucensis
Streptomyces l.
lucentensis
Nocardiopsis l.
Lucetina (p)
luciae
Desulfotomaculum l.
Lucibacterium harveyi (b)
luciferase
l. enzyme-based luminescence
system
lucifugus
Culex l.
Lucilia (p)
L. cuprina
L. illustris
Lucio
L. leprosy
L. reaction
lucipetus
Philophthalmus l.
lucivorax
Entomoplasma l.
Mycoplasma l.
Ludwig angina
lues
l. venerea
Lufyllin
lugdunensis
Staphylococcus l.
luggeri
Simulium l.
luglani
Culicoides l.
Lugol solution
Lukuni virus (LUKV)
LUKV
Lukuni virus
lumbar puncture (LP)
lumboperitoneal shunt
lumbrical

lumbrici
Monocystis l.
lumbricidal
lumbricide
lumbricoid
lumbricoides
Ascaris l.
lumbricosis
Lumbricus terrestris
luminal
l. agent
l. anisakidosis
l. infection
luminescens
Photorhabdus luminescens subsp. l.
Xenorhabdus l.
Luminetics ATP assay
luminosum
Entomoplasma l.
Mycoplasma l.
lumpy
l. jaw
l. jaw syndrome
l. skin disease
lunar periodicity
lunata
Curvularia l.
lunatus
Cochliobolus l.
lundensis
Pseudomonas l.
lung
air-conditioner l.
l. biopsy tissue
l. carcinoma
cavitary l.
cheese worker's l.
farmer's l.
malt worker's l.
mushroom-worker's l.
thresher's l.
unilateral hyperlucent l.
lungworms
lupi
Spirocerca l.
lupini
Rhizobium l.
lupinosa
porrigo l.
lupoid
l. hepatitis
l. leishmaniasis
lupus
l. anticoagulant
l. band test
l. erythematosus
uncomplicated l.
l. vulgaris

lurida
    Amycolatopsis orientalis subsp. *l.*
luridus
    Streptomyces l.
lurybayae
    Simulium l.
lusatiensis
    Defluvibacter l.
Luschka
    foramen of L.
    L. tonsil
lushana
    Lasiohelea l.
lusitaniae
    Borrelia l.
    Candida l.
    Clavispora l.
lusitanus
    Streptomyces l.
lutea
    Myceliophthora l.
Luteimonas mephitis (b)
luteinizing hormone (LH)
lutein/zeaxanthin
Luteococcus (b)
    L. *japonicus*
    L. *peritonei*
luteofluorescens
    Actinomadura l.
    Streptomyces l.
luteogriseus
    Streptomyces l.
luteola
    Auchmeromyia l.
    Chryseomonas l.
    Pseudomonas l.
luteolum
    Aureobacterium l.
    Microbacterium l.
    Pelodictyon l.
luteolus
    Agromyces l.
    Arthrobacter l.
    Cryptococcus l.
luteosporeus
    Streptomyces l.
luteovenus
    Culicoides l.
luteoverticillatum
    Streptoverticillium l.
luteoverticillatus
    Streptomyces l.

luteoviolacea
    Alteromonas l.
    Pseudoalteromonas l.
Luteovirus (v)
luteum
    Brevibacterium l.
    Curtobacterium l.
    Polyangium l.
luteus
    Methylobacter l.
    Methylococcus l.
    Micrococcus l.
    Nocardioides l.
    Rhodococcus l.
    Terracoccus l.
lutrae
    Dracunculus l.
    Staphylococcus l.
    Vagococcus l.
Luttrellia
lutzi
    Gigantorhynchus l.
    Psorophora l.
lutzianum
    Simulium l.
lutzii
    Anopheles l.
Lutzomyia (p)
    L. *fluviscutellata*
    L. *longipalpis*
    L. *peruensis*
Lutz-Splendore-Almeida disease
luzoniacum
    Eupenicillium l.
LV
    left ventricle
LVAD
    left ventricular assist device
L74V mutation
LVS
    live vaccine strain
LW
    laboratory worker
lwoffii
    Acinetobacter l.
lycopene
Lycoperdaceae
Lycoperdales
lycoperdonosis
Lycoperdon perlatum (f)
Lycopersicon esculentum
lycophora

L

NOTES

Lyderm
lydicus
    Streptomyces l.
lylae
    Micrococcus l.
Lymantria
    L. dispar
    L. ninayi virus
Lyme
    L. arthritis serology
    L. borreliosis
    L. borreliosis antibody
    L. disease (LD)
    L. disease antibody test
    L. disease immunoblot
    L. disease serology
    L. disease vaccine
lyme
    Leptospira inadai serovar *l.*
LYMErix
Lymnaea
lymph
    l. node basin
    l. node biopsy
    l. node culture
    l. varices
lymphadenitis
    acute febrile l.
    cervical l.
    diffuse l.
    focal mycobacterial l.
    mesenteric l.
    mycobacterial l.
    regional l.
    sclerosing l.
    submandibular l.
    suppurative granulomatous l.
    tuberculous l.
lymphadenopathy
    angioimmunoblastic l.
    benign l.
    generalized l.
    hilar l.
    inguinal l.
    mediastinal l.
    minor l.
    nonneoplastic l.
    persistent generalized l. (PGL)
    preauricular l.
    regional l.
lymphadenopathy-associated virus (LAV)
lymphangitidis
    Pasteurella l.
lymphangitis
lymphatic
    l. filariasis
    l. filariasis granuloma
    l. tuberculosis

lymph node
    draining l. n.
    enlarging l. n.
    inguinal l. n.
    paraaortic l. n.
    tumor-draining l. n. (TDLN)
lymphoblast
lymphoblastic leukemia
lymphoblastoid interferon
Lymphocryptovirus (v)
lymphocutaneous
    l. nodule
    l. sporotrichosis
Lymphocystivirus (v)
lymphocyte
    B l.
    CD4+ l.
    CD4 T l.
    CD8 T l.
    CIK l.
    l. count
    l. culture
    cytokine-induced killer l.
    cytotoxic T l. (CTL)
    l. depletion
    l. detected membrane antigen
      (LDMA)
    effector T l.
    peripheral blood l. (PBL)
    polyclonal B l.
    l. proliferation
    l. proliferation assay (LPA)
    l. subpopulation
    l. subset panel
    T-helper l.
    tumor-infiltrating l. (TIL)
lymphocyte-subset
lymphocytic
    l. choriomeningitis (LCM)
    l. choriomeningitis virus (LCMV)
    l. choriomeningitis virus group
    l. interstitial pneumonia
    l. meningitis
    l. meningoradiculitis
    l. pleocytosis
    l. pleocytosis
    l. proliferation assay (LPA)
lymphocytoma
    borrelial l.
lymphocytopenia
lymphocytosis
    atypical l.
    diffuse infiltrative l. syndrome
      (DILS)
    infectious l.
    peripheral blood CD8+ l.
    reactive l.
lymphocytosis-promoting factor

lymphogranuloma
l. venereum (LGV)
l. venereum conjunctivitis
l. venereum virus
lymphohistiocytic
lymphoid
l. aggregate
l. hyperplasia
l. interstitial pneumonia (LIP)
l. interstitial pneumonitis (LIP)
l. tissue
lymphokine-activated
l.-a. killer (LAK)
l.-a. killer cell
lympholytic
lymphoma
adult T-cell l. (ATL)
aggressive monoclonal l.
AIDS l.
AIDS-associated l.
AIDS-related l.
anaplastic large cell l.
B-cell l.
body cavity-based l. (BCBL)
Burkitt l.
Burkitt-like l.
central nervous system l.
cerebral l.
composite l.
cutaneous l.
cutaneous T-cell l. (CTCL)
effusion l.
extranodal l.
follicular non-Hodgkin l.
gastric l.
histiocytic l.
Hodgkin l.
immunoblastic l. (IBL)
intraocular l.
large cell l. (LCL)
large cell anaplastic l.
lymphoplasmocytoid l.
MALT l.
mantle cell l.
non-Hodgkin l. (NHL)
paranasal sinus l.
peripheral T-cell l.
plasmablastic l.
pleomorphic l.
polyclonal l.
primary brain l.

primary central nervous system l.
(PCNSL)
primary effusion l.
small noncleaved cell l. (SNC)
SNC l.
T-cell l.
lymphomatous meningitis
lymphopenia
CD4+ T l.
lymphophagocytosis
lymphophilum
Propionibacterium l.
lymphoplasmocytoid lymphoma
lymphoproliferation
lymphoproliferative
l. assay
l. disease
l. disorder
l. skin lesion
l. syndrome
l. virus group
lymphoreticular
lymphoreticular system
lyophilized
Lyphocin
L. Injection
lysin
lysine
l. decarboxylase
l. decarboxylase test
lysis
l. centrifugation
l. centrifugation method
l. centrifugation technique
Lysobacter (b)
L. antibioticus
L. brunescens
L. enzymogenes subsp. *cookii*
L. enzymogenes subsp. *enzymogenes*
L. gummosus
Lysobacteraceae
Lysobacterales
lysogen
lysogenesis
lysogenic
l. bacterium
l. induction
l. strain
lysogenization
lysogeny
lysosome
lysostaphin susceptibility test

L

NOTES

lysozyme
    l. test
Lyssavirus (v)
lytic
    l. infection
    l. lesion
    l. virus
lytica
    Cellulophaga l.
    Cytophaga l.
    Legionella l.

Lyticum (b)
    L. flagellatum
    L. sinuosum
lyticum
    Brevibacterium l.
    Sarcobium l.
Lytta vesicatoria
lyxosophila
    Candida l.

M
microfold
M cell
M concentration
M protein
M virus
M6 virus
M13 virus
M14 virus
M20 virus
MA
mycophenolic acid
Maalox H2 Acid Controller
MAAP
multiple arbitrary amplicon profiling
MAb-LA
monoclonal antibody-based latex
agglutination
MAC
Mycobacterium avium complex
MAC prophylaxis
macacae
Bacteroides m.
Bacteroides melaninogenicus subsp.
m.
Neisseria m.
Porphyromonas m.
Streptococcus m.
macaci
Entopolypoides m.
Macaua virus (MCAV)
macauensis
Amaricoccus m.
MacCallum-Goodpasture stain
MacCallum patch
Macchiavellos stain
MacConkey agar
maceachernii
Legionella m.
Tatlockia m.
macedonicus
Streptococcus m.
macedoniensis
Candida m.
macellaria
Callitroga m.
Cochliomyia m.
Musca m.
macerans
Bacillus m.
Cryptococcus m.
Paenibacillus m.
maceration
macestii
Desulfobacterium m.

macginleyi
Corynebacterium m.
machadoallisoni
Simulium m.
Machado-Guerreiro test
machardyi
Culicoides m.
machine
air filtration m.
Machlomovirus (v)
Machupo virus (MACV)
mackenziei
Ramichloridium m.
mackinnonii
Pyrenochaeta m.
macleodii
Alteromonas m.
Macluravirus (v)
macquariensis
Bacillus m.
Paenibacillus m.
macra
Actinomadura m.
Macracanthorhynchus hirudinaceus (p)
Macrobid
macrobiote
macrobroth dilution
macrocephala
Acrocarpospora m.
Macrococcus (b)
M. bovicus
M. carouselicus
M. caseolyticus
M. equipercicus
macrococcus
macroconidium
macrocyte
oval m.
macrocytic hyperchromic anemia
macrocytogenes
Azomonas m.
Azomonotrichon m.
Azotobacter m.
Macrodantin
macrogamete
macrogametocyte
macrogamont
macrogamy
macroglobulinemia
Waldenstrom m.
macrogoltabida
Sphingopyxis m.
macrogoltabidus
Sphingomonas m.
macrolide

M

macrolide-azalide
macromere
macromerozoite
macromolecule
    bacterial m.
Macromonas (b)
    M. bipunctata
    M. mobilis
macronucleus
    reniform m.
macronutrient
Macronyssidae
macroparasite
macrophage
    alveolar m.
    circulatory m.
    m. colony-stimulating factor (M-CSF)
    m. infectivity potentiator (mip)
    m. infectivity potentiator protein
    m. tropism
macrophage-tropic (M-tropic)
    m.-t. virus
Macrophoma (f)
    M. musae
    M. pinea
macropinosome
macrorchis
    Echinostoma m.
    Paragonimus m.
    Prosthogonimus m.
macrorestriction
macroscopic
    m. broth dilution test
    m. examination
    m. lesion
macrospora
    Sordaria m.
macrospore
Macrosporium tomato (f) (*See* **Alternaria**)
macrosporoideum
    Stemphylium m.
macrosporus
    Myxococcus m.
    Streptomyces m.
Macro-Vue RPR Card Test
mactans
    Latrodectus m.
macula
macular
    m. edema
    m. leprosy
    m. rash
maculatum
    Amblyomma m.
maculatus
    Spheroides m.

maculipes
    Anopheles m.
maculopapular
    m. rash
    m. skin lesion
maculopathy
    bull's-eye m.
maculosa
    Phytobdella m.
maculosum
    Mycoplasma m.
maculosus
    Plagiorchis m.
MACV
    Machupo virus
madagascariense
    Mycobacterium m.
madagascariensis
    Inermicapsifer m.
mad honey intoxication
Madrid virus (MADV)
Madura
    M. boil
    M. foot
    M. skull
madurae
    Actinomadura m.
Madurella (f)
    M. grisea
    M. mycetomatis
maduromycetoma
maduromycosis
MADV
    Madrid virus
mafenide
    m. acetate
magadiensis
    Halomonas m.
    Tindallia m.
magadii
    Natrialba m.
    Natronobacterium m.
magalhaesi
    Dirofilaria m.
Magan
Magendie
    foramen of M.
mageritense
    Mycobacterium m.
maggot
    cheese m.
    surgical m.
magna
    Fasciola m.
    Fascioloides m.
    Finegoldia m.
    Vahlkampfia m.

magnesium
    m. ammonium phosphate stone
    m. citrate
    m. salicylate
    m. sulfate
magnesium oxide
magnetic
    m. resonance imaging (MRI)
    m. stirrer
magnetic resonance (MR)
Magnetospirillum (b)
    M. gryphiswaldense
    M. magnetotacticum
magnetotacticum
    Aquaspirillum m.
    Magnetospirillum m.
magnifica
    Wohlfahrtia m.
magnivelare
    Tricholoma m.
magnoliae
    Candida m.
magnum
    Bifidobacterium m.
    Clostridium m.
    Desulfonema m.
    foramen m.
    omentum m.
magnus
    Cryptococcus m.
    Dactylogyrus m.
    Peptococcus m.
    Peptostreptococcus m.
magnusianum
    Cylindrocarpon m.
Magsal
Maguari virus (MAGV)
MAGV
    Maguari virus
mahii
    Halomethanococcus m.
    Methanohalophilus m.
Mahogany Hammock virus (MHV)
MAI
    Mycobacterium avium-intracellulare
    MAI bacteremia
    MAI complex
    MAI infection
maia
    Hemiluca m.
Main Drain virus (MDV)

Mainz
    Helicobacter sp. strain M.
mairii
    Pasteurella m.
maitotoxin
Majocchi granuloma
major
    m. agglutinin
    Babesia m.
    m. basic protein (MBP)
    Flectobacillus m.
    m. histocompatibility complex
      (MHC molecule, MHC)
    m. histocompatibility complex class
      I (MIIC-I)
    m. histocompatibility complex class
      II (MHC-II)
    Leishmania m.
    Monascus m.
    Simulium m.
majoricensis
    Procandida m.
majus
    Microdochium nivale var. *m.*
    Thiovulum m.
mal
    m. de Cayenne
    m. del pinto
    m. de Rio Cuarto virus
    m. de San Lazaro
    m. morado
    m. perforans
Malabar
    M. itch
    M. leprosy
malabarica
    phlegmasia m.
malabsorption
    m. syndrome
malabsorptive
    m. diarrhea
malachitica
    Actinomadura m.
malachitofuscus
    Streptomyces m.
malachitospinus
    Streptomyces m.
malacia
malady
malaise
Malakal virus (MALV)

M

NOTES

malar
  m. rash
malaria
  acute m.
  airport m.
  algid m.
  autochthonous m.
  benign tertian m.
  bilious remittent m.
  cerebral m.
  chronic m.
  m. comatosa
  double tertian m.
  dysenteric m.
  falciparum m.
  induced m.
  intermittent m.
  malariae m.
  malignant tertian m.
  monkey m.
  nonan m.
  pernicious m.
  m. prevention
  m. prophylaxis
  quartan m.
  quotidian m.
  relapsing m.
  remittent m.
  simian m.
  m. smear
  tertian m.
  therapeutic m.
  vivax m.
malariae
  m. malaria
  Plasmodium m.
malarial
  m. anemia
  m. cachexia
  m. crescent
  m. fever
  m. hemoglobinuria
  m. knob
  m. parasite
  m. paroxysm
  m. periodicity
  m. pigment
malariology
malariotherapy
malarious
Malarone
malassezi
Malassezia (f)
  M. folliculitis
  M. furfur
  M. pachydermatis
malathion
Malayan filariasis

malayensis
  Schistosoma m.
malayi
  Brugia m.
Malaysian typhoid
malaysiensis
  Streptomyces m.
Malbranchea (f)
  M. pulchella
  M. sclerotica
maleate
  azatadine m.
Malecot-type catheter
malefermentans
  Lactobacillus m.
malenominatum
  Clostridium m.
malformation
  congenital m.
  cortical gyral m.
mali
  Lactobacillus m.
  Sphingomonas m.
malicum
  Acetobacterium m.
malignancy
  cutaneous T-cell m.
  hematologic m.
  leptomeningeal m.
malignant
  m. ascites
  m. catarrhal fever
  m. catarrhal fever disease
  m. catarrh of cattle
  m. external otitis
  m. histiocytosis
  m. lymphocytic proliferation disease (MLPD)
  m. otitis externa
  m. tertian fever
  m. tertian malaria
  m. tertian malarial parasite
mallei
  Burkholderia m.
  Pseudomonas m.
Mallophaga
mallotivora
  Erwinia m.
malmoense
  Mycobacterium m.
malnourished
malnutrition
  protein-energy m.
malodoratus
  Enterococcus m.
malodorous discharge
malonate utilization test

malonatica
  Levinea m.
malonica
  Sporomusa m.
Malonomonas rubra (b)
Malpais Spring virus
malpighian tubule
MALT
  mucosa-associated lymphoid tissue
  mucosa-associated lymph tissue
  MALT lymphoma
Malta fever
maltaromicus
  Lactobacillus m.
maltese cross
MALToma
  mucosa-associated lymphoid tumor
maltophilia
  Pseudomonas m.
  Stenotrophomonas m.
  Xanthomonas m.
maltophilum
  Treponema m.
maltosa
  Candida m.
maltose fermentation test
malt worker's lung
malum venereum
MALV
  Malakal virus
Malvern analyzer
malyschevi
  Simulium m.
mamanpian
mammalian
  m. adenovirus
  m. binding lectin deficiency
  m. cell culture
  m. orthoreovirus (MRV)
  m. rotavirus
  m. type B oncovirus group
  m. type C retrovirus group
  m. type D retrovirus group
mammalitis
  bovine m.
mammillitis
  bovine herpes m.
  bovine ulcerative m.
  bovine vaccinia m.
mammography

Mammomonogamus (p)
  M. laryngeus
  M. nasicola
mammoplasty
Manawatu virus
Manawa virus (MWAV)
Manchurian fever
Mandelamine
mandelate
  methenamine m.
mandelii
  Pseudomonas m.
mandibular tuberculosis
Mandol
mandrillaris
  Balamuthia m.
manganicum
  Pedomicrobium m.
mange
  demodectic m.
  follicular m.
  sarcoptic m.
mangenotii
  Clostridium m.
mangiferae
  Dothiorella m.
  Nattrassia m.
mangrove fly
mania
manicata
  Fannia m.
manicatum
  Simulium m.
manicatus
  Dactylogyrus m.
manifestation
  atypical m.
  cutaneous m.
  musculoskeletal m.
  thoracic m.
manihotivorans
  Lactobacillus m.
Mannheimia (b)
  M. glucosida
  M. granulomatis
  M. haemolytica
  M. ruminalis
  M. varigena
mannitol
  m. fermentation
  m. fermentation test

M

NOTES

mannitolilytica
    Ralstonia m.
mannose fermentation test
manometer
Manson
    M. disease
    M. eye worm
    M. schistosomiasis
Mansonella (p)
    M. ozzardi
    M. perstans
    M. streptocerca
mansonelliasis
mansoni
    Exophiala m.
    Schistosoma m.
    Spirometra m.
Mansonia
    M. dyari
    M. perturbans
mansonii
    Zygosporium m.
Mansonioides
mansonoides
    Diphyllobothrium m.
    Spirometra m.
Mantel-Haenszel test
mantle cell lymphoma
Mantoux
    M. skin testing
    M. technique
manus
    tinea m.
manuum
    tinea m.
Mapap
maple bark disease
Mapputta virus (MAPV)
Maprik virus (MPKV)
Mapuera virus (MPRV)
MAPV
    Mapputta virus
maquilingensis
    Caldivirga m.
Maraba virus
Marafivirus (v)
Maranox
marasma
marasmic
Marburg
    M. fever
    M. virus (MARV, MBGV)
    M. virus disease
    M. virus group
marburgensis
    Methanothermobacter m.
Marburg-like viruses

marcescens
    Serratia m.
marcianae
    Alaria m.
Marcillin
Marco virus (MCOV)
Marcus-Gunn pupil
marcusii
    Paracoccus m.
Marek's disease-like viruses
margaretiae
    Eubacterium yurii subsp. *m.*
Margarinomyces (f)
Margarinos-Torres lesion
Margaropus winthemi (p)
marginal
    m. blepharitis
    m. excision
    m. gingiva
    m. resection
marginale
    Anaplasma m.
marginalis
    Pseudomonas m.
marginated chromatin
marginatum
    Clinostomum m.
    eczema m.
    erythema m.
    Hyalomma m.
marginatus
    Dermacentor m.
margrebowiei
    Schistosoma m.
mariae
    Aedes m.
marianensis
    Thermaerobacter m.
Maricaulis maris (b)
Marichromatium (b)
    M. gracile
    M. purpuratum
marijuana
marimammalium
    Actinomyces m.
marina
    Cytophaga m.
    Deleya m.
    Ectothiorhodospira m.
    Halomonas m.
    Methylarcula m.
    Methylophaga m.
    Microscilla m.
    Moritella m.
    Nitrospira m.
    Pirella m.
    Pirellula m.

Pseudomonas m.
Rhodopseudomonas m.
Marin County agent
Marinilabilia (b)
    M. agarovorans
    M. salmonicolor
Marinitoga camini (b)
Marinobacter (b)
    M. aquaeolei
    M. hydrocarbonoclasticus
Marinobacterium georgiense (b)
Marinococcus (b)
    M. albus
    M. halophilus
    M. hispanicus
marinoflava
    Cytophaga m.
Marinol
Marinomonas (b)
    M. communis
    M. mediterranea
    M. vaga
marinonascens
    Rhodococcus m.
marinorubra
    Serratia m.
Marinospirillum (b)
    M. megaterium
    M. minutulum
marinotypicum
    Flavobacterium m.
marinum
    Cyclobacterium m.
    Mycobacterium m.
    Rhabdochromatium m.
    Rhodobium m.
marinus
    Bacillus m.
    Bacillus globisporus subsp. *m.*
    Cryptococcus m.
    Dethiosulfovibrio m.
    Flectobacillus m.
    Hydrogenovibrio m.
    Mesophilobacter m.
    Methylobacter m.
    Prochlorococcus marinus subsp. *m.*
    Rhodothermus m.
    Staphylothermus m.
    Vibrio m.
maripaludis
    Methanococcus m.

maris
    Candida m.
    Caulobacter m.
    Colwellia m.
    Dietzia m.
    Maricaulis m.
    Oceanospirillum maris subsp. *m.*
    Planctomyces m.
    Propionigenium m.
    Rhodococcus m.
marismortui
    Bacillus m.
    Chromohalobacter m.
    Ectothiorhodospira m.
    Haloarcula m.
    Orenia m.
    Salibacillus m.
    Sporohalobacter m.
marisnigri
    Methanoculleus m.
    Methanogenium m.
maritima
    Candida m.
    Hippea m.
    Thermotoga m.
maritimus
    Culicoides m.
    Flexibacter m.
Marituba virus (MTBV)
maritypicum
    Microbacterium m.
marium
    Culicoides m.
marker
    genetic m.
    m. lesion
    surrogate m.
Marmoricola aurantiacus (b)
marmosetpox virus
marmot
marneffei
    penicilliosis m.
    Penicillium m.
maroniense
    Simulium m.
marquandii
    Paecilomyces m.
Marrakai virus (MARV)
marrow
    m. aplasia
    bone m. (BM)
    m. suppression

M

NOTES

Marseilles fever
Marshallagia marshalli (p)
marshalli
    Marshallagia m.
marsh fever
Marthritic
MARV
    Marburg virus
    Marrakai virus
marxi
    Ixodes m.
marxianus
    Kluyveromyces m.
    Saccharomyces m.
MAS
    mycobacteria antibiotic supplement
mashuense
    Streptoverticillium m.
mashuensis
    Streptomyces m.
mask
    Acnomel Acne M.
    Neutrogena Acne M.
    submicron m.
Mason-Pfizer monkey virus
masoucida
    Aeromonas salmonicida subsp. *m.*
mass
    adnexal m.
    body cell m. (BCM)
    fat-free m. (FFM)
    m. infection
    lean body m. (LBM)
    lean body muscle m.
    m. spectrometric analysis
    m. spectrometry
Massarinaceae
massasporeus
    Streptomyces m.
massiliae
    Rickettsia m.
Massilia timonae (b)
massiliensis
    Pelobacter m.
massive granulomatous orchitis
Masson
    M. body
    M. stain
Masson-Fontana silver stain
Mastadenovirus (v)
Mastigomycotina
Mastigophora
mastigote
mastitidis
    Corynebacterium m.
mastitis
    bovine m.

mastoiditis
    acute m.
Mastrevirus (v)
MAT
    microscopic agglutination test
matalense
    Trichosporon m.
matensis
    Streptomyces m.
material
    amorphous m.
    proteinaceous m.
maternal
    m. antibody
    m. chorioamnionitis
    m. immunity
    m. viremia
maternal-fetal HIV
mathranii
    Thermoanaerobacter m.
matritensis
    Citeromyces m.
matrixin
matrix metalloproteinase (MMP)
matruchoti
matruchotii
    Bacterionema m.
    Corynebacterium m.
Matruh virus (MTRV)
matsumotoense
    Catellatospora m.
    Micromonospora m.
matsuzakiense
    Dactylosporangium m.
matteabranchia
    Simulium m.
mattheei
    Schistosoma m.
mattogrossensis
    Anopheles m.
Matucare virus (MATV)
MATV
    Matucare virus
Maurer
    M. cleft
    M. dot
mauvecolor
    Streptomyces m.
Maxamine
Maxaquin
Maxenal
Maxifed
    M. DM
Maxifed-G
Maxiflor
maxillary sinusitis
maxima
    Sarcina m.

maximum
m. bactericidal dilution (MBD)
M. Strength Anbesol
M. Strength Desenex Antifungal
Cream
M. Strength Orajel
maximus
Dipetalogaster m.
Maxipime
Maxitrol
Maxivate Topical
Mayaro
M. virus (MAYV)
M. virus disease
maydis
Drechslera m.
Ustilago m.
Mayer
M. hematoxylin
M. mucicarmine stain
maynei
Euroglyphus m.
mayombei
Clostridium m.
MAYV
Mayaro virus
mazamorra
mazei
Methanococcus m.
Methanosarcina m.
Mazon Medicated Soap
Mazzotti
M. reaction
M. test
mazzottii
Borrelia m.
mbarigui
Simulium m.
MBC
bactericidal concentration
minimum bactericidal concentration
MBD
maximum bactericidal dilution
MBGV
Marburg virus
Mboke virus
MBP
major basic protein
MBZ
mebendazole
MCAV
Macaua virus

mcbrellneri
Brevibacterium m.
McCoy cell
mcginnisii
Exserohilum m.
McKee-Farrar
M.-F. prosthesis
M.-F. technique
mcmeekinii
Planococcus m.
Planomicrobium m.
MCOV
Marco virus
MCP
monocyte chemoattractant protein
m-cresyl acetate
M-CSF
macrophage colony-stimulating factor
MCT
medium-chain triglyceride
MD
microtube dilution
MD method
MD test
MDCV
Mojui Dos Campos virus
MDDC
monocyte-derived dendritic cell
MDM
minor-determinant mixture
MDOV
Monte Dourado virus
MDR
multidrug resistance
multidrug-resistant
multiple drug-resistant
MDR tuberculosis
MDRTB
multiple-drug resistant tuberculosis
MDS
myelodysplastic syndrome
MDV
Main Drain virus
MDXH210
Meaban virus (MEAV)
meal worm
measles
m. antibody
German m.
m. giant cell pneumonia
m. inclusion body encephalitis
m., mumps, rubella (MMR)

M

NOTES

measles *(continued)*
>   m., mumps, rubella vaccine
>   m. and rubella vaccine
>   m. and rubella vaccines, combined
>   tropical m.
>   m. virus
>   m. virus vaccine, live

measles-rinderpest-distemper virus group
measly
Measurin
meatal care
MEAV
>   Meaban virus

mebendazole (MBZ)
MEBV
>   Mount Elgon bat virus

mecA **gene**
mechanical
>   m. bladder outlet resistance
>   m. obstruction
>   m. vector

mechanism
>   defense m.
>   host defense m.

mechernichensis
>   *Thauera m.*

Mecistocirrus digitatus (p)
Meclan
>   M. Topical

meclocycline
>   m. sulfosalicylate

meconium
Mectizan
Meda-Cap
Medallion suture lens
Meda Tab
media *(pl. of* medium)
media
>   acute otitis m. (AOM)
>   *Aeromonas m.*
>   chronic otitis m.
>   otitis m.
>   tuberculous otitis m.

medial dysplasia
mediasiatica
>   *Francisella tularensis* subsp. *m.*

mediastinal
>   m. abscess
>   m. adenopathy
>   m. fibrosis
>   m. granuloma
>   m. histoplasmosis
>   m. lymphadenopathy
>   m. node

mediastinitis
>   fibrosing m.
>   hemorrhagic m.
>   suppurative m.

mediastinoscopy
>   cervical m.
>   left anterior m.

medicae
>   *Sinorhizobium m.*

medical
>   m. intensive care unit (MICU)
>   m. mycology
>   m. oncologist
>   m. subspecialist

medicalization
medicinalis
>   *Hirudo m.*

medicine
>   nuclear m. (NMR)
>   Reese's Pinworm M.
>   traditional Chinese m. (TCM)
>   tropical m.

Medihaler-Epi
Medihaler-Iso
Medina worm
medinensis
>   *Dracunculus m.*
>   *Fuellebornius m.*
>   *Gordius m.*
>   *Vena m.*

mediocidica
>   *Kitasatospora m.*

mediocidicum
mediocidicus
>   *Streptomyces m.*

mediolani
>   *Streptomyces m.*

mediolanus
>   *Agromyces m.*

mediopunctatus
>   *Anopheles m.*

mediosalina
>   *Roseospira m.*

mediovittata
>   *Aedes m.*

mediovittatum
>   *Simulium m.*

Mediplast Plaster
Mediport
Medipren
Medi-Quick Topical Ointment
mediterranea
>   *Marinomonas m.*

Mediterranean
>   M. erythematous fever
>   M. exanthematous fever
>   M. spotted fever

mediterranei
>   *Amycolatopsis m.*
>   *Halobacterium m.*
>   *Haloferax m.*

Nocardia m.
Vibrio m.
mediterraneum
  Mesorhizobium m.
  Rhizobium m.
mediterraneus
  Sulfitobacter m.
Medi-Tuss
medium, pl. **media**
  Acanthamoeba m.
  axenic m.
  Bacto-agar m.
  Bacto *Entamoeba* m.
  Balamuth aqueous egg yolk
    infusion m.
  Barbour-Stoenner-Kelly m.
  BG m.
  Boeck and Drbohlav Locke-egg-
    serum m.
  Bushley m.
  Chang m.
  Cleveland and Collier liver
    extract m.
  complete m.
  culture m.
  Czapek-Dox m.
  Diamond TYM m.
  Dorset culture egg m.
  Ellinghausen-McCollough-Johnson-
    Harris m.
  Endo m.
  Feinberg-Whittington m.
  Fildes m.
  Fletcher m.
  fluorescence-lactose-denitrification m.
    (FLN)
  Franz m.
  GLSH culture m.
  glucose, lactalbumin, serum, and
    hemoglobin culture m.
  Haemophilus test m. (HTM)
  Hirsch charcoal agar modified m.
  Johnson-Trussel m.
  Lash casein hydrolysate-serum m.
  Loeffler blood culture m.
  Lowenstein-Jensen culture m.
  Middlebrook 7H10 m.
  Middlebrook 7H11 m.
  modified whole-egg slant m.
  motility test m.
  Mueller-Hinton m.
  NNN m.

noninhibitory media
Novy-MacNeal-Nicolle m.
PLM-5 m.
Regan-Lowe m.
Roiron m.
Schneider *Drosophila* m.
selective m.
serum-casein-glucose-yeast
  extract m. (SCGYEM)
Simmons citrate m.
Stuart m.
Thayer-Martin m.
transport m.
Treponema m.
TY1-S-33 m.
TYSGM-9 m.
medium-chain triglyceride (MCT)
Medlar body
Medralone Injection
Medrol
  M. Oral
  M. Veriderm
medroxyprogesterone
  m. acetate (MPA)
medulla
  m. oblongata
MEE
  multilocus enzyme electrophoresis
meeki
  Eucocytis m.
mefloquine
  m. prophylaxis
Mefoxin
MEG
  metabolic, endocrine, and gastrointestinal
  MEG disorders
Megace
Megachytriaceae
Megacillin
  M. Susp
megacolon
  chagasic m.
  toxic m.
megaesophagus
megagamete
megakaryocyte
megakaryocytic
megaloblastic
  m. anemia
megalospore
Megalothrix (b)

M

NOTES

megalurus
    Philophthalmus m.
megamerozoite
Megamonas hypermegale (b)
meganucleus
Megaselia spiracularis
Megasphaera (b)
    M. cerevisiae
    M. elsdenii
megaspinosa
    Haemaphysalis m.
megaspore
megasporus
    Streptomyces m.
Megastoma (p) (*See* **Giardia lamblia**)
megastoma
    Habronema m.
megasyndrome
    chagasic m.
megaterium
    Bacillus m.
    Marinospirillum m.
Megatrichophyton (f)
    M. megnini
megestrol acetate
megistus
    Panstrongylus m.
meglumine antimonate
megnini
    Megatrichophyton m.
    Otobius m.
megninii
    Trichophyton m.
mehrai
    Artyfechinostomum m.
MEIA
    microparticle enzyme immunoassay
    microparticulate enzyme immunoassay
meibomian gland
meibomitis
Meig syndrome
Meiothermus (b)
    M. cerbereus
    M. chliarophilus
    M. ruber
    M. silvanus
Meissner plexus
mekongi
    Schistosoma m.
mel 1–3
    Meleagris adenovirus 1–3
Melacine
melaleucae
    Entomoplasma m.
    Mycoplasma m.
Melanconiaceae
Melanconiales

Melanconidaceae
melanesiensis
    Thermosipho m.
melanimon
    Aedes m.
melanin
melaninogenica
    Prevotella m.
melaninogenicus
    Bacteroides m.
    Bacteroides melaninogenicus subsp.
    m.
melanoderma
    parasitic m.
melanogaster
    Drosophila m.
Melanogastraceae
Melanogastrales
melanogenes
    Gluconobacter oxydans subsp. *m.*
    Streptomyces m.
melanoglossia
melanoma
    autologous m.
    cutaneous m.
    mucosal m.
Melanommataceae
Melanoplus sanguinipes
Melanosporaceae
melanosporofaciens
    Streptomyces m.
melanura
    Culiseta m.
Melao virus (MELV)
melarsoprol
melas
    Anopheles m.
mel B
meleagridis
    Cryptosporidium m.
    Eimeria m.
    Histomonas m.
    Mycoplasma m.
meleagris
    Agaricus m.
Meleagris adenovirus 1–3 (mel 1–3)
melena
Meleney synergistic gangrene
Meleny ulcer
melezitose fermentation test
meliae
    Pseudomonas m.
melibiose fermentation test
melibiosica
    Candida m.
melibiosus
    Lactobacillus curvatus subsp. *m.*

meliloti
  Rhizobium m.
  Sinorhizobium m.
melioidosis
  acute septicemic m.
Meliolaceae
melis
  Echinostoma m.
  Euparyphium m.
Melissococcus plutonius (b)
melitensis
  Brucella m.
Melittangium (b)
  M. alboraceum
  M. boletus
  M. lichenicola
melleus
  Culicoides m.
melliferum
  Spiroplasma m.
mellitus
  diabetes m.
  noninsulin-dependent diabetes m.
  (NIDDM)
Melogrammataceae
Meloidogyne (p)
  M. arenaria
  M. chitwoodi
  M. gramnicola
  M. hapla
  M. incognita
  M. javanica
  M. konaensis
melonis
  Xanthomonas m.
melophagi
  Wolbachia m.
Melophagus ovinus (p)
melphalan
melrosporus
  Streptomyces fervens subsp. m.
  Streptoverticillium fervens subsp. m.
MELV
  Melao virus
membranaefaciens
  Pichia m.
membrane
  amniotic m.
  artificial rupture of m.'s
  buccal m.
  bulging tympanic m.
  hyaline m.

mucous m.
premature rupture of m.'s (PROM)
rupture of m.'s (ROM)
spontaneous rupture of m.'s
tympanic m.
undulating m.
membranelle
membranifaciens
  Candida m.
membranoproliferative
  m. glomerulonephritis
membranous
  m. conjunctivitis
  m. glomerulonephritis
Memnionella (f)
memory
  B-cell m.
  m. B, T cell
  immune m.
  T-cell m.
men
  Anti-Acne Formula for M.
  men who have sex with m.
  (MSM)
Mcnadol
mendocina
  Pseudomonas m.
Mengo encephalitis
Mengovirus
Ménière disease
meningeal
  m. inflammation
  m. involvement
  m. irritation
  m. plague
  m. prophylaxis
  m. relapse
meningeal
meninges (*pl. of* meninx)
meningismus
meningitic
meningitidis
  Neisseria m.
meningitis
  aseptic m.
  bacterial pyogenic m.
  Candida m.
  cerebrospinal m.
  chemical m.
  cryptococcal m.
  eosinophilic m.
  epidemic cerebrospinal m.

M

NOTES

meningitis *(continued)*
    fungal m.
    gonococcal m.
    Haemophilus influenzae type b m.
    helminthic m.
    human pneumococcal m.
    Listeria m.
    listerial m.
    lymphocytic m.
    meningococcal m.
    Mollaret m.
    mumps m.
    nontuberculous m.
    pneumococcal m.
    postsurgical m.
    posttraumatic m.
    primary amebic m.
    protozoal m.
    pyogenic m.
    septic m.
    spirochetal m.
    tuberculous m.
    viral aseptic m.
meningococcal
    m. bacteremia
    m. conjunctivitis
    m. disease
    m. embolus
    m. meningitis
    m. vaccine
meningococcemia
    acute m.
meningococcus
meningoencephalitis
    acute primary hemorrhagic m.
    amebic m.
    chagasic m.
    eosinophilic m.
    herpetic m.
    primary amebic m. (PAM)
    primary amoebic m. (PAM)
    Toxoplasma gondii m.
    Trypanosoma cruzi m.
    zoster m.
meningomyelitis
Meningonema peruzzii (p)
meningoradiculitis
    lymphocytic m.
meningosepticum
    Chryseobacterium m.
    Flavobacterium m.
meningovascular
    m. involvement
    m. neurosyphilis
    m. syphilis
meninx, pl. **meninges**
meniscus, pl. **menisci**
Meniscus glaucopis (b)

Menomune-A/C/Y/W-135
Menopon
menorrhagia
menstrual toxic shock syndrome
    (MTSS)
mentagrophytes
    Trichophyton m.
mentation
    altered m.
Mentax
Mentezol
mepacrine stain
mepenzolate
meperidine
    m. HCl
mephitica
    Pseudomonas m.
mephitis
    Luteimonas m.
Mepron
    M. suspension
2-mercaptoethane sulfonate
2-mercaptoethanol
mercurator
    Aedes m.
mercuric
    m. chloride
    m. oxide
merdae
    Bacteroides m.
meridiana
    Halomonas m.
Meridian Merifluor kit
meridianum
    Eupenicillium m.
meridiei
    Desulfosporosinus m.
meridionale
    Simulium m.
Merifluor direct immunofluorescence
    detection system
merispore
meristematic
Meritec GC test
Mermet virus (MERV)
Mermis nigrescens (p)
Mermithidae
Mermithidea
merogenesis
merogenetic
merogony
meromyarian
Meronem
meront
meropenem
merosporangium
merotomy
merozoite

Merrem
    M. I.V.
merthiolate-formalin
merthiolate-iodine-formalin
meruoca
    Simulium m.
merus
    Anopheles m.
Meruvax II
MERV
    Mermet virus
merycicum
    Bifidobacterium m.
mesangial
mesangioproliferative
mesenteric
    m. adenitis
    m. adenopathy
    m. ischemia
    m. lymphadenitis
mesenterica
    Candida m.
mesenteroides
    Leuconostoc mesenteroides subsp. m.
mesenteron
mcsentery
mesna
Mesnex
Mesnieraceae
mesnili
    Chilomastix m.
Mesocestoides corti (p)
Mcsocestoididae
mesocricetorum
    Helicobacter m.
mesophaeum
    Hebeloma m.
Mesophelliaceae
mesophila
    Microbispora m.
    Thermomonospora m.
mesophilic
mesophilica
    Pseudomonas m.
mesophilicum
    Methylobacterium m.
Mesophilobacter marinus (b)
Mesoplasma (b)
    M. chauliocola
    M. coleopterae
    M. corruscae
    M. entomophilum

    M. florum
    M. grammopterae
    M. lactucae
    M. photuris
    M. pleciae
    M. seiffertii
    M. syrphidae
    M. tabanidae
Mesorhizobium (b)
    M. amorphae
    M. chacoense
    M. ciceri
    M. huakuii
    M. loti
    M. mediterraneum
    M. plurifarium
    M. tianshanense
Mesostigmata
mesothelial cell
mesothelioma
mesouviformis
    Thermomonospora m.
Mesozoa
messenger RNA (mRNA)
Mestatin
mestris
    Saccharomycodes m.
mesylatc
    delavirdine m. (DLV)
    nelfinavir m.
meta-analysis
metabiosis
metabolic
    m., endocrine, and gastrointestinal
      (MEG)
    m., endocrine, and gastrointestinal
      disorders
    m. products test
metabolism
    folate m.
Metacapnodiaceae
metacercaria
metacercarial antigen
metacestode
metachromatic
    m. body
    m. granule
metacryptozoite
metacyst
metadysentery
Metagonimus yokogawai (p)
metagrophytes

M

NOTES

metallic taste
metallicum
>   *Simulium m.*

metallicus
>   *Sulfolobus m.*

metallireducens
>   *Geobacter m.*

metalloproteinase
>   matrix m. (MMP)

Metallosphaera (b)
>   *M. prunae*
>   *M. sedula*

metamere
metameric
metamerism
metamorphose
metamorphosis
>   complete m.
>   holometabolous m.
>   incomplete m.

metamorphum
>   *Aquaspirillum m.*

Metamucil
metamyelocyte
metaphyseal
metaplasia
>   gastric m.
>   incomplete intestinal m.
>   intestinal m.
>   mucinous columnar m.
>   squamous m.

metapneumonic emphysema
Metapneumovirus (v)
Metarhizium (f)
>   *M. anisopliae*
>   *M. glutinosum*

Metasep
metastasis, pl. **metastases**
>   multiple synchronous
>   subcutaneous m.
>   skip m.
>   visceral m.

metastatic
>   m. infection

Metastigmata
metastrongyle
Metastrongylidae
Metastrongyloidea
Metastrongylus apri (p)
metatroph
metatrophic
Metavirus (v)
metazoa
>   trophoblastic m.

metazoonosis
Meted
meteori
>   *Agrobacterium m.*

meteorica
>   *Hydrotaea m.*

meteorism
meter
>   urine m.

metformin
>   m. hydrochloride

methadone
methanica
>   *Methanosarcina m.*
>   *Methylomonas m.*

Methanobacteriaceae
Methanobacteriales
Methanobacterium (b)
>   *M. alcaliphilum*
>   *M. arbophilicum*
>   *M. bryantii*
>   *M. congolense*
>   *M. defluvii*
>   *M. espanolae*
>   *M. formicicum*
>   *M. ivanovii*
>   *M. mobile*
>   *M. oryzae*
>   *M. palustre*
>   *M. ruminantium*
>   *M. subterraneum*
>   *M. thermoaggregans*
>   *M. thermoalcaliphilum*
>   *M. thermoautotrophicum*
>   *M. thermoflexum*
>   *M. thermoformicicum*
>   *M. thermophilum*
>   *M. uliginosum*
>   *M. wolfei*

Methanobrevibacter (b)
>   *M. arboriphilicus*
>   *M. curvatus*
>   *M. cuticularis*
>   *M. filiformis*
>   *M. oralis*
>   *M. ruminantium*
>   *M. smithii*

Methanocalculus (b)
>   *M. halotolerans*
>   *M. pumilus*

Methanococcaceae
Methanococcales
Methanococcoides (b)
>   *M. burtonii*
>   *M. methylutens*

Methanococcus (b)
>   *M. deltae*
>   *M. fervens*
>   *M. frisius*
>   *M. halophilus*
>   *M. igneus*
>   *M. infernus*

M. *jannaschii*
M. *maripaludis*
M. *mazei*
M. *thermolithotrophicus*
M. *vannielii*
M. *voltae*
M. *vulcanius*
Methanocorpusculaceae
Methanocorpusculum (b)
M. *aggregans*
M. *bavaricum*
M. *labreanum*
M. *parvum*
M. *sinense*
Methanoculleus (b)
M. *bourgensis*
M. *marisnigri*
M. *oldenburgensis*
M. *olentangyi*
M. *palmolei*
M. *thermophilus*
Methanofollis (b)
M. *liminatans*
M. *tationis*
methanogen
Methanogenium (b)
M. *aggregans*
M. *bourgense*
M. *cariaci*
M. *frigidum*
M. *frittonii*
M. *liminatans*
M. *marisnigri*
M. *olentangyi*
M. *organophilum*
M. *tationis*
M. *thermophilicum*
Methanohalobium evestigatum (b)
Methanohalophilus (b)
M. *halophilus*
M. *mahii*
M. *oregonense*
M. *portucalensis*
M. *zhilinae*
methanol
Methanolacinia paynteri (b)
methanolica
Acidomonas m.
Amycolatopsis m.
Pichia m.

methanolicus
Acetobacter m.
Bacillus m.
Methanolobus (b)
M. *bombayensis*
M. *siciliae*
M. *taylorii*
M. *tindarius*
M. *vulcani*
Methanomicrobiaceae
Methanomicrobiales
Methanomicrobium (b)
M. *mobile*
M. *paynteri*
Methanomicrococcus blatticola (b)
Methanoplanaceae
Methanoplanus (b)
M. *endosymbiosus*
M. *limicola*
M. *petrolearius*
Methanopyrus kandleri (b)
Methanosaeta (b)
M. *concilii*
M. *thermoacetophila*
Methanosarcina (b)
M. *acetivorans*
M. *barkeri*
M. *frisia*
M. *mazei*
M. *methanica*
M. *semesiae*
M. *siciliae*
M. *thermophila*
M. *vacuolata*
Methanosarcinaceae
methanosorbosa
Candida m.
Methanosphaera (b)
M. *cuniculi*
M. *stadtmanae*
Methanospirillum hungatei (b)
Methanothermaceae
Methanothermobacter (b)
M. *marburgensis*
M. *thermoautotrophicus*
M. *wolfei*
Methanothermus (b)
M. *fervidus*
M. *sociabilis*
Methanothrix (b)
M. *concilii*
M. *soehngenii*

M

NOTES

Methanothrix (continued)
    M. thermoacetophila
    M. thermophila
methantheline
methenamine
    m. hexamethylenetetramine
    m. hippurate
    m. mandelate
    m., phenyl salicylate, atropine, hyoscyamine, benzoic acid, and methylene blue
    m. silver stain (GMS)
methicillin
    factor essential for resistance to m. (*fem* factor)
    m. sodium
methicillin-resistant *Staphylococcus aureus* (**MRSA**)
methicillin-susceptible *Staphylococcus aureus* (**MSSA**)
methionine
methionotrophica
    Catellatospora citrea subsp. *m.*
methisoprinol
methocarbamol
method
    activated sludge m.
    auxanographic m.
    CMV early antigen FA m.
    CMV shell vial m.
    diffusion m.
    flotation m.
    genotypic typing m.
    HSV shell vial m.
    Hung m.
    intradermal m.
    Lancefield capillary precipitin m.
    Liborius m.
    lysis centrifugation m.
    MD m.
    microtube dilution m.
    multipuncture m.
    Porges m.
    prostatic localization m.
    Qbeta replicase m.
    rapid identification m. (RIM)
    serum bactericidal dilution m.
    sodium hydroxide digestion m.
    spiral gradient endpoint m.
    wick m.
    Wilson m.
method-*Neisseria*
    rapid identification m. (RIM-*Neisseria*)
methodology
methotrexate
methoxsalen

methoxybenzovorans
    Clostridium m.
methscopolamine
methyl
    m. alcohol
    m. red test
Methylarcula (b)
    M. marina
    M. terricola
methylbenzethonium chloride
methylcellulose
    gelatin, pectin, and m.
methylene
    m. blue
    m. blue stain
methylmalonic
Methylobacillus (b)
    M. flagellatus
    M. glycogenes
Methylobacter (b)
    M. agilis
    M. albus
    M. luteus
    M. marinus
    M. pelagicus
    M. psychrophilus
    M. whittenburyi
Methylobacterium (b)
    M. aminovorans
    M. chloromethanicum
    M. dichloromethanicum
    M. extorquens
    M. fujisawaense
    M. mesophilicum
    M. organophilum
    M. radiotolerans
    M. rhodesianum
    M. rhodinum
    M. thiocyanatum
    M. zatmanii
Methylocaldum (b)
    M. gracile
    M. lepidum
    M. szegediense
Methylocella palustris (b)
Methylococcaceae
Methylococcus (b)
    M. bovis
    M. capsulatus
    M. chroococcus
    M. luteus
    M. mobilis
    M. thermophilus
    M. vinelandii
    M. whittenburyi
Methylocystis (b)
    M. echinoides
    M. parvus

Methylomicrobium (b)
   M. *agile*
   M. *album*
   M. *pelagicum*
Methylomonas (b)
   M. *aurantiaca*
   M. *fodinarum*
   M. *methanica*
   M. *pelagica*
   M. *scandinavica*
Methylophaga (b)
   M. *marina*
   M. *sulfidovorans*
   M. *thalassica*
Methylophilus (b)
   M. *leisingeri*
   M. *methylotrophus*
Methylopila (b)
   M. *capsulata*
   M. *helvetica*
Methylorhabdus multivorans (b)
Methylosarcina (b)
   M. *fibrata*
   M. *quisquiliarum*
Methylosinus (b)
   M. *sporium*
   M. *trichosporium*
Methylosphaera hansonii (b)
methylotrophus
   Methylophilus m.
methylovorans
   Albibacter m.
methylovorum
   Hyphomicrobium m.
Methylovorus glucosotrophus (b)
methylpentosum
   Clostridium m.
methylphenidate
2-methyl-phosphonoformate
methylprednisolone
methylrosaniline chloride
methyltestosterone
4-methylumbelliferyl-beta-D-glucuronidase
  (MUG)
   -m.-D.-g. test
methylutens
   Methanococcoides m.
   Paracoccus m.
methysergide
Meticorten
Metimyd Ophthalmic
Metorchis conjunctus (p)

metorrhagia
metoxenous
metoxeny
Metras catheter
metrifonate
Metro
   M. IV
   M. I.V. Injection
Metrocream
MetroGel Topical
MetroGel-Vaginal
metromenorrhagia
metronidazole
metschnikovii
   Vibrio m.
Metschnikowia (f)
   M. *pulcherrima*
   M. *reukaufii*
   M. *zobellii*
Metschnikowiaceae
metyrosine
Meuse fever
mexicana
   Leishmania m.
   Psilocybe m.
Mexican spotted fever
mexicanum
   Simulium m.
mexicanus
   Desulfovibrio m.
   Paragonimus m.
Mexico virus
mexiletine
meyeri
   Actinomyces m.
   Leptospira m.
Mezlin
mezlocillin
MGIT
   mycobacteria growth indicator tube
MHA-TP
   microhemagglutination assay for
    Treponema pallidum
    MHA-TP test
MHC
   major histocompatibility complex
    MHC molecule
MHC-I
   major histocompatibility complex class I
MHC-II
   major histocompatibility complex class II

M

NOTES

MHV
Mahogany Hammock virus
MI
myocardial infarction
mibuna temperate virus
MIC
minimal inhibitory concentration
minimum inhibitory concentration
micaceus
Coprinus *m.*
Micatin Topical
Micavibrio admirandus (b)
micdadei
Legionella *m.*
Tatlockia *m.*
mice (*pl. of* mouse)
michiganense
Corynebacterium *m.*
michiganensis
Clavibacter michiganensis subsp. *m.*
Streptomyces *m.*
miconazole
m. cream
m. nitrate
m. suppository
MICRhoGAM
microabscess
eosinophilic m.
intraepidermal m.
microaerobion
microaerophil
microaerophile
microaerophilic
m. actinomycete
microaerophilism
microaerophilous
microaerophilum
Propionibacterium *m.*
microaneurysm
microangiopathy
conjunctival m.
HIV-induced m.
Microanthomyces alpinus (f)
Microascaceae
Microascales
Microascus trigonosporus (f)
Microbacteriaceae
Microbacterium (b)
M. *arabinogalactanolyticum*
M. *arborescens*
M. *aurantiacum*
M. *aurum*
M. *barkeri*
M. *chocolatum*
M. *dextranolyticum*
M. *esteraromaticum*
M. *flavescens*
M. *foliorum*

M. *halophilum*
M. *hominis*
M. *imperiale*
M. *keratanolyticum*
M. *ketosireducens*
M. *kitamiense*
M. *lacticum*
M. *laevaniformans*
M. *liquefaciens*
M. *luteolum*
M. *maritypicum*
M. *oxydans*
M. *phyllosphaerae*
M. *resistens*
M. *saperdae*
M. *schleiferi*
M. *terrae*
M. *terregens*
M. *testaceum*
M. *thalassium*
M. *trichothecenolyticum*
microbe
microbial
m. associates
M. Identification System (MIDI, MIS)
m. keratitis
m. persistence
m. susceptibility test
microbic
microbicide
vaginal m.
Microbilharzia variglandis (p)
microbiologic
microbiologist
Delft School of Dutch M.'s
microbiology
microbiotic
microbism
latent m.
Microbispora (b)
M. *aerata*
M. *amethystogenes*
M. *bispora*
M. *chromogenes*
M. *corallina*
M. *diastatica*
M. *echinospora*
M. *indica*
M. *karnatakensis*
M. *mesophila*
M. *parva*
M. *rosea* subsp. *aerata*
M. *rosea* subsp. *rosea*
M. *thermodiastatica*
M. *thermorosea*
M. *viridis*
microbroth dilution

Microbulbifer hydrolyticus (b)
microcephaly
microceras
    Dermatophagoides m.
Microcerebrus nunezi
Micrococcaceae
Micrococcus (b)
    M. agilis
    M. antarcticus
    M. halobius
    M. kristinae
    M. luteus
    M. lylae
    M. nishinomiyaensis
    M. roseus
    M. sedentarius
    M. varians
micrococcus, pl. **micrococci**
microconazole
microconidium, pl. **microconidia**
Microcyclus aquaticus (b)
microcyst
microcystic
microcytic
microdilution
    broth m.
    m. broth dilution test
    m. broth susceptibility test
    m. serum bactericidal test
    m. susceptibility testing
microdiskectomy
Microdochium (f)
    M. nivale
    M. nivale var. *majus*
Micro Drop yeast identification system
microellipsoides
    Saccharomyces m.
Microellobosporia (b)
    M. cinerea
    M. flavea
    M. grisea
    M. violacea
microembolization
microevolution
microfilaremia
microfilaria, pl. **microfilariae**
    nocturnal m.
    peripheral blood preparation for
      microfilariae
microfilarial sheath
microflavus
    Streptomyces m.

microflora
microfold (M)
    m. cell
microfusus
    Bacteroides m.
    Rikenella m.
microgamete
microgametocyte
microgamont
microgamy
microglial rod cell
microglobulin
micrograph
    electron m.
microhemagglutination
    m. assay
    m. assay for *Treponema pallidum*
      (MHA-TP)
    m. specific for *Treponema*
      pallidum
    m. test for *Treponema pallidum*
      (MHA-TP test)
microhematocrit
    m. capillary tube
    m. concentration
Micro-ID
    M.-I. system
microimmunofluorescence (MIF)
    m. test
microinfarction
Microlunatus phosphovorus (b)
micromerozoite
micrometer
    ocular m.
Micromonas micros (b)
Micromonospora (h)
    M. aurantiaca
    M. brunnea
    M. carbonacea
    M. carbonacea subsp. *aurantiaca*
    M. carbonacea subsp. *carbonacea*
    M. chalcea
    M. chersina
    M. coerulea
    M. echinospora
    M. echinospora subsp. *echinospora*
    M. echinospora subsp. *ferruginea*
    M. echinospora subsp. *pallida*
    M. gallica
    M. halophytica
    M. halophytica subsp. *halophytica*
    M. halophytica subsp. *nigra*

M

NOTES

Micromonospora (continued)
    M. *inositola*
    M. *matsumotoense*
    M. *nigra*
    M. *olivasterospora*
    M. *pallida*
    M. *purpurea*
    M. *purpureochromogenes*
    M. *rhodorangea*
    M. *rosaria*
Micromonosporaceae
micromotoscope
Micromycopsidaceae
Micronectriella
    M. *nivalis*
microNefrin
Micronema (p)
    M. *deletrix*
    Halicephalobus (M.)
microneme
micronemiasis
micronucleus
microorganism
    pathogenic m.
microparasite
microparticle enzyme immunoassay (MEIA)
microparticulate enzyme immunoassay (MEIA)
Micropeltidaceae
Microphallidae
microphthalmia
Micropolyspora (b)
    M. *angiospora*
    M. *brevicatena*
    M. *faeni*
    M. *internatus*
    M. *rectivirgula*
micropore
Micropruina glycogenica (b)
micropyle
micros
    Micromonas m.
    Peptostreptococcus m.
MicroScan
    M. gram-negative ID panel
    M. HNID Panel
    M. Negative COMBO type 5 system stem
    M. Pos IDENTIFICATION Panel
    M. Rapid Pos Combo Panel
    M. System
Microscilla (b)
    M. *marina*
microscope
    binocular dissecting m.
    dissecting m.

microscopic
    m. agglutination test (MAT)
    m. hematuria
microscopy
    acid-fast m.
    atomic force m.
    darkfield m.
    electron m. (EM)
    fluorescence m.
    immune electron m. (IEM)
    immunoelectron m.
    KOH m.
    light m.
    oil-immersion m.
    phase-contrast m.
    saline m.
    transmission electron m. (TEM)
    in vivo confocal m.
microsize
    griseofulvin m.
microslide culture
Microsphaera multipartita (b)
Microsphaeropsis (f)
Microspora
Microsporasida
Microsporea
microsporidia
microsporidial infection
microsporidian
    m. keratoconjunctivitis
microsporidiasis
microsporidiosis
    enteric m.
Microsporidium (p)
Microsporon (b)
Microsporum (f)
    M. *amazonicum*
    M. *audouinii*
    M. *audouinii* var. *langeronii*
    M. *audouinii* var. *rivalierii*
    M. *boullardii*
    M. *canis*
    M. *canis* var. *distortum*
    M. *cookei*
    M. *equinum*
    M. *ferrugineum*
    M. *flavescens*
    M. *fulvum*
    M. *gallinae*
    M. *gypseum*
    M. *japonicum*
    M. *nanum*
    M. *orientale*
    M. *persicolor*
    M. *racemosum*
    M. *vanbreuseghemii*
microsporus
    Rhizopus m.

microstoma
  Habronema m.
  Hymenolepis m.
microstomia
Microsulfon
Microtetraspora (b)
  M. africana
  M. angiospora
  M. fastidiosa
  M. ferruginea
  M. flexuosa
  M. fusca
  M. glauca
  M. helvata
  M. niveoalba
  M. polychroma
  M. pusilla
  M. recticatena
  M. roseola
  M. roseoviolacea
  M. rubra
  M. salmonea
  M. spiralis
  M. turkmeniaca
  M. tyrrhenii
  M. viridis
Microtheliopsidaceae
Microthyriaceae
Microthyriopsidaceae
microti
  Babesia m.
  Mycobacterium m.
  Mycoplasma m.
MicroTrak
  M. DFA
  M direct fluorescent antibody
    staining
  M. direct fluorescent-antibody test
Microtrombidium
microtube
  m. dilution (MD)
  m. dilution method
  m. dilution test
microtubule
  subpellicular m.
microvesicular steatosis
Microvirgula aerodenitrificans (b)
Microviridae
Microvirus (v)
microzoon
micturition

MICU
  medical intensive care unit
midazolam
Middelburg virus
Middlebrook
  M. 7H10 medium
  M. 7H11 medium
middle ear infection
midforceps
midge
MIDI
  Microbial Identification System
midlobular
Midol IB
midstream urine sample
midvoid urine specimen
Miescher tube
MIF
  microimmunofluorescence
migrans
  cutaneous larva m.
  erythema m. (EM)
  erythema chronicum m. (ECM)
  larva m.
  neural larva m.
  ocular larva m.
  spiruroid larva m.
  visceral larva m. (VLM)
migrating angioedema
migratoria
  Locusta m.
migulae
  Pseudomonas m.
migulanus
  Aneurinibacillus m.
  Bacillus m.
miharai
  Culicoides m.
Mikulicz
  M. cell
  M. syndrome
mikuniensis
  Kineosporia m.
mild
  silver protein, m.
miliary
  m. granulomatosis
  m. lesion
  m. nodule
  m. tuberculosis
miliary-appearing

M

NOTES

milieu
    acid m.
militaris
    Hydrotaea m.
milker's
    m. nodule
    m. nodule virus
milk proteolysis test
Miller-Fisher syndrome
milleri
    Candida m.
milletiae
    Erwinia m.
million
    infectious units per m. (IUPM)
    m. units (MU)
millipede
Millipore filter
milosensis
    Filobacillus m.
mimetica
    Anthomyia m.
mimicus
    Vibrio m.
Minatitlan virus (MNTV)
miner's disease
miniature scarlet fever
miniatus
    Argas m.
Mini-Dose
    HypRho-D M.-D.
mini-exon-derived
    m.-e.-d. ribonucleic acid gene
    m.-e.-d. RNA gene
Mini-Gamulin Rh
minilaparotomy
minimal inhibitory concentration (MIC)
minimum
    m. bactericidal concentration (MBC)
    Bifidobacterium m.
    m. inhibitory concentration (MIC)
    m. inhibitory concentration
      susceptibility test
minireovirus
Minitek
    M. Gram-Positive Panel
    M. *Neisseria* test
Mini-Tip Culturette
Minnal virus (MINV)
minnesotae
    Culiseta m.
Minocin
    M. IV Injection
    M. Oral
minocycline
    m. pleurodesis
minor
    Actinobacillus m.

    m. agglutinin
    Anopheles m.
    Lactobacillus m.
    Lagochilascaris m.
    m. lymphadenopathy
    Polyangium m.
    Thiocystis m.
    Thiorhodococcus m.
    Trichosporon m.
    Weissella m.
minor-determinant mixture (MDM)
minoxidil
Minoxigaine
Mintezol
minus
    Chromatium m.
    Cystobacter m.
    Ophiostoma m.
    m. sense-RNA genome
    Simulium m.
minusculum
    Simulium m.
minuta
    Hansenula m.
    Pichia minuta var. *m.*
    Rhodotorula m.
minute
    m. virus of canines (MVC)
    m. virus of mice (MVM)
minutella
    Phoma m.
minutisclerotica
    Chainia m.
minutiscleroticus
    Streptomyces m.
minutispora
    Phoma m.
minutisporangius
    Actinoplanes m.
minutissima
    Phomatospora m.
minutissimum
    Allochromatium m.
    Chromatium m.
    Corynebacterium m.
minutulum
    Marinospirillum m.
    Oceanospirillum m.
minutum
    Atopobium m.
    Eubacterium m.
    Thermoleophilum m.
    Treponema m.
minutus
    Lactobacillus m.
    Pseudocaedibacter m.
MINV
    Minnal virus

miosis
miotherma
    Petrotoga m.
mip
    macrophage infectivity potentiator
      mip protein
mira
    Planotetraspora m.
mirabilis
    Lautropia m.
    Proteus m.
    Streptomyces m.
    Sulfurococcus m.
miracidial immobilization test
miracidium
miracidium-hatching test
Mirim virus (MIRV)
miroungae
    Facklamia m.
mirum
    Actinosynnema m.
    Spiroplasma m.
MIRV
    Mirim virus
MIS
    Microbial Identification System
misakiensis
    Streptomyces m.
misdiagnosis
misionensis
    Streptomyces m.
misoprostol
mississippiensis
    Culicoides m.
missouriensis
    Actinoplanes m.
mist
    AsthmaHaler M.
    m. bacillus
    Bronitin M.
    Bronkaid M.
    Primatene M.
mitchellae
    Aedes m.
Mitchell River virus (MRV)
mite
    chigger m.
    dust m.
    follicle m.
    harvest m.
    itch m.
    m. typhus

mitigate
mitis
    Streptococcus m.
mitochondria
mitochondrial
    m. dysfunction
    m. toxicity
mitochondrion of hemoflagellate
mitogen
    m. response
mitogenic
    m. adherence lectin
    m. factor
mitomycin
Mitovirus (v)
mitoxantrone
mitral
    m. regurgitation
    m. stenosis
    m. valve
    m. valve prolapse
    m. valve prosthesis
Mitrazol
mitsuokai
    Catenibacterium m.
Mitsuokella (b)
    M. dentalis
    M. multacida
mixed
    m. aerobic and anaerobic abscess
    m. aerobic and anaerobic flora
    m. agglutination
    m. cellular Hodgkin disease
    m. cellularity
    m. chancre
    m. nail infection
    m. seborrheic-staphylococcal
      blepharitis
mixer
    vortex m.
mixta
    Pseudomonas m.
    Telluria m.
mixtum
    Prosimulium m.
mixture
    citric acid bladder m.
    minor-determinant m. (MDM)
    Vaseline-paraffin m.
mixtus
    Cellvibrio mixtus subsp. *m.*
Miyagawa body

M

NOTES

349

Miyagawanella (b)
miyamotoi
 Borrelia m.
miyazakii
 Paragonimus m.
mizutae
 Sphingobacterium m.
mizutaii
 Flavobacterium m.
MLEE
 multilocus enzyme electrophoresis
MLPD
 malignant lymphocytic proliferation
 disease
MLST
 multilocus sequence typing
MLV
 Mono Lake virus
MMLV
 Montana myotis leukoencephalitis virus
MMN
 multifocal motor neuropathy
M-mode echocardiography
MMP
 matrix metalloproteinase
MMR
 measles, mumps, rubella
 MMR vaccine
MMRSA
 mupirocin-resistant, methicillin-resistant
 Staphylococcus aureus
MM virus
MMWR
 Morbidity and Mortality Weekly Report
Mn936-77 virus
MNPV
 multiple nucleopolyhedrovirus
 Choristoneura fumiferana MNPV
 (CfMNPV)
 Orgyia pseudotsugata MNPV
 (OpMNPV)
MNTV
 Minatitlan virus
moatsii
 Mycoplasma m.
Mobala virus (MOBV)
mobaraense
 Streptoverticillium m.
mobaraensis
 Streptomyces m.
Mobidin
mobile
 Aminobacterium m.
 Carnobacterium m.
 Methanobacterium m.
 Methanomicrobium m.
 Mycoplasma m.
 Thermodesulfobacterium m.

mobilis
 Beijerinckia m.
 Desulfurococcus m.
 Ectothiorhodospira m.
 Heliobacillus m.
 Klebsiella m.
 Leptothrix m.
 Macromonas m.
 Methylococcus m.
 Nitrococcus m.
 Petrotoga m.
 Succinispira m.
 Thioflavicoccus m.
 Zymomonas mobilis subsp. m.
mobility
 electrophoretic m.
Mobiluncus (b)
 M. curtisii subsp. curtisii
 M. curtisii subsp. holmesii
 M. mulieris
MOBV
 Mobala virus
modality
 treatment m.
model
 mortality probability m.
modesticaldum
 Heliobacterium m.
modestius
 Thermocladium m.
Modestobacter multiseptatus (b)
modestohalophilus
 Lamprobacter m.
modestum
 Propionigenium m.
modicum
 Acholeplasma m.
modification
 Kopeloff m.
modified
 m. Kinyoun acid-fast stain
 m. oxidase test
 m. trichrome stain
 Uridon M.
 m. whole-egg slant medium
modifier
 biological response m. (BRM)
Modoc virus
MODS
 multiple organ dysfunction syndrome
modulation
 immune m.
Moeller decarboxylation test
Moellerella wisconsensis (b)
moerbista
 Wyeomyia m.
mofetil
 mycophenolate m.

Mogibacterium (b)
    M. pumilum
    M. timidum
    M. vescum
mogii
    Candida m.
mohave
    Culicoides m.
moiety
moist
    M. Again moisturizing gel
    m. desquamation
Moisturizer
    Betadine First Aid Antibiotics
    + M.
    First aid Antibiotics + M.
    Replens Vaginal M.
mojavensis
    Bacillus m.
Mojui Dos Campos virus (MDCV)
MOJUV
    Moju virus
Moju virus (MOJUV)
Mokola virus
molar
    mulberry m.
molare
    Mycoplasma m.
mold
    Alternaria m.
    Mucor m.
    pink bread m.
    ubiquitous saprophytic m.
molecular
    m. epidemiology
    M. Genetics Unit of the Institute
    of Biotechnology (ITQB)
    m. probe testing
    m. typing
molecule
    adhesion m.
    cellular adhesion m. (CAM)
    L-selectin m. (CD62L)
    MHC m.
        major histocompatibility complex
molecule-1
    endothelial leukocyte adhesion m.
    (ELAM-1)
    intercellular adhesion m. (ICAM-1)
    platelet endothelial cell
    adhesion m. (PECAM-1)
    vascular adhesion m. (VCAM-1)

molecule-2
    intercellular adhesion m. (ICAM-2)
molecule-3
    intercellular adhesion m. (ICAM-3)
molenkampi
    Prosthodendrium m.
molischianum
    Phaeospirillum m.
    Rhodospirillum m.
Moll
    gland of M.
mollaretii
    Yersinia m.
Mollaret meningitis
Mollicutes
mollis
    Culex m.
Mollisia fusca (f)
mollusc (*var. of* mollusk)
Mollusca
Molluscipoxvirus (v)
molluscum
    m. contagiosum
    m. contagiosum virus
mollusk, mollusc
molting
molybdites
    Chlorophyllum m.
mometasone furoate
monachus
    Labrys m.
monad
Monafed
    M. DM
monarthritis
Monascus (f)
    M. major
    M. pilosus
    M. ruber
    M. rubiginosus
Monazole-7
Monera
moneran
money pox
mongolense
    Rhizobium m.
Moniezia benedeni (p)
monilated
monilformis
    Gibberella m.
Monilia (f) (*See* **Candida**)

NOTES

moniliae
  Exophiala m.
monilial
moniliasis
Moniliella (f)
  M. suaveolens
moniliform
moniliforme
  Eubacterium m.
  Fusarium m.
Moniliformida
Moniliformidae
Moniliformis (p)
  M. moniliformis
moniliformis
  Armillifer m.
  Moniliformis m.
  Porocephalus m.
  Streptobacillus m.
Moniliformoidae
Monistat
  M. i.v. Injection
  M. Vaginal
Monistat-Derm Topical
monitoring
  Swan-Ganz m.
monkey
  m. kidney fibroblast monolayer
  m. malaria
  m. pox
monkeypox virus
Mono
  M. Lake virus (MLV)
monoarticular
monobiae
  Spiroplasma m.
Monoblepharidaceae
Monoblepharidales
Monocelis (p)
  M. lineata
  M. longiceps
monoceras
  Drechslera m.
  Setosphaeria m.
Monocercomonadidae
Monocercomonas (p)
  M. grassi
  M. ruminatium
Monocid
Monocillium (f)
monoclonal
  m. antibody
  m. antibody B291
  m. antibody-based latex
    agglutination (MAb-LA)
  m. antibody staining
  m. gammopathy

m. gammopathy of undetermined
  significance (MUGS)
m. lymphoproliferative syndrome
monoclonality
Monocystis lumbrici (p)
monocyte
  m. chemoattractant protein (MCP)
  m. tropic virus
monocyte-derived dendritic cell (MDDC)
monocytic ehrlichiosis
monocytogenes
  Listeria m.
monocytopenia
  transient m.
monocytosis
Monodictys nigrosperma (f)
Monodox
monoensis
  Culicoides m.
Monogenea
monogenesis
monogenetic
monogenous
Mono-Gesic
monohydrate
  cefadroxil m.
  cefalexin m.
  cephalexin m.
  doxycycline m.
monolayer
  human lung fibroblast m.
  monkey kidney fibroblast m.
monoleptic fever
monomycini
  Streptomyces m.
Mononegavirales
mononeuritis multiplex
mononeuropathy
  musculocutaneous m.
mononuclear
  m. cell infiltrate
  m. phagocyte
  m. phagocyte system
mononucleosis
  acute infectious m.
  EBV m.
  heterophil-negative m.
  infectious m. (IM)
  m. syndrome
mononucleosis-like syndrome
monopartite dsRNA mycovirus group
monophosphate
  adenine arabinoside m. (Ara-AMP)
  azidothymidine m. (AZTMP)
  cyclic adenosine m.
  cyclic guanine m. (cGMP)
  cyclic guanosine m.

fludarabine m.
nucleoside m.
monoplast
monoplastic
Monospot test
Monosticon Dri-Dot test
Monostoma arcuatum (p)
monostome
mono test
monotherapy
AZT m.
fluoroquinolone m.
intravesical BCG m.
nucleoside m.
Monotospora (f)
monotrichate
monotrichous
monoxenic culture
monoxenous
monozoic
montana
Candida m.
Montana myotis leukoencephalitis virus (MMLV)
montanense
Spiroplasma m.
montanensis
Rickettsia m.
montanus
Diamanus m.
Saccharomyces m.
Monte Dourado virus (MDOV)
monteilii
Pseudomonas m.
Montenegro skin test
Montezuma's revenge
Montgomery
M. County agent
M. County virus
monticola
Aedes m.
Montoyella (*See* **Treponema**)
M. nigra
Monurol
mood disorder
moon facies
Moorcroft agent
moorei
Amsacta m.
Solobacterium m.
Moorella (b)
M. glycerini

M. thermoacetica
M. thermoautotrophica
Mooren corneal ulcer
mooreparkense
Corynebacterium m.
Moore prosthesis
Mooser body
Mopeia virus
morado
mal m.
morae
Simulium m.
Moranyl
moravica
Legionella m.
moraviensis
Enterococcus m.
Moraxella (b)
M. anatipestifer
M. boevrei
M. (Branhamella) catarrhalis
M. (Branhamella) caviae
M. (Branhamella) cuniculi
M. (Branhamella) ovis
M. canis
M. caprae
M. equi
M. lincolnii
M. (Moraxella) atlantae
M. (Moraxella) bovis
M. (Moraxella) lacunata
M. (Moraxella) nonliquefaciens
M. (Moraxella) osloensis
M. (Moraxella) phenylpyruvica
M. saccharolytica
M. urethralis
Moraxellaceae
morbi
Catonella m.
morbidity
M. and Mortality Weekly Report (MMWR)
perioperative m.
m. rate
morbid obesity
morbilliform
m. eruption
m. rash
Morbillivirus (v)
morbillorum
Gemella m.
Streptococcus m.

M

NOTES

353

Morchellaceae
mordant
    iodine m.
    iron-alum m.
mordens
    Physaloptera m.
morel
    early false m.
    false m.
Morerastrongylus costaricensis (p)
Morgan bacillus (*See **Morganella**
  morganii*)
Morganella (b)
    M. morganii
    M. morganii subsp. *morganii*
    M. morganii subsp. *sibonii*
morgani
    Chordodes m.
morganii
    Morganella m.
    Morganella morganii subsp. *m.*
    Proteus m.
mori
Moriche virus (MORV)
moriokaense
    Mycobacterium m.
Moritella (b)
    M. japonica
    M. marina
    M. viscosa
    M. yayanosii
Morococcus cerebrosus (b)
morookaense
    Streptomyces m.
    Streptoverticillium m.
morookaensis
    Streptomyces m.
morphine
morphologic
    m. examination
    m. feature
morphotype
    bacterial m.
morrhuae
    Halococcus m.
morsitans
    Culiseta m.
    Glossina m.
mortality
    Pediatric Risk of M. (PRISM)
    m. probability model
    m. rate
Mortierellaceae
Mortierella wolfii (f)
mortiferum
    Fusobacterium m.

mortivallis
    Actinopolyspora m.
    Culicoides m.
mortuorum
    Cynomya m.
morum
    Acholeplasma m.
MoRu-Viraten
MORV
    Moriche virus
mor1 virus
mosaic wart
Mosco
moscoviensis
    Nitrospira m.
moshkovskii
    Entamoeba m.
Mosqueiro virus (MQOV)
mosquito
    anopheline m.
Mossman fever
Mossuril virus (MOSV)
MOSV
    Mossuril virus
moth-eaten appearance
mother
    antiretroviral-exposed m.
    m. colony
    m. cyst
    m. yaw
mother-to-child transmission (MTCT)
mother-to-fetus/infant transmission
motile
motility
    bacterial m.
    m. disturbance
    extraocular m.
    m. test
    m. test medium
motion sickness
motor conduction block
Motrin
    M. IB
    M. IB Sinus
    Junior Strength M.
MOTT
    mycobacteria other than *Mycobacterium
    tuberculosis*
mottling
moubata
    Ornithodoros m.
mount
    direct saline m.
    direct wet m.
    hanging-drop m.
    iodine m.
    KOH m.
    lactophenol cotton blue m.

nigrosin m.
saline wet m.
unstained saline m.
urine *Trichomonas* wet m.
vaginal wet m.
wet m.
Mount Elgon bat virus (MEBV)
mouse, pl. **mice**
    m. cytomegalovirus
    m. hepatitis
    m. mammary oncovirus
    minute virus of mice (MVM)
    m. neutralization test
    pneumonia virus of mice
mousepox virus
Mousse
    RID M.
mouth
    trench m.
Movat technique
movement
    ciliary m.
    protoplasmic m.
    saccadic eye m.
    streaming m.
moxalactam
    m. disodium
Moxalactum
Moxam
moxifloxacin
MP13 virus
MP15 virus
MPA
    medroxyprogesterone acetate
MPC
    mucopurulent cervicitis
M-PCR
    multiplex polymerase chain reaction
MPKV
    Maprik virus
MPM II
M-Prednisol Injection
MPRV
    Mapuera virus
MpV virus
MQOV
    Mosqueiro virus
MR
    magnetic resonance
MRI
    magnetic resonance imaging

mRNA
    messenger RNA
MRSA
    methicillin-resistant *Staphylococcus aureus*
        MRSA endocarditis
        mupirocin-resistant MRSA
MRV
    mammalian orthoreovirus
    Mitchell River virus
M-R-VAX II
MS2 virus
MSD Enteric Coated ASA
MSM
    men who have sex with men
MSP8 virus
MSSA
    methicillin-susceptible *Staphylococcus aureus*
MSTA Mumps
MSV virus
MTB
    Mycobacterium tuberculosis
        isoniazid-resistant MTB
        multidrug-resistant MTB
MTBV
    Marituba virus
MTCT
    mother-to-child transmission
M-tropic
    macrophage-tropic
    M-tropic virus
MTRV
    Matruh virus
MTSS
    menstrual toxic shock syndrome
MT virus
MU
    million units
Mucambo virus (MUCV)
mucate fermentation test
mucicarmine stain
mucidolens
    Pseudomonas m.
mucifaciens
    Corynebacterium m.
mucilaginosa
    Rothia m.
mucilaginosus
    Bacillus m.
    Stomatococcus m.
mucin clot test

M

NOTES

mucinosa
mucinous columnar metaplasia
mucin-secreting adenocarcinoma
mucitis
mucociliary
mucocutaneous
    m. candidiasis
    m. herpes simplex
    m. HSV lesion
    m. leishmaniasis
    m. relapse
    m. transmission
    m. vesicle
Muco-Fen-DM
Muco-Fen-LA
mucogenicum
    Mycobacterium m.
mucoid
    m. colony
    m. diarrhea
mucoides
    Trichosporon m.
mucolytic
Mucomyst
mucopurulent
    m. cervicitis (MPC)
    m. discharge
    m. endocervical exudate
    m. sputum
mucopus
    cervical m.
Mucor (f)
    M. circinelloides
    M. hiemalis
    M. javanicus
    M. mold
    M. racemosus
    M. ramosissimus
mucor
    Leucothrix m.
Mucoraceae
Mucorales
mucormycosis
    rhinocerebral m.
mucosa
    buccal m.
    Neisseria m.
    sinopulmonary m.
    vulval m.
mucosa-associated
    m.-a. lymphoid tissue (MALT)
    m.-a. lymphoid tumor (MALToma)
    m.-a. lymph tissue (MALT)
mucosae
    Lactobacillus m.
mucosal
    m. candidiasis
    m. disease virus

    m. disease virus group
    m. immunity
    m. leishmaniasis
    m. melanoma
    m. ulceration
mucosalis
    Campylobacter m.
    Campylobacter sputorum subsp. *m.*
Mucosil
mucositis
mucosus
    Desulfurococcus m.
mucous
    m. diarrhea
    m. membrane
    m. membrane chancre
    m. membrane chancroid
    m. patch
mucron
mucronata
    Bertiella m.
mucus
    rectal m.
MUCV
    Mucambo virus
Mudd Acne Cream
mud fever
Mudjinbarry virus
MUDV
    Munguba virus
Mueller-Hinton
    M.-H. agar
    M.-H. broth
    M.-H. medium
muelleri
    Aedes m.
    Simonsiella m.
Muellerius capillaris (p)
Muerto Canyon virus
MUG
    4-methylumbelliferyl-beta-D-
    glucoronidase test
    4-methylumbelliferyl-beta-D-
    glucuronidase
    MUG Disk
    MUG test
MUGS
    monoclonal gammopathy of
    undetermined significance
Muir Springs virus
mujiangensis
    Lasiohelea m.
mukohataei
    Haloarcula m.
mulaire lesion
mulberry molar
mule deer poxvirus

mulieris
> *Mobiluncus* m.

Mu-like viruses (v)

mulli
> *Contracaecum* m.

mulrennani
> *Culex* m.
> *Culicoides* m.

multacida
> *Mitsuokella* m.

multiacidus
> *Bacteroides* m.

multiannulatum
> *Ophiostoma* m.

multibacillary leprosy
multicentric Castleman disease
Multiceps (p) (*See* **Taenia**)
> M. *brauni*
> M. *gaigeri*
> M. *multiceps*
> M. *serialis*

multiceps
> *Multiceps* m.
> *Taenia* m.

multicolor
multidentatus
> *Culicoides* m.

multidermatomal
multidermatomeric herpes zoster
multidigit dactylitis
multidrug
> m. resistance (MDR)
> m. resistant virus

multidrug-resistant (MDR)
> m.-r. bacteria
> m.-r. MTB
> m.-r. TB

multifaceted
multifiliis
> *Ichthyophthirius* m.

multifocal
> m. extracutaneous sporotrichosis
> m. leukoencephalopathy
> m. motor neuropathy (MMN)

multiforme
> bullous erythema m.
> erythema m.
> *Eubacterium* m.

multiformis
> *Nitrosolobus* m.
> *Nitrosospira* m.

multigemmis
> *Candida* m.

multiglobuliferum
> *Oceanospirillum* m.

multigravida
multiinfarct dementia
multilobar
multilobular
multilocale
> *Acholeplasma* m.

multilocular hydatid cyst
multilocularis
> *Echinococcus* m.

multilocus
> m. enzyme electrophoresis (MEE, MLEE)
> m. enzyme electrophoresis analysis
> m. sequence typing (MLST)

multimammate
> m. papilloma virus
> m. rate

multinucleated giant cell
multiorgan
multipapillosa
> *Parafilaria* m.

multipara
> *Lachnospira* m.

multiparameter
multiparous
multipartita
> *Microsphaera* m.

multiple
> m. arbitrary amplicon profiling (MAAP)
> m. drug-resistant (MDR)
> m. fission
> m. myeloma
> m. nucleocapsid virus
> m. nucleopolyhedrovirus (MNPV)
> m. organ dysfunction syndrome (MODS)
> m. parasitism
> m. polyposis
> m. sclerosis
> m. sulfonamide
> m. synchronous subcutaneous metastasis

multiple-drug
> m.-d. regimen
> m.-d. resistant tuberculosis (MDRTB)

M

NOTES

multiplex
    mononeuritis m.
    m. polymerase chain reaction (M-PCR)
multiplex-PCR
multiplicative division
multipotens
    Desulfurella m.
multipunctatus
    Culicoides m.
multipuncture
    m. battery
    m. device
    m. method
multireferral health-service delivery
multiresinivorans
    Pseudomonas m.
multiresistant
multiseptatus
    Modestobacter m.
multisite
multispinosus
    Laelaps m. (See Plasmodium kochi)
Multitest
    M. CMI device
    M. CMI system
multivalent group B streptococcal polysaccharide-tetanus toxoid conjugate vaccine
multivariate
multivorans
    Burkholderia m.
    Dehalospirillum m.
    Desulfococcus m.
    Methylorhabdus m.
multivorum
    Acidiphilium m.
    Flavobacterium m.
    Sphingobacterium m.
multocida
    Pasteurella multocida subsp. *m.*
mumps
    m. encephalitis
    extrasalivary m.
    m. meningitis
    MSTA M.
    m. serology
    m. skin test antigen
    m. vaccine
    m. virus
    m. virus culture
    m. virus vaccine Jeryl Lynn strain
Mumpsvax
Munch-Petersen
    Christie, Atkins, and M.-P. (CAMP)

mundtii
    Enterococcus m.
Munguba virus (MUDV, MUNV)
municipale
    Thermocrispum m.
Munro abscess
MUNV
    Munguba virus
mupirocin
    m. calcium
mupirocin-resistant, methicillin-resistant *Staphylococcus aureus* (MMRSA)
mupirocin-resistant MRSA
mupirocin-resistant *Staphylococcus aureus*
mural
    m. thrombosis
murale
    Mycobacterium m.
    Williamsia m.
murdochii
    Serpulina m.
mureins
Murex
    M. *Candida albicans* test
    M. CMV DNA hybrid capture assay
muriaticus
    Tetragenococcus m.
muridarum
    Chlamydia m.
    Helicobacter m.
murinus
    Lactobacillus m.
    Streptomyces m.
muris
    Actinobacillus m.
    Cryptosporidium m.
    Ehrlichia m.
    Giardia m.
    Haemobartonella m.
    Hepatozoon m.
    Ixodes m.
    Mycoplasma m.
    Syphacia m.
murliniae
    Citrobacter m.
murmur
    Carey-Coombs m.
    insufficiency m.
    systolic regurgitant m.
Muromegalovirus (v)
murorum
    Acremonium m.
    Gliomastix m.

murrayi
>   *Deinococcus m.*
>   *Listeria m.*
Murray Valley encephalitis virus (MVE, MVEV)
Murre virus
Murutucu virus (MURV)
MURV
>   Murutucu virus
Mus
>   *Mus* adenovirus 1–2 (mus 1–2)
mus 1–2
>   *Mus* adenovirus 1–2
musae
>   *Candida m.*
>   *Laestadia m.*
>   *Macrophoma m.*
>   *Tritirachium m.*
Musca (p)
>   *M. autumnalis*
>   *M. domestica*
>   *M. domestica domestica*
>   *M. domestica vicina*
>   *M. macellaria*
muscae
>   *Entomophthora m.*
>   *Habronema m.*
>   *Staphylococcus m.*
muscaria
>   *Amanita muscaria* var. m.
muscarine
muscarinic cholinergic receptor
muscarinism
Muscidae
muscimol
Muscina
>   *M. dorsilinea*
>   *M. flukei*
>   *M. fulvacrura*
>   *M. levida*
>   *M. pascuorum*
>   *M. prolapsa*
muscle
>   m. biopsy
>   endocardium, vascular structures, interstitium of striated m. (EVI)
>   rectus femoris m.
Muscor
>   *M. ambiguus*
>   *M. herbariorum*
>   *M. indicus*
musculamine

musculocutaneous mononeuropathy
musculoskeletal
>   m. infection
>   m. manifestation
>   m. tuberculosis
mushroom
>   autumn skullcap m.
>   big laughing m.
>   death cap m.
>   destroying angel m.
>   fly agaric m.
>   fools' m.
>   gray pinkgill m.
>   green gill m.
>   horse m.
>   inky cap m.
>   jack o'lantern m.
>   little brown m. (LBM)
>   naked brimcap m.
>   panthercap m.
>   pepper bolete m.
>   m. poisoning
>   showy flamecap m.
>   sickener m.
>   smoothcap m.
>   sorrel webcap m.
>   sweat m.
>   tigertop m.
mushroom-worker's lung
mustelae
>   *Campylobacter m.*
>   *Campylobacter pylori* subsp. *m.*
>   *Helicobacter m.*
>   *Mycoplasma m.*
mut.
>   mutation
mutabilis
>   *Lecythophora m.*
>   *Nocardiopsis m.*
>   *Saccharothrix mutabilis* subsp. *m.*
>   *Streptomyces m.*
mutans
>   *Knemidocoptes m.*
>   m. streptococci
>   *Streptococcus m.*
mutant
>   auxotrophic m.
mutation (mut.)
>   resistance m.
mutilating leprosy
mutilation
>   genital m.

M

NOTES

mutiresistant *Staphylococcus aureus*
mutism
    akinetic m.
mutomycini
    Streptomyces m.
mutualism
mutualist
mutucuna
    Simulium m.
Mu virus
MVC
    minute virus of canines
MVE
    Murray Valley encephalitis virus
MVEV
    Murray Valley encephalitis virus
MVG-51 virus
M12 virus
M$_1$ virus
MVM
    minute virus of mice
MWAV
    Manawa virus
Myaderm
myagiana
    Bullera m.
myalgia
    epidemic m.
Myambutol
Myapap
myasthenia gravis
Mycelex
    M. Troche
Mycelex-7
Mycelex-G
mycelia (*pl. of* mycelium)
mycelia-derived antigen
mycelial
mycelian
mycelioid
Myceliophthora (f)
    M. lutea
    M. thermophila
mycelium, pl. **mycelia**
    aerial m.
    nonseptate m.
    septate m.
Myceloblastanon (f)
Mycelorrhizodes (f) (*See* **Candida**)
Mycenastraceae
mycete
mycetism
    m. cerebralis
    m. choliformis
    m. gastrointestinalis
    m. nervosa
    m. sanguinareus

Mycetocola (b)
    M. lacteus
    M. saprophilus
    M. tolaasinivorans
mycetoides
    Corynebacterium m.
mycetoma
    actinomycotic m.
    Brumpt white m.
    Carter black m. (*See* Madura foot)
    dermatophyte m.
    eumycotic m.
    Nicolle white m.
    Vincent white m.
    white m.
mycetomatis
    Madurella m.
Mychel-S
Mycifradin
    M. Sulfate
    M. Sulfate Oral
    M. Sulfate Topical
Myciguent
Mycitracin Topical
Myclo-Derm
Myclo-Gyne
mycobacteremia
mycobacteria
    m. antibiotic supplement (MAS)
    atypical m.
    m. culture
    m. growth indicator tube (MGIT)
    m. growth indicator tube system
    nontuberculous m. (NTM)
    m. other than *Mycobacterium*
      tuberculosis (MOTT)
    Runyon group I–IV m.
Mycobacteriaceae
mycobacterial
    m. abscess
    m. choroiditis
    m. culture
    disseminated nontuberculous m.
      (DNTM)
    m. infection
    m. lymphadenitis
    m. necrotizing pneumonia
mycobacteriosis
Mycobacterium (b)
    M. abscessus
    M. africanum
    M. agri
    M. aichiense
    M. alvei
    M. asiaticum
    M. aurum
    M. austroafricanum
    M. avium subsp. *avium*

M. *avium* complex (MAC)
M. *avium-intracellulare* (MAI)
M. *avium-intracellulare* complex
M. *avium* subsp. *paratuberculosis*
M. *avium* subsp. *silvaticum*
M. *bohemicum*
M. *bovis*
M. *branderi*
M. *brumae*
M. *celatum*
M. *chelonae*
M. *chelonae* abscess
M. *chelonae* subsp. *abscessus*
M. *chelonae* subsp. *chelonae*
M. *chitae*
M. *chlorophenolicum*
M. *chubuense*
M. *confluentis*
M. *conspicuum*
M. *cookii*
M. *diernhoferi*
M. *duvalii*
M. *elephantis*
M. *fallax*
M. *farcinogenes*
M. *flavescens*
M. *fortuitum* subsp.
   acetamidolyticum
M. *fortuitum-chelonae* complex
M. *fortuitum* subsp. *fortuitum*
M. *fortuitum* third biovar complex
M. *gadium*
M. *gastri*
M. *genavense*
M. *gilvum*
M. *goodii*
M. *gordonae*
M. *haemophilum*
M. *hassiacum*
M. *heckeshornense*
M. *heidelbergense*
M. *hiberniae*
M. *hodleri*
M. *interjectum*
M. *intermedium*
M. *intracellulare*
M. *komossense*
M. *kubicae*
M. *lentiflavum*
M. *leprae*
M. *lepraemurium*

M. *leprae*-stimulated lymphocyte
   transformation test
M. *madagascariense*
M. *mageritense*
M. *malmoense*
M. *marinum*
M. *microti*
M. *moriokaense*
M. *mucogenicum*
M. *murale*
M. *neoaurum*
M. *nonchromogenicum*
M. *novocastrense*
M. *obuense*
M. *parafortuitum*
M. *paratuberculosis*
M. *peregrinum*
M. phage lacticola
M. phage Leo
M. *phlei*
M. *porcinum*
M. *poriferae*
M. *pulveris*
M. *rhodesiae*
M. *scrofulaceum*
M. *senegalense*
M. *septicum*
M. *shimoidei*
M. *simiae*
M. *smegmatis*
M. *sphagni*
M. *szulgai*
M. *terrae*
M. *terrae-triviale* complex
M. *thermoresistibile*
M. *tokaiense*
M. *triplex*
M. *triviale*
M. *tuberculosis* (MTB)
M. *tuberculosis* subsp. *caprae*
M. *tuberculosis* detection
M. *tuberculosis* subsp. *tuberculosis*
M. *tusciae*
M. *ulcerans*
M. *vaccae*
M. *wolinskyi*
M. *xenopi*
mycobactin
mycobiotic agar
Mycobutin
Mycocaliciaceae
Mycocandida (f)

NOTES

Mycocentrospora acerina (f)
mycocide
Mycoderma (f)
mycoderma
    Candida m.
mycodermatitis
mycogastritis
Mycogen II Topical
mycoides
    Bacillus m.
    Mycoplasma mycoides subsp. *m.*
Mycokluyveria (f)
mycolic acid
Mycolog-II Topical
mycologist
mycology
    medical m.
Myconel Topical
mycophage
mycophenolate mofetil
mycophenolic acid (MA)
mycophilus
    Hypomyces m.
Mycoplana (b)
    M. bullata
    M. dimorpha
    M. ramosa
    M. segnis
Mycoplasma (b)
    M. adleri
    M. agalactiae
    M. agassizii
    M. alkalescens
    M. alligatoris
    M. alvi
    M. anatis
    M. anseris
    M. arginini
    M. arthritidis
    M. auris
    M. bovigenitalium
    M. bovirhinis
    M. bovis
    M. bovoculi
    M. buccale
    M. buteonis
    M. californicum
    M. canadense
    M. canis
    M. capricolum subsp. *capricolum*
    M. capricolum subsp.
     capripneumoniae
    M. caviae
    M. cavipharyngis
    M. citelli
    M. cloacale
    M. collis
    M. columbinasale

M. columbinum
M. columborale
M. conjunctivae
M. corogypsi
M. cottewii
M. cricetuli
M. crocodyli
M. cynos
M. dispar
M. edwardii
M. elephantis
M. ellychniae
M. equigenitalium
M. equirhinis
M. falconis
M. fastidiosum
M. faucium
M. felifaucium
M. feliminutum
M. felis
M. fermentans
M. flocculare
M. gallinaceum
M. gallinarum
M. gallisepticum
M. gallopavonis
M. gateae
M. genitalium
M. glycophilum
M. gypis
M. hominis
M. hominis bacteremia
M. hyopharyngis
M. hyopneumoniae
M. hyorhinis
M. hyosynoviae
M. imitans
M. incognitus
M. indiense
M. iners
M. infection
M. iowae
M. lactucae
M. lagogenitalium
M. leonicaptivi
M. leopharyngis
M. lipofaciens
M. lipophilum
M. lucivorax
M. luminosum
M. maculosum
M. melaleucae
M. meleagridis
M. microti
M. moatsii
M. mobile
M. molare
M. muris

M. mustelae
M. mycoides subsp. *capri*
M. mycoides subsp. *mycoides*
M. neurolyticum
M. opalescens
M. orale
M. ovipneumoniae
M. oxoniensis
M. penetrans
M. phocacerebrale
M. phocarhinis
M. phocidae
M. pirum
M. pneumonia
M. pneumoniae
M. primatum
M. pullorum
M. pulmonis
M. putrefaciens
M. salivarium
M. serology
M. simbae
M. somnilux
M. spermatophilum
M. spumans
M. sturni
M. sualvi
M. subdolum
M. synoviae
M. testudinis
M. T-strain
M. T-strain culture
M. verecundum
M. yeatsii

mycoplasma
m. disease

mycoplasmal
m. encephalitis
m. pharyngitis
m. pneumonia

Mycoplasmataceae
Mycoplasmatales
Mycoporaceae
mycosel agar
mycosis, pl. **mycoses**
m. cutis chronica
m. framboesioides
m. fungoides
m. intestinalis
ocular m.
pulmonary m.
systemic m.

Mycosphaerella (f)
M. tassiana
M. tulasnei
mycostatic
Mycostatin
mycotic
m. aneurysm
m. corneal ulcer disease
m. keratitis
Mycotorula (*See* **Candida**)
Mycotoruloides (f)
mycotoxicosis
mycotoxin
Myco-Triacet II
mycovirus
mydriasis
myelin basic protein
myelinolysis
myelitic enterovirus
myelitis
HTLV-1 m.
transverse m.
myelocyte
neutrophil m.
myelodysplasia
myelodysplastic
m. syndrome (MDS)
myeloencephalitis
myeloid
m. cell infiltration
m. leukemia
m. pool
myeloid/erythroid ratio
myeloma
multiple m.
plasma cell m.
myelomeningocele
myelopathy
acute transverse m. (ATM)
HTLV-1 m.
HTLV-1-associated m. (HAM)
tropical spastic paresis/HTLV-1-
associated m. (TSP/HAM)
myelophthisic anemia
myeloproliferative syndrome
myelosuppression
myelosuppressive therapy
myelotoxic drug
myelotoxicity
zidovudine-induced m.
myenteric plexus

M

NOTES

myiasis
    accidental m.
    African furuncular m.
    aural m.
    creeping m.
    human botfly m.
    intestinal m.
    nasal m.
    nosocomial m.
    ocular m.
    m. oestruosa
    subcutaneous m.
    tumbu dermal m.
    wound m.
Mykines virus (MYKV)
mykol
MYKV
    Mykines virus
Mylotarg
Myminic Expectorant
Myobiidae
myocardial
    m. disease
    m. infarction (MI)
myocarditis
    enteroviral m.
    interstitial m.
myocardotic
Myochrysine
myoclonic
    m. alien hand syndrome
    m. twitching
myoclonus
myocyte
    Anistchkow m.
myoglobinuria
myoid
D-**myoinositol 1,4,5,6-tetrakisphosphate**
MYO-**isositol fermentation test**
myometrial
myonecrosis
    clostridial m.
    nonclostridial anaerobic m.
myoneme
myopathy
myopericarditis
myositic
myositis
    acute m.
    crepitant m.
    epidemic m.
    m. purulenta
    m. purulenta tropica
    strep m.
    suppurative m.
    tropical m.
Myo-Triacet II
Myoviridae (v)

MY-PAP cervicovaginal lavage kit
Myphetane DC
myriad
Myriangiaceae
myringitis
    bullous m.
myringotomy
Myriodontium (f)
myrmecia
Myroides (b)
    M. odoratimimus
    M. odoratus
Myrothecium (f)
    M. cinctum
    M. leucotrichum
    M. roridum
    M. verrucaria
myrsinacearum
    Phyllobacterium m.
mysorens
    Arthrobacter m.
mystax
    Toxocara m.
mytili
    Vibrio m.
Mytilinidiaceae
Mytrex F Topical
Mytussin
    M. AC
    M. DAC
    M. DM
myxedema
Myxococcaceae
Myxococcales
myxococcoides
    Sporocytophaga m.
Myxococcus (b)
    M. coralloides
    M. disciformis
    M. flavescens
    M. macrosporus
    M. stipitatus
    M. virescens
    M. xanthus
myxofaciens
    Proteus m.
myxoma
    left atrial m.
    m. virus
    m. virus subgroup
myxomycete
Myxomycetes
Myxomycota
Myxospora
Myxosporea
Myxotrichum (f)
    M. cancellatum
    M. chartarum

M. deflexum
M. stipitatum
myxovirus

Myxozoa
M-Zole 7 Dual Pack

NOTES

M

N-9
nonoxynol-9
N-9 gel
N1 virus
N4 virus
N5 virus
naardenensis
Brettanomyces n.
naardensis
Dekkera n.
NAC
N-acetyl-cysteine
N-acetyl-cysteine (NAC)
***N*-acetylgalactosaminouronic acid**
***N*-acetylglucosamine fermentation test**
***N*-acetyl-L-cysteine-sodium hydroxide test (NALC test)**
***N*-acetylmuramic acid**
nadir
Nadopen-V
Nadostine
NADP⁺
nicotinamide adenine dinucleotide phosphate positive
NADP⁺ dependent malic enzyme
Nadsonia (f)
N. fulvescens var. elongata
N. fulvescens var. fulvescens
Naegleria (p)
N. aerobia
N. australiensis
N. fowleri
N. invadens
naeodendra
Candida n.
naeslundii
Actinomyces n.
nafate
cefamandole n.
Nafcil
N. Injection
nafcillin
n. sodium
Nafrine
naftifine
Naftin
nagana
Naganishia
naganishii
Streptomyces n.
naganoensis
Bacillus n.
Bacillus niacini
Leifsonia n.

nagasakiensis
Kitasatoa n.
nagelii
Lactobacillus n.
Nagler
N. reaction
N. test
nail
intramedullary fixation n.
Ony-Clear N.
ringworm of n.
Nair buffered methylene blue stain
nairi
Bivitellobilharzia n.
Nairobi
N. sheep disease virus (NSDV)
Nairovirus (v)
najae
Pentastoma n.
Nakalanga
N. dwarfism
N. syndrome
nakayamae
Sporolactobacillus nakayamae subsp. n.
naked brimcap mushroom
nakuruensis
Leptopsylla aethiopica n.
NALC test
Naldecon
N. DX Adult Liquid
N. Senior DX
N. Senior EX
Naldecon-EX Children's syrup
nalidixic
n. acid
n. acid test
Nallpen
N. Injection
name
trade n.
namibiensis
Thiomargarita n.
Namovirus (v)
nana
Endolimax n.
Hymenolepis n.
NANB
non-A, non-B
NANB hepatitis
nandrolone
n. decanoate
n. phenpropionate
nanellus
Culicoides n.

N

Nannizzia (f)
Nannocystis exedens (b)
Nanophyetidae
Nanophyetus (p)
    N. salmincola
    N. schikhobalowi
Nantucket knee
nanukayami
    n. fever
nanum
    Microsporum n.
nanus
    Culicoides n.
NAP
    P-nitro-alpha-acetylamino-beta-
    hydroxypropiophenone
    NAP test
naphthovorans
    Neptunomonas n.
Naprelan
Naprosyn
naproxen
Naranjal virus (NJLV)
narbonensis
    Streptomyces n.
narcissi
    Trichoderma n.
narcotic analgesic
Narnavirus (v)
narrow-spectrum agent
NAS
    Nasoule virus
Nasabid
nasal
    Bactroban N.
    Kondon's N.
    n. myiasis
    n. ora serrata
    n. septoplasty
    N. & Sinus Relief
    n. swab
    n. vestibule
nasale
    Schistosoma n.
nasalis
    Gasterophilus n.
NASBA
    nucleic acid sequence-band amplification
    nucleic acid sequence-based amplification
    NASBA HIV-1 RNA QT assay
NAS-BA
    nucleic acid sequence-based amplification
nashvillensis
    Streptomyces n.
nasicola
    Mammomonogamus n.
Nasik *Vibrio*

nasimurium
    Rothia n.
nasociliary
nasogastric (NG)
    n. tube
nasointestinal
nasolabial fold
Nasonex
nasoniae
    Arsenophonus n.
nasopharyngeal
    n. aspirate
    n. carcinoma
    n. culture
    n. leishmaniasis
    n. neoplasm
    n. swab
    n. wash
nasopharynx
nasorum
    Cryptosporidium n.
nasosinusoidal
nasotracheal aspiration
Nasoule virus (NAS)
Natacyn
    N. Ophthalmic
natalensis
    Candida n.
natamycin
natans
    Sphaerotilus n.
natatoria
    Blastomonas n.
    Sphingomonas n.
natatorius
    Blastobacter n.
National
    N. Academy of Sciences
    N. Committee on Clinical
      Laboratory Standards (NCCLS)
    N. Institute for Occupational Safety
      and Health (NIOSH)
    N. Institutes of Health (NIH)
    N. Nosocomial Infections
      Surveillance System (NNIS)
    N. Nosocomial Infection
      Surveillance (NNIS)
    N. Research Council
    N. Type Culture Collection
      (NTCC)
    N. Vaccine Advisory Committee
      (NVAC)
nativa
    Trichinella n.
native valve endocarditis
Natrialba (b)
    N. aegyptia
    N. asiatica

N. magadii
N. taiwanensis
natricina
    Physa n.
natriegens
    Beneckea n.
    Vibrio n.
Natrinema (b)
    N. pallidum
    N. pellirubrum
    N. versiforme
Natroniella acetigena (b)
Natronincola histidinovorans (b)
Natronobacterium (b)
    N. gregoryi
    N. magadii
    N. pharaonis
    N. vacuolatum
Natronococcus (b)
    N. amylolyticus
    N. occultus
natronolimnaea
    Dietzia n.
Natronomonas pharaonis (b)
Natronorubrum (b)
    N. bangense
    N. tibetense
Nattrassia mangiferae (f)
natural
    n. focus of infection
    n. hemolysin
    n. immunity
    n. killer (NK)
    n. killer cell
nausea
    epidemic n.
nautarum
    Legionella n.
nautica
    Pseudomonas n.
navarrensis
    Vibrio n.
Navarro virus (NAVV)
naviforme
    Fusobacterium n.
NAVV
    Navarro virus
Naxen
NBD
    necrotizing bowel disease
NBTE
    nonbacterial thrombotic endocarditis

NBV
    Nelson Bay orthoreovirus
NCCLS
    National Committee on Clinical
      Laboratory Standards
NCV
    non-cholera *Vibrio*
ND
    Congestac N.
Ndelle virus (NDEV)
NDEV
    Ndelle virus
NDOV
    Nyando virus
Ndumu virus (NDUV)
NDUV
    Ndumu virus
NDV
    Newcastle disease virus
NE-8D virus
neapolitana
    Thermotoga n.
neapolitanus
    Halothiobacillus n.
    Thiobacillus n.
near-infrared interactance (NIR)
Nebcin
    N. Injection
nebraskense
    Corynebacterium n
nebraskensis
    Clavibacter michiganensis subsp. *n.*
nebulizer
    jet-impeller n.
    pneumatic n.
nebulosum
    Simulium n.
NebuPent
    N. Inhalation
NEC
    necrotizing enterocolitis
necator
    Cupriavidus n.
Necator americanus (p)
necatrix
    Eimeria n.
necessarius
    Polynucleobacter n.
neck
    bull n.
    n. surgery
Neckar river virus (NRV)

N

NOTES

necrobiotic coagulum
necrogenes
 Fusobacterium n.*
necrolysis
 toxic epidermal n.
necroparasite
necrophilous
necrophorum
 Fusobacterium n.
 Fusobacterium necrophorum subsp.
  n.
necropsy
necrosis
 acute retinal n. (ARN)
 acute tubular n. (ATN)
 avascular n. (AVN)
 n. bacillus
 caseous n.
 fat n.
 full-thickness retinal n.
 hemorrhagic n.
 hepatocellular n.
 liquefaction n.
 progressive emphysematous n.
 progressive outer retinal n. (PORN)
 renal tubular n.
 varicella-zoster virus retinal n.
necrotic
 n. arachnidism
necroticans
 enteritis n.
necrotize
necrotizing
 n. amebic enterocolitis
 n. angiitis
 n. bowel disease (NBD)
 n. enterocolitis (NEC)
 n. fasciitis
 n. gingivostomatitis
 n. granulomatous inflammation
 n. infection
 n. inguinal adenopathy
 n. pneumonia
 n. retinitis
 n. soft-tissue infection (NSTI)
 n. stomatitis
 n. tonsillitis
 n. ulcerative gingivitis
 n. vasculitis
Necrovirus (v)
Nectonema
Nectonematoidea
Nectria (f)
 N. episphaeria
 N. haematococcus
 N. radicicola
Nectrioidaceae
Nectriopsis (f)

needle
 n. aspiration biopsy
 n. biopsy specimen
 n. culture
 n. exchange program
 Jamshidi n.
needlestick
nef gene
negative
 n. antigenemia
 gallium n.
 gram n.
negative-pressure box
negative-pressure isolation room
negevensis
 Simkania n.
NegGram
neghmei
 Anopheles franciscanus n.
neglectus
 Octomitus n.
Negri body
Neisseria (b)
 N. animalis
 BactiCard *N.*
 N. canis
 N. caviae
 N. cinerea
 N. cuniculi
 N. denitrificans
 N. dentiae
 N. elongata subsp. *elongata*
 N. elongata subsp. *glycolytica*
 N. flava
 N. flavescens
 N. gonorrhoeae
 N. gonorrhoeae culture
 N. gonorrhoeae DNA detection test
 N. gonorrhoeae susceptibility
  testing
 N. gonorrhoeae urethritis
 N. iguanae
 N. lactamica
 N. macacae
 N. meningitidis
 N. meningitidis vaccine
 N. mucosa
 N. mucosa endocarditis
 N. ovis
 N. perflava
 N. polysaccharea
 N. sicca
 N. subflava
 N. weaveri
Neisseria
Neisseriaceae
Neisseria-Haemophilus **Identification**
 (NHI)

Neisseria-Kwik test
neivai
> *Anopheles n.*

nelfinavir (NFV)
> n. mesylate

Nelson Bay orthoreovirus (NBV)
nelsoni
> *Trichinella n.*

Nemasol
nemathelminth
Nemathelminthes
nematicidal
nematicide
Nematocera
Nematoda
nematode
> anisakid n.
> trichuriid n.

nematodiasis
> cerebrospinal n.

Nematodirella longissimespiculata (p)
Nematodirus (p)
> *N. filicollis*
> *N. helvetianus*
> *N. spathiger*

nematoid
nematologist
nematology
Nematomorpha
nematophila
> *Xenorhabdus n.*

nematospermia
nemestrinae
> *Helicobacter n.*

nemodendra
> *Candida n.*

Neo
> N. Bace
> N. Citran Daycaps

Neoascaris vitulorum (p)
neoaurum
> *Mycobacterium n.*

neoceras
> *Fusarium n.*

Neochlamydia hartmannellae (b)
Neochordodes (p)
Neo-Cortef
> N.-C. Ophthalmic

Neocosmospora
> *N. vasinfecta*

NeoDecadron
> N. Ophthalmic
> N. Topical

Neoderm
Neo-Dexameth Ophthalmic
Neo-DM
neoendotheliazation
Neo-Estrone
neofagineus
> *Culicoides n.*

Neofed
neoformans
> *Cryptococcus n.*
> *Cryptococcus neoformans* var. *n.*
> *Filobasidiella n.*

Neo-fradin
> N.-f. Oral

neohemocyte
neomaculipalpus
> *Anopheles n.*

Neo-Metric
neomexicana
> *Cuterebra n.*

Neomixin Topical
neomontanus
> *Culicoides n.*

neomycin
> n., colistin, hydrocortisone, and
> thonzonium
> n. and polymyxin B
> n., polymyxin B, and
> dexamethasone
> n., polymyxin B, and gramicidin
> n., polymyxin B, and
> hydrocortisone
> n., polymyxin B, and prednisolone
> n. sulfate

neomycin/polymyxin/nalidixic acid
neonatal
> n. botulism
> n. herpes
> n. sepsis
> n. serum
> n. tetanus
> n. tuberculosis

neonate
neonatorium
> gonococcal ophthalmia n.
> herpes n.

neonatorum
> impetigo n.

N

NOTES

neonatorum *(continued)*
    noma n.
    ophthalmia n. (ON)
Neopap
neoplasia
    anal intraepithelial n.
    cervical intraepithelial n. (CIN)
    cervical invasive n. (CIN)
    EBV-associated lymphoid n.
    intraepithelial n.
neoplasm
    anogenital n.
    nasopharyngeal n.
neoplastic
    n. lesion
neoplasticum
    Gongylonema n.
neopropionicum
    Clostridium n.
neopterin
Neorickettsia helminthoeca (b)
Neosartorya fischeri (f)
Neospora canimum (p)
Neosporin
    N. Cream
    N. G.U. Irrigant
    N. Ophthalmic Ointment
    N. Ophthalmic solution
    N. Topical Ointment
neosquamocolumnar junction
Neo-Synephrine 12 Hour Nasal solution
Neo-Tabs
    N.-T. Oral
neoteny
Neotestudina rosatii (f)
neotomae
    Brucella n.
Neotopic
Neotricin HC Ophthalmic Ointment
Neotrombicula autumnalis (p)
neotype
    n. culture
    n. strain
Neo-Zol
nepalensis
    Catenuloplanes n.
nephrectomy
nephridium
nephritis
    acute interstitial n.
    acute tubulointerstitial n.
    interstitial n.
    tubular interstitial n.
    tubulointerstitial n.
nephritogenic
nephrocalcinosis
nephrogenic diabetes insipidus

nephrolithiasis
nephromegaly
Nephronex
nephropathia
    n. epidemica
nephropathy
    HIV-associated n. (HIVAN)
    quartan malarial n.
    reflux n.
nephrosis
    hemoglobinuric n.
nephrotic syndrome
nephrotoxic
    n. agent
nephrotoxicity
Nepovirus (v)
neptunium
    Hyphomicrobium n.
    Hyphomonas n.
Neptunomonas naphthovorans (b)
Nepuyo virus (NEPV)
NEPV
    Nepuyo virus
nereida
    Beneckea n.
nereis
    Vibrio n.
nerve
    long thoracic n.
    optic n.
    trigeminal n.
nervosa
    mycetism n.
Nesotriatoma
    N. flavida
nested PCR
Nesterenkonia halobia (b)
nesterenkovii
    Brachybacterium n.
Nestrex
nest of von Brunn
net
    n. anabolism
    n. catabolism
    Pap N.
neteri
    Cedecea n.
Netilmicin
Netivot virus
Netromycin
netropsis
    Streptomyces n.
    Streptoverticillium n.
Network
    HIV Vaccine Efficacy Trials N.
      (HIVNET)
    HIV Vaccine Trials N. (HVTN)

Neufeld
    N. capsular test
    N. reaction
neuii
    Actinomyces neuii subsp. *n.*
Neupogen Injection
neural
    n. growth factor
    n. larva migrans
    n. leprosy
    n. tube defect (NTD)
neuralgia
    postherpetic n.
    trigeminal n.
neuraminidase
neuridine
neuritic
neuritis
    acute n.
    brachial n.
    cranial n.
    experimental allergic n.
    optic n.
    peripheral n.
    sciatic n.
neuroblastoma
neuroborreliosis
neurobrucellosis
neurocysticercosis
neurodevelopmental
neurodevelopmental assessment
neuroendocrine
neurogenic
    n. bladder
neuroimaging
neuroleptic
    n. malignant syndrome (NMS)
neurologic
    n. dysfunction
neurolysis
    toxic epidermal n.
neurolyticum
    Mycoplasma n.
neuromuscular
    n. blockade
    n. paralysis
neuron
    lower motor n. (LMN)
    upper motor n. (UMN)
neuronal vacuolation
neuroophthalmologic
neuroparasitosis

neuropathia
    n. epidemica
neuropathic ulceration
neuropathy
    brachial plexus n.
    cranial n.
    diabetic n.
    multifocal motor n. (MMN)
    peripheral n.
    sensory n.
neurophagia
neuropil
neuropsychologic testing
neuroretinitis
Neurospora (f)
    N. crassa
    N. sitophila
neurosurgery
neurosyphilis
    meningovascular n.
    parenchymatous n.
    tertiary n.
neurotoxic
    n. shellfish poisoning (NSP)
neurotoxic cascade
neurotoxin
    botulinum n.
neurotoxoplasmosis
neurotropism
neurovirulence
neustonensis
    Porphyrobacter n.
neutralization test
Neutrexin
    N. Injection
Neutrogena
    N. Acne Mask
    N. Healthy Scalp Anti-Dandruff
    N. On-The-Spot Acne Lotion
    N. T/Derm
    N. T/Gel
neutropenia
    chemotherapy-induced n.
    cyclic n.
neutropenic
    n. enterocolitis
    n. fever
    n. host
    n. patient
neutrophil
    n. band
    n. chemotaxis

N

NOTES

neutrophil *(continued)*
    n. leukocyte count
    n. myelocyte
neutrophilia
neutrophilic
    n. infiltration
    n. pleocytosis
neutrophilus
    Thermoproteus n.
nevadensis
    Aedes n.
nevi (*pl.* of nevus)
Nevinny
    basophilic halo of N.
Nevirapine
nevirapine (NVP)
Nevskia ramosa (b)
nevus, pl. **nevi**
    spider n.
new
    n. combination
    N. Minto virus (NMV)
    N. World leishmaniasis
    N. York virus
Newcastle disease virus (NDV)
New-Durabolic
newer rifamycin
nexile
    Clostridium n.
neyagawaensis
    Streptomyces n.
NF Cough Syrup with Codeine
NFV
    nelfinavir
NG
    nasogastric
    NG tube
Ngaingan virus (NGAV)
Ngari virus (NRIV)
NGAV
    Ngaingan virus
N.G.T. Topical
NGU
    nongonococcal urethritis
NH
    nursing home
NHI
    Neisseria-Haemophilus Identification
NHL
    non-Hodgkin lymphoma
ni
    Trichoplusia n.
niacin accumulation test
niacini
    Bacillus n.
nickel and dime lesion
Niclocide
niclosamide

Nicolle white mycetoma
nicolli
    Spelotrema n.
nicotianae
    Arthrobacter n.
nicotinamide
    n. adenine dinucleotide
    n. adenine dinucleotide phosphate
    n. adenine dinucleotide phosphate
      positive (NADP$^+$)
    n. adenine dinucleotide phosphate
      positive dependent malic enzyme
    n. nucleoside
nicotinovorans
    Arthrobacter n.
nicrescens
    Prevotella n.
NidaGel
NIDDM
    noninsulin-dependent diabetes mellitus
nidulans
    Aspergillus n.
    Emericella n.
Nidulariaceae
Nidulariales
nidus
Niesslia (f)
nifedipine
nifurtimox
niger
    Aspergillus n.
    Catenuloplanes n.
    Ceratophyllus n.
    Culicoides n.
    Peptococcus n.
    Streptomyces n.
night
    Actifed Allergy Tablet (N.)
    N. Cast R
    n. soil
    n. sweat
Nighttime
    Baby N.
nigra
    Chainia n.
    Micromonospora n.
    Micromonospora halophytica subsp.
      n.
    Montoyella n.
    pityriasis n.
    tinea n.
nigrapulchrituda
    Beneckea n.
nigrescens
    Hyphelia n.
    Mermis n.
    Streptomyces n.
    Trichoderma n.

nigricans
    Azotobacter nigricans subsp. *n.*
    Herpetosiphon n.
    Lewinella n.
nigriceps
    Anthomyia n.
nigricoxum
    Simulium n.
nigrifaciens
    Alteromonas n.
    Pseudoalteromonas n.
    Streptomyces n.
nigrificans
    Carnimonas n.
    Desulfotomaculum n.
nigrifluens
    Brenneria n.
    Erwinia n.
nigripalpus
    Culex n.
nigripes
    Aedes n.
    Didymium n.
nigripulchritudo
    Vibrio n.
nigritarsis
    Anopheles n.
nigromaculis
    Aedes n.
nigrosin
    n. mount
    n. preparation
nigrosperma
    Monodictys n.
Nigrospora sphaerica (f)
nigrovittatus
    Tabanus n.
NIH
    National Institutes of Health
niigataensis
    Aminobacter n.
Nikolsky sign
nilotica
    Limnatis n.
nil per os (NPO)
Nilstat
nimbus
    Anopheles n.
nimipressuralis
    Enterobacter n.
    Erwinia n.
nimodipine

nimorazole
ninayi
NIOSH
    National Institute for Occupational Safety
    and Health
NIP
    nonspecific interstitial pneumonitis
Nipah virus
niphadopsis
    Aedes n.
niphandrodes
    Gregarina n.
nipponensis
    Ixodes n.
nipponicum
    Aquaspirillum itersonii subsp. *n.*
    Gnathostoma n.
Nique virus (NIQV)
NIQV
    Nique virus
NIR
    near-infrared interactance
niridazole
nishinomiyaensis
    Dermacoccus n.
    Micrococcus n.
nishizawae
    Pasteuria n.
nit
nitazoxanide
nitens
    Anocentor n.
nitida
    Gordonia n.
    Segmentina n.
nitidus
    lichen n.
nitrate
    butoconazole n.
    n. disk test
    econazole n.
    gallium n.
    n. to gas
    gas from n.
    miconazole n.
    n. reducer
    n. reduction test
    silver n. ($AgNO_3$)
nitrate-negative strain
nitratis
    Thialkalivibrio n.

N

NOTES

nitrativorans
    Comamonas n.
nitratophila
    Candida n.
nitratus
    Agromyces cerinus subsp. *n.*
nitrification
nitrite
    amyl n.
    n. reduction test
    urine n.
nitritigenes
    Actinomadura n.
nitritireducens
    Stenotrophomonas n.
nitritogenes
    Eubacterium n.
P-nitro-alpha-acetylamino-beta-hydroxypropiophenone (NAP)
Nitrobacter (b)
    N. alkalicus
    N. hamburgensis
    N. vulgaris
    N. winogradskyi
Nitrobacteraceae
Nitrocefin
    N. disk test
    N. testing
Nitrococcus mobilis (b)
Nitrocystis (*See* **Nitrobacter**)
nitrofigilis
    Arcobacter n.
    Campylobacter n.
nitrofural
nitrofuran
    n. derivative
nitrofurantoin
nitrofurazone
nitrogen
    blood urea n. (BUN)
    blood urea n./creatinine (BUN/Cr)
    liquid n.
nitrogen-rich
nitroglycerin
nitroimidazole
    n. derivative
nitrophenolicus
    Nocardioides n.
p-nitrophenylglycerol (PNPG)
nitroreducens
    Pseudomonas n.
Nitrosococcus (b)
    N. nitrosus
    N. oceani
Nitrosogloea (b) (*See* **Nitrobacter**)
Nitrosolobus multiformis (b)
Nitrosomonas europaea (b)

Nitrosospira (b)
    N. briensis
    N. multiformis
    N. tenuis
Nitrospina gracilis (b)
Nitrospira (b)
    N. marina
    N. moscoviensis
nitrosporeus
    Streptomyces n.
nitrosus
    Nitrosococcus n.
Nitschkiaceae
nivale
    Fusarium n.
    Leucosporidium n.
    Microdochium n.
nivalis
    Lanosa n.
    Micronectriella n.
nivea
    Fennellia n.
    Thiothrix n.
niveoalba
    Microtetraspora n.
niveoruber
    Streptomyces n.
niveus
    Aspergillus n.
    Streptomyces n.
Nix
    N. Creme Rinse
nizatidine
Nizoral
    N. A-D Shampoo
NJLV
    Naranjal virus
njovera
NK
    natural killer
      NK cell
Nkolbisson virus (NKOV)
NKOV
    Nkolbisson virus
NK-Spore Ophthalmic Ointment
NMR
    nuclear medicine
      NMR scan
NMS
    neuroleptic malignant syndrome
NMTSS
    nonmenstrual toxic shock syndrome
NMV
    New Minto virus
NM1 virus
NNIS
    National Nosocomial Infections Surveillance System

National Nosocomial Infection
  Surveillance
NNN medium
NNRTI
  nonnucleoside reverse transcriptase
  inhibitor
noackiae
  Buttiauxella n.
nobeli
  Plagiorchis n.
noboritoensis
  Streptomyces n.
Nocardia (b)
  N. abscessus
  N. africana
  N. amarae
  N. autotrophica
  N. brain abscess
  N. brasiliensis
  N. brevicatena
  N. calcarea
  N. carnea
  N. cellulans
  N. coeliaca
  N. corynebacterioides
  N. crassostreae
  N. culture
  N. cyriacigeorgici
  N. farcinica
  N. flavorosea
  N. globerula
  N. hydrocarbonoxydans
  N. mediterranei
  N. nova
  N. orientalis
  N. otitidiscaviarum
  N. paucivorans
  N. petroleophila
  N. pinensis
  N. pseudobrasiliensis
  N. restricta
  N. rugosa
  N. salmonicida
  N. saturnea
  N. seriolae
  N. sulphurea
  N. transvalensis
  N. uniformis
  N. vaccinii
  N. veterana
nocardia
Nocardiaceae

nocardiasis
nocardioform
  n. bacteria
Nocardioidaceae
Nocardioides (b)
  N. albus
  N. aquaticus
  N. fastidiosus
  N. jensenii
  N. luteus
  N. nitrophenolicus
  N. plantarum
  N. pyridinolyticus
  N. simplex
Nocardiopsis (b)
  N. africana
  N. alba
  N. alba subsp. *prasina*
  N. alborubida
  N. antarctica
  N. coeruleofusca
  N. dassonvillei subsp. *albirubida*
  N. dassonvillei subsp. *dassonvillei*
  N. dassonvillei subsp. *prasina*
  N. flava
  N. halophila
  N. kunsunensis
  N. listeri
  N. longispora
  N. lucentensis
  N. mutabilis
  N. prasina
  N. synnemataformans
  N. syringae
  N. trehalosei
  N. tropica
nocardiosis
nocturia
nocturnal
  n. microfilaria
  n. periodicity
nodal
  n. fever
  n. rhythm
Nodamura
  N. virus
nodatum
  Eubacterium n.
Nodaviridae
Nodavirus (v)
node
  atrioventricular n.

NOTES

node *(continued)*
    n. involvement
    lymph n. *(See* lymph node)
    mediastinal n.
    Osler n.
    sinoatrial n.
nodosa
    infantile periarteritis n.
    polyarteritis n.
    trichomycosis n.
nodososetosus
    Arachnomyces n.
nodosum
    erythema n.
    Fervidobacterium n.
nodosus
    Bacteroides n.
    Dichelobacter n.
    Streptomyces n.
nodovanous
nodular
    n. body
    n. disease
    n. eosinophilic panniculitis
    n. infiltrate
    n. leprosy
    n. lesion
    n. lymphoid hyperplasia
nodularis
    trichomycosis n.
nodule
    Aschoff n.
    cavitating pulmonary n.
    granulomatous n.
    lymphocutaneous n.
    miliary n.
    milker's n.
    noncavitating pulmonary n.
    oxyuris n.
    pulmonary n.
    subcutaneous n.
    ulcerative subcutaneous n.
nodulectomy
Nodulisporium (f)
noei
    Anopheles franciscanus n.
nogalater
    Streptomyces n.
noguchii
    Leptospira n.
nogueirai
    Simulium n.
noire
    tache n.
nojiriensis
    Streptomyces n.
Nola virus
Nolex LA

noma
    n. neonatorum
nomenclatural type
nomenclature
    binary n.
    linnaean system of n.
non-ABC hepatitis
nonadherence
nonadherent
non-A-E hepatitis
non-*Aeruginosa* pseudomonad
non-A-G hepatitis
No-Name Dandruff Treatment
nonan malaria
non-A, non-B (NANB)
    non-A, non-B hepatitis
    non-A, non-B hepatitis virus
nonbacterial
    n. diarrhea
    n. infection
    n. thrombotic endocarditis (NBTE)
nonbullous impetigo
nonbursate
noncardiogenic pulmonary edema
noncaseating
    n. granuloma
    n. granulomatous disease
noncavitating pulmonary nodule
noncellular
non-cholera *Vibrio* (NCV)
nonchromogenicum
    Mycobacterium n.
nonchromogens
nonclostridial anaerobic myonecrosis
noncoliform
nonconjugative plasmid
noncultivable
noncytolytic virus
nondermatophyte fungus
nondescript macular
nondiastaticum
    Streptosporangium n.
nondisseminated cutaneous leishmaniasis
Non-Drowsy
    Comtrex Maximum Strength N.-D.
    Contac Cold N.-D.
    Drixoral N.-D.
nondysenteric
nonencapsulated
nonenterococcal
nonenteropathogenic virus
nonenveloped
    n. virus
nonfasting glucose
nonfermentans
    Hansenula n.
    Pichia minuta var. *n.*
nonfermentative

nonfermenting
nonfilarial elephantiasis
nongonococcal
    n. septic arthritis
    n. urethritis (NGU)
nonhemolytic streptococcus
non-HIV chronic gingivitis
non-Hodgkin lymphoma (NHL)
nonhormonal
nonicteric
nonimmune
    n. agglutination
    n. hydrops
noninfectious
    n. disease complication
    n. urethritis
noninflammatory
    n. diarrhea
    n. myopathy
noninhibitory media
noninsulin-dependent diabetes mellitus
    (NIDDM)
nonjudgmental
nonlipophilic *Corynebacterium*
nonliquefaciens
    Moraxella (Moraxella) n.
    Pseudomonas n.
nonlytic virus
nonmalignant adenoidal hypertrophy
nonmenstrual toxic shock syndrome
    (NMTSS)
nonmotile
    n. pleomorphic bacillus
nonmucoid
nonneoplastic lymphadenopathy
nonnephrotic-range proteinuria
nonnucleoside
    n. reverse transcriptase inhibitor
      (NNRTI, NRTI)
    n. RT inhibitor
nonnutrient agar plate
nonoccluded baculovirus
nonoliguric
Nonomuraea (b)
    N. africana
    N. angiospora
    N. dietzii
    N. fastidiosa
    N. ferruginea
    N. flexuosa
    N. helvata
    N. longicatena

    N. polychroma
    N. pusilla
    N. recticatena
    N. roseola
    N. roseoviolacea subsp. *carminata*
    N. roseoviolacea subsp.
      roseoviolacea
    N. rubra
    N. salmonea
    N. spiralis
    N. turkmeniaca
nonopiate
nonoxynol
nonoxynol-9 (N-9)
nonparalytic polio
nonpathogenic
    n. spirochetal
nonphotochromogen
nonpigment-producing acid-fast bacillus
nonpitting edema
nonpneumonic
nonpolio enterovirus
nonproductive
nonprogressive
nonpruritic
nonreactive dermatitis
nonreproducible
nonscarring alopecia
nonseptate mycelium
nonsexual generation
non-small cell lung cancer (NSCLC)
nonspecific
    n. interstitial pneumonitis (NIP,
      NSIP)
    n. vaginosis
non-spore-forming
    n.-s.-f. bacteria
nonsporulating
nonsteroidal
    n. antiinflammatory
    n. antiinflammatory agent (NSAIA)
    n. antiinflammatory drug (NSAID)
nonsuppurative
nonsurgically
nonsynchronous budding
nonsyncytium-inducing (NSI)
nontoxigenic
nontreponemal
    n. genital ulcer disease
    n. serologic test
    n. syphilis test

N

NOTES

nontuberculous
  n. meningitis
  n. mycobacteria (NTM)
  n. pneumonia
nontypeable *Haemophilus influenzae*
nontyphi
  n. *Salmonella* bacteremia
nontyphoidal
  n. salmonella infection
  n. *Salmonella* species
  n. salmonellosis
nonulcerative disease
nonvenereal syphilis
nonviable
nonviral hepatitis
No Pain-HP
nopporoensis
  Hyalopus n.
norbensis
  Saccharomyces n.
nordeoxyguanosine
norepinephrine
norfloxacin
norimbergensis
  Burkholderia n.
  Pandoraea n.
Noritate
  N. Cream
normal
  n. antitoxin
  n. gut flora
  n. pressure hydrocephalus
normoblast
normocellular
normochromic
normocytic normochromic anemia
normoinsulinemia
noroestensis
  Anopheles n.
Noroxin
  N. Oral
Norplant
Nor-tet Oral
North
  N. American blastomycosis
  N. Asian tick typhus
  N. Queensland tick fever
Northway virus (NORV)
nortriptyline
NORV
  Northway virus
norvegensis
  Candida n.
  Pichia n.
norvegica
  Candida n.
  Thermodesulforhabdus n.

norvegicum
  Desulfomicrobium n.
norvegicus
  Dinophysis n.
Norvir
Norwalk
  N. agent
  N. gastroenteritis
  N. virus
Norwalk-like
  N.-l. agent
Norway itch
Norwegian scabies
Nosema (p)
  N. algerae
  N. bombycis
  N. connori
  N. lophii
  N. whitei
nosema disease
Nosematidae
Nosematidida
nosocomial
  n. bacteremia
  n. eye infection
  n. gastroenteritis
  n. infective endocarditis
  n. keratitis
  n. myiasis
  n. pathogen
  n. pneumonia
  n. retinochoroiditis
  n. rotavirus infection
  n. salmonellosis
  n. urinary tract infection
  n. viral conjunctivitis
nosocominal infection
nosomycosis
nosophora
  Oncomelania n.
nosophyte
Nosopsyllus fasciatus (p)
nostras
  piedra n.
Nostrilla
notatum
  Simulium n.
noterae
  Acetoanaerobium n.
Notezine
notiale
  Simulium n.
notifiable infectious disease
Notoedres cati (p)
noursei
  Streptomyces n.
nova
  Nocardia n.

Novacet Topical
novaecaesareae
    Streptomyces n.
Novahistex
    N. DM
    N. DM Expectorant
Novahistine
    N. DM
    N. DM Expectorant
novamexicanus
    Culicoides n.
Novamoxin
Nova Perfecting Lotion
Novasen
Novatoxyl
novella
    Starkeya n.
novellus
    Thiobacillus n.
novel pathogen
novicida
    Francisella n.
    Francisella tularensis biogroup *n.*
Novirhabdovirus (v)
Novo-AZT
Novobetamet
novobiocin
    n. resistance
    n. susceptibility test
novobiosepticus
    Staphylococcus hominis subsp. *n.*
novocastrense
    Mycobacterium n.
Novo-Cefaclor
Novo-Chlorocap
Novo-Cimetine
Novo-Cloxin
Novo-Doxylin
Novo-Famotidine
Novo-Furan
Novo-Gesic
Novo-Ketoconazole
Novo-Lexin
Novo-Naprox
Novo-Nidazol
Novo-Norfloxacin
Novo-Pen-VK
Novo-Pranol
Novo-Prednisolone
Novo-Profen
Novo-Ranidine
Novo-Rythro Encap

Novo-Salmol
Novo-Soxazole
Novosphingobium (b)
    N. aromaticivorum
    N. capsulatum
    N. roseae
    N. stygiae
    N. subarcticum
    N. subterraneae
Novo-Sucralate
Novo-Tetra
Novo-Trimel
Novo-Triphyl
Novo-Zolamide
novyi
    Clostridium n.
Novy and MacNeal blood agar
Novy-MacNeal-Nicolle medium
noxia
    Selenomonas n.
NP-27
NPO
    nil per os
n-propanol
NR
    Organidin NR
    Tussi-Organidin DM NR
NRIV
    Ngari virus
NRTI
    nonnucleoside reverse transcriptase
      inhibitor
    nucleoside analog reverse transcriptase
      inhibitor
    nucleoside reverse transcriptase inhibitor
NRV
    Neckar river virus
NSAIA
    nonsteroidal antiinflammatory agent
NSAID
    nonsteroidal antiinflammatory drug
NSCLC
    non-small cell lung cancer
NSDV
    Nairobi sheep disease virus
NSI
    nonsyncytium-inducing
NSIP
    nonspecific interstitial pneumonitis
NSP
    neurotoxic shellfish poisoning

N

NOTES

NSTI
    necrotizing soft-tissue infection
NTAV
    Ntaya virus
Ntaya virus (NTAV)
NTCC
    National Type Culture Collection
NTD
    neural tube defect
NTM
    nontuberculous mycobacteria
nt-1, -2 virus
NTZ Long Acting Nasal solution
NU10
    Pseudomonas aeruginosa N.
Nu-Amoxi
Nu-Ampi
    N.-A. Trihydrate
NuBasics
Nu-Cephalex
nuchal
    n. rigidity
Nu-Cimet
nuclear
    n. medicine (NMR)
    n. medicine scan
    n. polyhedrosis virus
nucleated
    n. red blood cell
nucleatum
    Fusobacterium nucleatum subsp. *n.*
nuclei
nuclei (*pl. of* nucleus)
nucleic
    n. acid amplification
    n. acid amplification test
    n. acid hybridization
    n. acid hybridization analysis
    n. acid hybridization test
    n. acid probe
    n. acid probe assay
    n. acid sequence-band amplification
        (NASBA)
    n. acid sequence-based amplification
        (NASBA, NAS-BA)
nucleocapsid
nucleolus, pl. **nucleoli**
Nucleophaga
Nucleopolyhedrovirus (v)
nucleopolyhedrovirus
    multiple n. (MNPV)
    single n. (SNPV)
Nucleopore filter
Nucleorhabdovirus (v)
nucleoside
    n. analog
    n. analog reverse transcriptase
        inhibitor (NRTI)

    n. monophosphate
    n. monotherapy
    nicotinamide n.
    n. reverse transcriptase inhibitor
        (NRTI)
**nucleoside-associated mitochondrial
    toxicity**
nucleotide
    n. analog
    n. sequence analysis
nucleotide reverse transcriptase inhibitor
nucleus, pl. **nuclei**
    basal n.
    basket n.
    gametic n.
    germ n.
    gonad n.
    reproductive n.
    somatic n.
    trophic n.
NucliSens
    N. test
    N. testing
Nu-Cloxi
Nucofed
    N. Pediatric Expectorant
Nu-Cotrimox
Nucotuss
Nudibaculovirinae
nudiseta
    Synthesiomyia n.
nudiventrus
    Dissonus n.
Nu-Doxycycline
Nu-Famotidine
Nugent score
Nugget virus (NUGV)
NUGV
    Nugget virus
Nu-Ibuprofen
Nu-Ketocon
null hypothesis
nulliparity
numerical taxonomy
Numzitdent
Numzit Teething
Nu-Naprox
nunestovari
    Simulium n.
nunezi
    Microcerebus n.
nuneztovari
    Anopheles n.
Nu-Pen-VK
Nuprin
Nu-Prochlor
Nu-Propranolol

Nu-Ranit
nursing home (NH)
Nu-Tetra
Nutracort Topical
nutrient agar
nutrition
    parenteral n.
    total parenteral n. (TPN)
nutritionally variant streptococcus (NVS)
Nutrol A D
Nuttallia obscurata
NVAC
    National Vaccine Advisory Committee
NVP
    nevirapine
NVS
    nutritionally variant streptococcus
Nyaderm
Nyando virus (NDOV)
nycticoracis
    Cathaemasia n.

Nyctotheridae
Nyctotherus (p)
    N. cordiformis
    N. ovalis
Nydrazid
nymph
nymphaerum
    Dichotomophthoropsis n.
nymphal
nyssa
    Simulium n.
nystagmus
nystatin
    n. solution
    topical n.
    n. and triamcinolone
nystatin-resistant *Candida rugosa*
Nystat-Rx
Nystex
Nytrel filter

NOTES

N

O

O agglutinin
O colony

O:5

Yersinia enterocolitica biotype 1,
serotype O.

O/129

vibriostatic agent O.

O087 virus
o6 virus
oakridgensis

Legionella o.

Oak-Vale virus
O.A.S.I.S. Blood Culture System
oatmeal-tomato paste agar
OB

occult blood

obamensis

Rhodothermus o.

Obermeier spirillum
obesity

morbid o.
truncal o.

obesum

Simulium o.

Obesumbacterium (b)

O. proteus

obeum

Ruminococcus o.

objective synonym
obligate

o. aerobe
o. anaerobe
o. intracellular parasite
o. intracellular protozoan

obliterans

endarteritis o.

obliterative endarteritis
oblongata

medulla o.

obnubilation
Obodhiang virus
oboediens

Acetobacter o.
Gluconacetobacter o.

obovatum

Phialemonium o.

obovoideum

Ramichloridium o.

obscurata

Nuttallia oN.

obscuriglobus

Gemmata o.

obscuripennis

Anthomyia o.
Culicoides o.

obscurus

Geodermatophilus o.

obsoletus

Culicoides o.

obstetric factor
obstructing bronchial aspergillosis
obstruction

bile duct o.
bladder neck o.
high-grade extrahepatic biliary o.
mechanical o.

obstructive uropathy
obtundation
obtunded
obtusa

Holospora o.

obtusisporum

Cylindrocarpon o.

obtusum

Arthroderma o.

obuense

Mycobacterium o.

obuensis

Rhodococcus o.

obvelata

Syphacia o.

obvelatus

Cosmocephalus o.

obviating
OC

oral contraceptive

Oc1r virus
occidentalis

Anopheles o.
Dermatocentor o.
Pogonomyrmex o.

occluded baculovirus
Occlusal
Occlusal-HP Liquid
occlusion

hyaline glomerular o.

occlusive vasculitis
occult

o. blood (OB)
o. blood test
o. filariasis

occulta

Wyeomyia o.

occultum

Pyrodictium o.

occultus

Natronococcus o.

O

Occupational Safety and Health Administration (OSHA)

oceanense
> Desulfofrigus o.

oceani
> Nitrosococcus o.

oceanicum
> Clostridium o.

Oceanimonas (b)
> O. baumannii
> O. doudoroffii

oceanitis
> Hyphomonas o.

oceanosedimentum
> Flavobacterium o.

Oceanospirillum (b)
> O. beijerinckii subsp. beijerinckii
> O. beijerinckii subsp. pelagicum
> O. commune
> O. hiroshimense
> O. jannaschii
> O. japonicum
> O. kriegii
> O. linum
> O. maris subsp. hiroshimense
> O. maris subsp. maris
> O. maris subsp. williamsae
> O. minutulum
> O. multiglobuliferum
> O. pelagicum
> O. pusillum
> O. vagum

Oceanside virus
ocellus
ochracea
> Capnocytophaga o.
> Chainia o.
> Leptothrix o.

ochraceiscleroticus
> Streptomyces o.

ochraceum
> Simulium o.

ochraceus
> Aspergillus o.
> Bacteroides o.

ochratoxin
> o. A

ochripes
> Anthomyia o.

Ochrobactrum (b)
> O. anthropi
> O. grignonense
> O. intermedium
> O. tritici

Ochroconis (f)
> O. constricta
> O. gallopavum
> O. humicola

Ochromobactrum anthropii (b)
Ockelbo
> Sindbis virus subtype O.
> O. virus

OCP
> Onchocerciasis Control Program
> oral contraceptive pill

ocreata
> Amanita o.

Octadecabacter (b)
> O. antarcticus
> O. arcticus

octapeptide
> cyclic o.

Octavianiaceae
octavius
> Anaerococcus o.
> Peptostreptococcus o.

octenidine
Octicair Otic
Octomitidae
Octomitus (p)
> O. intestinalis
> O. neglectus

octreodile
octreotide
> o. acetate

octulosonic acid
OcuClear Ophthalmic
Ocuflox Ophthalmic
Ocugram
ocular
> o. amoebic keratitis
> o. cysticercosis
> o. cytology
> o. infection
> o. larva migrans
> o. larva migrans granuloma
> o. micrometer
> o. mycosis
> o. myiasis
> o. onchocerciasis
> o. sparganosis
> o. syphilis
> o. toxoplasmosis
> o. trachoma
> o. tuberculosis
> o. zoster

oculata
> Gordiacea o.

oculi
> Acholeplasma o.

oculifera
> Anthomyia o.

oculogenital disease
oculoglandular tularemia
oculo-hominis
> Phoma o.-h.

oculomotor nerve palsy
Ocu-Merox
Ocumycin
Ocusulf-10 Ophthalmic
Ocutricin
    O. Ophthalmic solution
    O. Topical Ointment
Oddi
odds ratio (OR)
odintsovae
    Candida o.
odontogenic
    o. infection
odontolyticus
    Actinomyces o.
Odontotremataceae
odor
    amine o.
odoratimimus
    Myroides o.
odoratum
    Flavobacterium o.
odoratus
    Myroides o.
odorifer
    Streptomyces o.
odorifera
    Serratia o.
subsp. *odorifera*
    Erwinia carotovora subsp. *odorifera*
odoriferum
    Pectobacterium carotovorum subsp.
    o.
odorimutans
    Anaerovorax o.
odorus
    Sporobolomyces o.
Odrenisrou virus (ODRV)
ODRV
    Odrenisrou virus
odynophagia
Oedaleus senegalensis
oeni
    Oenococcus o.
Oenococcus oeni (b)
oenos
    Leuconostoc o.
Oerskovia (b)
    O. turbata
    O. xanthineolytica
oesophagostomiasis
Oesophagostominae

Oesophagostomum (p)
    O. apiostomum
    O. bifurcum
    O. columbianum
    O. dentatum
    O. quadrispinulatum
    O. radiatum
    O. venulosum
Oestridae
oestrids
Oestrilin
oestrosis
oestruosa
    myiasis o.
Oestrus ovis (p)
Off-Ezy
ofloxacin
Ogawa
    Vibrio cholerae O1 biotype El Tor
     serotype O.
    Vibrio cholerae serotype *O.*
oguniense
    Pyrobaculum o.
OHFV
    Omsk hemorrhagic fever virus
ohioensis
    Isospora o.
OHL
    oral hairy leukoplakia
ohmeri
    Endomycopsis o.
    Pichia o.
ohwakuensis
    Sulfurisphaera o.
OIA
    optimal immunoassay
oidia
Oidiodendron cerealis (f)
oidiomycin
Oidium (f)
oidium
oiketorakras
    Anopheles o.
oil
    BAL in O.
    castor o.
    coal tar, lanolin, and mineral o.
    soybean o.
Oil-Free Acne Wash
oil-immersion microscopy
ointment
    A and D O.

O

NOTES

ointment *(continued)*
    AK-Spore H.C. Ophthalmic O.
    Antibiotic O.
    Baby's Own O.
    Cormax O.
    Cortisporin Ophthalmic O.
    Cortisporin Topical O.
    Medi-Quick Topical O.
    Neosporin Ophthalmic O.
    Neosporin Topical O.
    Neotricin HC Ophthalmic O.
    NK-Spore Ophthalmic O.
    Ocutricin Topical O.
    Panscol O.
    Salacid O.
    Septa Topical O.
    Terak Ophthalmic O.
    Terramycin w/Polymyxin B
      Ophthalmic O.
    Whitfield o.
Oita 296 virus
OK-432
okadaic acid
okeanokoites
    Flavobacterium o.
    Planococcus o.
    Planomicrobium o.
okenii
    Chromatium o.
Okhotskiy virus (OKHV)
OKHV
    Okhotskiy virus
oklahomensis
    Culicoides o.
Okola virus (OKOV)
OKOV
    Okola virus
OKT3 murine monoclonal antibody
olamine
    ciclopirox o.
oldenburgensis
    Methanoculleus o.
Old World leishmaniasis
oleaceus
    Saccharomyces o.
olearium
    Sporobacterium o.
Oleavirus (v)
olecranon bursitis
olentangyi
    Methanoculleus o.
    Methanogenium o.
oleophila
    Candida o.
oleovorans
    Pseudomonas o.
oleronius
    Bacillus o.

olfactory spread
olidum
    Cylindrocarpon o.
Olifantsvlei virus (OLIV)
Oligacanthorhynchidae
oligarthrus
    Echinococcus o.
Oligella (b)
    O. ureolytica
    O. urethralis
oligoarticular
oligoclonal band
oligohydramnios
oligomenorrhea
oligosaccharide
    sialic acid-containing o.
oligospermia
oligospora
    Actinomadura o.
    Arthobotrys o.
oligosymptomatic
Oligotropha carboxidovorans (b)
oligotrophica
    Agromonas o.
oliguria
oliogoarthritis
oliterans
    balanitis xerotica o.
OLIV
    Olifantsvlei virus
olivacea
    Chainia o.
olivaceiscleroticus
    Streptomyces o.
olivaceoviridis
    Streptomyces o.
olivaceum
    Coniosporium o.
olivaceus
    Streptomyces o.
olivapovliticus
    Alkalibacterium o.
olivasterospora
    Micromonospora o.
olivatrum
olivochromogenes
    Streptomyces o.
olivomycini
    Streptomyces o.
    Streptoverticillium o.
olivoreticuli
    Streptomyces olivoreticuli subsp. *o.*
    Streptoverticillium olivoreticuli
      subsp. *o.*
    Streptoverticillium olivoreticuli
      subsp. *o.*
olivoreticulum

olivoverticillatum
>   Streptoverticillium o.
olivoverticillatus
>   Streptomyces o.
olivoviridis
>   Streptomyces o.
Ollulanus tricuspis (p)
Olpidiaceae
Olpidiopsidaceae
omega-3 fatty acid
Omega Cohort
Omegatetravirus (v)
omentum
>   o. magnum
omeprazole
omiyaensis
>   Streptomyces o.
Omnicef
Omniflox
OmniHIB
>   O. vaccine
Omnipen
Omnipen-N
omnivorous
OMOV
>   Omo virus
Omo virus (OMOV)
omphalitis
Omphalospora (f)
Omphalotus illudens (f)
Omsk
>   O. hemorrhagic fever
>   O. hemorrhagic fever virus
>   (OHFV)
ON
>   ophthalmia neonatorum
Oncet
Onchocerca (p)
>   O. cervicalis
>   O. gibsoni
>   O. gutturosa
>   O. volvulus
onchocerciasis
>   ocular o.
Onchocerciasis Control Program (OCP)
onchocercid
Onchocercidae
Onchocercinae
onchocercoma
onchocercosis
onchodermatitis
oncogene

oncogenesis
oncogenic
oncologist
>   medical o.
Oncomelania
>   O. nosophora
>   O. quadrasi
oncosphere
>   o. embryo
OncoTICE
oncovirus
>   mouse mammary o.
>   porcine type C o.
oneidensis
>   Shewanella o.
one-stop shop
Onguent
>   Antibiotique O.
Onicola spirula (p)
ONNV
>   O'nyong-nyong virus
onset
>   sexual o.
Onychocola canadensis (f)
onychomycosis
Ony-Clear
>   O.-C. Nail
>   O.-C. Spray
Onygenaceae
O'nyong-nyong
>   O.-n. fever
>   O.-n. virus (ONNV)
oogonium
ookinete
Oomycetes
oomycosis
oophorectomy
oophoritis
oortii
>   Corynebacterium o.
Oospora granulosa (f)
oosporangium
oospore
ootype
Opa
>   opacity
>   Opa protein
>   Opa typing
opaca
>   Wohlfahrtia o.
opacification

O

NOTES

opacities
opacity (Opa)
    corneal o.
    o. protein
opacus
    Rhodococcus o.
opalescens
    Mycoplasma o.
opalinifrons
    Simulium o.
open reading frame (ORF)
open-wedge biopsy specimen
operating room (OR)
opercula (*pl. of* operculum)
operculated
operculate egg
operculum, pl. **opercula**
Opherophtera brumata
Ophiobolus heterosporus
Ophiostoma (f)
    O. bacillisporum
    O. distortum
    O. minus
    O. multiannulatum
    O. piceae
    O. piliferum
    O. triangulosporum
Ophiostomataceae
Ophiostomatales
Ophiovirus (v)
Ophryoscolecidae
Ophthacet
ophthalmia
    Egyptian o.
    granular o.
    o. neonatorum (ON)
Ophthalmic
    Achromycin O.
    AK-Chlor O.
    AK-Cide O.
    AK-Neo-Dex O.
    AK-Poly-Bac O.
    AK-Sulf O.
    AKTob O.
    AK-Tracin O.
    Alomide O.
    Bleph-10 O.
    Blephamide O.
    Cetamide O.
    Cetapred O.
    Chibroxin O.
    Chloroptic O.
    Chloroptic-P O.
    Ciloxan O.
    Genoptic S.O.P. O.
    Gentacidin O.
    Gentak O.
    Ilotycin O.

    Isopto Cetamide O.
    Isopto Cetapred O.
    Metimyd O.
    Natacyn O.
    Neo-Cortef O.
    NeoDecadron O.
    Neo-Dexameth O.
    OcuClear O.
    Ocuflox O.
    Ocusulf-10 O.
    Ophthochlor O.
    Polysporin O.
    Polytrim O.
    Pred-G O.
    Quixin O.
    Sodium Sulamyd O.
    Sulf-10 O.
    TobraDex O.
    Tobrex O.
    Tomycine O.
    Vasocidin O.
    Vasosulf O.
    Vira-A O.
    Viroptic O.
    Visine L.R. O.
ophthalmic/topical
    erythromycin (ophthalmic/topical)
ophthalmicus
    herpes zoster o.
    zoster o.
ophthalmic zoster
ophthalmoganglionary complex
ophthalmomycosis
ophthalmomyiasis
ophthalmoplegia
ophthalmoscope
ophthalmoscopy
    direct o.
    indirect o.
Ophtho-Chloram
Ophthochlor Ophthalmic
Ophthocort
Ophtho-Sulf
opiate
    o. antispasmodic
opisthomastigote
opisthorchiasis
opisthorchid
Opisthorchiida
Opisthorchiidae
Opisthorchioidea
Opisthorchis (p)
    O. felineus
    O. tenuicollis
    O. viverrini
opisthotonic posture
opisthotonus

OpMNPV
> *Orgyia pseudotsugata* MNPV

opportunist

opportunistic
> o. pathogen
> o. systemic fungal infection

opsonic
> o. defect

opsonin
> immune o.

opsonization

opsonophagocytosis assay

optic
> o. atrophy tremor
> o. chiasm
> o. disc
> o. disk edema
> o. nerve
> o. neuritis

optic chiasm

optimal immunoassay (OIA)

Optimyxin
> O. Plus

optochin

Optochin susceptibility test

OPV
> oral polio vaccine
> oral poliovirus vaccine

OPV-Sabin vaccine

OR
> odds ratio
> operating room

Orabase
> O. HCA Topical
> Kenalog in O.
> O. Plain

Orabase-B

Orabase-O

Orajel
> Baby O.
> Maximum Strength O.
> O. Maximum Strength
> O. Perioseptic

oral
> Aristocort O.
> Atolone O.
> o. attenuated poliomyelitis virus vaccine
> Bio-Tab O.
> o. candidiasis
> o. candidosis
> o. cavity tuberculosis

CeeNU O.
Ceftin O.
Celestone O.
Cipro O.
Cleocin HCl O.
Cleocin Pediatric O.
Coly-Mycin S O.
o. contraceptive (OC)
o. contraceptive pill (OCP)
o. contrast
Decadron O.
Delta-Cortef O.
o. donovanosis
Dynacin O.
o. erosive lichen planus
Estrace O.
Flagyl O.
Gly-Oxide O.
o. hairy leukoplakia (OHL)
o. infection
Kenacort O.
Lamisil O.
o. lesion
Loniten O.
Medrol O.
Minocin O.
Mycifradin Sulfate O.
Neo-fradin O.
Neo-Tabs O.
Noroxin O.
Nor-tet O.
Panmycin O.
PediaCare O.
Pediapred O.
o. polio vaccine (OPV)
o. poliovirus vaccine (OPV)
Prelone O.
Protostat O.
Proxigel O.
o. rehydration
o. rehydration solution (ORS)
Rifadin O.
Rimactane O.
Robitet O.
o. squamous cell carcinoma
Sumycin O.
o. suspension
terbinafine (o.)
Terramycin O.
Tetracap O.
o. thrush
triamcinolone (inhalation, o.)

O

NOTES

oral *(continued)*
    o. ulceration
    Unipen O.
    Uri-Tet O.
    Vancocin O.
oral-dental
orale
    Desulfomicrobium o.
    Mycoplasma o.
oralis
    Bacteroides o.
    Kingella o.
    Methanobrevibacter o.
    Prevotella o.
    Streptococcus o.
orange
    acridine o. (AO)
    o. cast
Orasept
Orasol
Orasone
Orbenin
orbiculare
orbiscindens
    Clostridium o.
orbit
orbital
    o. abscess
    o. apex syndrome
    o. cellulitis
    o. infection
    o. tuberculosis
orbitale
    Simulium o.
Orbivirus (v)
orbivirus
orchiococcus
orchitis
    massive granulomatous o.
Orcytes rhinoceros
ordalii
    Vibrio o.
order
Ordrine AT Extended Release Capsule
oregonense
    Methanohalophilus o.
oregonensis
    Candida o.
    Culicoides o.
    Heliothrix o.
orellanine
orellanus
    Cortinarius o.
Orenia (b)
    O. marismortui
    O. salinaria
    O. sivashensis

orenii
    Halothermothrix o.
ORF
    open reading frame
orf
    o. virus
    o. virus subgroup
organ
    reproductive o.'s
organelle
    cell o.
organelles
    paired o.
organic arsenical
Organidin NR
organism
    aerobic facultatively anaerobic o.
    Aerococcus-like o. (ALO)
    BCG o.
    Campylobacter-like o. (CLO)
    community-acquired o.
    eukaryotic o.
    fastidious o.
    gram-negative o.
    gram-positive o.
    hypothetical mean o. (HMO)
    pleomorphic o.
    pleuropneumonia-like o.'s (PPLO)
organism-host interaction
Organization
    Bulletin of World Health O.
    Joint Commission on Accreditation
      of Healthcare O.'s (JCAHO)
    Pan American Health O.
organoid
organomegaly
organophilum
    Methanogenium o.
    Methylobacterium o.
organotrophum
    Pyrobaculum o.
organotropic
organotropism
organotropy
organotypic culture
organovorum
    Acidiphilium o.
Orgyia pseudotsugata **MNPV (OpMNPV)**
Oribaculum catoniae (b)
Oriboca virus (ORIV)
oriental
    o. cholangiohepatitis
    o. ringworm
    o. schistosomiasis
    o. sore
    o. ulcer

orientale
    Gongylonema o.
    Microsporum o.
orientalis
    Amycolatopsis orientalis subsp. *o.*
    Atherigona o.
    Issatchenkia o.
    Nocardia o.
    Streptomyces o.
    Vibrio o.
Orientia tsutsugamushi (b)
orientis
    Desulfosporosinus o.
    Desulfotomaculum o.
    Rhodobium o.
Orientobilharzia
orificial tuberculosis
origin
    fever of unknown o. (FUO)
    unknown o.
Original
    Doan's, O.
Orimune
orinoci
    Streptomyces o.
    Streptoverticillium o.
oris
    Bacteroides o.
    cancrum o.
    Lactobacillus o.
    Prevotella o.
orisratti
    Streptococcus o.
oritzi
    Gigantorhynchus o.
ORIV
    Oriboca virus
Oriximina virus (ORXV)
orleanensis
    Acetobacter o.
    Acetobacter aceti subsp. *o.*
Ornade-DM
ornate
Ornex Cold
Ornex-DM
ornidazole
Ornidyl
    O. Injection
Ornithidorus (p)
ornithine
    o. deaminase
    o. test

Ornithinicoccus hortensis (b)
Ornithinimicrobium humiphilum (b)
ornithinolytica
    Klebsiella o.
Ornithobacterium rhinotracheale (b)
Ornithobilharzia (p)
    O. canaliculata
    O. intermedia
    O. pricei
Ornithodoros (p)
    O. erraticus
    O. hermsi
    Ornithodoros moubata
    O. parkeri
    O. rudis
    O. savignyi
    O. talaje
    O. tholozani
    O. turicata
    O. venezuelensis
    O. verrucosus
Ornithonyssus (p)
    O. bacoti
    O. bursa
    O. sylviarum
ornithosis virus
oroanal contact
Oro-Clense
orofacial odontogenic infection
orogenital
orolabial herpes
oronasal junction
oropharyngeal
    o. anthrax
    o. aphthae
    o. candidiasis
    o. lesion
    o. mucosa
    o. tularemia
oropharynx
Oropouche virus (OROV)
oroticum
    Clostridium o.
OROV
    Oropouche virus
Oroya fever
orphan
    enteric cytopathic human o.
    (ECHO)
    enteric cytopathogenic human o.
    (ECHO)
    o. virus

O

NOTES

ORS
oral rehydration solution
ORSA
oxacillin-resistant *Staphylococcus aureus*
Ortho-Dienestrol Vaginal
Orthohepadnavirus (v)
Orthomyxoviridae
orthomyxovirus
orthopnea
Orthopoxvirus (v)
orthopoxvirus
OrthoProbe assay
Orthoptera
Orthoreovirus (v)
orthoreovirus
  avian o.
  mammalian o. (MRV)
  Nelson Bay o. (NBV)
orthostasis
orthostatic
  o. dizziness
  o. syncope
orthostatic hypotension
ortizi
  Simulium o.
Orungo virus (ORUV)
ORUV
  Orungo virus
ORXV
  Oriximina virus
oryzae
  Aspergillus o.
  Azospira o.
  Bullera o.
  Methanobacterium o.
  Tritirachium o.
  Xanthomonas o.
Oryzavirus (v)
oryzihabitans
  Flavimonas o.
  Pseudomonas o.
os
  nil per os (NPO)
Oscillochloris (b)
  O. chrysea
  O. trichoides
Oscillospira guilliermondii (b)
osculatum
  Contracaecum o.
oseltamir
oseltamivir .
O-serotype
OSHA
  Occupational Safety and Health
  Administration
oshimae
  Picrophilus o.

oshimai
  Thermus o.
Osler node
osloensis
  Moraxella (Moraxella) o.
osmotic
ossamyceticus
  Streptomyces hygroscopicus subsp.
  o.
OSSAV
  Ossa virus
Ossa virus (OSSAV)
osseous hydatid cyst
ossification
  heterotopic o.
osteitis
  acne-pustulosis-hyperostosis-o.
osteoarthritis
  dystrophic o.
osteoarthropathy
  hypertrophic o. (HOA)
osteoarticular
  o. candidiasis
  o. sporotrichosis
  o. tuberculosis
osteochondritis
osteomalacia
osteomyelitis
  Aspergillus o.
  Candida o.
  candidal o.
  chronic diffuse sclerosing o.
  Kingella kingae o.
  pelvic o.
  sternal o.
  tuberculous o.
  vertebral o.
osteonecrosis
osteopathy
  diabetic o.
osteopenia
osteoporosis
osteoradionecrosis
ostertagi
  Ostertagia o.
Ostertagia (p)
  O. circumcincta
  O. ostertagi
  O. trifurcata
Ostertagiinae
ostreatus
  Pleurotus o.
Ostropales
oswaldoi
  Anopheles o.
otae
  Arthroderma o.

Otic
    Acetasol HC O.
    AK-Spore H.C. O.
    AntibiOtic O.
    Bacticort O.
    Cipro HC O.
    Coly-Mycin O.
    Cortatrigen O.
    Cortisporin O.
    Cortisporin-TC O.
    O. Domeboro
    Dri-Ear O.
    Drotic O.
    Ear-Eze O.
    LazerSporin-C O.
    Octicair O.
    Otic-Care O.
    OtiTricin O.
    Otobiotic O.
    Otocort O.
    Otomycin-HPN O.
    Otosporin O.
    Pediotic O.
    Swim-Ear O.
    UAD O.
    VoSol HC O.
Otic-Care Otic
oticus
    herpes zoster o.
otitidis
    Brevibacterium o.
    Turicella o.
otitidiscaviarum
    Nocardia o.
otitis
    acute suppurative o.
    Alloiococcus o.
    o. externa
    Haemophilus influenzae o.
    malignant external o.
    o. media
    syphilitic o.
otitis media
OtiTricin Otic
otobiosis
Otobiotic Otic
Otobius (p)
    O. lagophilus
    O. megnini
Otocort Otic
otocyst
Otodectes cysnotis (p)

otodectic
Otofuke agent
otolaryngologic
Otomycin-HPN Otic
otomycosis
Otosporin Otic
otosyphilis
ototoxicity
Otrivin
Ouango virus (OUAV)
OUAV
    Ouango virus
OUBIV
    Oubi virus
Oubi virus (OUBIV)
oulora
    Prevotella o.
oulorum
    Bacteroides o.
Ourem virus
Ourmiavirus (v)
ousairani
    Culicoides o.
outbreaks
    foodborne o.
OV
    oyster virus
ova (*pl. of* ovum)
ovale
    Pseudeurotium o.
    Trichosporon o.
ovalis
    Candida o.
    Nyctotherus o.
    Quinella o.
oval macrocyte
ovalocyte
ovarian
    o. failure
    o. tuberculosis
    o. vein thrombosis
ovata
    Sporomusa o.
ovatus
    Bacteroides o.
overdistention
overnight Giemsa stain
overwintering
ovi 1–6
    ovine adenovirus 1–6
Ovide
    O. Topical

O

NOTES

oviedoi
  Simulium o.
ovina
  Eimeria o.
ovine
  o. AAV virus
  o. adenovirus 1–6 (ovi 1–6)
ovinus
  Melophagus o.
oviparous
ovipneumoniae
  Mycoplasma o.
oviposit
oviposition
ovipositor
O1 virus
ovis
  Anaplasma o.
  Bovicola o.
  Brucella o.
  Chorioptes o.
  Cysticercus o.
  Damalina o.
  Eperythrozoon o.
  Helcococcus o.
  Moraxella (Branhamella) o.
  Neisseria o.
  Oestrus o.
  Psorergates o.
  Psoroptes o.
  Streptococcus o.
  Taenia o.
  Tetratrichomonas o.
ovoid
ovoides
  Trichosporon o.
ovolarviparous
ovolyticus
  Flexibacter o.
O-V Staticin
ovum, pl. ova
  ova and parasites
  ova and parasites examination
owensensis
  Caldicellulosiruptor o.
owl's eye inclusion
owyheensis
  Culicoides o.
OX-19
  Proteus O.
ox
  ox bot
  ox warble
Oxacillin
oxacillin
  o. sodium
oxacillin-resistant *Staphylococcus aureus*
  (ORSA)

oxalatica
  Ralstonia o.
oxalaticus
  Ammoniphilus o.
oxalicum
  Clostridium o.
oxalicus
  Oxalophagus o.
oxaliferum
  Achromatium o.
oxalivorans
  Ammoniphilus o.
Oxalobacter (b)
  O. formigenes
  O. vibrioformis
Oxalophagus oxalicus (b)
oxamicus
  Desulfovibrio vulgaris subsp. *o.*
oxamniquine
Oxandrin
oxandrolone
oxazolidinone
Oxgall media culture
oxiconazole
oxidase
  o. reaction
  o. test
oxidation
oxidative
oxidative-fermentative test
oxidative phosphorylation
oxide
  ethylene o. (ETO)
  mercuric o.
  zinc o.
oxidoreducens
  Eubacterium o.
Oxistat
  O. Topical
OXN-100P virus
OXN-52P virus
Oxobacter pfennigii (b)
Oxoid Signal System
oxolinic acid
oxoniensis
  Mycoplasma o.
Oxsoralen
Oxsoralen-Ultra
oxtriphylline
Oxy
  O. Control
  O. Deep Pore
  O. Medicated Pads
  O. Night Watch
  O. Power Pads
  O. 10 Wash

Oxy-5
    O. Advanced Formula for Sensitive
    Skin
    O. Tinted
**Oxy-10 Advanced Formula for Sensitive
  Skin**
oxyclinae
    Desulfovibrio o.
oxycodone
oxydans
    Arthrobacter o.
    Brevibacterium o.
    Gluconobacter oxydans subsp. *o.*
    Microbacterium o.
Oxyderm
oxygen
    hyperbaric o.
oxygenation
Oxy-Hood
Oxyl
    H 2 O.
oxymetazoline
    o. hydrochloride
oxymetholone
oxysporum
    Cladosporium o.
    Fusarium o.

oxytetracycline
    o. and hydrocortisone
    o. and polymyxin B
oxytoca
    Klebsiella o.
oxyuriasis
oxyuricide
oxyurid
Oxyurida
Oxyuridae
Oxyuris (p)
    O. incognita
    O. vermicularis
oxyuris
    o. nodule
Oxyuroidea
oyapockense
    Simulium o.
oyster virus (OV)
ozaenae
    Klebsiella o.
    Klebsiella pneumoniae subsp. *o.*
ozaenia
ozzardi
    Mansonella o.

NOTES

O

φH-like viruses
P034
P-450
    cytochrome P.
p24
    p. antigen
    p. antigenemia
    p. viral protein
P107 virus
P1-like viruses
P1 virus
P22-like viruses
P22 virus
P2-like viruses
P2 virus
P335 virus
P45 virus
PA
    protective antigen
P450-3A
    cytochrome P.
P-a-1 virus
PA-2 virus
pabuli
    Bacillus p.
    Paenibacillus p.
pacemaker endocarditis
pachydermatis
    Malassezia p.
pachypus
    Atherix p.
Pachysolen tannophilus (f)
pacifica
    Deleya p.
    Halomonas p.
    Wuchereria p.
pacificensis
    Psychrobacter p.
pacificum
    Carboxydibrachium p.
    Diphyllobothrium p.
pacificus
    Alcaligenes p.
    Ignicoccus p.
    Ixodes p.
    Thermococcus p.
Pacis
pack
    interferon alfa-2b and ribavirin
      combination p.
    M-Zole 7 Dual P.
    ribavirin combination p.
paclitaxel
Pacora virus (PCAV)

PACTG
    Pediatric AIDS Clinical Trial Group
    Protocol
pactum
    Streptomyces p.
Pacui virus (PACV)
PACV
    Pacui virus
pad
    Bichat fat p.
    Clearasil P.'s
    Oxy Medicated P.'s
    Oxy Power P.'s
Padebact GC OMNI test
padenii
    Chlamydoabsidia p.
padwickii
    Trichoconis p.
Paecilomyces (f)
    P. fumusoroseu
    P. javanicus
    P. lilacinus
    P. marquandii
    P. variotii
    P. viridis
Paederus
    P. dermatitis
    P. gemellus
Paenibacillus (b)
    P. alginolyticus
    P. alvei
    P. amylolyticus
    P. apiarius
    P. azotofixans
    P. borealis
    P. campinasensis
    P. chibensis
    P. chondroitinus
    P. curdlanolyticus
    P. dendritiformis
    P. durus
    P. glucanolyticus
    P. gordonae
    P. granivorans
    P. illinoisensis
    P. kobensis
    P. koreensis
    P. larvae
    P. larvae subsp. *larvae*
    P. larvae subsp. *pulvifaciens*
    P. lautus
    P. lentimorbus
    P. macerans
    P. macquariensis
    P. pabuli

P

Paenibacillus (continued)
    P. peoriae
    P. polymyxa
    P. popilliae
    P. pulvifaciens
    P. thiaminolyticus
    P. validus
PAF
    platelet-activating factor
PAGE
    polyacrylamide gel electrophoresis
Page ameba saline
PAGE-SS
    polyacrylamide gel electrophoresis with
    silver stain
Paget disease
pahangi
    Brugia p.
Pahayokee virus (PAHV)
PAHV
    Pahayokee virus
Pahvant
    P. Valley fever
    P. Valley plague
pain
    P. Aid Free
    crescendo p.
    hemorrhagic p.
    pleuritic p.
    pleuritic chest p.
    referred p.
painful articular syndrome
Pain-HP
    No P.-H.
paint
    salicylic and lactic acid p. (SAL)
PAIR
    puncture, aspiration, injection, and
    reaspiration
    PAIR procedure
paired organelles
pajaroello
    p. tick
Pak
    Pharmacy Pill P.
Palaeacanthocephala
Palaeococcus (b)
    P. ferrophilus
Palaron
palearctica
    Francisella tularensis biogroup *p.*
    Yersinia enterocolitica subsp. *p.*
Palestina virus (PLSV)
palestinensis
    Acanthamoeba p.
palindromic rheumatism

palisading
    p. epithelioid cell
    p. rod
palivizumab
pallens
    Aedes fulvus p.
    Prevotella p.
palleronii
    Actinoplanes p.
    Hydrogenophaga p.
    Pseudomonas p.
pallescens
    Cochliobolus p.
    Curvularia p.
palliation
palliative
pallida
    Crataerina p.
    Isosphaera p.
    Micromonospora p.
    Micromonospora echinospora subsp.
    p.
    Pilimelia columellifera subsp. *p.*
pallidipes
    Glossina p.
pallidula
    Glaciecola p.
pallidum
    DFA tissue test for *Treponema p.*
    (DFAT-TP)
    direct fluorescent antibody
    examination for *Treponema p.*
    (DFA-TP)
    microhemagglutination assay for
    Treponema p. (MHA-TP)
    microhemagglutination specific for
    Treponema p.
    microhemagglutination test for
    Treponema p. (MHA-TP test)
    Natrinema p.
    Treponema p.
pallidus
    Bacillus p.
    Synosternus p.
palmae
    Acholeplasma p.
    Zymobacter p.
palmaris
    tinea nigra p.
palmar-plantar erythrodysesthesia
palmar rash
palmellina
    trichomycosis p.
palmerae
    Culicoides p.
palmioleophila
    Candida p.

palmitate
  clofazimine p.
palmitatis
  Desulfuromonas p.
palmolei
  Methanoculleus p.
palpalis
  Glossina p.
palpebrae
palpebral
  p. edema
palpebrarum
  pediculosis p.
palpitation
palsy
  Bell p.
  cranial nerve p.
  facial p.
  oculomotor nerve p.
paludal
  p. fever
paludigena
  Candida p.
paludosa
  Tipula p.
paludosum
  Acetobacterium p.
Paludrine
palustre
  Methanobacterium p.
palustris
  Kocuria p.
  Methylocella p.
  Rhodopseudomonas p.
  Ruminococcus p.
PALV
  Palyam virus
Palyam virus (PALV)
PAM
  primary amebic meningoencephalitis
  primary amoebic meningoencephalitis
pametensis
  Helicobacter p.
Pamine
pamoate
  pyrantel p.
pampoikilus
  Culicoides p.
Pamprin IB
Panadol
panamensis
  Leishmania p.

Pan American Health Organization
panaritium digiti
pancarditis
pancolitis
pancreatic
  p. abscess
  p. amylase
  p. enzyme
  p. exocrine
  p. pseudocyst
  p. sepsis
  p. transplantation
  p. tuberculosis
pancreaticum
  Eurytrema p.
pancreatitis
  biliary p.
  hemorrhagic p.
panculture
pancuronium
pancytopenia
  transient p.
pandemic
Pandoraea (b)
  P. apista
  P. norimbergensis
  P. pnomenusa
  P. pulmonicola
  P. sputorum
panel
  ABI AnIDENT p.
  cellular immune p.
  Haemophilus-Neisseria
    identification p.
  HNID p.
  lymphocyte subset p.
  MicroScan gram-negative ID p.
  MicroScan HNID P.
  MicroScan Pos
    IDENTIFICATION P.
  MicroScan Rapid Pos Combo P.
  Minitek Gram-Positive P.
  respiratory p.
  Sceptor P.
panencephalitis
  progressive rubella p.
  subacute sclerosing p. (SSPE)
Paneolus foenisicii (f)
Pangola stunt virus
panhypopituitarism
Panicovirus (v)
panipenem

NOTES

P

401

panis
  Lactobacillus p.
Panmycin Oral
pannicola
  Chrysosporium p.
panniculitis
  cold p.
  nodular eosinophilic p.
pannorus
  Geomyces p.
pannus
panophthalmitis
PanOxyl-AQ
PanOxyl Bar
Panretin
Panscol
  P. Lotion
  P. Ointment
pansporoblast
pansporoblastic
Panstrongylus
  P. megistus
pantelleriensis
  Halomonas p.
panthercap mushroom
pantherina
  Amanita p.
p24 antigen
p24 antigenemia
Pantoea (b)
  P. agglomerans
  P. ananatis
  P. citrea
  P. dispersa
  P. punctata
  P. stewartii subsp. *indologenes*
  P. stewartii subsp. *stewartii*
  P. terrea
pantomorphia
pantomorphic
pantothenticus
  Bacillus p.
  Virgibacillus p.
pantotropha
  Thiosphaera p.
pantotrophus
  Paracoccus p.
panuveitis
PAP
  preoperative antimicrobial prophylaxis
Pap
  Papanicolaou
  Pap Net
  Pap stain
papago
  Aedes p.
Papanicolaou (Pap)

P. smear
P. stain of sputum
paper
  p. mill worker's disease
  Whatman No. 541 filter p.
papillae corona glandis
papillary
  p. hypertrophy
  p. stenosis
papilledema
Papillibacter cinnamivorans (b)
papilliferum
  hidradenoma p.
papilligerum
  Contracaecum p.
papillitis
papilloma
  conjunctival p.
  zymotic p.
papillomaform wart
papillomatosis
  hirsutoid p.
  recurrent respiratory p.
papillomatous skin lesion
Papillomavirus (v)
papillomavirus
  human p. (HPV)
  p. infection
Paplex
PapMV
Papovaviridae
papovavirus
pappataci fever
Pap smear
papular
  p. acrodermatitis
  p. eruption
  p. fever
  p. lesion
  p. rash
Papulaspora equi (f)
papule
  erythematous hyperpigmented p.
  pearly coronal p.
  pearly penile p.
papulonecrotic tuberculid
papulonodular rash
papulopustule
papulosis
  bowenoid p.
papulosquamous skin lesion
papyrosolvens
  Clostridium p.
paraaminosalicylic acid (PAS)
paraaortic lymph node
parabasal
  p. body
  p. filament

Parabasalidea
parabrevis
>   Bacillus p.
>   Brevibacillus p.

parabuchneri
>   Lactobacillus p.

paracasei
>   Lactobacillus paracasei subsp. p.

paracentesis
>   abdominal p.
>   p. fluid cytology
>   therapeutic p.

Parachlamydia acanthamoebae (b)
parachlorometaxylenol
paracholera
Parachordodes (p)
>   P. pustulosus
>   P. tolosanus
>   P. violaceus

Parachordodinae
Paracoccidioidaceae
paracoccidioidal granuloma
Paracoccidioides (f)
>   P. brasiliensis
>   P. lithogenes

paracoccidioidin
paracoccidioidomycosis (PCM)
Paracoccus (b)
>   P. alcaliphilus
>   P. alkenifer
>   P. aminophilus
>   P. aminovorans
>   P. carotinifaciens
>   P. denitrificans
>   P. halodenitrificans
>   P. kocurii
>   P. marcusii
>   P. methylutens
>   P. pantotrophus
>   P. solventivorans
>   P. thiocyanatus
>   P. versutus

paracochleata
>   Kitasatospora p.

paracochleatus
>   Streptomyces p.

paracolon bacillus
paraconglomeratum
>   Brachybacterium p.

paraconjugatus
>   Caedibacter p.

Paracraurococcus ruber (b)

paracrine
>   p. cytokine

paracuniculus
>   Haemophilus p.

paradigm
paradisiaca
>   Brenneria p.
>   Erwinia p.

paradoxical
paradoxum
>   Clostridium p.

paradoxus
>   Acetobacter pasteurianus subsp. p.
>   Alcaligenes p.
>   Listerella p.
>   pulsus p.
>   Saccharomyces p.
>   Streptomyces p.
>   Variovorax p.

paradysentery bacillus
paraensi
>   Echinostoma p.

paraensis
>   Culicoides p.

paraffin-embedded
Parafilaria multipapillosa
paraflagella
paraflagellate
paraflagellum
parafortuitum
>   Mycobacterium p.

parafrenal abscess
paragallinarum
>   Haemophilus p.

paragonimiasis
>   abdominal p.
>   cerebral p.

Paragonimidae
Paragonimus (p)
>   P. africanus
>   P. heterotremus
>   P. kellicotti
>   P. macrorchis
>   P. mexicanus
>   P. miyazakii
>   P. skrjabini
>   P. uterobilateralis
>   P. westermani

Paragonimus **granuloma**
Paragordiinae
Paragordius varius (p)

NOTES

P

paraguay
    Trichosporon p.
paraguayense
    Simulium p.
parahaemolytica
    Beneckea p.
parahaemolyticus
    Haemophilus p.
    Vibrio p.
parainfluenza
    p. 3
    p. type 1, 2, 3
    p. type 4A
    p. type 4B
    p. virus
    p. virus antigen
    p. virus culture
    p. virus serology
parainfluenzae
    Haemophilus p.
    Haemophilus p. biotype II
    parainfluenza virus type 1–4
parakefiri
    Lactobacillus p.
parakeratosis
Paralactobacillus selangorensis (b)
Paralephostrongylus (p)
paraleprosis
paralimentarius
    Lactobacillus p.
paraluis-cuniculi
paraluiscuniculi
    Treponema p.
paralysis, pl. **paralyses**
    flaccid p.
    immune p.
    neuromuscular p.
    tick p.
paralyssa
paralytic
    p. ileus
    p. polio
    p. poliomyelitis
    p. shellfish poisoning (PSP)
paramastigote
Paramatta agent
Paramecium
    P. aurelia
    P. bursaria
    P. caudatum
    P. coli
    P. putrinum
    P. trichium
paramesenteroides
    Leuconostoc p.
    Weissella p.
paramethasone acetate
Paramoeba

Paramphistomatidae
Paramphistomatoidea
paramphistomiasis
Paramphistomum (p)
Paramushir virus (PMRV)
Paramyxoviridae
Paramyxovirinae
Paramyxovirus
paramyxovirus
paranasal
    p. sinus
    p. sinus lymphoma
Paraná virus (PARV)
paranense
    Simulium p.
paraneoplastic
Para-pak fecal collection kit
paraparesis
    HTLV-1-associated
        myelopathy/tropical spastic p.
        (HAM/TSP)
    topical spastic p.
    tropical spastic p.
parapaucimobilis
    Sphingomonas p.
paraperfringens
    Clostridium p.
parapertussis
    Bordetella p.
paraphrohaemolyticus
    Haemophilus p.
paraphrophilus
    Haemophilus p.
parapiliferus
    Culicoides p.
paraplantarum
    Lactobacillus p.
paraplegia
    Pott p.
paraplegic
parapneumonic effusion
Parapoxvirus (v)
parapoxvirus
paraproteinemia
parapsilosis
    Candida p.
parapunctipennis
    Anopheles p.
    Anopheles p. parapunctipennis
paraputrificum
    Clostridium p.
pararama
pararugosa
    Candida p.
pararugosum
    Trichosporon p.
Parasaccharomyces (f)

parasanguis
    Streptococcus p.
Parascaris equorum (p)
parasite
    accidental p.
    apicomplexan p.
    autistic p.
    autochthonous p.
    blood smear for malarial p.'s
    commensal p.
    euroxenous p.
    facultative p.
    filarial p.
    gastrointestinal p.
    helminthic p.
    heterogenetic p.
    heteroxenous p.
    incidental p.
    inquiline p.
    intracellular p.
    malarial p.
    malignant tertian malarial p.
    obligate intracellular p.
    ova and p.'s
    protozoan p.
    quartan p.
    specific p.
    spurious p.
    stenoxous p.
    temporary p.
    tertian p.
    trypanosomal p.
    urine for p.'s
    urine ova and p.'s
parasite-host ecosystem
parasitemia
    p. stage
    Trypanosoma cruzi p.
parasitic
    p. cyst
    p. disease
    p. endophthalmitis
    p. flatworm
    p. gastroenteritis
    p. hemoptysis
    p. infection
    p. keratitis
    p. melanoderma
    p. thyroiditis
parasitica
    Phialophora p.

parasiticidal
parasiticide
parasiticum
    eczema p.
    Polyangium p.
Parasitiformes
parasitism
    ectopic p.
    multiple p.
parasitivorax
    Cheyletiella p.
parasitize
parasitized erythrocyte
parasitocenose
parasitogenesis
parasitogenic
parasitoid
parasitological
parasitologist
parasitology
parasitome
parasitophorous vacuole
parasitosis
    delusional p.
parasitotropic
parasitotropism
parasitotropy
parastrongylosis
Parastrongylus cantonensis (p)
parasuis
    Haemophilus p.
parasympathetic
paratenesis
paratenic host
parathyroid hormone (PTH)
Paratorulopsis
Paratorulosis banhegyii
paratrophic
paratuberculosis
    Mycobacterium p.
    Mycobacterium avium subsp. p.
paratyphi
    Salmonella p.
paratyphoid
    p. bacillus (*See Salmonella*
        enteritidis)
    p. bacteria (*See Salmonella*
        enteritidis)
    p. fever
parauberis
    Streptococcus p.

NOTES

P

paravaccinia
　p. virus
　p. virus infection
Parazoa
parazoon
pardi
　Trichosporon p.
Parechovirus (v)
paredis
　Treponema socranskii subsp. *p.*
Paregle aestiva
paregoric
parenchyma
parenchymal
　p. cell
parenchymatic liver disease
parenchymatous
　p. involvement
　p. neurosyphilis
Parendomyces
parent cyst
parenteral
　p. antibiotic
　Coly-Mycin M P.
　p. morphine
　p. nutrition
　p. therapy
parenteral/aqueous
　penicillin G (p./a.)
parenterally transmitted non-A non-B hepatitis (PT-NANBH)
parenteric fever
paresis
　up-gaze p.
paresthesia
　circumoral p.
　perioral p.
Parinaud
　P. oculoglandular syndrome
parisiensis
　Legionella p.
parkeri
　Borrelia p.
　Ornithodoros p.
　Rickettsia p.
Parkinson disease
Parmulariaceae
parnassum
　Simulium p.
Parodiopsidaceae
paromomycin
paromomycinus
　Streptomyces rimosus subsp. *p.*
parontospora
　Planomonospora parontospora subsp. *p.*
paronychia
　herpetic p.

parooensis
　Conglomeromonas largomobilis subsp. *p.*
　Skermanella p.
Paroo River virus (PRV)
parotid
　p. gland
　p. gland tuberculosis
parotiditis
　epidemic p.
parotitis
paroxetine
paroxysm
　malarial p.
paroxysmal
　p. cold hemoglobinuria
　p. stage
parrot
　p. disease
　p. fever
Parry Creek virus
pars
　p. plana vitrectomy
　p. planitis
parthenogenesis
partial
　p. agglutinin
　p. motor seizure
　p. prophylaxis
particeps
　Culiseta p.
particle
　coronavirus-like p. (CVLP)
　Dane p.
　kappa p.
　single-shelled p.
　virus p.
　virus-like p. (VLP)
Partitiviridae
Partitivirus (v)
parturient
Partuss LA
parumapertus
　Dermacentor p.
PARV
　Paraná virus
parva
　Emmonsia p.
　Emmonsia parva var. *p.*
　Leptospira p.
　Microbispora p.
parvisporogenes
　Streptomyces p.
　Streptoverticillium p.
Parvobacteriaceae
Parvolex
parvo-like virus
Parvoviridae

Parvovirus (v)
parvovirus
    p. B19
    p. B19 DNA
    p. B19 IgG antibody
    p. B19 IgM antibody
    bovine p.
    p. B19 serology
    feline p.
    goose p.
    human p.
    lapine p.
    porcine p.
parvula
    Veillonella p.
    Veillonella p. subsp. *parvula*
    Veillonella p. subsp. *rodentium*
parvulum
    Atopobium p.
parvulus
    Pediococcus p.
    Peptostreptococcus p.
    Streptococcus p.
    Streptomyces p.
parvum
    Acholeplasma p.
    Aquabacterium p.
    Chrysosporium p.
    Chrysosporium parvum var. *p.*
    cryptosporidiosis p.
    Cryptosporidium p.
    Diphyllobothrium p.
    Eperythrozoon p.
    Haplosporangium p.
    Methanocorpusculum p.
    Roseospirillum p.
    Treponema p.
parvus
    Anopheles p.
    Anopheles parapunctipennis
    Methylocystis p.
    Streptomyces p.
Paryphostomum sufrartyfex (p)
PAS
    paraaminosalicylic acid
    periodic acid-Schiff
    periodic acid-Schiff stain
    PAS stain
P.A.S.
    sodium P.
pascens
    Arthrobacter p.

pascui
    Clostridium p.
pascullei
    Legionella pneumophila subsp. *p.*
pascuorum
    Muscina p.
paspali
    Azorhizophilus p.
Passalurus ambiguus (p)
passive
    p. agglutination
    p. hemagglutination test
    p. immunity
    p. immunization
    p. immunoprophylaxis
pasteri
    Gigantorhynchus p.
Pasteur
    Louis P.
Pasteurella (b)
    P. aerogenes
    P. anatis
    P. avium
    P. bettyae
    P. caballi
    P. canis
    P. dagmatis
    P. gallicida
    P. gallinarum
    P. granulomatis
    P. haemolytica
    P. langaaensis
    P. lymphangitidis
    P. mairii
    P. multocida subsp. *gallicida*
    P. multocida subsp. *multocida*
    P. multocida subsp. *septica*
    P. pestis (*See Yersinia pestis*)
    P. pneumotropica
    P. species taxon 16
    P. stomatis
    P. testudinis
    P. trehalosi
    P. ureae
    P. volantium
pasteurella
Pasteurellaceae
Pasteurelleae
pasteurellosis
pasteuri
    Staphylococcus p.

NOTES

P

Pasteuria (b)
  P. nishizawae
  P. penetrans
  P. ramosa
  P. thornei
Pasteuriaceae
pasteurianum
  Clostridium p.
pasteurianus
  Acetobacter p.
pasteurii
  Bacillus p.
  Lactosphaera p.
  Ruminococcus p.
  Sporosarcina p.
Pastia
  P. line
  P. sign
pastorianus
  Saccharomyces p.
pastoris
  Pichia p.
  Prochlorococcus marinus subsp. *p.*
PATAV
  Pata virus
Pata virus (PATAV)
patch
  MacCallum p.
  mucous p.
  PediaPatch Transdermal P.
  sandy p.
  scrotal T p.
  Testoderm TTS p.
  Trans-Plantar Transdermal P.
  Trans-Ver-Sal Transdermal P.
Pate d'Unna
patei
  Brugia p.
patersoni
  Anopheles franciscanus p.
Pathilon
pathocidicus
  Streptomyces albus subsp. *p.*
Pathocil
pathogen
  Agency for Toxic Substances and
    Disease Registry, Airborne P.'s
  enteric p.
  Legionella-like amebal p.
  nosocomial p.
  novel p.
  opportunistic p.
  single-host p.
  specific p.
pathogen-directed
pathogenesis
  viral p.

pathogenic
  p. microorganism
  p. strain
pathogenicity
pathognomic
pathognomonic
pathology
pathophysiology and natural history
Pathum Thani virus (PTHV)
patient
  ambulatory p.
  HIV-infected p.
  neutropenic p.
  penicillin-allergic p.
patient-centered
patient-specific
Patois virus (PATV)
patterned homeopathy
PATV
  Patois virus
paucibacillary
  p. leprosy
paucimobilis
  Pseudomonas p.
  Sphingomonas p.
Paucimonas lemoignei (b)
paucisymptomatic
paucity
paucivorans
  Acetothermus p.
  Aminomonas p.
  Dolosicoccus p.
  Fusibacter p.
  Nocardia p.
  Sporomusa p.
  Zymophilus p.
paucula
  Ralstonia p.
Paul-Bunnell test
paunch
  protease p.
paurometabola
  Tsukamurella p.
paurometabolum
  Corynebacterium p.
Pautrier abscess
pavlovskyi
  Ixodes p.
PAV virus
Paxillaceae
Paxillus involutus (f)
Paxton disease
paynei
  Simulium p.
paynteri
  Methanolacinia p.
  Methanomicrobium p.
PB-1 virus

PBC
    protected brush catheter
PBCV-1 virus
PBL
    peripheral blood lymphocyte
PBMC
    peripheral blood mononuclear cell
PBP
    penicillin-binding protein
PBP1 virus
PBS1 virus
PbV
    Penicillium brevicompactum virus
        PbV virus
PC84 virus
PCA
    protected catheter aspirate
PCAV
    Pacora virus
PCE
PCEC rabies vaccine
Pc-fV
    Penicillium cyaneo-fulvum virus
        Pc-fV virus
PCM
    paracoccidioidomycosis
PCNSL
    primary central nervous system
    lymphoma
PCP
    Pneumocystis carinii pneumonia
        PCP prophylaxis
PCR
    polymerase chain reaction
        Amplicor PCR
        PCR amplification test
        arbitrary-primed PCR (AP-PCR)
        PCR combined with single-strand
          conformation polymorphism (PCR-
          SSCP)
        competitive PCR (cPCR)
        PCR fragment analysis
        PCR immunoassay
        inter-repeat PCR (IR-PCR)
        nested PCR
        quantitative competitive PCR (QC-
          PCR)
        repetitive element-based PCR
        repetitive extragenic palindromic
          PCR (REP-PCR)
        Roche Amplicore PCR
        semiquantitative PCR

        ultrasensitive quantitative PCR
        PCR with arbitrary primer (AP-
          PCR)
PCR-enzyme immunoassay
PCR-ISH
    polymerase chain reaction in situ
    hybridization
PCR-RFLP analysis
PCR-SSCP
    PCR combined with single-strand
    conformation polymorphism
PcV
    Penicillium chrysogenum virus
        PcV virus
PD
    peritoneal dialysis
PDH
    progressive disseminated histoplasmosis
PE
    Pseudomonas exotoxin
        Guiatuss PE
        Halotussin PE
PE1 virus
peacockii
        Rickettsia p.
peak
        p. blood level
        p. plasma concentration
pealeana
        Shewanella p.
pearly
        p. coronal papule
        p. penile papule
Peaton virus
PECAM-1
    platelet endothelial cell adhesion
    molecule-1
peccator
        Culex p.
pechumani
        Culicoides p.
Pecluvirus (v)
pecorum
        Chlamydia p.
        Chlamydophila p.
        Gasterophilus p.
pecosensis
        Culicoides p.
pectenicida
        Vibrio p.
pectenotoxin
pectinate

NOTES

P

Pectinatus (b)
    P. cerevisiiphilus
    P. frisingensis
pectinis
    Cristispira p.
pectinolytica
    Aeromonas salmonicida subsp.
      pectinolytica
pectinophilus
    Bacteroides p.
pectinoschiza
    Lachnospira p.
pectinovora
    Cytophaga p.
pectinovorum
    Flavobacterium p.
    Treponema p.
pectin sugar
Pectobacterium (b)
    P. cacticida
    P. carnegieana
    P. carotovorum subsp. *atrosepticum*
    P. carotovorum subsp.
      betavasculorum
    P. carotovorum subsp. *carotovorum*
    P. carotovorum subsp. *odoriferum*
    P. carotovorum subsp. *wasabiae*
    P. chrysanthemi
    P. cypripedii
    P. rhapontici
pectoris
    unstable angina p.
pecuarum
    Cnephia p.
pedal edema
pedalis
    Linognathus p.
Pedameth
PediaCare Oral
Pediacof
Pedialyte
PediaPatch Transdermal Patch
Pediapred Oral
Pedia-Profen
pediatric
    P. AIDS Clinical Trial Group
      Protocol (PACTG)
    Benylin P.
    Calmylin P.
    Cleocin P.
    Codamine P.
    P. Cough syrup
    Cycofed P.
    Fedahist Expectorant P.
    Hycomine P.
    p. intensive care unit (PICU)
    P. Risk of Mortality (PRISM)
    Robitussin P.

Pediatrix
Pediazole
pedicellata
    Drechslera p.
    Setosphaeria p.
Pedicinus ancoratus (p)
Pedi-Cort V Creme
pedicular
pediculation
pediculatus
    Chondromyces p.
pediculi
pediculicide
Pediculidae
Pediculoides (p) (*See* **Pyemotes**)
    P. ventricosus
pediculoides
    dermatitis p.
pediculosis
    p. capitis
    p. corporis
    p. palpebrarum
    p. pubis
    p. vestimenti
pediculous
Pediculus (p)
    P. humanus
    P. humanus capitis
    P. humanus corporis
    P. humanus humanus
pediculus
Pedi-Dri Topical Powder
Pediococcus (b)
    P. acidilactici
    P. damnosus
    P. dextrinicus
    P. halophilus
    P. inopinatus
    P. parvulus
    P. pentosaceus
    P. urinaeequi
pedioforme
    Thiolamprovum p.
pedioformis
    Amoebobacter p.
Pediotic Otic
Pedi-Pro Topical
pedis
    dermatomycosis p.
    tinea p.
Pedituss
Pedobacter (b)
    P. africanus
    P. heparinus
    P. piscium
    P. saltans
pedogenesis

Pedomicrobium (b)
    P. americanum
    P. australicum
    P. ferrugineum
    P. manganicum
    P. podsolicum
pedrosoi
    Fonsecaea p.
    Hormodendron p.
pedum
    Contracaecum p.
pedunculated lesion
PedvaxHIB
    P. vaccine
peenash
PEEP
    positive end-expiratory pressure
peer-support program
pefloxacin
PEG
    percutaneous endoluminal gastrostomy
    percutaneous endoscopic gastrostomy
       PEG tube
Pegohylemyia seneciella (p)
Pegomya affinis
pegylated
    p. interferon
    p. liposomal-encapsulated
      doxorubicin
PEIA assay
PEJ
    percutaneous endoscopic jejunostomy
pelagia
    Beneckea p.
    Listonella p.
pelagica
    Methylomonas p.
pelagicum
    Methylomicrobium p.
    Oceanospirillum p.
    Oceanospirillum beijerinckii subsp.
      p.
pelagicus
    Methylobacter p.
pelagius
    Vibrio p.
Pelamoviriod (v)
Pelczaria aurantia (b)
Pelger-Huet anomaly
peliliouensis
    Culicoides p.

peliosis
    bacillary p. (BP)
Pelistega europaea (b)
pellagra-associated dermatitis
pellagroid dermatitis
pellet
    Testopel P.
pelletieri
    Actinomadura p.
pellicle
pellicular
pelliculosa
    Candida p.
pellirubrum
    Natrinema p.
Pelobacter (b)
    P. acetylenicus
    P. acidigallici
    P. carbinolicus
    P. massiliensis
    P. propionicus
    P. venetianus
Pelodera (p)
    P. strongyloides
    P. teres
Pelodictyon (b)
    P. clathratiforme
    P. luteolum
    P. phaeoclathratiforme
    P. phaeum
pelophila
    Thiomicrospira p.
pelophilus
    Propionibacter p.
Pelospora glutarica (b)
pelta
Peltasteraceae
peltata
    Candida p.
Peltopycnidiaceae
pelvic
    p. actinomycosis
    p. brim
    p. cellulitis
    p. inflammatory disease (PID)
    p. osteomyelitis
    p. thrombophlebitis
pemphigoid
    bullous p.
pemphigus
    p. antibody
    p. contagiosum

NOTES

P

penaeicida
> *Vibrio p.*

penciclovir

pendens
> *Amoebobacter p.*
> *Thermofilum p.*
> *Thiocapsa p.*

peneaus

Penecort Topical

penetrans
> *Mycoplasma p.*
> *Pasteuria p.*
> *Sarcopsylla p.*
> *Tunga p.*

penetrating
> p. keratoplasty
> p. wound

Penetrex

Penglobe

penguinpox virus

penicillatum
> *Trichosporon p.*

penicillin
> p. allergy skin testing
> amino p.
> antipseudomonad p.
> p. aqueous
> aqueous crystalline p. G
> aqueous procaine p. G (APPG)
> benzathine p.
> benzathine p. G
> broad-spectrum p.
> crystalline p.
> p. disk test
> p. G
> p. G benzathine
> p. G benzathine and procaine
>   combined
> p. G (parenteral/aqueous)
> p. G procaine
> isoxazolyl p.
> penicillinase-resistant p. (PRP)
> phenoxymethyl p.
> potassium p. G (KPG)
> procaine p.
> procaine p. G
> p. skin test
> p. V
> p. V potassium

penicillin-allergic patient

penicillinase
> p. test

penicillinase-producing
> p.-p. gonococci (PPNG)
> p.-p. *Neisseria gonorrhoeae* (PPNG)
> p.-p. organisms susceptibility testing

penicillinase-resistant penicillin (PRP)

penicillin-binding protein (PBP)

penicillin-resistant pneumococcus

penicilliosis
> disseminated p.
> p. marneffei

Penicillium (f)
> *P. brevicompactum* virus (PbV)
> *P. chrysogenum*
> *P. chrysogenum* virus (PcV)
> *P. citrinum*
> *P. commune*
> *P. cyaneo-fulvum* virus (Pc-fV)
> *P. decumbens*
> *P. expansum*
> *P. funiculosum*
> *P. griseofulvum*
> *P. janthinellum*
> *P. marneffei*
> *P. purpurogenum*
> *P. rugulosum*
> *P. stoloniferum* F virus (PsV-F)
> *P. stoloniferum* S virus (PsV-S)
> *P. verruculosum*

penicilloides
> *Aspergillus p.*
> *Gliocladium p.*

penicilloyl
> p. polylysine (PPL)
> p. polylysine skin test

penicillus

penile
> p. condyloma
> p. gangrene
> p. tuberculosis

penis
> autoamputation of p.
> lateral fixation of p.

Penlac

penneri
> *Proteus p.*

pennies
> copper p.

pennivorans
> *Fervidobacterium p.*

penobscotensis
> *Simulium p.*

Pentacarinat Injection

Pentafuside

Pentakine

pentalagi
> *Haemaphysalis p.*

Pentam-300 Injection

pentamidine
> aerosolized p.
> p. isethionate

Pentamycetin

pentapeptide

Pentastoma najae (p)

pentastomiasis

Pentastomida
pentaticum
Pentatrichomonas hominis (p)
pentavalent
    p. antimonial
    p. antimony-containing compound
    p. gas gangrene antitoxin
pentazocine
pentosaceus
    Bacteroides p.
    Pediococcus p.
pentosovorans
    Anaerofilum p.
Pentostam
pentosus
    Lactobacillus p.
pentoxifylline
Pentratrichomonas hominis
Pentrax
Pen.Vee K
pen VK
peoriae
    Bacillus p.
    Paenibacillus p.
Pepcid
    P. AC Acid Controller
    P. RPD
pepper bolete mushroom
Peptamen
peptic
    p. ulcer
    p. ulcer disease (PUD)
peptide
    p. antibiotic
peptide-specific T cell
peptidivorans
    Clostridium p.
peptidoglycan
    p. synthesis
peptidolytica
    Pseudoalteromonas p.
peptidovorans
    Dethiosulfovibrio p.
Pepto-Bismol
Peptococcaceae
Peptococcus (b)
    P. asaccharolyticus
    P. glycinophilus
    P. heliotrinreducens
    P. indolicus
    P. magnus
    P. niger

    P. prevotii
    P. saccharolyticus
Peptol
peptone
peptonic
Peptoniphilus (b)
    P. asaccharolyticus
    P. harei
    P. indolicus
    P. ivoii
    P. lacrimalis
peptonophilus
    Thermoactinomyces p.
    Thermococcus p.
Peptostreptococcus (b)
    P. anaerobius
    P. asaccharolyticus
    P. barnesae
    P. harei
    P. heliotrinreducens
    P. hydrogenalis
    P. indolicus
    P. ivorii
    P. lacrimalis
    P. lactolyticus
    P. magnus
    P. micros
    P. octavius
    P. parvulus
    P. prevotii
    P. productus
    P. tetradius
    P. vaginalis
peracetic acid
percent of the periphery that has ciliary activity (PPCA)
percolatus
    Rhodococcus p.
percutaneous
    p. cholangiography
    p. drainage
    p. endoluminal gastrostomy (PEG)
    p. endoluminal gastrostomy tube
    p. endoscopic gastrostomy (PEG)
    p. endoscopic jejunostomy (PEJ)
    p. liver biopsy
    p. needle aspiration
    p. needle aspiration biopsy
    p. transhepatic cholangiography (PTCA)
percutaneously
    p. placed line

NOTES

P

peregrinum
  Aquaspirillum peregrinum subsp. *p.*
  Mycobacterium p.
perenne
  Clostridium p.
perfect
  p. fungus
  p. stage
  p. state
Perfectoderm Gel
perfectomarina
  Pseudomonas p.
perfilievii
  Ancalochloris p.
perflava
  Neisseria p.
perflavum
  Simulium p.
perfoetens
  Fusobacterium p.
perfoliata
  Anoplocephala p.
perfoliatus
  Echinochasmus p.
perforans
  Coniosporium p.
  mal p.
perforated
  p. duodenal ulcer
perforation
  bowel p.
  large-bowel p.
perforin
perfringens
  Clostridium p.
perfusion
  hyperthermic antiblastic p. (HAP)
  hyperthermic isolated limb p.
    (HILP)
periadenitis
perianal
  p. condylomata
  p. streptococcal cellulitis
periapical
  p. abscess
periappendiceal abscess
periarticular
pericardial
  p. effusion
  p. fluid cytology
  p. friction rub
  p. tuberculosis
pericardiocentesis
pericardiotomy
pericarditis
  tuberculous p.
pericardium
Periconia (f)

pericyst
Pericystales
Peridex
  P. Oral Rinse
perilobular
perinasal skin
perinatal
  p. transmission
perineal
  p. lesion
  p. MRSA colonization
  p. pruritus
  P. Skin Cleanser
perinephrial leukocytosis
perinephric abscess
Perinet virus (PERV)
perineum
perinuclear halo
PerioChip
Periochip
periocular
  p. infection
  p. skin
period
  incubation p.
  latent p.
  prepatent p.
periodic
  p. acid-Schiff (PAS)
  p. acid-Schiff stain (PAS)
  p. filariasis
  p. sharp wave complex (PSWC)
periodicity
  diurnal p.
  filarial p.
  lunar p.
  malarial p.
  nocturnal p.
  subperiodic p.
periodontal
  p. abscess
  p. disease
periodonticum
  Fusobacterium p.
periodontii
  Centipeda p.
periodontitis
  localized juvenile p. (LJP)
PerioGard
perionyx
perioperative
  p. morbidity
perioral
  p. paresthesia
periorbital
  p. cellulitis
  p. edema

Perioseptic
    Orajel P.
Periostat
periosteum
periostitis
peripapillary
peripartum
peripheral
    p. arterial catheter
    p. arteries and veins ultrasound
    p. atherosclerosis
    p. blood CD8$^+$ lymphocytosis
    p. blood lymphocyte (PBL)
    p. blood lymphocyte analysis
    p. blood mononuclear cell (PBMC)
    p. blood preparation for
      microfilariae
    p. blood stem cell infusion
    p. blood stem cell transplant
    p. coin lesion
    p. edema
    p. eosinophilia
    p. fat wasting
    p. intravenous catheter
    p. leukocytosis
    p. lipoatrophy
    p. lipodystrophy
    p. neuritis
    p. neuropathy
    p. osteoarticular tuberculosis
    p. smear
    p. T-cell lymphoma
    p. visual field loss
peripherally inserted central catheter
  (PICC)
peripheral neuropathy
Periplanata
periplast
periportal fibrosis
perirectal
peristalsis
peristoma
peristomal
peristome
peristomium
perithecium
peritoneal
    p. dialysis (PD)
    p. fluid
    p. fluid cytology
peritonei
    Luteococcus p.

peritoneum
peritonitis
    bacterial p.
    Brucella melitensis p.
    Candida p.
    CAPD-associated p.
    fungal p.
    spontaneous p.
    spontaneous bacterial p. (SBP)
    tuberculous p.
peritonsillar
peritracheal gland
peritrichal
Peritrichida
peritrichous
periurethral
    p. abscess
periurinary
perivascular
    p. cuffing
    p. infiltration
    p. pattern
perivasculitis
periventricular
perlatum
    Lycoperdon p.
Perles
    Tessalon P.
permanent
    p. cardiac pacemaker infection
    p. stained smear examination
Permapen
permeability
permeable
permethrin
Permount
pernicious
    p. anemia
    p. malaria
pernix
    Aeropyrum p.
Pernox
perolens
    Lactobacillus p.
perometabolis
    Thiobacillus p.
    Thiomonas p.
peromysci
    Bartonella p.
    Grahamella p.
Peronsporaceae

NOTES

P

peroris
  Streptococcus p.
**peroxidase-antiperoxidase
  immunocytochemical stain**
peroxide
  benzoyl p.
  carbamide p.
  erythromycin and benzoyl p.
  hydrogen p.
  vaporized hydrogen p. (VHP)
Peroxin A5, A10
peroxydans
  Acetobacter p.
perplexens
  Anopheles p.
Persa-Gel
persarum
  Dracunculus p.
Persian relapsing fever
persica
  Borrelia p.
  Cellulomonas p.
  Lewinella p.
  Wolbachia p.
persicina
  Erwinia p.
Persicobacter diffluens (b)
persicolor
  Arthroderma p.
  Microsporum p.
  Trichophyton p.
persicus
  Argas p.
  Herpetosiphon p.
persistence
  microbial p.
**persistent generalized lymphadenopathy
  (PGL)**
persister
personality change
personal protective equipment (PPE)
personatus
  Reduvius p.
Personnelle
  P. Contre le Rhume
  P. DM
person-to-person transmission
person with AIDS (PWA)
perstans
  acrodermatitis p.
  Dipetalonema p.
  Mansonella p.
persulcatus
  Ixodes p.
PERT
  P. assay
pertactin (PRN)

pertenue
  Treponema p.
  Treponema pallidum subsp. p.
pertinax
  Simulium p.
Pert Plus
pertucinogena
  Pseudomonas p.
perturbans
  Mansonia p.
Pertussin
  P. CS
  P. ES
pertussis
  Bordetella p.
  diphtheria, tetanus toxoids and
    acellular p. (DTaP)
  p. exotoxin
  p. serology
  p. toxin (PT)
  whole-cell p.
pertussis-like syndrome
peruana
  verruca p.
  verruga p.
peruensis
  Lutzomyia p.
Peruvian
  P. tarantula
  P. wart
peruviana
  Leishmania p.
peruzzii
  Meningonema p.
PERV
  Perinet virus
peryassui
  Anopheles p.
pes febricitans
pest
Pestalotiopsis (f)
peste-des-petits-ruminants virus
pestifera
  Epicauta p.
pestis
  Pasteurella p. (See Yersinia pestis)
  Yersinia p.
Pestivirus (v)
PET
  positron emission tomography
petechia, pl. **petechiae**
petechial
  p. exanthem
  p. hemorrhage
  p. rash
petersoni
  Simulium p.
petit mal seizure

petraea
> *Geotoga p.*

Petri
> P. dish
> P. dish culture

Petriellidium (f)

petrii
> *Bordetella p.*

petrohuensis
> *Candida p.*

petrolearius
> *Methanoplanus p.*

petroleophila
> *Nocardia p.*
> *Pseudonocardia p.*

Petrotoga (b)
> P. *miotherma*
> P. *mobilis*

peucetius
> *Streptomyces p.*

peus
> *Culex p.*

Peyronellaea (f)

Peyronie disease

Pezizaceae

Pezizales

PFA
> foscarnet
> phosphonoformic acid

Pfeiffer bacillus

PfEMP-1
> *Plasmodium falciparum* erythrocyte
> membrane protein-1

Pfennigia purpurea (b)

pfennigii
> *Clostridium p.*
> *Oxobacter p.*
> *Syntrophobacter p.*
> *Thiocapsa p.*
> *Thiococcus p.*

PFGE
> pulsed-field gel electrophoresis
> PFGE type IIa

Pfiesteria-**associated syndrome**

Pfiesteria piscicida

Pfizerpen
> P. G

Pf1, Pf2, Pf3 virus

PFT
> pulmonary function test

P/G
> Fulvicin P/G

PGAV
> Pongola virus

PGL
> persistent generalized lymphadenopathy

PH
> Propa PH

pH
> pH slip
> pH testing
> vaginal pH

PHA
> phytohemagglutinin

Phacidiaceae

phacidiomorpha
> *Didymella p.*
> *Glomerella p.*

Phadebact
> P. coagglutination test
> P. GC OMNI test
> P. *Haemophilus influenzae* type b
> COA test
> P. *Haemophilus* test

Phaenicia (p)
> P. *cuprina*
> P. *sericata*

Phaeoannellomyces elegans (f)

phaeobacteroides
> *Chlorobium p.*

phaeochromogenes
> *Streptomyces p.*

phaeoclathratiforme
> *Pelodictyon p.*

Phaeococcomyces catenatus (f)

phaeofaciens
> *Streptomyces p.*

phaeohyphomycosis
> systemic p.

phaeohyphomycotic cyst

phaeomuriformis
> *Sarcinomyces p.*

phaeomycotic cyst

phaeopurpureus
> *Streptomyces p.*

Phaeosclera dematioides (f)

Phaeoscopulariopsis (f)

phaeospermum
> *Arthrinium p.*

Phaeosphaeriaceae

Phaeospirillum (b)
> P. *fulvum*
> P. *molischianum*

NOTES

P

Phaeotheca (f)
    P. *fissurella*
    P. *triangularis*
Phaeotrichaceae
Phaeotrichoconis crotalatiae (f)
phaeovibrioides
    Chlorobium p.
phaeoviridis
    Streptomyces p.
phaeum
    Pelodictyon p.
    Thermacetogenium p.
phage
    beta p.
    defective p.
    rod-shaped p.
    SpV4-type p.
    p. typing
    p. with contractile tail
    p. with double capsid
    p. with long noncontractile tail
    p. with short tail
phagedenic chancroid
phagocyte
    dust p.
    mononuclear p.
    pigmented p.
phagocytic
    p. cell
phagocytize
phagocytophila
    Ehrlichia p.
phagocytosis
Phallaceae
Phallales
phalloides
    Amanita p.
phalloidin
phallolysin
Phanatuss Cough syrup
Phanerochaete chrysosporium (f)
Phaneropsolus bonnei (p)
phanerozoite
PHA-P
    phytohemagglutinin-P
pharaonis
    Halobacterium p.
    Natronobacterium p.
    Natronomonas p.
pharmacodynamic
pharmacokinetic
pharmacologic
pharmacologic acumen
pharmacotherapy
Pharmacy Pill Pak
Pharminil DM
Pharmitussin DM

pharyngeal
    p. gonorrhea
    p. tularemia
pharyngis
    Streptococcus constellatus subsp. *p.*
pharyngitis
    acute p.
    arcanobacterial p.
    exudative p.
    GABHS p.
    gonococcal p.
    group A beta-hemolytic
      streptococcal p.
    mycoplasmal p.
    streptococcal p.
pharyngoconjunctival fever
pharyngoconjunctivitis
pharyngomycosis
pharyngotonsillitis
    streptococcal p.
pharynx
    posterior p.
Phascolarctobacterium faecium (b)
phase
    cardiopulmonary p.
    convalescent p.
    lag p.
    logarithmic p.
    prodromal p.
    stationary p.
phase-contrast
    p.-c. lens
    p.-c. microscopy
phaseoli
    Rhizobium p.
    Xanthomonas p.
phasmid
Phasmidia
Phelloriniaceae
Phenadex Senior
Phenameth DM
phenazinium
    Burkholderia p.
    Pseudomonas p.
phenazopyridine
    p. hydrochloride
    sulfamethiazole p.
    sulfamethoxazole and p.
    sulfisoxazole and p.
Phenergan
    P. VC With Codeine
    P. With Dextromethorphan
Phenhist Expectorant
phenobarbital
    hyoscyamine, atropine, scopolamine,
      and p.
phenobarbitone
phenol

phenol-chloroform extraction
phenolic
phenolica
    Desulfobacula p.
phenolicum
    Desulfobacterium p.
phenomenon, pl. **phenomena**
    Eagle p.
    Koebner p.
    prozone p.
    quellung p.
    Raynaud p.
    Splendore-Hoeppli p.
    Twort-d'Herelle p.
Phenosense assay
phenothiazine
phenotype
    cytolytic p.
    syncytium-inducing p.
    temperature-sensitive p.
phenotypic
    p. assay
    p. drug resistance
    p. testing
phenotyping
phenoxybenzamine
phenoxymethylpenicillin
phenoxymethyl penicillin
phenpropionate
    nandrolone p.
phentolamine
phenylalanine
    p. deaminase production
    p. deaminase test
phenylbutazone
phenylephrine
    guaifenesin, phenylpropanolamine,
      and p.
    sulfacetamide and p.
Phenylfenesin L.A.
phenylketonuria
Phenylobacterium immobile (b)
phenylpropanolamine
    caramiphen and p.
    guaifenesin and p.
    hydrocodone and p.
phenylpyruvica
    Moraxella (Moraxella) p.
phenylpyruvicus
    Psychrobacter p.
phenyltoloxamine, phenylpropanolamine,
    and acetaminophen

phenytoin
Pherazine
    P. VC w/ Codeine
    P. w/DM
    P. With Codeine
Phialemonium (f)
    P. curvatum
    P. obovatum
phialoconidium
Phialophora (f)
    P. americana
    P. bubakii
    P. parasitica
    P. radicicola 2-2-A virus
    P. richardsiae
    P. verrucosa
phialophore-type conidiophore
Philippine capillariasis
philippinense
    Kibdelosporangium p.
philippinensis
    Actinoplanes p.
    Capillaria p.
philippinese
    Eupenicillium p.
philodendri
    Hansenula p.
    Pichia p.
philomiragia
    Francisella p.
    Yersinia p.
Philophthalmidae
Philophthalmus (p)
    P. gralli
    P. hegeneri
    P. lucipetus
    P. megalurus
Philosamia ricini
phlebitis
    septic p.
    suppurative peripheral p.
Phlebotomidae
phlebotomine
phlebotomist
Phlebotomus (p)
    Culicoides phlebotomus
phlebotomus
    p. fever
    p. fever virus
    p. fly
    p. sandfly
phlebotomy

NOTES

P

Phlebovirus (v)
phlegmasia malabarica
phlegmon
    emphysematous p.
    gas p.
phlegmonous
    p. cellulitis
    p. reaction
phlei
    Mycobacterium p.
Phleogenaceae
Phlyctidiaceae
Phnom Penh bat virus (PPBV)
phobia
    fever p.
phocacerebrale
    Mycoplasma p.
phocae
    Arcanobacterium p.
    Atopobacter p.
    Corynebacterium p.
    Streptococcus p.
Phocanema decipiens (p)
phocarhinis
    Mycoplasma p.
phocidae
    Mycoplasma p.
Phocoenobacter uteri (b)
phoeniceum
    Spiroplasma p.
phoeniciae
    Aedes p.
Phoma (f)
    P. cava
    P. cruris-hominis
    P. eupyrena
    P. glomerata
    P. herbarum
    P. hibernica
    P. minutella
    P. minutispora
    P. oculo-hominis
    P. sorghina
Phomatospora minutissima (f)
Phome aspidieticola
phoresis
Phoridae
Phormia regina (p)
Phormidium
    P. autumnale
    P. laminosum
    P. valderianum
phormii
    Fusarium p.
phorozoon
phosalacinea
    Kitasatospora p.

phosalacineus
    Streptomyces p.
phospate
    calcium magnesium ammonium p.
phosphatase
    alkaline p.
    serum alkaline p.
phosphate
    acetyl p.
    Aralen Phosphate With
      Primaquine P.
    chloroquine p.
    Cleocin P.
    clindamycin p.
    Decadron P.
    nicotinamide adenine dinucleotide p.
    primaquine p.
    triple p.
phosphazid
phosphodiesterase
phosphokinase
    creatine p. (CPK)
phospholipase C
phospholipid
Phosphonavir
phosphonoformate
    trisodium p.
phosphonoformic acid (PFA)
phosphoprotein
phosphoreum
    Photobacterium p.
phosphorylation
phosphorylcholine
phosphotungstic acid destain
phosphovorus
    Microlunatus p.
photoautotroph
photoautotrophic
Photobacterium (b)
    P. belozerskii
    P. damselae subsp. *damselae*
    P. damselae subsp. *piscicida*
    P. fischeri
    P. histaminum
    P. iliopiscarium
    P. leiognathi
    P. logei
    P. phosphoreum
    P. profundum
photobacterium, pl. **photobacteria**
photobiotic
photochromogenic
photocoagulation
    laser p.
photodynamic therapy
photogen
photogenesis
photogenic

photoheterotroph
photoheterotrophic
photometricum
    Rhodospirillum p.
photophobia
photophore
photoreactivation
Photorhabdus (b)
    P. asymbiotica
    P. luminescens subsp. *akhurstii*
    P. luminescens subsp. *laumondii*
    P. luminescens subsp. *luminescens*
    P. temperata
photuris
    Mesoplasma p.
Phragmobasidiomycetidae
Phragmopelthecaceae
phthalocyanine
Phthirus pubis (p)
PHV
    Prospect Hill virus
Phycodnavirus (v)
Phycomycetes
phycomycetosis
phycomycosis
    rhinocerebral p.
Phyllachoraceae
Phyllobacterium (b)
    P. myrsinacearum
    P. rubiacearum
Phyllocontin
phylloides (p)
    Demodex p.
phyllosphaerae
    Microbacterium p.
Phyllosticta (f)
phylogenetic
    p. tree
phylogeny
Physa
    P. natricina
    P. rivalis
Physaloptera (p)
    P. caucasica
    P. mordens
    P. praeputialis
    P. rara
physalopteriasis
Physalopteridae
Physalopterinae
Physalopteroidea
Physalospora (f)

Physarales
Physarum pusillum (f)
physellae
    Trichobilharzia p.
physicochemical
physiology
    Score for Neonatal Acute P.
    (SNAP)
physiotherapy
Physocephalus sexalatus (p)
Physodermataceae
Physosporella höhn (f)
Phytobdella (p)
    P. lineata
    P. maculosa
Phytoflagellata
phytohemagglutinin (PHA)
phytohemagglutinin-P (PHA-P)
phytoid
Phytomastigina
Phytomastigophorasida
Phytomastigophorea
phytophagy
Phytoreovirus (v)
PI
    protease inhibitor
pian bois
PIAV
    Picola virus
pica
PICC
    peripherally inserted central catheter
Picchini
    P. syndrome
piceae
    Ophiostoma p.
Pichia (f)
    P. alcoholophila
    P. angusta
    P. anomala
    P. bispora
    P. burtonii
    P. canadensis
    P. capsulata
    P. carsonii
    P. cellobiosa
    P. ciferrii
    P. farinosa
    P. fermentans
    P. finlandica
    P. glucozyma
    P. guilliermondii

NOTES

P

Pichia (continued)
    P. *haplophila*
    P. *henricii*
    P. *holstii*
    P. *jadinii*
    P. *lindnerii*
    P. *membranaefaciens*
    P. *methanolica*
    P. *minuta* var. *minuta*
    P. *minuta* var. *nonfermentans*
    P. *norvegensis*
    P. *ohmeri*
    P. *pastoris*
    P. *philodendri*
    P. *pini*
    P. *polymorpha*
    P. *quercuum*
    P. *rhodanensis*
    P. *sargentensis*
    P. *stipitis*
    P. *strasburgensis*
    P. *subpelliculosa*
    P. *toletana*
    P. *trehalophila*
    P. *vini*
    P. *xylosa*
Pichinde virus (PICV)
pickettii
    Burkholderia p.
    Pseudomonas p.
    Ralstonia p.
picobirnavirus
Picola virus (PIAV)
picolinophilus
    Arthrobacter p.
picorna-parvo-like agent
Picornaviridae
picornavirus
Picrophilus (b)
    P. *oshimae*
    P. *torridus*
pictipennis
    Anopheles p.
pictipes
    Simulium p.
pictorum
    Pseudomonas p.
PICU
    pediatric intensive care unit
PICV
    Pichinde virus
PID
    pelvic inflammatory disease
piechaudii
    Achromobacter p.
    Alcaligenes p.
piedra
    black p.

    p. nostras
    white p.
Piedraiaceae
Piedraia hortae (f)
pifanoi
    Simulium p.
pigment
    malarial p.
    p. production test
pigmented phagocyte
pignaliae
    Candida p.
pigra
    Desulfomonas p.
pigrum
    Dolosigranulum p.
PIH
    pregnancy-induced hypertension
PIIBNV6-C virus
PIIBNV6 virus
PI-induced hyperlipidemia
pilae
    Knemidocoptes p.
pili
    F p.
    R p.
piliated gonococcus
piliferum
    Ophiostoma p.
piliferus
    Culicoides p.
piliforme
    Clostridium p.
Pilimelia (b)
    P. *anulata*
    P. *columellifera* subsp. *columellifera*
    P. *columellifera* subsp. *pallida*
    P. *terevasa*
pill
    birth control p. (BCP)
    Doan's Backache P.'s
    oral contraceptive p. (OCP)
pillar
    tonsillar p.
Pillotina (b)
    P. *calotermitidis*
Pilobolaceae
pilosa
    Cavernicola p.
pilosicoli
    Brachyspira p.
    Serpulina p.
pilosum
    Corynebacterium p.
    Simulium p.
pilosus
    Culex p.

Monascus p.
Streptomyces p.
Pima
Pimelobacter (b)
    P. jensenii
    P. simplex
    P. tumescens
pimozide
pinea
    Macrophoma p.
pinensis
    Chitinophaga p.
    Nocardia p.
pinetorium
    Eupenicillium p.
pini
    Candida p.
    Pichia p.
piniformis
    Skermania p.
pink bread mold
pinkeye
pinocytosis
Pinoyella simii
Pin-Rid
pinta
pintid
pinto
    mal del p.
pintoi
    Simulium p.
pinworm
    p. preparation
    p. vaginitis
Pin-X
pioglitazone
pionips
    Aedes p.
Piophila casei (p)
Piophilidae
piperacillin
    p. and tazobactam sodium
piperacillin+tazobactam
piperatus
    Boletus p.
piperazine
    p. citrate
    p. solution
piperi
    Simulium p.
pipestem fibrosis
pipette

pipetting
pipiens
    Culex p.
pipientis
    Wolbachia p.
Pipracil
Piptocephalidaceae
Pirella (b)
    P. marina
    P. staleyi
Pirellula (b)
    P. marina
    P. staleyi
Pirenella conica (f)
Piricauda (f)
piriform
Piroplasma donovani (p)
Piroplasmasina
Piroplasmida
Piroplasmorida
piroplasmosis
piroxicam
pirum
    Mycoplasma p.
PIRYV
    Piry virus
Piry virus (PIRYV)
piscicida
    Pfiesteria p.
    Photobacterium damselae subsp. *p.*
    Pseudoalteromonas p.
piscicola
    Carnobacterium p.
    Lactobacillus p.
piscifermentans
    Staphylococcus p.
pisciphila
    Exophiala p.
Piscirickettsia salmonis (b)
piscium
    Haemophilus p.
    Lactococcus p.
    Pedobacter p.
    Sphingobacterium p.
    Trichosporon p.
pisi
    Xanthomonas p.
pisiformis
    Cysticercus p.
    Taenia p.
piston-pump inhibitor

NOTES

pit
clathrin-coated p.
Pithoascaceae
Pithoascus langeronii (f)
Pithomyces (f)
P. atro-olivaceus
P. chartarum
Pitrex
pittsburghensis
Legionella p.
Pittsburgh pneumonia agent
pituitary
p. gland
p. tuberculosis
pituitosa
Sphingomonas p.
pityriasis
p. capitis
p. folliculorum
p. nigra
p. rosea
p. versicolor
Pityrosporum (f)
pivampicillin
pivotal
Pixuna virus (PIXV)
PIXV
Pixuna virus
pizza-pie fundus
PKS
pulmonary Kaposi sarcoma
PL-1 virus
placei
Haemonchus p.
placentae
abruptio p.
placenta previa
placidus
Ferroglobus p.
Plagiorchiida
Plagiorchioidea
Plagiorchis (p)
P. maculosus
P. nobeli
plague
p. bacillus
bubonic p.
cutaneous p.
duck p.
meningeal p.
Pahvant Valley p.
pneumonic p.
septicemic p.
sylvatic p.
p. vaccine
plain
Orabase P.
tetanus toxoid p.

planci
Acanthaster p.
Planctomyces (b)
P. bekefii
P. brasiliensis
P. guttaeformis
P. hajdui
P. limnophilus
P. maris
P. stranskae
Planctomycetaceae
Planctomycetales
plane
fascial p.
p. wart
planitis
pars p.
plankter
plankton
planktonic
p. algae
Planobispora (b)
P. longispora
P. rosea
Planococcus (b)
P. alkanoclasticus
P. citreus
P. halophilus
P. kocurii
P. mcmeekinii
P. okeanokoites
Planomicrobium (b)
P. koreense
P. mcmeekinii
P. okeanokoites
Planomonospora (b)
P. alba
P. parontospora subsp. antibiotica
P. parontospora subsp. parontospora
P. sphaerica
P. venezuelensis
Planopolyspora crispa (b)
Planorbis
Planotetraspora mira (b)
plant agglutinin
plantar
p. rash
p. wart
plantarii
Burkholderia p.
Pseudomonas p.
plantarum
Curtobacterium p.
Lactobacillus p.
Lactococcus p.
Nocardioides p.
Streptococcus p.

planticola
>*Klebsiella p.*
>*Rauoltella p.*

planus
>lichen p.
>oral erosive lichen p.

plaque
>atheromatous p.
>bacterial p.
>bacteriophage p.
>p. neutralization technique
>prion protein scrapie isoform-
>   reactive p. (PrP^{Sc}-reactive plaque)
>PrP^{Sc}-reactive p.
>>prion protein scrapie isoform-
>>   reactive plaque
>p. reduction neutralization assay
>p. sporotrichosis

plaque-like
Plaquenil
plasma
>p. anti-SEA antibody concentration
>p. cell
>p. cell balanitis
>p. cell deciduitis
>p. cell infiltrate
>p. cell myeloma
>p. cortisol concentration
>P. Exchange/Sandoglobulin Guillain-
>   Barró Syndrome Trial Group
>fresh frozen p. (FFP)
>p. glucose
>p. HIV load
>p. HIV RNA concentration
>p. HIV RNA level
>p. lactate
>p. lipid concentration
>p. retinol level
>p. selenium level
>p. viral burden
>p. viral level
>p. viral load (PVL, pVL)
>p. viremia

plasmablastic lymphoma
plasmacytic interstitial nephritis
plasmacytoma
plasmacytosis
plasma-derived
plasmapheresis
Plasmaviridae
Plasmavirus (v)

plasmid
>p. analysis
>bacteriocinogenic p.
>conjugative p.
>F p.
>infectious p.
>nonconjugative p.
>p. pattern analysis (PPA)
>p. profile
>p. profiling
>resistance p. (R-plasmid)
>transmissible p.

plasmodial
Plasmodiidae
Plasmodiophorales
Plasmodiophoromycetes
Plasmodium (p)
>*P. berghei*
>*P. cynomolgi*
>*P. falciparum*
>*P. falciparum* erythrocyte membrane
>   protein-1 (PfEMP-1)
>*P. knowlesi*
>*P. kochi*
>*P. malariae*
>*P. ovale*
>*P. vivax*

Plasmodium-opsonizing antibody
plasmotomy
Plaster
>Mediplast P.
>Sal-Acid P.

plastic-embedded
plastic envelope culture
plastid
plate
>nonnutrient agar p.
>Presumpto p.
>stigmal p.

platelet
>p. count
>p. endothelial cell adhesion
>   molecule-1 (PECAM-1)
>p. transfusion

platelet-activating factor (PAF)
platelet-neutralization
platensis
>*Coprothermobacter p.*
>*Streptomyces p.*

plating
Platinol
Platinol-AQ

NOTES

P

platyhelix
    Spiroplasma p.
platyhelminth
Platyhelminthes
Platynosomum fastosum (p)
platyurus
    Helicotylenchus p.
plauti
    Fusobacterium p.
plautii
    Eubacterium p.
PLAV
    Playas virus
Playas virus (PLAV)
plebeius
    Vaginulus p.
pleciae
    Mesoplasma p.
plecoglossicida
    Pseudomonas p.
pleconaril
Plectomycetes
Plectosphaerella cucumerina (f)
plectridium
Plectrovirus
pleiomorpha
    Acrocarpospora p.
Pleistophora hyphessobryonchis
Pleistophorida
pleocytosis
    cerebrospinal fluid p.
    CSF p.
    eosinophilic p.
    lymphocytic p.
    neutrophilic p.
Pleomassariaceae
pleomorpha
    Cryptomyces p.
pleomorphic
    p. lymphoma
    p. organism
    p. phage virus
pleomorphus
    Streptococcus p.
Pleosporaceae
Pleospora herbarum (f)
plerocercoid
    p. larva
Plesiomonas shigelloides (b)
plethysmography
    BodPod p.
    strain-gauge p.
    whole-body p.
pleural
    p. aspirate
    p. effusion
    p. empyema
    p. fluid

    p. fluid cytology
    p. fluid tap
    p. pH level
    p. tuberculosis
pleuristriatus
    Culex p.
pleurisy
    epidemic diaphragmatic p.
    serofibrinous p.
    tuberculous p.
pleuritic
    p. chest pain
    p. pain
pleurodesis
    doxycycline p.
    minocycline p.
pleurodynia
    epidemic p.
pleurogenous
Pleurophoma pleurospora (f)
Pleurophragmium (f)
pleuropneumoniae
    Actinobacillus p.
    Haemophilus p.
pleuropneumonia-like organisms (PPLO)
pleuropulmonary
    p. amebiasis
pleurospora
    Pleurophoma p.
Pleurotus (f)
    P. columbinus
    P. ostreatus
    P. pulmonarius
    P. sapidus
plexicaudatum
    Eubacterium p.
plexus
    Auerbach p.
    Batson p.
    choroid p.
    Meissner p.
    myenteric p.
plicatilis
    Spirochaeta p.
plicatus
    Streptomyces p.
PLM-5 medium
PLMVd
PLSV
    Palestina virus
plumbeum
    Hyalomma p.
plumbism
plumosus
    Chironomus p.
pluranimalium
    Arcanobacterium p.
    Streptococcus p.

pluricolorescens
    Streptomyces p.
plurifarium
    Mesorhizobium p.
pluripotent
pluriseptata
    Drechslera p.
plus
    Clearasil B.P. P.
    Compound W P.
    Duramist P.
    Ionil-T P.
    Optimyxin P.
    Pert P.
    P & S P.
    Quinsana P.
    p. sense-RNA genome
    P. Sinus
    Soluver P.
    Tri-Tannate P.
Pluteacaea
Pluteus (f)
plutonius
    Melissococcus p
pluvialis
pluvialis
    Anthomyia p.
    Haematopota p.
plymuthica
    Serratia p.
PMC
    pseudomembranous colitis
PMEA
    adefovir
      Bis-POM PMEA
PML
    progressive multifocal
      leukoencephalopathy
PMN
    polymorphonuclear leukocyte
      agranular PMN
PMNL
    polymorphonuclear leukocyte
PMRV
    Paramushir virus
PMS-Amantadine
PMS-Conjugated Estrogens
PMS-Dexamethasone
PMS-Erythromycin
PMS-Isoniazid
PMS-Lindane
PMS-Nystatin

PMS-Prochlorperazine
PMS-Pseudoephedrine
PMS-Pyrazinamide
PMS-Sucralfate
PMS-Tobramycin
PMV 1–9
    avian paramyxovirus virus 1–9
pneumatic nebulizer
pneumaticum
    Prosthecomicrobium p.
pneumobacillus
pneumococcal
    p. bacteremia
    p. capsular polysaccharide (CPS)
    p. capsular polysaccharide antigen
    p. infection
    p. meningitis
    p. sepsis
    p. surface adhesin A
    p. surface antigen A
    p. vaccine
    7-valent p. conjugate vaccine
pneumococcosis
pneumococcus, pl. **pneumococci**
    Fraenkel p.
    penicillin-resistant p.
Pneumocystis (f)
    P. carinii
    P. carinii choroiditis
    P. carinii pneumonia (PCP)
    P. carinii test
    P. jiroveci
pneumocystosis
    extrapulmonary p. (EPP)
    p. granulomatosa
pneumoencephalography
pneumolysin (SPN)
Pneumomist
pneumomycosis
pneumonia
    abattoir-associated p.
    adenoviral p.
    aspiration p.
    atypical p.
    bacterial pneumococcal p.
    bronchiolitis obliterans-organizing p.
      (BOOP)
    Candida p.
    p. cavitation
    chronic eosinophilic p. (CEP)
    chronic fibrocavitary p.
    CMV p.

NOTES

P

pneumonia *(continued)*
  community-acquired p.
  community-acquired bacterial p.
    (CAP)
  diffuse interstitial p. (DIP)
  embolic p.
  focal p.
  Friedländer p.
  gram-negative p.
  Haemophilus influenzae p.
  Hecht p.
  hematogenous p.
  influenza p.
  interstitial plasma cell p.
  Klebsiella p.
  lobar p.
  lymphocytic interstitial p.
  lymphoid interstitial p. (LIP)
  measles giant cell p.
  mycobacterial necrotizing p.
  Mycoplasma p.
  mycoplasmal p.
  necrotizing p.
  nontuberculous p.
  nosocomial p.
  Pneumocystis carinii p. (PCP)
  primary atypical p.
  sepsis p.
  staphylococcal p.
  streptococcal p.
  varicella p.
  p. virus of mice
  walking p.
  woolsorter's p.
pneumoniae
  Chlamydia p.
  Chlamydophila p.
  drug-resistant *Streptococcus* p.
  drug-susceptible *Streptococcus* p.
  Klebsiella p.
  Klebsiella pneumoniae subsp. *p.*
  Mycoplasma p.
  Streptococcus p.
pneumonic
  p. infiltrate
  p. plague
  p. tularemia
pneumonitis
  chlamydial p.
  chronic interstitial p.
  CMV p.
  eosinophilic p.
  fibrinopurulent p.
  granulomatous p.
  hemorrhagic p.
  hypersensitivity p.
  interstitial p.
  lymphoid interstitial p. (LIP)

  nonspecific interstitial p. (NIP,
    NSIP)
  radiation p.
  rheumatoid p.
pneumonococcal
pneumonococcus
Pneumonyssoides caninum (p)
Pneumonyssus (p)
  P. caninum
  P. simicola
Pneumopent
pneumopericarditis
pneumophila
  Legionella pneumophila subsp. *p.*
pneumosintes
  Bacteroides p.
  Dialister p.
Pneumoslide
pneumothorax
pneumotropica
  Pasteurella p.
Pneumovax
  P. 23
Pneumovirinae
Pneumovirus (v)
pnomenusa
  Pandoraea p.
PNPG
  p-nitrophenylglycerol
PNU-140690
Pnu-Imune
  P.-I. 23
PO$_4$
  chloroquine P.
poae
  Leifsonia p.
POCkit HSV-2 Rapid Test
podagra
Podaxaceae
Podaxales
Pod-Ben-25
Podocon-25
Podofilm
podofilox
Podofin
podophyllin
  p. resin
  p. and salicylic acid
podophyllotoxin
podophyllum resin
Podospora
  P. anserina
  P. leporina
podosterni
  Simulium p.
Podoviridae
podsolicum
  Pedomicrobium p.

podzolicus
> *Cryptococcus p.*

Pogonomyrmex
> *P. occidentalis*
> *P. rugosus*

POHS
> presumed ocular histoplasmosis
> syndrome

poinarii
> *Xenorhabdus p.*
> *Xenorhabdus nematophila* subsp. *p.*

poinsettiae
> *Corynebacterium p.*

point
> Erb p.

point-prevalent survey (PPS)

poison
> protoplasmic p.

poisoning
> amnesic shellfish p. (ASP)
> bacterial food p.
> ciguatera fish p.
> diarrheic shellfish p. (DSP)
> diarrhetic shellfish p.
> fish p.
> food p.
> fugu p.
> grayanotoxin p.
> histamine p.
> kinkoti bean p.
> mushroom p.
> neurotoxic shellfish p. (NSP)
> paralytic shellfish p. (PSP)
> pufferfish p.
> pyrrolizidine alkaloid p.
> red kidney bean p.
> salmon p.
> *Salmonella* food p.
> scombroid p.
> shellfish p.
> staphylococcal food p.
> *Staphylococcus* food p.
> tetradon p.
> toadstool p.

Polaribacter (b)
> *P. filamentus*
> *P. franzmannii*
> *P. glomeratus*
> *P. irgensii*

Polaromonas vacuolata (b)

polar ring

pole
> posterior p.

polecki
> *Entamoeba p.*

Pol-encoded

Polerovirus (v)

polio
> nonparalytic p.
> paralytic p.
> p. vaccine (IPV)
> vaccine-related paralytic p.

polioencephalitis
> p. infectiva

poliomyelitis
> abortive p.
> acute anterior p.
> acute bulbar p.
> bulbar p.
> paralytic p.
> p. virus

poliovirus
> p. 1
> p. antibody
> p. culture
> p. hominis
> human p.
> human p. 1, 2
> inactivated p.
> p. serology
> p. type 2 Lansing strain
> p. vaccine
> p. vaccine
> wild-type p.

polka fever

Pollenia
> *P. rudis*

polonica
> *Bilharziella p.*

polyacrylamide
> p. gel electrophoresis (PAGE)
> p. gel electrophoresis with silver
> stain (PAGE-SS)

polyadenylation signal

Polyadnaviridae

polyanetholesulfonate
> sodium p. (SPS)

Polyangiaceae

Polyangium (b)
> *P. aureum*
> *P. cellulosum*
> *P. fumosum*
> *P. luteum*

NOTES

P

Polyangium (*continued*)
P. minor
P. parasiticum
P. rugiseptum
P. sorediatum
P. spumosum
P. vitellinum
polyanions
polyantibiotic
polyarteritis
p. nodosa
polyarthritis
epidemic p.
Ross River p.
polyarthropathy
acute symmetric p.
polyarticular
p. arthritis
polychemotherapy
polychroma
Actinomadura p.
Microtetraspora p.
Nonomuraea p.
polychromogenes
Arthrobacter p.
Streptomyces p.
Polycidin
Polycillin
Polycillin-N
polyclonal
p. antibody
p. B lymphocyte
p. lymphoma
p. lymphoproliferative syndrome
polycystic
p. echinococcosis
p. hydatid disease
p. kidney disease
Polycytella hominis (f)
polycythemia
polydactylitis
Polyderm
polydioxanone
polydipsia
Polydnaviridae
polyendosporus
Anaerobacter p.
polyene
polyether
polygalacturonate
quinidine p.
Polygam
P. S/D
polyhedrosis
Poly-Histine CS
polyhydramnios
polyhydroxylated cyclic hydrocarbon

polyisoprenivorans
Gordonia p.
polyleptic fever
polylysine
penicilloyl p. (PPL)
polymastigote
polymenorrhea
polymerase
p. chain reaction (PCR)
p. chain reaction in situ
hybridization (PCR-ISH)
p. gamma
RNA-dependent DNA p.
polymerization
polymicrobial
p. bacteremia
p. endocarditis
p. infection
p. soiling
polymicrobian
polymitus
polymixin B
polymorpha
Gregarina p.
Hansenula p.
Hyphomonas p.
Pichia p.
Sporichthya p.
polymorphic infiltration
Polymorphidae
polymorphism
amplicon fragment length p.
(AFLP)
PCR combined with single-strand
conformation p. (PCR-SSCP)
restriction fragment length p.
(RFLP)
single-strand conformation p.
(SSCP)
polymorphonuclear
p. cell
p. leukocyte (PMN, PMNL)
p. pleocytosis
polymorphum
Aquaspirillum p.
Fusarium p.
Fusobacterium nucleatum subsp. p.
polymorphus
Caseobacter p.
Flexibacter p.
Polymox
polymyalgia rheumatica
polymyarian
polymyositis
idiopathic p.
p. syndrome

polymyxa
>> Bacillus p.
>> Paenibacillus p.

polymyxin
>> p. B
>> p. B and hydrocortisone
>> p. B sulfate
>> p. E

polynesiensis
>> Aedes p.

polyneuropathy
>> sensory p.

Polynucleobacter (b)
>> P. necessarius

polynucleotide vaccine

Polyomavirus (v)

polyomavirus
>> p. BK
>> BKV human p.
>> JC p.

polyp
>> colonic p.
>> villous p.

Polypaecilum insolutum (f)

polypapilloma

polypectomy snare

polypeptide
>> endothelial-monocyte activating p.
>> II (EMAP II)

polyphaga
>> Acanthamoeba p.

polyphagia

polypharmaceutic

polypharmacy

Polyplax (p)

polyploidy

Polyporaceae

polyposis
>> colonic p.
>> multiple p.

polypragmatus
>> Bacteroides p.

Poly-Pred Ophthalmic suspension

polypropylene

polyprotein
>> Gag p.
>> Gag-Pol p.

polyradiculitis
>> ascending p.

polyradiculoneuritis
>> postinfective p.

polyradiculopathy

polyribosyl-ribitol-phosphate (PRP)

polysaccharea
>> Neisseria p.

polysaccharide
>> p. capsule
>> pneumococcal capsular p. (CPS)
>> p. synthesis test

polysaccharolyticum
>> Clostridium p.
>> Fusobacterium p.
>> Thermoanaerobacterium p.

polyserositis
>> tuberculous p.

polyspora
>> Crenothrix p.
>> Sydowia p.

Polysporin
>> P. Ophthalmic
>> P. Topica

Polystigmatales

Polystomellaceae

Polytar

polytene chromosome

polytetrafluorethylene (PTFE)

Polytopic

Polytracin

polytricha
>> Chryseomonas p.

Polytrim
>> P. Ophthalmic

polytropus
>> Ilyobacter p.

polyurethane

polyuria

polyvalent
>> antivenin Crotalidae p.
>> p. gas gangrene antitoxin
>> p. pneumococcal polysaccharide
>> vaccine

polyvinyl
>> p. alcohol (PVA)
>> p. chloride (PVC)

polyzoic

pomaceae
>> Zymomonas mobilis subsp. p.

pombe
>> Schizosaccharomyces p.

pomona
>> Leptospira interrogans serovar p.

pomorum
>> Acetobacter p.

NOTES

P

Pomovirus (v)
Pondocillin
pongine herpesvirus 2
Pongola virus (PGAV)
ponos
Ponteves virus (PTVV)
Pontiac fever
pontiacus
    Sulfitobacter p.
pontis
    Lactobacillus p.
pontomedullary
pool
    Lim Benyesh-Melnick intersecting antiserum p.
    myeloid p.
poonensis
    Chainia p.
    Streptomyces p.
popilliae
    Bacillus p.
    Paenibacillus p.
    Rickettsiella p.
popliteal ultrasound
popoffii
    Aeromonas p.
populeti
    Clostridium p.
populi
    Candida p.
    Xanthomonas p.
porci
    Eimeria p.
porcine
    p. adenovirus 1–6
    p. astrovirus 1–11
    p. circovirus
    p. enteric calcivirus
    p. enterovirus 1–11
    p. hemagglutinating encephalomyelitis virus
    p. parvovirus
    p. rubulavirus
    p. transmissible gastroenteritis
    p. transmissible gastroenteritis virus
    p. type C oncovirus
    p. xenograft
porcinum
    Mycobacterium p.
porcinus
    Actinobacillus p.
    Streptococcus p.
Pore
    Oxy Deep P.
Porges method
Poria (f)
Porifera

poriferae
    Mycobacterium p.
PORN
    progressive outer retinal necrosis
porocephaliasis
Porocephalida
Porocephalidae
porocephalosis
Porocephalus
    P. armillatus
    P. crotali
    P. moniliformis
poroconidium
pororicense
    Haplographium p.
porospore
porphyria
    p. cutanea tarda
Porphyrobacter (b)
    P. neustonensis
    P. tepidarius
Porphyromonas (b)
    P. asaccharolytica
    P. cangingivalis
    P. canoris
    P. cansulci
    P. catoniae
    P. circumdentaria
    P. crevioricanis
    P. endodontalis
    P. gingivalis
    P. gingivicanis
    P. gulae
    P. levii
    P. macacae
    P. salivosa
porrigo
    p. favosa
    p. furfurans
    p. lupinosa
    p. scutulata
Port-a-Cath
portal
    p. hypertension
    p. tract
portio
    cervical p.
    p. vaginalis
Porton virus
portoricensis
    Aedes p.
portucalensis
    Methanohalophilus p.
portulacae
    Dichotomophthora p.
Posadas disease
Posadasia (f)

positive
>biologic false p. (BFP)
>p. end-expiratory pressure (PEEP)
>gram p.
>indole p.
>nicotinamide adenine dinucleotide phosphate p. (NADP⁺)
>p. predictive value (PPV)
>Rh p.
>trace p.

positron emission tomography (PET)
posoensis
>Culicoides p.

Pospiviroid (v)
postabortal
>p. endometritis
>p. infection

postanginal sepsis
postencephalitis syndrome
postenteritis reactive arthritis
posterior
>p. fornix
>p. fossa syndrome
>p. pharynx
>p. pole
>p. segment
>p. superior iliac spine (PSIS)
>p. tongue
>p. urethral valve

postexposure
>p. prevention
>p. prophylaxis

postgatei
>Desulfobacter p.

postherpetic neuralgia
posthysterectomy cellulitis
postinfectious
>p. encephalomyelitis
>p. eosinophilia
>p. leukoencephalitis

postinfective polyradiculoneuritis
postinflammatory pigmentation
post-kala azar dermal leishmaniasis
postmenopausal
postoperative
postpartum
>p. bacteremia
>p. endometritis (PPE)

postpolio syndrome
postprostatectomy
postsalpingitis infertility

poststreptococcal
>p. acute glomerulonephritis
>p. AGN

postsurgical
>p. meningitis

posttransfusion
>p. hepatitis (PTH)
>p. purpura

posttransplantation lymphoproliferative disorder (PTLD)
posttransplant lymphoproliferative disorder (PTLD)
posttraumatic meningitis
postulate
>Koch p.

postulated
posture
>decorticate p.
>opisthotonic p.

potassium
>p. alum
>amoxicillin and clavulanate p.
>benzylpenicillin p.
>p. dichromate solution
>p. hydroxide (KOH)
>p. hydroxide stain
>p. hydroxide testing
>p. hydroxide wet mount preparation
>p. iodide
>P. Iodide Enseals
>p. penicillin G (KPG)
>penicillin V p.
>ticarcillin and clavulanate p.
>total body p. (TBK)

potato virus Y
potency
potent
>p. antiretroviral therapy
>p. protease inhibitor

potential
>p. exposure
>somatosensory evoked p. (SSEP)

potentiate
potentiator
>macrophage infectivity p. (mip)

Potexvirus (v)
Potomac fever
potronii
>Acremonium p.

Pott
>P. disease
>P. paraplegia

NOTES

P

433

Potyvirus (v)
pouch culture
poulsonii
 Spiroplasma p.
poultryman's itch
poultry rotavirus
poverty
povidone-iodine aqueous solution
POVT
 puerperal ovarian vein thrombosis
Powassan
 P. virus (POWV)
 P. virus encephalitis
Powder
 Absorbine Antifungal Foot P.
 Lotrimin AF Spray P.
 Pedi-Dri Topical P.
 Zeasorb-AF P.
POWV
 Powassan virus
pox
 money p.
 monkey p.
Poxviridae
poxvirus
 California harbor seal p.
 p. of Coleoptera
 p. of Diptera
 p. of Lepidoptera and Orthoptera
 mule deer p.
pp65 antigenemia
PP7 virus
PP8 virus
PPA
 plasmid pattern analysis
PPBV
 Phnom Penh bat virus
PPCA
 percent of the periphery that has ciliary
 activity
PPD
 purified protein derivative
 5 tuberculin unit strength purified protein
 derivative
  PPD test
  Tine Test PPD
PPE
 personal protective equipment
 postpartum endometritis
PPH
 primary pulmonary hypertension
PPI
 proton pump inhibitor
PPL
 penicilloyl polylysine
  PPL skin test
PPLO
 pleuropneumonia-like organisms

PPNG
 penicillinase-producing gonococci
 penicillinase-producing *Neisseria*
  gonorrhoeae
PPS
 point-prevalent survey
PPV
 positive predictive value
 Precarious Point virus
PR
 protease
  PR chemotherapy
  PR inhibitor
PR3 virus
PR4 virus
PR64FS virus
PR772 virus
practice
 Advisory Committee on
  Immunization P.'s (ACIP)
 good manufacturing p. (GMP)
practitioner
 infection control p. (ICP)
praeacuta
 Tissierella p.
praeacutus
 Bacteroides p.
praecisus
praecox
 Streptomyces p.
praeputialis (p)
 Physaloptera p.
praevalens
 Halanaerobium p.
Pragia fontium (b)
Prague strain Rous sarcoma virus
 (PRSV)
prairie itch
pramoxine
pranobex
 inosine p.
prasina
 Nocardiopsis p.
 Nocardiopsis alba subsp. *p.*
 Nocardiopsis dassonvillei subsp. *p.*
prasinopilosus
 Streptomyces p.
prasinosporus
 Streptomyces p.
Prasinovirus (v)
prasinus
 Streptomyces p.
Prauserella rugosa (b)
prausnitzii
 Fusobacterium p.
pravastatin
praziquantel

PRCA
    pure red cell aplasia
prealbumin
preantibiotic era
preauricular
    p. lymphadenopathy
Precarious Point virus (PPV)
precaution
    standard p.
Precef
precipitate
    keratic p.
precipitation
    immune p.
precipitin
    immunodiffusion tube p. (IDTP)
    p. test
    tube p. (TP)
precursor
    p. B cell
    p. pool
Pred
    Liquid P.
Pred-G Ophthalmic
predictive value
prednicarbate
Prednicen-M
prednisolone
    chloramphenicol and p.
    p. and gentamicin
    neomycin, polymyxin B, and p.
    sulfacetamide and p.
    p. (systemic)
Prednisol TBA Injection
prednisone
    p. acetate
preeclampsia
preferred agent
pregnancy
    ectopic p.
pregnancy-induced hypertension (PIH)
prehospitalization
prehybridization
Preisz-Nocard bacillus (*See*
    Corynebacterium pseudotuberculosis)
preleukemia
Prelone Oral
Premarin
premature rupture of membranes
    (PROM)
prematurity
premenopausal

Premier *Helicobacter pylori* **assay**
Premphase
Prempro
premunition
prenatal/congenital
preoperative
    p. antimicrobial prophylaxis (PAP)
prep
    KOH p.
    wet p.
preparation
    cerebrospinal fluid India ink p.
    crush p.
    Cryptococcus p.
    cytocentrifuge p.
    Enterobius vermicularis p.
    filariasis peripheral blood p.
    germicidal p.
    India ink p.
    KOH p.
    nigrosin p.
    pinworm p.
    potassium hydroxide wet mount p.
    Scholl Athlete's Foot P.'s
    touch p.
    Trichomonas vaginalis wet p.
    trypanosomiasis peripheral blood p.
    Tzanck p.
    wet mount p.
prepatent period
Pre-pen skin test
prepubertal
prepuce
prereduced
preretinal
Prescription Strength Desenex
preseptal cellulitis
preseptal/orbital cellulitis
pressor support
pressure
    continuous positive airway p.
      (CPAP)
    intracranial p.
    positive end-expiratory p. (PEEP)
presumed ocular histoplasmosis
    syndrome (POHS)
presumptive diagnosis
Presumpto plate
preterm
pretibial
    p. fever
    p. rash

NOTES

P

pretiosum
    Actinosynnema pretiosum subsp. *p.*
Pretoria virus (PREV)
pretoriensis
    Saccharomyces p.
Pretz-D
PREV
    Pretoria virus
Prevacid
prevalence
Prevent
    Gaviscon P.
prevention
    Centers for Disease Control and P.
      (CDCP)
    malaria p.
    postexposure p.
    urinary tract infection p.
    varicella-zoster p.
preventive treatment
Preveon
preveon
Prevex
    P. B
    P. Diaper Rash Cream
    P. HC
previa
    placenta p.
Prevnar
Prevotella (b)
    P. albensis
    P. bivia
    P. brevis
    P. bryantii
    P. buccae
    P. buccalis
    P. corporis
    P. dentalis
    P. denticola
    P. disiens
    P. enoeca
    P. heparinolytica
    P. intermedia
    P. loescheii
    P. melaninogenica
    P. nicrescens
    P. oralis
    P. oris
    P. oulora
    P. pallens
    P. ruminicola
    P. ruminicola subsp. *brevis*
    P. ruminicola subsp. *ruminicola*
    P. tannerae
    P. veroralis
    P. zoogleoformans
prevotii
    Anaerococcus p.

    Peptococcus p.
    Peptostreptococcus p.
pricei
    Ornithobilharzia p.
prick test
Priftin
Prilosec
primaevus
    Leptoconops p.
primaquine
    chloroquine and p.
    p. and chloroquine
    p. phosphate
primary
    p. amebic meningitis
    p. amebic meningoencephalitis
      (PAM)
    p. amoebic meningoencephalitis
      (PAM)
    p. atypical pneumonia
    p. brain lymphoma
    p. central nervous system
      lymphoma (PCNSL)
    p. coccidioidomycosis
    p. effusion lymphoma
    p. growth hormone deficiency
    p. infection
    p. meningococcal conjunctivitis
    p. occult bacteremia
    p. progressive lung disease
    p. prophylaxis
    p. pulmonary histoplasmosis
    p. pulmonary hypertension (PPH)
    p. screw worm
    p. septicemia
    p. syphilis
    p. tuberculosis
    p. viremia
primary syphilis
Primatene Mist
primate T-lymphotropic virus 1, 2, 3
Prima Toxin A enzyme immunoassay
primatum
    Mycoplasma p.
Primaxin
primer
    PCR with arbitrary p. (AP-PCR)
    sequence-specific DNA p. (SSDP)
primerite
primigravida
primiparous
primite
primordium
    genital p.
Primsol
Principen
Prioderm

prion
- p. disease
- p. protein (PrP)
- p. protein normal isoform (PrP^c)
- p. protein scrapie isoform (PrP^{Sc})
- p. protein scrapie isoform-reactive plaque (PrP^{Sc}-reactive plaque)

priority
- law of p.

PRISM
- Pediatric Risk of Mortality

pristinamycin

PRN
- pertactin

Pro-Amox

proatherogenic

probacteriophage
- defective p.

Pro-Banthine

probe
- acridine ester-labeled nucleic acid p.
- chlamydia p.
- DNA p.
- *Legionella* DNA p.
- nucleic acid p.
- p. test

probenecid
- ampicillin and p.

probiosis

probiotic

problematic

Probstymayria vivipara (p)

procainamide

procaine
- p. benzylpenicillin
- p. penicillin
- penicillin G p.
- p. penicillin G

Procandida
- *P. albicans*
- *P. grubyii*
- *P. langeronii*
- *P. majoricensis*
- *P. stellatoidea*
- *P. tamarindii*
- *P. tropicalis*

Procaryotae

procaryote

procaryotic

procedure
- hanging-drop p.

loop electrosurgical excisional p. (LEEP)
- PAIR p.
- puncture, aspiration, injection, and reaspiration p.
- transurethral prostate p. (TURP)

procellaris
- *Anthomyia procellaris*

procercoid

Procerovum varium (p)

process
- host-immune p.

Prochloraceae

Prochlorales

ProChlorax

Prochlorococcus (b)
- *P. marinus* subsp. *marinus*
- *P. marinus* subsp. *pastoris*

Prochloron didemni (b)

Prochlorothrix (b)
- *P. hollandica*

Prochlorotrichaceae

prochlorperazine

Procrit

proctitis

proctocolectomy

proctocolitis

proctodeal

proctodeum

proctoscopic examination

proctoscopy

procyonis
- *Baylisascaris* p.
- *Belascaris* p.
- *Gnathostoma* p.

prodexargenteum
- *Simulium* p.

prodromal
- p. labor
- p. phase
- p. stage

prodrome

production
- antibody p.
- hydrogen sulfide p.
- phenylalanine deaminase p.
- urease p.

productus
- *Peptostreptococcus* p.
- *Ruminococcus* p.

proerythrocyte

NOTES

P

Profen
    P. II
    P. II DM
    P. LA
professional
    infection control p. (ICP)
profile
    blood cell p.
    hepatitis B p.
    plasmid p.
    protein p.
    T-cell p.
profiling
    biochemical p.
    multiple arbitrary amplicon p.
    (MAAP)
    plasmid p.
profound thrombocytopenia
profundum
    Photobacterium p.
profundus
    Archaeoglobus p.
    Desulfovibrio p.
    Thermococcus p.
progenitalis
    herpes p.
progenitor
    p. cell
    erythroid p.
    hematopoietic p.
progeny virus
progesterone
progestin implant
proglottid
proglottina
    Davainea p.
proglottis
prognosis
program
    AIDS Drug Assistance P. (ADAP)
    drug-maintenance p.
    educational p.
    needle exchange p.
    Onchocerciasis Control p. (OCP)
    peer-support p.
    United Nations AIDS Control p.
    (UNAIDS)
progressive
    p. bacterial synergistic
    p. cleavage
    p. disseminated histoplasmosis
    (PDH)
    p. emphysematous necrosis
    p. multifocal leukoencephalopathy
    (PML)
    p. outer retinal necrosis (PORN)
    p. rubella panencephalitis
progressive-stage disease

proguanil
    atovaquone and p.
    p. and atovaquone
ProHIBIT vaccine
proinflammatory cytokine
Prokaryotae
prokaryote
prokaryotic
    p. bacteria
prolapsa
    Muscina p.
prolapse
    mitral valve p.
    rectal p.
Prolastin
proliferation
    amastigote p.
    p. assay
    basaloid p.
    glial p.
    lymphocyte p.
proliferative dermatitis
proliferatum
    Fusarium p.
prolificans
    Scedosporium p.
Prolinoborus fasciculus (b)
prolixus
    Rhodnius p.
prolonged
    p. acute hepatitis
    p. diarrhea
Proloprim
PROM
    premature rupture of membranes
promastigote
promethazine
    p. and codeine
    p. and dextromethorphan
    p., phenylephrine, and codeine
Promethist With Codeine
Prometh VC With Codeine
Promicromonospora (b)
    P. citrea
    P. enterophila
    P. sukumoe
promoter
    core p.
promyelocyte
pronormoblast
    giant p.
Pronto Shampoo
Prontosil
proomii
    Virgibacillus p.
propafenone
propagated

propamidine
    p. isothionate
Propanthel
propantheline
Propa PH
propensity
prophage
    defective p.
prophylactic
    p. antianaerobe chemotherapy
    p. antibiotic
prophylaxis
    antibiotic p.
    antimicrobial p.
    MAC p.
    malaria p.
    mefloquine p.
    meningeal p.
    partial p.
    PCP p.
    postexposure p.
    preoperative antimicrobial p. (PAP)
    primary p.
    rabies p.
    secondary p.
propinquum
    Corynebacterium p.
propionate
    testosterone p.
Propionibacter (b)
    P. pelophilus
Propionibacteriaceae
Propionibacterium (b)
    P. acidipropionici
    P. acnes
    P. avidum
    P. cyclohexanicum
    P. freudenreichii subsp.
      freudenreichii
    P. freudenreichii subsp. *shermanii*
    P. granulosum
    P. innocuum
    P. jensenii
    P. lymphophilum
    P. microaerophilum
    P. propionicus
    P. thoenii
propionica
    Arachnia p.
    Desulfurella p.
    Smithella p.

propionicum
    Clostridium p.
propionicus
    Desulfobulbus p.
    Pelobacter p.
    Propionibacterium p.
Propioniferax innocua (b)
Propionigenium (b)
    P. maris
    P. modestum
Propionispira arboris (b)
Propionispora vibrioides (b)
Propionivibrio dicarboxylicus (b)
propofol
proportional susceptibility testing
propoxyphene
propranolol
propria
    lamina p.
proptosis
propylene glycol diacetate
Prorazin
Proscar
proscolex
Prosimulium
    P. hirtipes
    P. mixtum
Prosostomata
ProSpect
    P. *Cryptosporidium* microtiter assay
Prospect Hill virus (PHV)
prostacyclin
prostaglandin E
Prostaphlin
prostatectomy
    cystoscopic p.
prostate-specific antigen (PSA)
prostatic
    p. abscess
    p. fluid culture
    p. hypertrophy
    p. localization method
prostatitis
prostatodynia
Prosthecobacter (b)
    P. debontii
    P. dejongeii
    P. fusiformis
    P. vanneervenii
Prosthecochloris aestuarii (b)
Prosthecomicrobium (b)
    P. enhydrum

NOTES

P

439

Prosthecomicrobium (continued)
  P. hirschii
  P. litoralum
  P. pneumaticum
Prosthenorchis elegans (p)
prosthesis, pl. prostheses
  genitourinary p.
  Groningen voice p.
  indwelling voice p.
  McKee-Farrar p.
  mitral valve p.
  Moore p.
  Robbins voice p.
  voice p.
prosthetic
  p. valve dysfunction
  p. valve endocarditis (PVE)
Prosthodendrium molenkampi (p)
Prosthogonimus macrorchis (p)
Prostigmata
prostitution
prostoserdovii
proteamaculans
  Serratia proteamaculans subsp. *p.*
protean
protease (PR)
  endosomal p.
  p. inhibitor (PI)
  p. paunch
protease-sparing regimen
protected
  p. brush catheter (PBC)
  p. catheter aspirate (PCA)
  p. specimen brush (PSB)
protective antigen (PA)
Proteeae
protein
  antibiotic p.
  antiviral p.
  choline-binding p.
  circumsporozoite p.
  C-reactive p. (CRP)
  CSF p.
  cytoadherent p.
  EBNA-1 p.
  p. fever
  gp120/160 viral p.
  gp41 viral p.
  heat shock p. (HSP)
  herpesvirus p.
  HIV viral p.
  immune p.
  23-kDa p.
  p. kinase R
  M p.
  macrophage infectivity
    potentiator p.
  major basic p. (MBP)

  mip p.
  monocyte chemoattractant p. (MCP)
  myelin basic p.
  Opa p.
  opacity p.
  penicillin-binding p. (PBP)
  prion p. (PrP)
  p. profile
  p24 viral p.
  p. S deficiency
  p. serine
  S100 glial p.
  Tamm-Horsfall p.
  tau p.
  thrombospondin-related adhesive p.
  total p.
  viral p.
protein-1
  insulinlike growth factor binding p.
    (IGFBP-1)
  Plasmodium falciparum erythrocyte
    membrane p. (PfEMP-1)
proteinaceous
  p. material
proteinase
protein-energy malnutrition
protein-II
  histidine-rich p.-I. (HRP-II)
protein-losing enteropathy
proteinosis
  alveolar p.
proteinuria
proteoclasticum
  Clostridium p.
proteoclasticus
  Caloramator p.
proteoglycan
proteolytic
proteolytica
  Aeromonas hydrophila subsp. *p.*
proteolyticum
  Clostridium p.
  Trichosporon p.
proteolyticus
  Coprothermobacter p.
  Deinococcus p.
  Thermobacteroides p.
  Vibrio p.
Proteus (b)
  P. hauseri
  P. inconstans
  P. inconstans subgroup A
  P. inconstans subgroup B
  P. mirabilis
  P. morganii
  P. myxofaciens
  P. OX-19
  P. OXK agglutinin titer

P. *penneri*
P. *rettgeri*
P. *vulgaris*
proteus
Obesumbacterium p.
Prothazine-DC
prothionamide
prothoracic gland
prothrombin
p. time (PT)
p. time and partial thromboplastin
time (PT/PTT)
protist
Protista
protobe
protobiology
protocol
immunosuppressed p. (ISP)
Pediatric AIDS Clinical Trial
Group P. (PACTG)
protofilament
Protogastraceae
protogonoplasm
protomerite
Protomonas (b)
P. extorquens
Protomycetaceae
Protomycetales
proton
p. magnetic resonance spectroscopy
p. pump inhibitor (PPI)
protonymph
protooncogene
Protophallaceae
protophormiae
Arthrobacter p.
Brevibacterium p.
protopianoma
protoplasmic
p. movement
p. poison
protoplast
protoporphyrin
protoscolex, pl. **protoscolices**
protospore
Protostat Oral
Protostrongylus rufescens (p)
Protostheca (f)
P. *wickerhamii*
P. *zopfii*
Protothecosis

protothecosis
disseminated p.
prototroph
prototrophic
p. strain
Protozoa
protozoa (*pl. of* protozoon)
protozoal
p. infection
p. meningitis
protozoan
p. cyst
p. infection
obligate intracellular p.
p. parasite
protozoiasis
protozoicide
protozoologist
protozoology
protozoon, pl. **protozoa**
protozoophage
Protrin
Proventil
P. HFA
Provera
Providencia (b)
P. *alcalifaciens*
P. *friedericiana*
P. *heimbachae*
P. *rettgeri*
P. *rustigianii*
P. *stuartii*
proviral
p. HIV RNA level
p. load
provirus
HTLV-1 p.
provocans
Aedes p.
provocative challenge
prowazekii
Rickettsia p.
proxetil
cefpodoxime p.
Proxigel Oral
proximal
p. tibia
p. weakness
prozone phenomenon
PRP
penicillinase-resistant penicillin
polyribosyl-ribitol-phosphate

NOTES

P

PrP
  prion protein
PrP^{Sc}
  prion protein scrapie isoform
PrP^c
  prion protein normal isoform
PRP-D vaccine
PRP-OMPC vaccine
PrP^{Sc}-reactive plaque
PRP-T vaccine
PRR1 virus
PRSV
  Prague strain Rous sarcoma virus
pruinosum
  Simulium p.
  Sporotrichum p.
prunae
  Metallosphaera p.
pruni
  Sphingomonas p.
prunicolor
  Streptomyces p.
pruritic
pruritus
  p. ani
  perineal p.
  vaginal p.
  p. vulvae
  vulvar p.
PRV
  Paroo River virus
prydzensis
  Pseudoalteromonas p.
Prymnesiovirus (v)
PS4 virus
PS8 virus
PSA
  prostate-specific antigen
psammoticus
  Streptomyces p.
PSB
  protected specimen brush
PSE
  Entex P.
  Guaifenex P.
pseudalcaliphilus
  Bacillus p.
Pseudallescheria (f)
  P. angusta
  P. boydii
  P. ellipsoidea
  P. fusoidea
  P. shearii
pseudallescheriasis
pseudallescheriosis
  pulmonary p.

Pseudaminobacter (b)
  P. defluvii
  P. salicylatoxidans
Pseudamphistomum truncatum (p)
pseudarthrosis
pseudelminth
Pseudeurotiaceae
Pseudeurotium ovale (f)
pseudoalba
  Bullera p.
pseudoalcaligenes
  Pseudomonas p.
  Pseudomonas pseudoalcaligenes
  subsp. *p.*
Pseudoalteromonas (b)
  P. antarctica
  P. atlantica
  P. aurantia
  P. carrageenovora
  P. citrea
  P. denitrificans
  P. distincta
  P. elyakovii
  P. espejiana
  P. haloplanktis
  P. haloplanktis subsp. *tetraodonis*
  P. luteoviolacea
  P. nigrifaciens
  P. peptidolytica
  P. piscicida
  P. prydzensis
  P. rubra
  P. tetraodonis
  P. tunicata
  P. ulvae
  P. undina
Pseudoamycolata halophobica (b)
pseudoaneurysm
pseudoappendicitis
pseudoavium
  Enterococcus p.
pseudobacteremia
pseudobrasiliensis
  Nocardia p.
pseudobubo
Pseudobutyrivibrio ruminis (b)
Pseudocaedibacter (b)
  P. conjugatus
  P. falsus
  P. minutus
Pseudo-Car DM
pseudocatenulatum
  Bifidobacterium p.
pseudocelom
Pseudochaetosphaeronema (f)
  P. larense
Pseudococcidioides (f)
Pseudocochliobolus (f)

pseudocowpox virus
pseudocyst
 pancreatic p.
pseudodiphtheria
pseudodiphtheriticum
 Corynebacterium p.
pseudodiverticulosis
 esophageal intramural p.
pseudodysentery
pseudoechinosporeus
 Streptomyces p.
pseudoephedrine
 acetaminophen, dextromethorphan,
  and p.
 acrivastine and p.
 chlorpheniramine and p.
 p. and dextromethorphan
 diphenhydramine and p.
 guaifenesin and p.
 p. hydrochloride
 hydrocodone and p.
 p. and ibuprofen
 triprolidine and p.
pseudoepidemic
pseudoepitheliomatous hyperplasia
pseudoerysipelas
pseudoexiguum
 Simulium p.
pseudofelineus
 Amphimerus p.
pseudofirmus
 Bacillus p.
pseudoflava
 Hydrogenophaga p.
 Pseudomonas p.
Pseudofrin
Pseudofusarium (f)
Pseudo-Gest Plus tablet
pseudoglanders
pseudogout
pseudogriseolus
 Streptomyces p.
Pseudohansenula (f)
pseudohypertrophy
pseudohypha
pseudohyphae
pseudointermedia
 Candida p.
pseudolambica
 Candida p.
pseudolepromatous leishmaniasis
pseudolipolytica

pseudolithiasis
 biliary p.
pseudolongum
 Bifidobacterium pseudolongum var.
  p.
Pseudolynchia
 P. canariensis
pseudolysogenic strain
pseudomaculipes
 Anopheles p.
pseudomallei
 Burkholderia p.
 p. group
 Pseudomonas p.
pseudomembrane
pseudomembranous
 p. candidiasis
 p. cheilitis
 p. colitis (PMC)
 p. colitis toxin assay
 p. lesion
pseudomesenteroides
 Leuconostoc p.
Pseudomicrodochium (f)
 P. fusarioides
 P. suttonii
pseudomonad
 non-*Aeruginosa* p.
 Stutzeri group of p.'s
Pseudomonadaceae
Pseudomonadales
Pseudomonadeae
Pseudomonas (b)
 P. abietaniphila
 P. acidovorans
 P. aeruginosa
 P. aeruginosa bacteremia
 P. aeruginosa NU10
 P. agarici
 P. alcaligenes
 P. alcaliphila
 P. aminovorans
 P. amygdali
 P. andropogonis
 P. anguilliseptica
 P. antimicrobica
 P. asplenii
 P. aurantiaca
 P. aureofaciens
 P. avellanae
 P. avenae subsp. *avenae*
 P. avenae subsp. *citrulli*

NOTES

P

Pseudomonas (continued)
P. avenae subsp. konjaci
P. azotoformans
P. balearica
P. beijerinckii
P. beteli
P. boreopolis
P. brassicacearum
P. cannabina
P. carboxydohydrogena
P. caricapapayae
P. caryophylli
P. cattleyae
P. cepacia
P. chlororaphis
P. cichorii
P. cissicola
P. citronellolis
P. cocovenenans
P. corrugata
P. delafieldii
P. diminuta
P. doudoroffii
P. echinoides
P. elongata
P. exotoxin (PE)
P. exotoxin A
P. facilis
P. ficuserectae
P. flava
P. flavescens
P. flectens
P. fluorescens
P. fragi
P. frederiksbergensis
P. fulva
P. fuscovaginae
P. gelidicola
P. geniculata
P. gessardii
P. gladioli
P. glathei
P. glumae
P. graminis
P. halophila
P. hibiscicola
P. huttiensis
P. indigofera
P. iners
P. jessenii
P. kilonensis
P. lanceolata
P. lemoignei
P. libanensis
P. lundensis
P. luteola
P. mallei
P. maltophilia

P. mandelii
P. marginalis
P. marina
P. meliae
P. mendocina
P. mephitica
P. mesophilica
P. migulae
P. mixta
P. monteilii
P. mucidolens
P. multiresinivorans
P. nautica
P. nitroreducens
P. nonliquefaciens
P. oleovorans
P. oryzihabitans
P. palleronii
P. paucimobilis
P. perfectomarina
P. pertucinogena
P. phage chi-6 virus
P. phenazinium
P. pickettii
P. pictorum
P. plantarii
P. plecoglossicida
P. pseudoalcaligenes
P. pseudoalcaligenes subsp. citrulli
P. pseudoalcaligenes subsp. konjaci
P. pseudoalcaligenes subsp.
    pseudoalcaligenes
P. pseudoflava
P. pseudomallei
P. putida
P. putida biotype B
P. pyrrocinia
P. radiora
P. resinovorans
P. rhodesiae
P. rhodos
P. rubrilineans
P. rubrisubalbicans
P. saccharophila
P. savastanoi
P. septicemia
P. solanacearum
P. species ASO
P. spinosa
P. stanieri
P. straminea
P. stutzeri
P. synxantha
P. syringae
P. syringae subsp. savastanoi
P. syringae subsp. syringae
P. syzygii
P. taeniospiralis

P. taetrolens
P. testosteroni
P. thivervalensis
P. tolaasii
P. tremae
P. vancouverensis
P. veronii
P. vesicularis
P. viridiflava
P. woodsii
pseudomonic acid A
Pseudomonilia (f0
pseudomutans
 Caedibacter p.
pseudomycelium
Pseudomycoderma (f)
pseudomycoides
 Bacillus p.
pseudonecrophorum
 Fusobacterium p.
Pseudo-nitzschia
 P.-n. fraudulenta
 P.-n. pungens
Pseudonocardia (b)
 P. alni
 P. asuccharolytica
 P. autotrophica
 P. azurea
 P. compacta
 P. halophobica
 P. hydrocarbonoxydans
 P. petroleophila
 P. saturnea
 P. spinosa
 P. sulfidoxydans
 P. thermophila
Pseudonocardiaceae
pseudoparasite
pseudoparenchyma
Pseudophaeotrichum (f)
pseudophyllid
Pseudophyllidea
pseudoplantarum
 Lactobacillus casei subsp. *p.*
pseudopod
pseudopodium, pl. **pseudopodia**
 hyaline p.
pseudopunctipennis
 Anopheles p.
pseudorabies virus
Pseudoramibacter alactolyticus (b)

pseudorobustus
 Helicotylenchus p.
pseudoseizure
Pseudosphaeriaceae
pseudospiralis
 Trichinella p.
Pseudostertagia bullosa (p)
Pseudoterranova decipiens (p)
pseudotibiamaculatus
 Anopheles p.
pseudotropicalis
 Candida p.
pseudotubercle
pseudotubercular yersiniosis
pseudotuberculosis
 Corynebacterium p.
 Yersinia p.
pseudotumor
 amebic p.
 p. cerebri
 colonic p.
pseudovenezuelae
 Streptomyces p.
Pseudovirus (v)
pseudovulgure
 Streptosporangium p.
Pseudoxanthomonas (b)
 P. broegbernensis
psidii
 Erwinia p
Psilobotrys (t)
psilocin
Psilocybe
 P. cubensis
 P. mexicana
psilocybin
Psilorchis hominis (p)
Psilostomatidae
PSIS
 posterior superior iliac spine
psittaci
 Chlamydia p.
 Chlamydophila p.
 Giardia p.
 Lactobacillus p.
psittacinepox virus
psittacosis
 p. inclusion body
 p. virus
psoas abscess
Psorcon
psorelcosis

NOTES

P

Psorergates (p)
    P. bos
    P. ovis
    P. simplex
psoriasiform
psoriatic arthritis
psoriGel
Psorion Topical
Psorophora
    P. cyanescens
    P. ferox
    P. horrida
    P. lutzi
Psoroptes ovis (p)
psoroptic acariasis
Psoroptidae
Psoroptoidea
Psorospermium (p)
PSP
    paralytic shellfish poisoning
P & S Plus
P&S Shampoo
PST virus
PSV
    Punta Salinas virus
PsV-F
    Penicillium stoloniferum F virus
PS17 virus
PsV-S
    Penicillium stoloniferum S virus
PSWC
    periodic sharp wave complex
psychiatric disease
Psychoda alternata (p)
Psychodinae
psychoeducational
psychological dynamics
psychosis
psychotropic
Psychrobacter (b)
    P. frigidicola
    P. glacincola
    P. immobilis
    P. pacificensis
    P. phenylpyruvicus
    P. urativorans
psychroerythraea
    Colwellia p.
Psychroflexus (b)
    P. gondwanensis
    P. torquis
psychrolactophilus
    Arthrobacter p.
Psychromonas antarctica (b)
psychrophila
    Candida p.
    Cytophaga p.

    Desulfotalea p.
    Sporosarcina p.
psychrophile
psychrophilic
psychrophilum
    Aquaspirillum p.
    Cryobacterium p.
    Flavobacterium p.
psychrophilus
    Bacillus p.
    Flexibacter p.
    Methylobacter p.
psychrosaccharolyticus
    Bacillus p.
Psychroserpens burtonensis (b)
psychrotropica
    Colwellia p.
psyllium
PT
    pertussis toxin
    prothrombin time
PT11 virus
PTB virus
PTCA
    percutaneous transhepatic
    cholangiography
pteronyssinus
    Dermatophagoides p.
pterotermitidis
    Hollandina p.
pterygium, pl. **pterygia**
Pterygodermatites dipodomis (p)
Pterygota
PTFE
    polytetrafluorethylene
PTH
    parathyroid hormone
    posttransfusion hepatitis
pthiriasis
    p. capitis
    p. corporis
    p. pubis
PTHV
    Pathum Thani virus
PTLD
    posttransplantation lymphoproliferative
    disorder
    posttransplant lymphoproliferative
    disorder
PT-NANBH
    parenterally transmitted non-A non-B
    hepatitis
ptosis
PT/PTT
    prothrombin time and partial
    thromboplastin time
PTV
    Punta Toro virus

PTVV
 Ponteves virus
ptyseos
 Tatumella p.
pubic
 p. lice
 p. louse
pubis
 pediculosis p.
 Phthirus p.
 pthiriasis p.
Puchong virus (PUCV)
puctisporus
PUCV
 Puchong virus
PUD
 peptic ulcer disease
pudenda
 granuloma p.
 ulcerating granuloma of p.
pudendal ulcer
pudendi
 granuloma p.
pudibunda
 Dasychira p.
Pueblo Viejo virus
puerperal
 p. endometritis
 p. fever
 p. ovarian vein thrombosis (POVT)
 p. sepsis
puerperium
puffball
pufferfish poisoning
Puffin Island virus
pugetense
 Simulium p.
pugetii
 Cycloclasticus p.
puicherrima (f)
 Capronia p.
pulchella
 Malbranchea p.
pulcher
 Streptomyces p.
pulcherrima
 Candida p.
 Metschnikowia p.
pulchrum
 Gongylonema p.
Pulex simulans (p)

pulicans
 purpura p.
pulicicide
Pulicidae
pullatus
 Aedes p.
pulldown assay
pullorum
 Aegyptianella p.
 Bifidobacterium p.
 Helicobacter p.
 Mycoplasma p.
pullulans
 Aureobasidium p.
 Pullularia p.
 Trichosporon p.
Pullularia
 P. fermentans var. *benedekii*
 P. jeanselmei
 P. pullulans
 P. werneckii
pullulate
pullulation
pulmonale
 cor p.
pulmonarius
 Pleurotus p.
pulmonary
 p. actinomycosis
 p. amebic abscess
 p. anthrax
 p. aspergilloma
 p. cryptococcosis
 p. cryptosporidiosis
 p. dirofilariasis
 p. distomiasis
 p. embolus
 p. endarteritis
 p. function test (PFT)
 p. hemorrhage
 p. histoplasmosis
 p. infection
 p. Kaposi sarcoma (PKS)
 p. mycosis
 p. nodule
 p. pseudallescheriosis
 p. sporotrichosis
 p. tuberculosis
pulmonic
pulmonicola
 Pandoraea p.

NOTES

P

447

pulmonis
  Mycoplasma p.
  Tsukamurella p.
Pulmophylline
pulsed-field gel electrophoresis (PFGE)
pulsellum
pulsus
  p. alternans
  p. paradoxus
pulveraceus
  Streptomyces p.
pulvereri
  Staphylococcus p.
pulveris
  Mycobacterium p.
pulverulentum
  Simulium p.
pulvifaciens
  Bacillus p.
  Paenibacillus p.
  Paenibacillus larvae subsp. p.
pulvinate
pulvule
  Cinobac P.'s
  Co-Pyronil 2 P.'s
  Ilosone P.'s
  Seromycin P.'s
pumilio
  Haplorchis p.
pumilum
  Mogibacterium p.
pumilus
  Bacillus p.
  Methanocalculus p.
pump
  intraaortic balloon p.
punch
  p. biopsy
  sclerocorneal p.
punched-out
punctal
  p. occlusion
  p. scarring
punctata
  Aeromonas punctata subsp. p.
  Haemaphysalis p.
  Pantoea p.
punctate
  p. keratitis
  p. keratopathy
punctifer
  Tabanus p.
punctimacula
  Anopheles p.
punctipennis
  Anopheles p.
punctodes
  Aedes p.

punctulatus
  Anopheles p.
puncture
  p., aspiration, injection, and
    reaspiration (PAIR)
  p., aspiration, injection, and
    reaspiration procedure
  lumbar p. (LP)
  p. wound of foot
pungens
  Pseudo-nitzschia p.
punicea
  Candida p.
  Glaciecola p.
puniceum
  Clostridium p.
puniceus
  Streptomyces p.
Punta
  P. Salinas virus (PSV)
  P. Toro virus (PTV)
pupa
pupil
  Argyll Robertson p.
  Marcus-Gunn p.
Pupipara
pupiparous
pure
  p. culture
  p. red cell aplasia (PRCA)
Puri-Clens
purified protein derivative (PPD)
purinolyticum
  Clostridium p.
Puritan-Bennett Cascade humidifier
purpeofuscus
  Streptomyces p.
purpura
  p. fulminans
  hemolytic uremic
    syndrome/thrombotic
    thrombocytopenia p. (HUS/TTP)
  Henoch p.
  Henoch-Schönlein p.
  idiopathic thrombocytopenic p.
    (ITP, ITTP)
  immune thrombocytopenic p. (ITP)
  posttransfusion p.
  p. pulicans
  thrombocytopenic p.
  thrombotic thrombocytopenic p.
    (TTP)
  vasculitic p.
purpurascens
  Epicoccum p.
  Streptomyces p.

purpuratum
>> *Chromatium* p.
>> *Marichromatium* p.

purpurea
>> *Claviceps* p.
>> *Kitasatoa* p.
>> *Micromonospora* p.
>> *Pfennigia* p.
>> *Sarracenia* p.

purpureipes
>> *Aedes* p.

purpureochromogenes
>> *Micromonospora* p.

purpureum
>> *Tritirachium* p.

purpureus
>> *Amoebobacter* p.
>> *Rhinoestrus* p.
>> *Rhodocyclus* p.
>> *Streptomyces* p.

purpuric

purpurogena
>> *Chainia* p.

purpurogeneiscleroticus
>> *Streptomyces* p.

purpurogenum
>> *Penicillium* p.

purulence

purulent
>> p. conjunctivitis
>> p. discharge
>> p. endocervical exudate
>> p. enterocolitis
>> p. gonococcal arthritis

purulenta
>> myositis p.

Purus virus (PURV)

PURV
>> Purus virus

purvisi
>> *Cyclodontostomum* p.

pus
>> anchovy sauce p.
>> p. cell
>> culture of p.
>> frank p.

pushchinoensis
>> *Anoxybacillus* p.

pusilla
>> *Actinomadura* p.
>> *Microtetraspora* p.
>> *Nonomuraea* p.

pusillum
>> *Brevibacterium* p.
>> *Curtobacterium* p.
>> *Oceanospirillum* p.
>> *Physarum* p.

pusillus
>> *Culicoides* p.
>> *Rhizomucor* p.

pusio
>> *Fannia* p.

pustula
>> *Candida* p.

pustular
>> p. acrodermatitis
>> p. center
>> p. dermatitis
>> p. lesion
>> p. syphilid

pustule
>> acneiform p.

pustulosus
>> *Parachordodes* p.

putative

putei
>> *Desulfotomaculum* p.

putida
>> *Pseudomonas* p.

putidus
>> *Thermoactinomyces* p.

putredinis
>> *Bacteroides* p.

putrefaciens
>> *Alteromonas* p.
>> *Clostridium* p.
>> *Mycoplasma* p.
>> *Shewanella* p.

putrefaction

putrefactive

putrescentiae
>> *Tyrophagus* p.

putridiconchylium
>> *Aquaspirillum* p.

putrificum
>> *Clostridium* p.

putrinum
>> *Paramecium* p.

Puumala virus (PUUV)

PUUV
>> Puumala virus

PVA
>> polyvinyl alcohol
>> PVA fixative

NOTES

P

449

PVC
    polyvinyl chloride
PVE
    prosthetic valve endocarditis
    late PVE
PVF K
PVL, pVL
    plasma viral load
P-V-Tussin
PWA
    person with AIDS
Pychodnaviridae
Pycnothyriaceae
Pycnothyriales
pyelitis
pyelogram
    infusion p.
    intravenous p. (IVP)
pyelonephritis
pyelonephritogenic
Pyemotes (p)
    P. tritici
Pyemotidae
Pyernochaeta (f)
Pygidiopsis summa (p)
pylori
    Campylobacter p.
    Helicobacter p.
Pym fever
pyococcus
pyocyanic
pyocyanin
    p. test
pyoderma
    chancriform p.
    p. gangrenosum
pyodermatous infection
pyogenes
    Actinomyces p.
    Arcanobacterium p.
    Bacteroides p.
    Corynebacterium p.
    Streptococcus p.
pyogenes-like
pyogenic
    p. bacterium
    p. beta-hemolytic *Streptococcus*
    p. cholangitis
    p. exudate
    p. fever
    p. infection
    p. liver abscess
    p. meningitis
pyogranulomatous
pyomelanin
pyomyositis
    tropical p.
Pyopen

pyosalpinx
pyoverdin test
PYR
    pyrrolidonyl arylamidase
    PYR test
PyR
    L-pyrrolidonyl-beta-naphthylamide
    PyR substrate
Pyral
    Jaa P.
pyrantel
    p. pamoate
pyrazinamidase test
pyrazinamide (PZA)
    rifampin, isoniazid, and p.
pyrazinoic acid amide
pyrazinoquinoline
pyrazolone
Pyrenidiaceae
Pyrenochaeta (f)
    P. mackinnonii
    P. romeroi
    P. unguis-hominis
pyrenoid
Pyrenophora (f)
Pyrenothricaceae
pyrethrin
    p.s and piperonyl butoxide
pyrexia
pyridinivorans
    Rhodococcus p.
pyridinolyticus
    Nocardioides p.
Pyridium
pyridoxal
pyridoxine
pyrifoliae
    Erwinia p.
pyriform
    p. apparatus
pyriformis
    Tetrahymena p.
pyrimethamine
pyrimethamine-sulfadoxine
Pyrinex Pediculicide Shampoo
pyrinus
    Enterobacter p.
Pyrinyl
    P. II Liquid
    P. Plus Shampoo
pyrithione zinc
Pyrobaculum (b)
    P. aerophilum
    P. arsenaticum
    P. islandicum
    P. oguniense
    P. organotrophum

Pyrococcus (b)
    P. furiosus
    P. glycovorans
    P. horikoshii
    P. woesei
Pyrodictium (b)
    P. abyssi
    P. brockii
    P. occultum
pyrogen
    endogenous p.
pyrogenes
    Leptospira interrogans serovar *p.*
pyrogenic
Pyroglyphidae
Pyrolobus (b)
    P. fumarii
pyrophilus
    Aquifex p.

pyrophosphate dihydrate crystal
pyrrocinia
    Burkholderia p.
    Pseudomonas p.
pyrrole
pyrrolidonyl
    p. arylamidase (PYR)
    p. arylamidase test
pyrrolizidine
    p. alkaloid
    p. alkaloid intoxication
    p. alkaloid poisoning
pyruvate kinase deficiency
Pythiaceae
Pythium insidiosum
pyuria
Pyxidiophoraceae
PZA
    pyrazinamide

NOTES

P

Q

Q
- Q fever
- Q fever serology
- Q fever vaccine
- Q Test Strep

QAC
- quaternary ammonium compound

Qalyub virus (QYBV)

QBC
- quantitative buffy coat
- QBC malaria tube
- QBC technique

Qbeta
- Q. probe amplification
- Q. replicase method

QC-PCR
- quantitative competitive PCR
- quantitative competitive polymerase chain reaction

qinghaosu

quadplate

quadrasi
- Oncomelania q.

quadrata
- Haloarcula q.

quadrifidum
- Arthroderma q.
- Simulium q.

quadrimaculatus
- Anopheles q.

quadripertusus
- Haematopinus q.

quadrispinulatum
- Oesophagostomum q.

quadristrigatum
- Simulium q.

quadrivittatum
- Simulium q.

quadruple therapy

qualitative
- q. RNA PCR assay

quantification
- viral load q.

Quantiplex
- Q. HCV-RNA Assay
- Q. HIV-1 RNA assay

quantitative
- q. assay
- q. bDNA
- q. buffy coat (QBC)
- q. buffy coat malaria tube
- q. buffy coat technique
- q. competitive PCR (QC-PCR)
- q. competitive polymerase chain reaction (QC-PCR)

- q. culture
- q. human herpesvirus 6 IgG antibody
- q. human herpesvirus 6 IgM antibody
- q. immunoglobulin analysis

quartan
- double q.
- q. fever
- q. malaria
- q. malarial nephropathy
- q. parasite
- triple q.

quasispecies

quateirensis
- Legionella q.

quaternary
- q. ammonium compound (QAC)

quebecense
- Simulium q.

Queensland
- Q. fruit fly virus
- Q. tick typhus

quellung
- q. phenomenon
- q. reaction
- q. test

quercicolum
- Clostridium q.

quercicolus
- Dendrosporobacter q.

quercina
- Brenneria q.
- Erwinia q.

quercitrusa
- Candida q.

quercuum
- Candida q.
- Pichia q.

query fever

Queyrat
- erythroplasia of Q.

Quibron

Quibron-T/SR

quickeanum
- Trichophyton equinum var. q.

quiescence

quiescent

quinacrine HCl

Quinaglute

Quinalan

Quinella ovalis (b)

quinghaosu

Quinidex

453

quinidine
    q. gluconate
    q. polygalacturonate
    q. sulfate
quinii
    Clostridium q.
quinine
    q. dihydrochloride
    q. sulfate
quinlivanii
    Legionella q.
quinolone
Quinora
quinovora
    Serratia proteamaculans subsp. *q.*
quinquefasciatus
    Culex q.
Quinsana Plus
quinsy
quintana
    Bartonella q.
    Rochalimaea q.

quintan fever
quintile
Quinton and Groshong catheter
Quinton-Scribner external arteriovenous shunt
quinupristin
    q. and dalfopristin
quinuprostin-dafopristin
quisquiliarum
    Methylosarcina q.
Quixin Ophthalmic
quorum sensing
quotidian
    q. fever
    q. malaria
Qβ virus
QYBV
    Qalyub virus

R
 R. & C Shampoo
 R. pili
 R. virus
R17 virus
R1-Myb virus
R23 virus
R34 virus
39R861
 Escherichia coli 39R861
R5 virus
RA
 rubella vaccine RA 27/3
RA-1 virus
Rabavert
rabbit
 r. coronavirus
 r. fever
 r. fever antibody
rabies
 r. detection
 r. encephalitis
 r. immunoglobulin (RIG)
 r. neutralizing antibody
 r. prophylaxis
 r. vaccine adsorbed (RVA)
 r. vaccine induced encephalomyelitis
 r. viral culture
 r. virus
 r. virus group
 r. virus vaccine
racemicus
 Sporolactobacillus nakayamae subsp.
 r.
racemochromogenes
 Streptomyces r.
racemose
 r. cyst
racemosum
 Arthroderma r.
 Microsporum r.
 Syncephalastrum r.
racemosus
 Cysticercus r.
 Mucor r.
racenisi
 Simulium r.
rachoui
 Anopheles r.
racquet hypha
radial
 r. diffusion
 r. immunodiffusion (RID)
radiation
 r. pneumonitis

radiatum
 Oesophagostomum r.
radiatus
 Argas r.
radicicola
 Cylindrocarpon r.
 Nectria r.
radicidentis
 Actinomyces r.
radiculitis
radiculomyelitis
radiculomyeloencephalitis
radiculomyelopathy
radiculoneuronitis
rudingae
 Actinomyces r.
radioactive iodine
radioallergosorbent test (RAST)
radiobacter
 Agrobacterium r.
 Rhizobium r.
radiodurans
 Deinococcus r.
radiofrequency generator
radiographic study
radioimmunoassay (RIA)
 double antibody r.
radioimmunoblot assay (RIBA)
radioimmunoprecipitation analysis
radioimmunotherapy
radiolabeled tracer
radiolucent
Radiomycetaceae
radionuclide
 r. bone scan
radiophilus
 Deinococcus r.
radiopugnans
 Deinococcus r.
radiora
 Pseudomonas r.
radioresistens
 Acinetobacter r.
radiorespirometry typing
radiosensitive
radiosurgery
 gamma knife r.
radiotherapy
 external beam r.
 x-ray r.
radiotolerans
 Arthrobacter r.
 Methylobacterium r.
 Rubrobacter r.

RADIV
  Radi virus
Radi virus (RADIV)
RADT
  rapid antigen-detection test
raffinolactis
    Lactococcus r.
    Streptococcus r.
raffinose fermentation test
raffinosivorans
    Zymophilus r.
raffinosus
    Enterococcus r.
ragsorter's disease
Rahnella aquatilis (b)
railenensis
    Candida r.
Raillietiella (p)
Raillietina (p)
    R. asiatica
    R. celebensis
    R. garrisoni
raillietiniasis
Rainey corpuscle
raising
    straight leg r.
rale
Ralstonia (b)
    R. basilensis
    R. eutropha
    R. gilardii
    R. mannitolilytica
    R. oxalatica
    R. paucula
    R. pickettii
    R. solanacearum
rameus
    Streptomyces r.
Ramichloridium (f)
    R. cerophilum
    R. mackenziei
    R. obovoideum
    R. schulzeri
ramigera
    Zoogloea r.
ramoplanin
ramosa
    Mycoplana r.
    Nevskia r.
    Pasteuria r.
ramosi
    Anopheles evansae r.
ramosissimus
    Mucor r.
ramosum
    Clostridium r.
    Erythromicrobium r.

ramosus
    Agromyces r.
    Arthrobacter r.
Ramsay Hunt syndrome
Ramularia destructiva (f)
ramulosus
    Streptomyces r.
ramulus
    Eubacterium r.
ranarum
    Basidiobolus r.
Ranavirus (v)
random
    r. amplified polymorphic DNA
      (RAPD)
    r. urine
rangeli
    Anopheles r.
    Simulium r.
    Trypanosoma r.
rangoon
    Streptomyces r.
rangoonensis
    Streptomyces r.
ranitidine
    r. bismuth citrate
    r. hydrochloride
Ranke complex
Ranson criteria
Raoultella (b)
rapamycin
RAPD
    random amplified polymorphic DNA
Raphidascaris (p)
Raphidomonadea (p)
RapID
    R. ANA II System
    R. NH system
    R. onE system
rapid
    r. antigen-detection test (RADT)
    r. broth system
    r. carbohydrate degradation test
    r. carbohydrate utilization test
    r. CMV isolation
    r. dipstick test
    r. fermentation test
    r. HSV isolation
    r. identification method (RIM)
    r. identification method-*Neisseria*
      (RIM-*Neisseria*)
    r. latex agglutination test
    R. NF Plus system
    r. plasma reagent (RPR)
    r. plasma reagent test
    r. plasma reagin (RPR)
    r. plasma reagin circle card test
      (RPR-CT)

R

r. plasma reagin test
r. streptococcal antigen test
RapiDEC
R. aurease test
R. Staph
R. Staph test
rapidicrescens
Thiobacillus r.
rara
Caenorhabditis r.
Physaloptera r.
Rarobacter (b)
R. faecitabidus
R. incanus
rash
antitoxin r.
arthropod-borne viral arthritis
and r.
Diaper R.
hemorrhagic r.
macular r.
maculopapular r.
malar r.
morbilliform r.
palmar r.
papular r.
papulonodular r.
petechial r.
plantar r.
pretibial r.
vesicopustular r.
vesicular r.
r. viral culture
Rasmussen
R. aneurysm
R. disease
R. encephalitis
raspberry tongue
RAST
radioallergosorbent test
rat
r. bite fever
r. coronavirus
r. cytomegalovirus
r. lung fluke
r. mite dermatitis
r. rotavirus
r. virus (RV)
rate
erythrocyte sedimentation r. (ESR)
fatality r.
glomerular filtration r. (GFR)

morbidity r.
mortality r.
multimammate r.
rathayi
Clavibacter r.
Corynebacterium r.
Rathayibacter r.
Rathayibacter (b)
R. iranicus
R. rathayi
R. toxicus
R. tritici
ratio
albumin-to-globulin r.
CD4:CD8 r.
CD4+:CD8+ r.
helper cell/suppressor r.
leukocyte/epithelial cell r.
myeloid/erythroid r.
odds r. (OR)
surface area to volume r. (SA/V)
T4/T8 r.
VAT:TAT r.
visceral abdominal fat to total
abdominal fat ratio
visceral abdominal fat to total
abdominal fat r. (VAT:TAT ratio)
waist:hip r. (WHR)
ratti
Streptococcus r.
Strongyloides r.
Veillonella r.
Veillonella alcalescens subsp. r.
Rauoltella
R. plunticola
R. terrigena
rauschi
Acanthocephalus r.
ravautii
Candida r.
ray fungus
Raynaud phenomenon
rayon swab
Raza virus
Razdan virus (RAZV)
RAZV
Razdan virus
RB
reticulate body
RBC
red blood cell
RBC index

NOTES

RBUV
  Rochambeau virus
RBV
  Rio Bravo virus
rDNA
  recombinant DNA
REA
  restriction endonuclease analysis
  restriction enzyme analysis
reactant
  acute phase r.
reaction
  Abbott LCx ligase chain r.
  abscess-granulomatous r.
  acute phase r. (APR)
  adverse drug r.
  allergic r.
  allograft r.
  Arthus r.
  cholera-red r.
  cross r.
  downgrading r.
  false-negative r.
  fibroblastic r.
  focal r.
  granulomatous r.
  Herxheimer r.
  hypersensitivity r.
  id r.
  IgE-mediated r.
  JH r.
  lepra type-1, -2 r.
  ligase chain r. (LCR)
  Lucio r.
  Mazzotti r.
  multiplex polymerase chain r. (M-PCR)
  Nagler r.
  Neufeld r.
  oxidase r.
  phlegmonous r.
  polymerase chain r. (PCR)
  quantitative competitive polymerase chain r. (QC-PCR)
  quellung r.
  receptor-ligand-type r.
  reversal r.
  reverse transcriptase polymerase chain r. (RT-PCR)
  Roche Amplicore polymerase chain r.
  Schwartzman r.
  in situ polymerase chain r. (IS-PCR)
  Weil-Felix r.
reactivated
  r. Chagas disease
  r. tuberculosis

reactivation
reactive
  r. arthritis
  r. astrogliosis
  r. dermatitis
  r. enzyme immunoassay
  r. hyperemia
  r. lymphocytosis
reactivity
  immune r.
  skin test r.
  variant tuberculin r.
READ
  restriction endonuclease analysis
reagent
  acid-Schiff r.
  Ehrlich r.
  rapid plasma r. (RPR)
  sulfation r.
reagin
  rapid plasma r. (RPR)
  r. screen test (RST)
  unheated serum r. (USR test)
reaginic test
reaspiration
  puncture, aspiration, injection, and r. (PAIR)
reassortant
  r. virus
Rebeteol
Rebetron
rebetron
rebound
  r. hyperemia
  r. of plasma HIV RNA level
  r. tenderness
  viral load r.
  virologic r.
recalcitrant
  r. pustular acrodermatitis
receptor
  acetylcholine r.
  B-cell r.
  beta-adrenergic r.
  C-C chemokine r., CCR5
  CD4+ r.
  chemokine r.
  C-X-C chemokine r., CXCR4
  high affinity antigen r.
  histamine-2 r. (H_2R)
  5-HT3 r. antagonist
  low affinity antigen r.
  muscarinic cholinergic r.
  r. protein tyrosine kinase (RPTK)
  T-cell r. (TCR, TcR)
receptor-ligand-type reaction
receptor-mediated endocytosis
recidivan

recidivans
  leishmaniasis r.
recifei
  Acremonium r.
recifensis
  Streptomyces r.
reciprocally
reclusa
  Loxosceles r.
Recombigen HIV 1/2 assay
recombinant
  r. antigen
  r. consensus interferon
  r. DNA (rDNA)
  r. expressed vaccine
  r. factor VIII
  r. HIV-1 latex agglutination test
  r. human growth hormone (rhGH)
  r. human interleukin-3 (rhIL-3)
  r. immunoblot assay (RIBA)
  r. interferon alfa-2b
  intertypic r.
  r. strain
  r. tumor necrosis factor alpha
    (rTNFα)
  r. vaccinia virus
  r. virus assay (RVA)
  r. VV
recombination
  genetic r.
Recombivax
  R. HB
  R. Hepatitis B
reconditum
  Dipetalonema r.
recrudescence
recrudescent
  r. infection
  r. louse-borne typhus
  r. typhus fever
recta
  Wolinella r.
rectal
  r. mucus
  r. prolapse
  r. swab
rectale
  Eubacterium r.
recticatena
  Actinomadura r.
  Microtetraspora r.
  Nonomuraea r.

rectilineatus
  Actinoplanes r.
rectiverticillatum
  Streptoverticillium r.
rectiverticillatus
  Streptomyces r.
rectiviolaceus
  Streptomyces r.
rectivirgula
  Faenia r.
  Micropolyspora r.
  Saccharopolyspora r.
rectocolitis
rectum
  Clostridium r.
rectus
  Campylobacter r.
  r. femoris muscle
recurrens
  herpes simplex r.
recurrent
  r. aspiration
  r. colitis
  r. cutaneous abscess
  r. fever
  r. HSV labialis
  r. infection
  r. pyogenic abscess
  r. respiratory papillomatosis
recurrentis
  Borrelia r.
recurva
  Triatoma r.
recurvatum
  Echinoparyphium r.
recurvatus
  Cokeromyces r.
red
  beefy r.
  r. blood cell (RBC)
  r. blood cell transfusion
  r. cell aplasia
  r. cell cast
  r. cell enzymopathy
  r. cell fragmentation
  r. eye
  r. fever
  r. kidney bean poisoning
  r. man syndrome (RMS)
  r. mouth bacterium
redia
red-orange discoloration

R

NOTES

reduced-dose chemotherapy
reducer
    nitrate r.
Redutemp
reduviid, reduvid
    r. bug
Reduviidae
Reduvius personatus
REE
    resting energy expenditure
Reed Ranch virus
Reed-Sternberg cell
Reed-Sternberg-like cell
reemergence
Reese's Pinworm Medicine
reevesi
    Culex r.
    Culicoides r.
referred pain
reflex
    deep tendon r. (DTR)
    gag r.
reflexus
    Argas r.
reflux
    acid r.
    r. esophagitis
    gastroesophageal r. (GER)
    r. nephropathy
    vesicourethral r.
Regan-Lowe medium
regensburgei
    Yokenella r.
regensis
    Streptomyces r.
regimen
    antimicrobial dosing r.
    clarithromycin/ethambutol r.
    dosing r.
    multiple-drug r.
    protease-sparing r.
    streptomycin-containing anti-TB r.
    trimodality r.
    usual adult r.
regina
    Phormia r.
region
    apocrine r.
    hypodense r.
    ringworm of genitocrural r.
regional
    r. adenitis
    r. lymphadenitis
    r. lymphadenopathy
registry
    AIDS r.
    antiretroviral pregnancy r.
Regitine

regression
    tumor r.
regularis
    Actinoplanes r.
    Ampullariella r.
regulon
regurgitant
regurgitation
    aortic r.
    mitral r.
rehydration
    oral r.
Reiter
    R. disease
    R. syndrome
relapse
    mucocutaneous r.
relapsing
    r. fever
    r. hepatitis B
    r. malaria
relative
    r. immunity
    r. risk (RR)
release
    compassionate r.
Relenza
Reliavac drain
relief
    Cold Medication Daytime R.
    Dayquil Sinus with Pain R.
    Nasal & Sinus R.
    Vicks DayQuil Sinus Pressure &
        Congestion R.
reliquens
    Hysterothylacium r.
Remel test
remission
    transient complete hematologic r.
remittent
    r. malaria
    r. malarial fever
remitting fever
remover
    Scholl Wart R.
    Wart R.
rempeli
    Aedes r.
Remune
Renacidin
renal
    r. amyloidosis
    r. calculus
    r. candidiasis
    r. colic
    r. dialysis
    r. dysfunction
    r. failure

R

r. tuberculosis
r. tubular cast
r. tubular necrosis
r. ultrasound
renale
Corynebacterium r.
Dioctophyma r.
Renibacterium salmoninarum (b)
reniform macronucleus
Renoquid
Renova
Rentamine
reorient
Reoviridae
Reovirus
reovirus
channel catfish r. (CRV)
chub r.
coho salmon r.
Tench r.
turbot r.
r. virus subgroup
reovirus-like agent
repand
repeat
genomic r.
repeated
r. exposure
r. respiratory infection
repens
Dirofilaria r
Eurotium r.
repetitive
r. element-based PCR
r. extragenic palindromic PCR
(REP-PCR)
replacement
fluid r.
Replens
R. Vaginal Moisturizer
repleta
Drosophila r.
replicate organism direct agar contact
(RODAC-TM)
replication
self-sustaining sequence r. (3SR)
viral r.
replication-competent retrovirus assay
replicator system stem
Report
Morbidity and Mortality Weekly R.
(MMWR)

REP-PCR
repetitive extragenic palindromic PCR
rep-PCR
reproduction
asexual r.
reproductive
r. nucleus
r. organs
ReProtect
reptans
Aspergillus r.
requirement
immunization r.
RES
reticuloendothelial system
Rescaps-D S.R. Capsule
Rescriptor
rescue
stem cell r.
r. therapy
Research
Agency for Health Care Policy
and R.
HIV Epidemiology R. (HER)
resection
marginal r.
wedge r.
reservoir
r. host
r. of infection
vitelline r.
residual volume
resin
cholestyramine r.
podophyllin r.
podophyllum r.
resiniphila
Zoogloea r.
resinovorans
Pseudomonas r.
resinovorum
Flavobacterium r.
resistance
antimycotic r.
beta-lactamase-mediated r.
colonization r.
constitutive r.
functional bladder outlet r.
r. gene
H1-type plasmid-encoded r.
insulin r.
mechanical bladder outlet r.

NOTES

461

resistance *(continued)*
    multidrug r. (MDR)
    r. mutation
    novobiocin r.
    phenotypic drug r.
    r. plasmid (R-plasmid)
resistant
    azole r.
Resistencia virus (RTAV)
resistens
    Aureobacterium r.
    Microbacterium r.
resistogram
resistomycificus
    Streptomyces r.
resorption
    fetal r.
Respa-DM, -GF
Respaire-120 SR
Respaire-60 SR
Respa-1st
Respbid
RespiGam
Respihaler
    Dexacort Phosphate in R.
respiratory
    r. alkalosis
    r. anthrax
    r. chain
    r. cryptosporidiosis
    r. enteric orphan virus
    r. excursion
    r. infection virus
    r. isolation implementation
      efficiency (RIIE)
    r. isolation implementation
      sensitivity (RIIS)
    r. mucosa
    r. panel
    r. secretion
    r. syncytial virus (RSV)
    r. syncytial virus group
    r. syncytial virus immune globulin
      (RSVIG, RSV-IGIV)
    r. tract
    r. tract infection
    r. virus
Respirgard II nebulizer
Respirovirus (v)
response
    antitumor r.
    attenuated fever r.
    cell-mediated immune r.
    cellular immune r.
    CMI r.
    Communicable Disease Surveillance
      and R. (CSR)
    end-of-treatment r.

    F-wave r.
    host r.
    humoral r.
    IgG r.
    IgM r.
    immune r.
    late phase r.
    mitogen r.
    secondary T-cell r.
    sustained r.
    systemic inflammatory r.
    virologic r.
Restan virus (RESV)
rest body
resting energy expenditure (REE)
restless leg syndrome
restricta
    Nocardia r.
restriction
    r. endonuclease analysis (REA,
      READ)
    r. endonuclease assay
    r. enzyme analysis (REA)
    r. fragment length polymorphism
      (RFLP)
    r. fragment length polymorphism
      technique
restrictus
    Aspergillus r.
    Azovibrio r.
    Dehalobacter r.
restuans
    Culex r.
resurgent
resuscitation
    fluid r.
RESV
    Restan virus
resveratrol
Resyl
retbaense
    Desulfohalobium r.
reticulate body (RB)
reticulatus
    Dermacentor r.
reticuli
    Streptomyces r.
reticuliscabiei
    Streptomyces r.
reticulitermitidis
    Clevelandina r.
reticulocyte
reticuloendothelial
    r. blockade
    r. system (RES)
reticuloendotheliosis virus
reticulohistiocytosis
    congenital self-healing r.

reticulonodular
- r. infiltration
- r. radiograph

reticulum

retina
- tuberculosis of the r.

retinal
- r. arteritis
- r. detachment
- r. exudation
- r. pigment epithelium (RPE)

Retin-A Micro Topical

retinitis
- bornavirus r.
- CMV r.
- cytomegalovirus r.
- necrotizing r.

retinoblastoma

retinochoroiditis
- bilateral r.
- nosocomial r.

9-*cis*-retinoic acid

retinoic acid

retinoid

retinopathy
- HIV r.
- hypertensive r.

retinyl acetate

Retisol-A

Retortamonadida

Retortomonas intestinalis

retraction
- intercostal r.

retroauricular

retroinfection

retroorbital headache

retroperitoneal
- r. abscess
- r. fibrosis
- r. ultrasound

retropharyngeal abscess

retropubic urethropexy

retrospective

retrosternal

Retrovir

Retroviridae

retrovirus
- human r.
- squirrel monkey r.
- viper r.

rettgeri
- *Proteus r.*
- *Providencia r.*

reukaufii
- *Candida r.*
- *Metschnikowia r.*

reuszeri
- *Bacillus r.*
- *Brevibacillus r.*

reuteri
- *Lactobacillus r.*

revenge
- Montezuma's r.

reversal reaction

reverse
- r. CAMP test
- r. passive hemagglutination assay
- r. transcriptase (RT)
- r. transcriptase inhibitor (RTI)
- r. transcriptase polymerase chain reaction (RT-PCR)
- r. transcriptase primer extension (RTPE)
- r. transcriptase primer extension analysis

reversed
- r. passive hemagglutination (RPHA)
- r. passive latex agglutination
- r. passive latex particle agglutination (RPLA)

reverse-osmosis (RO)

Reversol

Rev gene

revolutum
- *Echinostoma r.*

Reye syndrome

RF
- rheumatoid factor

RFLP
- restriction fragment length polymorphism
- RFLP technique

RFLP-based subtyping

RFV
- Royal Farm virus

rGCSF

R-Gel

rGM-CSF
- granulocyte/macrophage colony-stimulating factor

rgp160
- r. vaccine

NOTES

RGV
  Rio Grande virus
Rh
  Gamulin Rh
  Mini-Gamulin Rh
  Rh positive
Rhabdiasoidea
Rhabditella
  R. axei
Rhabditida
Rhabditidae
rhabditiform
  r. larva
Rhabditis (p)
  R. terricola
Rhabditis-like
Rhabditoidea
Rhabditoides inermis
Rhabdochromatium marinum (b)
rhabdoformis
  Desulfobulbus r.
rhabdomyolysis
rhabdomyosarcoma
Rhabdophora
Rhabdoviridae
rhabdovirus
  hirame r.
  snakehead r.
  ulcerative disease r.
Rhadinovirus (v)
rhagii
  Candida r.
Rhagionidae
rhamnolipid
rhamnosa
  Kineosporia r.
rhamnosum
  Brachybacterium r.
rhamnosus
  Lactobacillus r.
  Lactobacillus casei subsp. *r.*
rhapontici
  Erwinia r.
  Pectobacterium r.
Rh$_O$(D) immune globulin
rhenobacensis
  Rhodopseudomonas r.
rheologic
rheotaxis
rheotropism
rhesus
  r. rotavirus-tetravalent vaccine
rheumatic
  r. fever
  r. valvulitis
rheumatica
  polymyalgia r.

rheumatic heart disease
  scarlatina r.
rheumatism
  palindromic r.
  Shanghai r.
rheumatogenicity
rheumatogenic streptococcal strain
rheumatoid
  r. arthritis
  r. factor (RF)
  r. pneumonitis
rheumatologic
rhGH
  recombinant human growth hormone
rhIL-3
  recombinant human interleukin-3
rhinaria
  Linguatula r.
Rhindocladium (f)
rhinitis
  acute viral r.
  allergic r.
  atrophic r.
  chronic atrophic r.
  viral r.
rhinocerebral
  r. infection
  r. mucormycosis
  r. phycomycosis
rhinoceros
  Orcytes r.
Rhinocladiella (f)
  R. aquaspersa
  R. atrovirens
Rhinocladium (f)
rhinoestrosis
Rhinoestrus purpureus (p)
rhinomucormycosis
rhinorrhea
  cerebrospinal r.
rhinoscleroma
rhinoscleromatis
  Klebsiella r.
  Klebsiella pneumoniae subsp. *r.*
rhinosporidiosis
Rhinosporidium seeberi
Rhinosyn-DMX
Rhinosyn Liquid
Rhinosyn-PD Liquid
Rhinosyn-X Liquid
rhinotracheale
  Ornithobacterium r.
rhinotracheitis
  infectious bovine r.
Rhinotrichum (f)
Rhinovirus (v)
rhinovirus
  r. 1B

bovine r.
bovine r. 1–2
human r. 1–100
human r. 1A
rhipicephali
    Rickettsia r.
Rhipicephalinae
Rhipicephalus (p)
    R. *appendiculatus*
    R. *sanguineus*
Rhipidiaceae
Rhizidiaceae
Rhizidiomyces (f)
Rhizidiomyces virus
Rhizidiomycetaceae
Rhizidiovirus (v)
Rhizobacter (b)
Rhizobiaceae
Rhizobium (b)
    R. *ciceri*
    R. *etli*
    R. *fredii*
    R. *galegae*
    R. *gallicum*
    R. *giardinii*
    R. *hainanense*
    R. *huakuii*
    R. *huautlense*
    R. *japonicum*
    R. *leguminosarum*
    R. *loti*
    R. *lupini*
    R. *mediterraneum*
    R. *meliloti*
    R. *mongolense*
    R. *phaseoli*
    R. *radiobacter*
    R. *rhizogenes*
    R. *rubi*
    R. *tianshanense*
    R. *trifolii*
    R. *tropici*
    R. *undicola*
    R. *vitis*
    R. *yanglingense*
Rhizoctonia (f)
rhizogenes
    Agrobacterium r.
    Rhizobium r.
rhizoid
Rhizomonas suberifaciens (b)
Rhizomucor pusillus (p)

rhizophila
    Kineosporia r.
    Kocuria r.
rhizoplast
Rhizopoda
rhizopodia
Rhizopogonaceae
rhizopterin
Rhizopus (f)
    R. *arrhizus*
    R. *microsporus*
    R. *stolonifer*
rhizosphaerae
    Agromyces r.
rhizosphera
    Gordonia r.
Rhizothyriaceae
rhodamine stain
rhodanensis
    Pichia r.
Rhodanobacter lindaniclasticus (b)
rhodesiae
    Mycobacterium r.
    Pseudomonas r.
Rhodesian
    R. sleeping sickness
    R. trypanosomiasis
rhodesianum
    Methylobacterium r.
rhodesiense
    Trypanosoma brucei r.
rhodina
    Botryosphaeria r.
rhodinum
    Methylobacterium r.
rhodnii
    Rhodococcus r.
Rhodnius prolixus (p)
Rhodobaca bogoriensis (b)
Rhodobacter (b)
    R. *adriaticus*
    R. *azotoformans*
    R. *blasticus*
    R. *capsulatus*
    R. *euryhalinus*
    R. *sphaeroides*
    R. *sulfidophilus*
    R. *veldkampii*
Rhodobacteriaceae
Rhodobium (b)
    R. *marinum*
    R. *orientis*

R

NOTES

rhodochrous
    Rhodococcus r.
Rhodocista centenaria (b)
Rhodococcus (b)
    R. aichiensis
    R. aurantiacus
    R. bronchialis
    R. chlorophenolicus
    R. chubuensis
    R. coprophilus
    R. corallinus
    R. equi
    R. erythropolis
    R. fascians
    R. globerulus
    R. koreensis
    R. luteus
    R. marinonascens
    R. maris
    R. obuensis
    R. opacus
    R. percolatus
    R. pyridinivorans
    R. rhodnii
    R. rhodochrous
    R. roseus
    R. ruber
    R. rubropertinctus
    R. sputi
    R. terrae
    R. zopfii
Rhodocyclus (b)
    R. gelatinosus
    R. purpureus
    R. tenuis
Rhodoferax (b)
    R. antarcticus
    R. fermentans
Rhodomicrobium (b)
    R. vannielii
Rhodomyces (f)
Rhodopila globiformis (b)
Rhodoplanes (b)
    R. elegans
    R. roseus
Rhodopseudomonas (b)
    R. acidophila
    R. adriatica
    R. blastica
    R. capsulata
    R. gelatinosa
    R. globiformis
    R. julia
    R. marina
    R. palustris
    R. rhenobacensis
    R. rosea
    R. rutila

    R. sphaeroides
    R. sulfidophila
    R. sulfoviridis
    R. viridis
rhodorangea
    Micromonospora r.
rhodos
    Pseudomonas r.
Rhodospira trueperi (b)
Rhodospirillaceae
Rhodospirillales
Rhodospirillum (b)
    R. centenum
    R. fulvum
    R. molischianum
    R. photometricum
    R. rubrum
    R. salexigens
    R. salinarum
    R. sodomense
    R. tenue
Rhodosporidium (f)
Rhodothalassium salexigens (b)
Rhodothermus (b)
    R. marinus
    R. obamensis
Rhodotorula (f)
    R. glutinis
    R. minuta
    R. rubra
rhodotoxin
Rhodovibrio (b)
    R. salinarum
    R. sodomensis
Rhodovulum (b)
    R. adriaticum
    R. euryhalinum
    R. iodosum
    R. robiginosum
    R. strictum
    R. sulfidophilum
RhoGAM
RhoIGIV
Rholosone
rhombencephalitis
rhombi
    Arthrobacter r.
Rhoprolene
Rhoprosone
Rhume
    Personnelle Contre le R.
rhusiopathiae
    Erysipelothrix r.
rhysodes
    Acanthamoeba r.
rhythm
    gallop r.
    nodal r.

Rhytismataceae
Rhytismatales
RIA
    radioimmunoassay
RIBA
    radioimmunoblot assay
    recombinant immunoblot assay
ribadeneirai
ribavirin
    r. combination pack
ribeiroi
    Trichosporon r.
riboflavin
riboflavina
    Devosia r.
ribonuclease
    r. H (RNaseH)
ribonucleic acid (RNA)
riboprinting
riboprobe
    antisense r.
ribose fermentation test
ribosomal
    r. ribonucleic acid (rRNA)
    r. RNA
ribotyping
    Enterobacter cloacae r.
rice
    r. itch
    r. starch
rice-Tween agar
Rich
    Cyto R.
richardii
    Leminorella r.
richardsiae
    Phialophora r.
richteri
    Solenopsis r.
ricini
    Philosamia r.
ricinus
    Ixodes r.
Rickettsia (b)
    R. *aeschlimannii*
    R. *africae*
    R. *akari*
    R. *australis*
    R. *bellii*
    R. *canadensis*
    R. *conorii*
    R. *felis*

R. *helvetica*
R. *honei*
R. infection
R. *japonica*
R. *massiliae*
R. *montanensis*
R. *parkeri*
R. *peacockii*
R. *prowazekii*
R. *rhipicephali*
R. *rickettsii*
R. *rickettsii* serology
R. *sennetsu*
R. *sibirica*
R. *slovaca*
R. *tsutsugamushi*
R. *typhi*
rickettsia
rickettsial
    r. disease
    r. infection
Rickettsiales
rickettsialpox
Rickettsieae
Rickettsiella (b)
    R. *chironomi*
    R. *grylli*
    R. *popilliae*
    R. *stethorae*
rickettsii
    Rickettsia r.
rickettsioses
rickettsiosis
    vesicular r.
Rictularia (f)
Rictularioidea
RID
    radial immunodiffusion
    RID Mousse
    RID Shampoo
Ridenol
riegelii
    Corynebacterium r.
Riemerella (b)
    R. *anatipestifer*
    R. *columbina*
rifabutin
    r.-associated uveitis
    r. plus delavirdine
    r. plus efavirenz
    r. plus nevirapine

R

NOTES

Rifadin
R. Injection
R. Oral
Rifamate
rifampicin
rifampin (RMP)
r. and isoniazid
r., isoniazid, and pyrazinamide
rifampin-impregnated catheter
rifamycin
rifamycini
Actinomadura cremea subsp. *r.*
rifapentine
r. rimantadine
Rifater
rIFN-A
Rift
R. Valley fever
R. Valley fever virus (RVFV)
RIG
rabies immunoglobulin
riggsi
Culicoides r.
right-sided endocarditis
right ventricular hypertrophy (RVH)
rigidity
decerebrate r.
nuchal r.
rigidum
Acetofilamentum r.
Hysterothylacium r.
RIIE
respiratory isolation implementation
efficiency
RIIS
respiratory isolation implementation
sensitivity
Rikenella microfusus (b)
RIM
rapid identification method
Rimactane
R. Oral
rimae
Atopobium r.
Lactobacillus r.
rimantadine
rifapentine r.
RIM-*Neisseria*
rapid identification method-*Neisseria*
RIM-*Neisseria* test
rimosus
Streptomyces rimosus subsp. *r.*
rinderpest virus
ring
beta-lactam r.
r. chromosome
Liesegang r.

polar r.
signet r.
ring-enhancing
r.-e. lesion
ringworm
r. of beard
black-dot r.
r. of body
crusted r.
r. of foot
r. of genitocrural region
honeycomb r.
r. of nail
oriental r.
r. of scalp
scaly r.
Tokelau r.
Rinse
Nix Creme R.
Peridex Oral R.
Rio
R. Bravo virus (RBV)
R. Grande cichlid virus
R. Grande virus (RGV)
R. Segunda virus
riparia
Actinokineospora r.
riparius
Aedes r.
rishiriensis
Streptomyces r.
risk
relative r. (RR)
risk-reduction
risticii
Ehrlichia r.
risus sardonicus
ritonavir (RTV)
lopinavir and r.
r. plasma level
r. soft gel cap
ritonavir-indinavir
ritonavir-saquinavir
Ritter disease
rivadeneirai
Anopheles r.
rivalierii
Microsporum audouinii var. *r.*
rivalis
Physa r.
rivasi
Simulium r.
Rivasone
river blindness
riverine tsetse fly
rivolta
Isospora r.

R

rivuli
> *Simulium* r.

rLFN-alpha-2

RML-105355 virus

RMP
> rifampin

RMS
> red man syndrome

RMSF
> Rocky Mountain spotted fever

RMV virus

RNA
> ribonucleic acid
>> expanded range HIV-1 RNA
>> RNA genome
>> hepatitis C viral RNA
>> HIV-1 RNA
>> ribosomal RNA
>> RNA tumor virus
>> RNA viral load

RNA-based assay

RNA-dependent DNA polymerase

RNaseH
> ribonuclease H

RNase L 2'-5' oligoadenylate synthetase

RO
> reverse-osmosis

Robafen
> R. AC, CF, DM

Robaxin

Robbins voice prosthesis

Robicillin VK

Robidex

Robidrine

Robigesic

robiginosum
> *Rhodovulum* r.

Robinul
> R. Forte

Robitet Oral

Robitussin
> R. A-C
> R. Cough Calmers
> R. Pediatric
> R. Pediatric Cough & Cold
> R. Severe Congestion Liqui-Gels

Robitussin-CF

Robitussin-DAC

Robitussin-DM

Robitussin-PE

robusta
> *Candida* r.

robustum
> *Ketogulonicigenium* r.

robustus
> *Gordius* r.

Rocephin

Rochalimaea (b)
> R. elizabethae
> R. henselae
> R. quintana
> R. vinsonii

Rochambeau virus (RBUV)

Roche
> R. Amplicore PCR
> R. Amplicore polymerase chain reaction

rochei
> *Streptomyces* r.

Rocio
> R. virus (ROCV)

Rocky
> R. Mountain spotless fever
> R. Mountain spotted fever (RMSF)
> R. Mountain spotted fever serology

ROCV
> Rocio virus

rod
> Auer r.
> basal r.
> beaded r.
> germinal r.
> gram-negative r.
> gram-positive r.
> palisading r.

RODAC-TM
> replicate organism direct agar contact

rodentium
> *Citrobacter* r.
> *Helicobacter* r.
> *Staphylococcus sciuri* subsp. *r.*
> *Veillonella* r.

rodhaini
> *Cordylobia* r.
> *Schistosoma* r.

rod-shaped phage

roentgenogram

roentgenographic

RO-Eyewash

Rofact

Roferon-A

Rogaine Topical

RO-Gentycin

Rogitine

NOTES

rogosae
  Lactobacillus r.
rohdei
  Yersinia r.
Roiron medium
roll
  r. tube
  r. tube culture
ROM
  rupture of membranes
Romaña sign
Roman fever
Romanovsky stain
Romberg sign
romeroi
  Pyrenochaeta r.
Rondamine-DM Drops
Rondec-DM
rondoni
  Anopheles r.
room
  operating r. (OR)
RO-Predphate
roridum
  Myrothecium r.
rorotaense
  Simulium r.
rosa
  Sphingomonas r.
rosacea
  acne r.
rosaria
  Micromonospora r.
rosatii
  Neotestudina r.
rose
  r. bengal staining
  r. bengal test
  r. fever
  r. handler's disease
  r. spot
rosea
  Bactoderma r.
  Chainia r.
  Hysterolecitha r.
  Kocuria r.
  Microbispora rosea subsp. *r.*
  Planobispora r.
  Rhodopseudomonas r.
  Thiocapsa r.
  Thiopedia r.
roseae
  Novosphingobium r.
Roseateles depolymerans (b)
Roseburia cecicola (b)
rosei
  Saccharomyces r.

Roseibium (b)
  R. denhamense
  R. hamelinense
roseiflava
  Sphingomonas r.
Roseinatronobacter thiooxidans (b)
roseiscleroticus
  Streptomyces r.
Roseivivax (b)
  R. halodurans
  R. halotolerans
Rosellinia (f)
rosellus
  Hypomyces r.
Rosenbach
  erysipeloid of R.
rosenbergii
  Hyphomonas r.
Roseobacter (b)
  R. algicola
  R. denitrificans
  R. gallaeciensis
  R. litoralis
Roseococcus thiosulfatophilus (b)
roseodiastaticus
  Streptomyces r.
roseoflavus
  Streptomyces r.
roseofulvus
  Streptomyces r.
roseogriseum
  Acremonium r.
roseola
  Actinomadura r.
  epidemic r.
  r. infantum
  Microtetraspora r.
  Nonomuraea r.
  r. subitum
roseola-like eruption
roseoliform exanthem
roseolilacinus
  Streptomyces r.
Roseolovirus (v)
roseolus
  Flexibacter r.
  Streptomyces r.
Roseomonas (b)
  R. cervicalis
  R. fauriae
  R. gilardii
roseopersicina
  Lamprocystis r.
  Thiocapsa r.
roseosalivarius
  Hymenobacter r.
Roseospira mediosalina (b)
Roseospirillum parvum (b)

roseosporus
    Streptomyces r.
Roseovarius tolerans (b)
roseoverticillatum
    Streptoverticillium r.
roseoverticillatus
    Streptomyces r.
roseoviolacea
    Actinomadura r.
    Microtetraspora r.
    Nonomuraea r. subsp. *roseoviolacea*
roseoviolaceus
    Streptomyces r.
roseoviridis
    Streptomyces r.
rosette
roseum
    Clostridium r.
    Dactylosporangium r.
    Streptosporangium r.
    Thermomicrobium r.
    Tritirachium r.
roseus
    Amoebobacter r.
    Craurococcus r.
    Micrococcus r.
    Rhodococcus r.
    Rhodoplanes r.
    Salinicoccus r.
rosiglitazone
Ross
    R. River fever
    R. River polyarthritis
    R. River virus (RRV)
rossensis
    Colwellia r.
rossianum
    Thermonema r.
rossii
    Actinobacillus r.
rostella
rostellum
    armed r.
    unarmed r.
rostratum
    Exserohilum r.
Rotatest
Rotavirus (v)
rotavirus
    adult diarrhea r. (ADRV)
    attenuated human r.
    avian r.

    r. gastroenteritis
    group C r.
    r. groups A, B, C
    human r.
    mammalian r.
    poultry r.
    r. rapid detection
    rat r.
    sheep r.
Rothia (b)
    R. dentocariosa
    R. mucilaginosa
    R. nasimurium
Roth spot
Rotocaps
    Ventolin R.
rotundatum
    Trichosporon r.
rotundus
    Desmodus r.
Roubac
rough
    r. colony
Rouhex-G
roundworm
    large r.
Rounox
Rouphylline
Rous sarcoma virus
route
    fecal-oral r.
rouxii
    Saccharomyces r.
Rovamycine
rowbothamii
    Legionella r.
roxithromycin
Royal Farm virus (RFV)
royreba
    Acanthamoeba r.
RPD
    Pepcid R.
RPE
    retinal pigment epithelium
RPHA
    reversed passive hemagglutination
RPLA
    reversed passive latex particle
    agglutination
R-plasmid
    resistance plasmid

NOTES

RPR
  rapid plasma reagent
  rapid plasma reagin
    RPR CARD test
    RPR titer
RPR-CT
  rapid plasma reagin circle card test
RPTK
  receptor protein tyrosine kinase
RPV virus
RR
  relative risk
RR66 virus
rRNA
  ribosomal ribonucleic acid
    rRNA sequence analysis
RRV
  Ross River virus
RRV-TV vaccine
RSSE
  Russian spring-summer encephalitis
RSSEV
  Russian spring-summer encephalitis virus
RST
  reagin screen test
RSV
  respiratory syncytial virus
    RSV antigen
    RSV culture
    RSV serology
    RSV testing
    RSV titer
RSVIG
  respiratory syncytial virus immune
  globulin
RSV-IGIV
  respiratory syncytial virus immune
  globulin
RT
  reverse transcriptase
    RT inhibitor
    RT virus
RTAV
  Resistencia virus
RT codon 69
RTI
  reverse transcriptase inhibitor
rTNFα
  recombinant tumor necrosis factor alpha
RT-PCR
  reverse transcriptase polymerase chain
  reaction
    competitive RT-PCR (cRT-PCR)
RTPE
  reverse transcriptase primer extension
    RTPE analysis
RTV
  ritonavir

rub
  pericardial friction r.
rubella
  r. antibody
  congenital r.
  IgG antibody to r.
  IgM antibody to r.
  measles, mumps, r. (MMR)
  r. and measles vaccine
  r. serology
  r. vaccine RA 27/3
  r. virus
  r. virus culture
  r. virus vaccine, live
rubelliform
rubeola
ruber
    Flexibacter r.
    Meiothermus r.
    Monascus r.
    Paracraurococcus r.
    Rhodococcus r.
    Streptomyces r.
    Thermocrinis r.
    Thermus r.
rubi
    Agrobacterium r.
    Rhizobium r.
rubiacearum
    Phyllobacterium r.
rubida
    Amycolatopsis r.
    Triatoma r.
rubidaea
    Serratia r.
rubidus
    Hyostrongylus r.
rubiginosohelvolus
    Streptomyces r.
rubiginosum
    Simulium r.
rubiginosus
    Monascus r.
    Streptomyces r.
Rubivirus (v)
rubor
rubra
    Actinomadura r.
    Alteromonas r.
    Basipetospora r.
    Chainia r.
    Malonomonas r.
    Microtetraspora r.
    Nonomuraea r.
    Pseudoalteromonas r.
    Rhodotorula r.
    Rugamonas r.
    Spirillospora r.

rubradiris
  Streptomyces achromogenes subsp. *r.*
rubratoxin
rubrifaciens
  Acidisphaera r.
  Brenneria r.
  Erwinia r.
rubrilineans
  Pseudomonas r.
rubrilucens
  Legionella r.
Rubrimonas cliftonensis (b)
rubrireticuli
  Streptomyces r.
rubrisubalbicans
  Herbaspirillum r.
  Pseudomonas r.
rubrithorax
  Simulium r.
Rubrivivax gelatinosus (b)
Rubrobacter (b)
  R. radiotolerans
  R. xylanophilus
rubrobrunea
  Actinomadura r.
rubrobrunneus
  Aspergillus r.
rubrochlorinus
  Streptomyces r.
rubrofasciata
  Triatoma r.
rubrogriseus
  Streptomyces r.
rubropertincta
  Gordonia r.
rubropertinctus
  Rhodococcus r.
rubrorugosus
rubroverticillatus
  Streptomyces r.
rubrum
  Acidiphilium r.
  Rhodospirillum r.
rubtzovi
  Simulium r.
Rubulavirus (v)
rubulavirus
  porcine r.
ruckeri
  Yersinia r.

rudis
  Ornithodoros r.
  Pollenia r.
Rudivirus (v)
rudolphii
  Contracaecum r.
Ruegeria (b)
  R. algicola
  R. atlantica
  R. gelatinovorans
rufescens
  Protostrongylus r.
rufulus
  Scopulariopsis r.
rufus
  Streptomyces libani subsp. *r.*
Rugamonas rubra (b)
rugatobispora
  Actinomadura r.
rugglesi
  Simulium r.
rugiseptum
  Polyangium r.
rugopelliculosa
  Candida r.
rugosa
  Amycolatopsis r.
  Candida r.
  Nocardia r.
  nystatin-resistant *Candida r.*
  Prauserella r.
rugosum
  Trichosporon r.
rugosus
  Pogonomyrmex r.
rugulosum
  Penicillium r.
ruhlandii
  Achromobacter r.
  Alcaligenes r.
ruminalis
  Mannheimia r.
ruminantium
  Bifidobacterium r.
  Cowdria r.
  Eubacterium r.
  Methanobacterium r.
  Methanobrevibacter r.
  Selenomonas ruminantium subsp. *r.*
ruminatium
  Monocercomonas r.

NOTES

R

ruminicola
>*Bacteroides ruminicola* subsp. *r.*
>*Prevotella r.*
>*Prevotella ruminicola* subsp. *r.*

ruminis
>*Acetitomaculum r.*
>*Desulfotomaculum r.*
>*Lactobacillus r.*
>*Pseudobutyrivibrio r.*
>*Succiniclasticum r.*

Ruminobacter amylophilus (b)
Ruminococcus (b)
>*R. albus*
>*R. bromii*
>*R. callidus*
>*R. flavefaciens*
>*R. gnavus*
>*R. hansenii*
>*R. hydrogenotrophicus*
>*R. lactaris*
>*R. obeum*
>*R. palustris*
>*R. pasteurii*
>*R. productus*
>*R. schinkii*
>*R. torques*

rumoiensis
>*Vibrio r.*

Runella slithyformis (b)
Runyon
>R. classification of nontuberculous mycobacteria
>R. group I–IV mycobacteria

ruoffiae
>*Ignavigranum r.*

rupestre
>*Hyphelia r.*

rupia
rupture
>cardiac r.
>r. of membranes (ROM)

rural cutaneous leishmaniasis
Russell
>R. body
>R. viper

russelli
>*Vahlkampfia r.*

russensis
>*Dethiosulfovibrio r.*

Russian
>R. spring-summer encephalitis (RSSE)
>R. spring-summer encephalitis (Eastern subtype)
>R. spring-summer encephalitis virus (RSSEV)
>R. spring-summer encephalitis (Western subtype)
>R. tick-borne encephalitis

russii
>*Fusobacterium r.*

Russulaceae
Russula emetica (f)
Russulales
rust
rustigianii
>*Providencia r.*

rusty sputum
rutgersensis
>*Glycomyces r.*
>*Streptomyces rutgersensis* subsp. *r.*

rutila
>*Rhodopseudomonas r.*

Ru-Tuss
>R.-T. DE
>R.-T. Expectorant

RV
>rat virus

RVA
>rabies vaccine adsorbed
>recombinant virus assay

RVFV
>Rift Valley fever virus

RVH
>right ventricular hypertrophy

R$_1$ virus
R$_2$ virus
Ryan stain
ryckmani
>*Culicoides r.*

Rymed
Rymed-TR
Rymovirus (v)
Ryna-C Liquid
Ryna-CX
Ryna Liquid
Rynatuss Pediatric suspension

S
Svedburg unit
S-1153
S-60
S100 glial protein
S13 virus
S-2L virus
S-4L virus
S-6 virus
SA
Sinutab SA
Targel SA
SA10 virus
SA12 virus
sabaudiense
Spiroplasma s.
saber
s. shin
s. tibia
Sabia virus
Sabin-Feldman dye test
Sabin vaccine
Sabouraud agar
Sabouraudites (f)
SABOV
Sabo virus
Sabo virus (SABOV)
Saboya virus (SABV)
Sabulin
saburreum
Eubacterium s.
SABV
Saboya virus
sac
lacrimal s.
sacbrood virus
saccade
saccadic eye movement
saccari
Xanthomonas s.
sacchari
Amycolatopsis s.
Fusarium s.
Gluconacetobacter s.
Thermoactinomyces s.
Saccharobacter fermentatus (b)
Saccharococcus (b)
S. caldoxylosilyticus
S. thermophilus
saccharolytica
Moraxella s.
saccharolyticum
Clostridium s.

Halanaerobium saccharolyticum
subsp. s.
Thermoanaerobacterium s.
saccharolyticus
Caldicellulosiruptor s.
Enterococcus s.
Halococcus s.
Haloincola saccharolyticus subsp. s.
Peptococcus s.
Staphylococcus s.
Streptococcus s.
Saccharomonospora (b)
S. azurea
S. cyanea
S. glauca
S. viridis
S. xinjiangensis
Saccharomyces (f)
S. bailii
S. bayanus
S. bisporus
S. capensis
S. carlsbergensis
S. cerevisiae
S. cerevisiae var. ellipsoideus
S. delbrueckii
S. fermentati
S. florentinus
S. fragilis
S. heterogenicus
S. hienipiensis
S. inusitatus
S. italicus
S. kluyveri
S. krusei (See Candida krusei)
S. lactis
S. marxianus
S. microellipsoides
S. montanus
S. norbensis
S. oleaceus
S. paradoxus
S. pastorianus
S. pretoriensis
S. rosei
S. rouxii
S. uvarum
Saccharomycetaceae
Saccharomycetales
Saccharomycodes
S. mestris
Saccharomycopsis
S. synnaedendra

S

saccharophila
  Cytophaga s.
  Pseudomonas s.
saccharophilum
  Flavobacterium s.
  Halonatronum s.
  Treponema s.
Saccharopolyspora (b)
  S. erythraea
  S. gregorii
  S. hirsuta subsp. hirsuta
  S. hirsuta subsp. kobensis
  S. hirsuta subsp. taberi
  S. hordei
  S. rectivirgula
  S. spinosa
  S. spinosporotrichia
  S. taberi
  S. thermophila
Saccharothrix (b)
  S. aerocolonigenes
  S. aerocolonigenes subsp.
    aerocolonigenes
  S. aerocolonigenes subsp.
    staurosporea
  S. albidocapillata
  S. australiensis
  S. coeruleofusca
  S. coeruleoviolacea
  S. cryophilis
  S. espanaensis
  S. flava
  S. longispora
  S. mutabilis subsp. capreolus
  S. mutabilis subsp. mutabilis
  S. syringae
  S. tangerinus
  S. texasensis
  S. violacea
  S. waywayandensis
saccharovorum
  Halobacterium s.
  Halorubrobacterium s.
  Halorubrum s.
Sachsia
sacroiliac joint
sacroiliitis
sacrum
saddleback
  s. caterpillar
  s. fever curve
saeculare
  Bifidobacterium s.
Safe Tussin 30
SAF fixative
safranin
  s. stain

SAFV
  Saint-Floris virus
saginata
  Taenia s.
  taeniasis s.
sagitta
  Dipus s.
Sagittula stellata (b)
Sagiyama virus (SAGV)
Sagrahamala (f)
saguaro cactus virus (SgCV)
SAGV
  Sagiyama virus
SAH
  subarachnoid hemorrhage
saheli
  Sinorhizobium s.
saimiri
  herpesvirus s. (HVS)
saimiriine herpesvirus 1
Saint-Floris virus (SAFV)
sainthelensi
  Legionella s.
saitoana
  Candida s.
sakazakii
  Enterobacter s.
sake
  Candida s.
sakei
  Lactobacillus s.
  Lactobacillus s. subsp. *sakei*
Sakhalin virus (SAKV)
Saksenaeaceae
Saksenaea vasiformis (f)
SAKV
  Sakhalin virus
SAL
  salicylic and lactic acid paint
Salac
Salacid Ointment
Sal-Acid Plaster
salamae
  Salmonella choleraesuis subsp. *s.*
Salanga virus (SGAV)
salbutamol
salegens
  Flavobacterium s.
  Salegentibacter s.
Salegentibacter salegens (b)
Salehabad virus (SALV)
Saleto-200, -400
salexigens
  Bacillus s.
  Chromatium s.
  Chromohalobacter s.
  Desulfovibrio s.
  Halochromatium s.

Rhodospirillum s.
Rhodothalassium s.
Salibacillus s.
Salflex
Salgesic
Salibacillus (b)
    S. marismortui
    S. salexigens
salicin fermentation test
salicinius
    Lactobacillus salivarius subsp. *s.*
salicis
    Brenneria s.
    Erwinia s.
salicylate
    choline s.
    magnesium s.
    sodium s.
salicylatoxidans
    Pseudaminobacter s.
salicylic
    s. acid and lactic acid
    s. acid and propylene glycol
    s. and benzoic acid compound
    s. and lactic acid paint (SAL)
salida
    Candida s.
salifodinae
    Halococcus s.
salthi
    Culicoides s.
Saliject
salina
    Artemisia s.
    Deleya s.
    Halomonas s.
    Streptimonospora s.
salinaria
    Orenia s.
salinarium
    Halobacterium s.
salinarius
    Culex s.
    Culicoides s.
    Halanaerobacter s.
salinarum
    Rhodospirillum s.
    Rhodovibrio s.
saline
    s. agglutinin
    isotonic s.
    s. microscopy

Page ameba s.
    s. wet mount
salinestris
    Azotobacter s.
Salinicoccus (b)
    S. hispanicus
    S. roseus
Salinivibrio (b)
    S. costicola subsp. *costicola*
    S. costicola subsp. *vallismortis*
salivaria
salivarium
    Mycoplasma s.
salivarius
    Lactobacillus salivarius subsp. *s.*
    Streptococcus s.
salivary
    s. amylase
    s. gland disease
    s. gland tuberculosis
salivation
salivosa
    Porphyromonas s.
salivosus
    Bacteroides s.
Salk vaccine
salmanticensis
    Candida s.
salmincola
    Nanophyetus s.
    Troglotrema s.
salmon
    s. poisoning
    S. River virus
salmonea
    Actinomadura s.
    Microtetraspora s.
    Nonomuraea s.
Salmonella (b)
    antimicrobial-resistant *S.*
    S. arizonae
    S. arthritis
    S. bongori
    S. choleraesuis subsp. *bongori*
    S. choleraesuis subsp. *choleraesuis*
    S. choleraesuis subsp. *diarizonae*
    S. choleraesuis subsp. *houtenae*
    S. choleraesuis subsp. *indica*
    S. choleraesuis subsp. *salamae*
    S. contamination
    S. enteritidis
    S. food poisoning

NOTES

477

Salmonella *(continued)*
 S. O antigen test
 S. paratyphi
 S. septicemia
 S. typhi
 S. typhimurium
Salmonelleae
salmonellosis
 nontyphoidal s.
 nosocomial s.
salmoneum
 Acrodontium s.
salmonicida
 Aeromonas salmonicida subsp. *s.*
 Nocardia s.
 Vibrio s.
salmonicolor
 Cytophaga s.
 Marinilabilia s.
 Sporidiobolus s.
 Sporobolomyces s.
salmoninarum
 Renibacterium s.
 Vagococcus s.
salmonis
 Exophiala s.
 Piscirickettsia s.
 Streptomyces s.
 Streptoverticillium s.
salmostica
 Cryptobia s.
salomonis
 Helicobacter s.
salpingitis
 acute gonococcal s.
 gonococcal s.
salpingo-oophoritis
salsalate
Salseb
Salsitab
salsuginis
 Halanaerobium s.
salt
 bile s.
 bismuth s.
 chaotropic s.
 s. sensitivity
 s. tolerance test
 s. water associated skin gangrene
  sepsis
saltans
 Bodo s.
 Pedobacter s.
saltonensis
 Culicoides s.
saltwater-related wound
SALV
 Salehabad virus

salvage
 s. chemotherapy
 s. highly active antiretroviral
  therapy (SHAART)
 s. therapy
Salve
 Callus S.
Sal Vieja virus (SVV)
samboni
 Simulium s.
sample
 first-void urine s.
 FVU s.
 midstream urine s.
sampling
 bone marrow s.
sampsonii
 Streptomyces s.
Samsonia erythrinae (b)
San
 S. Angelo virus (SAV)
 S. Joaquin fever
 S. Juan virus (SJV)
 S. Perlita virus (SPV)
sanchezi
 Argas s.
sancti
 Flexibacter s.
sanctielii
 Anopheles s.
sanctuary site
sand
 s. flea
 hydatid s.
Sandaracinobacter sibiricus (b)
sandfly
 s. fever
 s. fever Naples virus (SFNV)
 s. fever Sicilian virus (SFSV)
 s. fever and Uukuniemi virus
  group
 s. fever virus
 phlebotomus s.
Sandjimba virus (SJAV)
Sandoglobulin
sandramycini
 Kribbella s.
sandworm
sandy patch
sanfranciscensis
 Lactobacillus s.
Sango virus (SANV)
Sanguibacter (b)
 S. *inulinus*
 S. *keddieii*
 S. *suarezii*
sanguinareus
 mycetism s.

sanguineum
  Simulium s.
sanguineus
  Allodermanyssus s.
  Diaptomus s.
  Rhipicephalus s.
sanguinicola
  Aerococcus s.
sanguinipes
  Melanoplus s.
sanguinis
  Gemella s.
  Globicatella s.
  Sphingomonas s.
  Streptococcus s.
sanguisuga
  Culicoides s.
  Triatoma s.
sanguivorous
sannanensis
  Streptomyces s.
santamariae
  Candida s.
Santarem virus (STMV)
santarosai
  Leptospira s.
Santa Rosa virus (SARV)
santicrucis
  Legionella s.
santjacobensis
  Candida s.
Santosai temperate virus
SANV
  Sango virus
São Paulo fever
saperconazole
saperdae
  Aureobacterium s.
  Brevibacterium s.
  Curtobacterium s.
  Microbacterium s.
saphenous homograft
saphenum
  Eubacterium s.
sapidus
  Pleurotus s.
sapomandens
  Desulfotomaculum s.
saponavida
  Syntrophomonas wolfei subsp. s.

sapovorans
  Desulfovibrio s.
  Syntrophomonas s.
sapphire II virus
sapphirina
  Uranotaenia s.
Sapporo
  S. agent
  S. virus
Sapporo-like viruses (v)
sapporonense
  Streptoverticillium s.
sapporonensis
  Streptomyces s.
saprobe
saprobic
saprogen
saprogenic
Saprolegniaceae
Saprolegniales
saprophilous
saprophilus
  Mycetocola s.
saprophyte
  facultative s.
saprophytic
  s. aspergillosis
  s. fungus
  s. hypha
saprophyticus
  Staphylococcus saprophyticus subsp.
  s.
Saprospira grandis (b)
saprozoic
saprozoonosis
SAPS II
saquinavir (SQV)
  s. hard gel capsule
  s. HGC
  s. soft gelatin capsule
Saraca virus (SRAV)
Sarcina (b)
  S. maxima
  S. ventriculi
sarcine
Sarcinomyces phaeomuriformis (f)
Sarcinosporon inkin (f)
Sarcobium (b)
  S. lyticum
Sarcocystidae
Sarcocystis (p)
  S. bovifelis

S

NOTES

Sarcocystis (continued)
    S. hominis
    S. suihominis
    S. tenella
sarcocystis
sarcocystosis
sarcode
Sarcodina
sarcoidosis
    active s.
sarcoma
    AIDS-related Kaposi s.
    granulocytic s.
    Kaposi s. (KS)
    pulmonary Kaposi s. (PKS)
    soft tissue limb s.
Sarcomastigophora
sarconeme
Sarcophaga (p)
    S. argyrostoma
Sarcophagidae
Sarcopsylla penetrans (p)
Sarcopsyllidae
Sarcoptes (p)
    S. hominis
    S. scabei var. *humani*
    S. scabiei
sarcoptic
    s. acariasis
    s. mange
sarcoptid
Sarcoptidae
Sarcoptiformes
Sarcoptoidea
sardiniensis
    Clostridium s.
sardonicus
    risus s.
sargentensis
    Pichia s.
sargramostim
Sarna HC
Sarracenia purpurea
Sarracenomyia
sartgoformum
    Clostridium s.
SARV
    Santa Rosa virus
sashimi
SAS software for statistical analysis
SAStid Plain Therapeutic Shampoo and Acne Wash
SAT1
    Aphthovirus S.
SAT2
    Aphthovirus S.
SAT3
    Aphthovirus S.

satellite
    s. cell
    s. colony
    s. lesion
Sathuperi virus (SATV)
Satinique Anti-Dandruff
saturated
    s. mercuric chloride
    s. solution of potassium iodide (SSKI)
saturnea
    Amycolata s.
    Nocardia s.
    Pseudonocardia s.
Saturnia pavonia **virus**
saturnus
    Hansenula s.
SATV
    Sathuperi virus
satyri
    Bertia s.
Saumarez Reef virus (SREV)
saundersi
    Culicoides s.
sausage-roll nerve thickening
SAV
    San Angelo virus
SA/V
    surface area to volume ratio
savanna tsetse fly
savastanoi
    Pseudomonas s.
    Pseudomonas syringae subsp. *s.*
savignyi
    Ornithodoros s.
savonica
    Candida s.
sawgrass virus (SAWV)
SAWV
    sawgrass virus
sawyeri
    Anopheles argyritarsis s.
saxitoxin
SBP
    spontaneous bacterial peritonitis
SC
    hemoglobin SC
scabei
Scabene
scabetic mite
scabicide
scabiei
    Sarcoptes s.
    Streptomyces s.
scabies
    crusted s.
    Norwegian s.
    Streptomyces s.

scalaris
> *Fannia s.*

scalded skin syndrome

scale
> Chalder Fatigue S.
> HIV Dementia S. (HDS)
> Karnofsky Performance S.
> Zubrod performance s.

scalp
> Hair and S.
> s. infection
> ringworm of s.

Scalpicin Topical

scaly ringworm

scan
> bone s.
> computed tomography brain s.
> (CT)
> gallium abscess s.
> gallium tumor s.
> indium-labeled white blood cell s.
> indium leukocyte s.
> NMR s.
> nuclear medicine s.
> radionuclide bone s.
> soft tissue s.
> technetium s.
> three-phase bone s.
> V/Q s.
> whole-body bone s.

Scandinavian housewife disease

scandinavica
> *Methylomonas s.*

scanloni
> *Culicoides s.*

scapula

scapularis
> *Aedes s.*
> *Ixodes s.*

scarlatina rheumatica

scarlatiniform
> s. eruption

scarlet
> s. fever
> s. fever antitoxin
> s. fever toxin A

scarring
> corneal s.
> punctal s.

scatologenes
> *Clostridium s.*

scatophagy

SCAV
> Sunday Canyon virus

SCC
> squamous cell cancer

Scedosporium (f)
> *S. apiospermum*
> *S. prolificans*

Sceptor
> S. Panel
> S. System

SCGYEM
> serum-casein-glucose-yeast extract
> medium

SCH 56592

schaalii
> *Actinobaculum s.*

Schaedler agar

schatavii
> *Candida s.*

Schaudinn fixative solution

Scheinpharm Triamcine-A

Schenck disease

schenckii
> *Sporothrix s.*

scheremetewskyi
> *Dermatophagoides s.*

schikhobalowi
> *Nanophyetus s.*

Schilling test

Schineria larvae (b)

schinkii
> *Ruminococcus s.*

Schistocerca gregaria

schistocyte

schistocytosis

Schistosoma (p)
> *S. bovis*
> *S. curassoni*
> *S. haematobium*
> *S. incognitum*
> *S. indicum*
> *S. intercalatum*
> *S. japonicum*
> *S. malayensis*
> *S. mansoni*
> *S. margrebowiei*
> *S. mattheei*
> *S. mekongi*
> *S. nasale*
> *S. rodhaini*
> *S. sinensium*

NOTES

S

Schistosoma (continued)
    S. spindale
    S. suis
schistosomal
    s. dermatitis
Schistosomatidae
Schistosomatium douthitti (p)
Schistosomatoidea
schistosome
    s. cercaria
    s. egg-hatching test
    s. granuloma
schistosomiasis
    Asiatic s.
    bladder s.
    cerebrospinal s.
    ectopic s.
    hepatosplenic s.
    intestinal s.
    Manson s.
    oriental s.
    urinary s.
    urogenital s.
schistosomulum
Schistotaenia srivastavai (p)
Schizoblastosporion (f)
    S. henrici
    S. starkeyi
schizogenesis
schizogony
schizomycete
schizomycetic
schizont
    tissue s.
schizonticide
Schizophora
schizophrenia
Schizophyllaceae
Schizophyllum commune (f)
schizopinax
    Aedes s.
Schizopyrenida
Schizosaccharomyces pombe (f)
Schizothyriaceae
Schizotrypanum (p) (*See* **Trypanosoma**)
schizozoite
schlegelii
    Bacillus s.
schleiferi
    Aureobacterium s.
    Microbacterium s.
    Staphylococcus schleiferi subsp. *s.*
Schlichter test
schmidlei
    Thioploca s.
schmidtmummi
    Simulium s.

Schmorl bacillus (*See* **Fusobacterium necrophorum**)
Schneider *Drosophila* **medium**
schneideri
    Elaeophora s.
schoenleinii
    Trichophyton s.
Scholl
    S. Athlete's Foot Preparations
    S. Wart Remover
    S. Zino
schtitka
    Eubacterium yurii subsp. *s.*
schubertii
    Aeromonas s.
Schüffner
    S. dots
    S. granule
schulzeri
    Ramichloridium s.
Schwartzia succinivorans (b)
Schwartzman reaction
Schwarz vaccine
sciatic neuritis
Sciences
    National Academy of S.
scindens
    Clostridium s.
scintigraphy
    biliary s.
    bone s.
scissiparity
sciuri
    Staphylococcus sciuri subsp. *s.*
sciurobia
    Leptopsylla s.
Sclavo-PPD solution
Sclavo Test-PPD
sclera, pl. **sclerae**
scleral
    s. buckle
    s. icterus
scleritis
sclerocorneal punch
Sclerodermataceae
Sclerodermatales
sclerose
sclerosing
    s. agent
    s. cholangitis
    s. keratitis
    s. lymphadenitis
sclerosis
    amyotrophic lateral s.
    multiple s.
sclerotherapy
    variceal s.

sclerotialus
>   *Streptomyces s.*

sclerotica
>   *Malbranchea s.*

sclerotic body

Sclerotinaceae

sclerotiorum
>   *Aspergillus s.*

sclerotium

scoleces (*pl. of* scolex)

scoleciasis

scoleciform

Scolecobasidium (f)
>   *S. terreum*
>   *S. tshawytschae*

scolecoid

scolecology

scolex, pl. **scolices, scoleces**

Scolopendra gigantea

scomber
>   *Cystoopsis s.*

scombroid
>   s. poisoning

scombrotoxin

SCOPE
>   Surveillance and Control of Pathogens of Epidemiologic Importance

scophthalmi
>   *Vibrio s.*

scophthalmum
>   *Chryseobacterium s.*
>   *Flavobacterium s.*

scopolamine

Scopulariopsis (f)
>   *S. asperula*
>   *S. fusca*
>   *S. koningii*
>   *S. rufulus*

score
>   acute physiology and chronic health evaluation s. (APACHE II score)
>   APACHE II s.
>   acute physiology and chronic health evaluation score
>   Karnofsky Performance S.
>   Knodell s.
>   S. for Neonatal Acute Physiology (SNAP)
>   Nugent s.
>   Simplified Acute Physiology S.
>   vaginal flora s.

scorpii
>   *Bothriocephalus s.*

scorpion

Scorpiones

Scotch
>   S. tape swab
>   S. tape test

scotiae
>   *Actinobacillus s.*

scotochromogens

scotoductus
>   *Thermus s.*

scotoma, pl. **scotomata**

scotti
>   *Leucosporidium s.*

Scot-Tussin
>   S.-T. DM Cough Chasers
>   S.-T. Senior Clear

scrapie

scraping
>   conjunctival s.
>   corneal s.
>   cytobrush s.
>   skin s.

scratch test

screen
>   Bac-T S.
>   strep s.
>   urine bacteria s.
>   urine bacterial s.

screening
>   s. culture
>   cytologic s.

screwworm, screw worm
>   s. fly

Scribner and Thomas shunt

ScrMV

scrofula

scrofulaceum
>   *Mycobacterium s.*

scrofuloderma

scrotal
>   s. abscess
>   s. T patch

scrub
>   Exidine S.
>   s. typhus

scruff

sculpturatus
>   *Centruroides s.*

scurf

NOTES

scutellaris
 Aedes s.
scutifer
 Cyclops s.
Scutigera
scutistriatum
 Simulium s.
scutular
scutulata
 porrigo s.
scutulum
scutum
SCV
 Sixgun City virus
Scytalidium (f)
 S. dimidiatum
 S. hyalinum
 S. infestans
 S. japonicum
 S. lignicola
SD
 seborrheic dermatitis
 WinRho SD
S/D
 Gammagard S/D
 Polygam S/D
SD1 virus
SDA
 strand displacement amplification
SDD
 selective decontamination of the digestive
 tract
 selective digestive decontamination
SDNV
 Serra do Navio virus
SDS-PAGE
 sodium dodecyl sulfate-polyacrylamide
 gel electrophoresis
sd virus
Se
 selenium
seabather's eruption
sea louse
sealpox virus
seal worm
seatworm
sebaceous
Sebaldella termitidis (b)
Sebcur
Sebcur/T
sebi (f)
 Wallemia s.
Sebizon Topical Lotion
seborrhea
seborrheic
 s. dermatitis (SD)
 s. keratosis
Sebulex

Sebulon
Secernentea
secnidazole
secondary
 s. bacterial infection
 s. glaucoma
 s. host
 s. prophylaxis
 s. screw worm
 s. syphilis
 s. T-cell response
 s. viremia
Secotiaceae
secretion
 cervicovaginal s.
 growth hormone s.
 respiratory s.
 syndrome of inappropriate
 antidiuretic hormone s. (SIADH)
 vaginal s.
secretory diarrhea
secretory-excretory antigen
section
 cesarean s. (C-section)
secular
SED
 semielemental diet
sedative-hypnotic drug
Sedatuss DM
sedentarius
 Kytococcus s.
 Micrococcus s.
sediment
 urine s.
sedimentation/centrifugation technique
sedimentation technique
sedis
 incertae s.
sedlakii
 Citrobacter s.
sedula
 Metallosphaera s.
seeberi
 Rhinosporidium s.
seed
 s. hematogenously
seeding of joint
seeligeri
 Listeria s.
segment
 posterior s.
segmental atelectasis
segmented
segmenter
Segmentina nitida
segmenting body
segnis
 Caulobacter s.

Haemophilus s.
Leptopsylla s.
Mycoplana s.
seiffertii
    Acholeplasma s.
    Mesoplasma s.
seizure
    s. disorder
    partial motor s.
    petit mal s.
sejunctus
    Aspergillus s.
selangorensis
    Paralactobacillus s.
Seldane
selection
    antibiotic s.
selective
    s. decontamination of the digestive
      tract (SDD)
    s. digestive decontamination (SDD)
    s. IgG subclass deficiency
    s. intestinal decontamination (SID)
    s. medium
    s. serotonin receptor blocker
selenatis
    Thauera s.
Selenihalanaerobacter (b)
    S. shriftii
selenitrireducens
    Bacillus s.
selenium (Se)
    s. sulfide
Selenomonas (b)
    S. acidaminovorans
    S. artemidis
    S. dianae
    S. flueggei
    S. infelix
    S. lacticifex
    S. lipolytica
    S. noxia
    S. ruminantium subsp. *lactilytica*
    S. ruminantium subsp. *ruminantium*
    S. sputigena
Seletar virus (SELV)
self-inoculation
self-limited
    s.-l. HBsAg-positive infection
    s.-l. hepatitis B surface antigen-
      positive infection
self-limiting

self-replicating
self-sustaining sequence replication
    (3SR)
Seliberia stellata (b)
Selsun
    S. Blue
    S. Blue Shampoo
    S. Gold for Women
SELV
    Seletar virus
semen
    s. viral load
semesiae
    Methanosarcina s.
Semichon acid carmine stain
semielemental diet (SED)
semilogarithmic
seminale
    Corynebacterium s.
seminis
    Actinobacillus s.
semipermeable
semiquantitative
    s. culture (SQC)
    s. culture technique
    s. occult blood
    s. PCR
semirecumbent
semisynthetic
semitectum
    Fusarium s.
Semliki Forest virus (SFV)
Semprex-D
Sena Madureira virus (SMV)
senarmontii
    Stibiobacter s.
Sendai virus
seneciella
    Pegohylemyia s.
Senecio longilobus
senegalense
    Halanaerobium saccharolyticum
      subsp. *s.*
    Mycobacterium s.
senegalensis
    Auchmeromyia s.
    Curvularia s.
    Haloincola saccharolyticus subsp. *s.*
    Leptosphaeria s.
    Oedaleus s.
senescent erythrocyte

S

NOTES

senezii
　　Desulfovibrio s.
SENIC
　　Study on Efficacy of Nosocomial
　　　Infection Control
senior
　　Phenadex S.
　　s. synonym
sennetsu
　　Ehrlichia s.
　　Rickettsia s.
Sennetsu fever
sensing
　　quorum s.
Sensititre
　　S. System
sensitive/less
　　s. sensitive enzyme immunoassay
　　s. sensitive enzyme immunoassay
　　　testing
sensitivity
　　antibiotic s.
　　respiratory isolation
　　　implementation s. (RIIS)
　　salt s.
sensitization
　　active s.
　　cross s.
sensitized
　　s. cell
　　s. culture
sensorineural
sensorium
sensory
　　s. neuropathy
　　s. polyneuropathy
sensu
　　s. lato
　　s. stricto
Sential
seoi
　　Gymnophalloides s.
Seoul
　　S. virus (SEOV)
　　S. virus infection
seoulensis
　　Fibricola s.
　　Streptomyces s.
SEOV
　　Seoul virus
sepedonicum
　　Corynebacterium s.
sepedonicus
　　Clavibacter michiganensis subsp. *s.*
Sepedonium (f)
Sepik virus (SEPV)
sepsis, pl. **sepses**
　　biliary s.

catheter-related s. (CRS)
central line s.
dog bite s.
fulminant s.
group B streptococcal s. (GBS)
Haemophilus influenzae s.
s. inflammatory syndrome
intraabdominal s.
intravascular catheter-acquired s.
intravenous line s.
line s.
neonatal s.
pancreatic s.
pneumococcal s.
s. pneumonia
postanginal s.
puerperal s.
salt water associated skin
　gangrene s.
splenectomy-related s.
Stomatococcus mucilaginosus s.
s. syndrome
Septata intestinalis (p)
septate mycelium
Septa Topical Ointment
septatum
　　Streptoverticillium s.
septatus
　　Streptomyces s.
septentrionale
　　Contracaecum s.
septic
　　s. arthritis
　　s. bursitis
　　s. cholangitis
　　s. dactylitis
　　s. embolization
　　s. meningitis
　　s. nonsuppurative thrombophlebitis
　　s. pelvic thrombophlebitis
　　s. phlebitis
　　s. scarlet fever
　　s. shock
　　s. shock-like syndrome
　　s. thrombosis
septica
　　Pasteurella multocida subsp. *s.*
septic arthritis
septicemia
　　bacterial s.
　　Candida s.
　　canine bite-associated s.
　　catheter-related s. (CRS)
　　chronic s.
　　community-acquired s.
　　Enterobacter cloacae s.
　　gonococcal s.
　　hemorrhagic s.

primary s.
Pseudomonas s.
Salmonella s.
s. treatment
septicemic
s. plague
Septi-Chek
S.-C. AFB system
S.-C. blood culture
S.-C. Blood Culture System
septicum
Clostridium s.
Mycobacterium s.
Septobasidiaceae
Septobasidiales
Septobasidium cokeri (f)
septoplasty
nasal s.
Septra
S. DS
septum
sepulcralis
Hypomyces s.
SEPV
Sepik virus
sequanensis
Candida s.
sequela, pl. **sequelae**
s. of influenza
Sequels
Diamox S.
sequence
HIV-1 genomic s.
insertion s.
viral nucleotide s.
sequence-independent single primer amplification (SISPA)
sequence-specific DNA primer (SSDP)
sequencing
s. analysis
HIV-1 gene s.
sequential antibiotic therapy
sequentially
Sequinavir
Sequivirus (v)
sequoiosis
sera (*pl. of* serum)
serebans
seregans
Hallella s.
serendipitously

serialis
Multiceps s.
Taenia s.
seriatum
Simulium s.
sericata
Phaenicia s.
series
Dismuke s.
serine
protein s.
seringue
seriolae
Nocardia s.
seriolicida
Enterococcus s.
SERO
serologic typing
seroconversion
seroconverter
serodeconvert
serodiagnosis
Serodia-Myco II test
seroepidemiological
serofast
serofibrinous pleurisy
serogroup
serogrouping
serologic
s. assay
s. enzyme immunoassay
s. syphilis
s. test
s. testing
s. test for syphilis (STS)
s. typing (SERO)
serological
serology
Bordetella pertussis s.
borreliosis s.
Chlamydia pneumoniae s.
Chlamydia psittaci s.
CMV s.
Coxsackie B virus s.
Coxsackie virus s.
cryptococcal antigen s.
Cryptococcus s.
CSF cryptococcal antigen s.
EBV virus s.
Ehrlichia s.
Entamoeba histolytica s.
fungal s.

S

NOTES

serology *(continued)*
    hantavirus s.
    HBV s.
    Helicobacter pylori s.
    hepatitis B s.
    hepatitis C s.
    hepatitis D s.
    hepatitis E s.
    herpes zoster s.
    histoplasmosis s.
    HIV-1 s.
    IgG s.
    infectious mononucleosis s.
    influenza A, B s.
    Legionella s.
    Leptospira s.
    Lyme arthritis s.
    Lyme disease s.
    mumps s.
    Mycoplasma s.
    parainfluenza virus s.
    parvovirus B19 s.
    pertussis s.
    poliovirus s.
    Q fever s.
    Rickettsia rickettsii s.
    Rocky Mountain spotted fever s.
    RSV s.
    rubella s.
    serum cryptococcal antigen s.
    sporotrichosis s.
    syphilis s.
    TORCH s.
    Toxoplasma s.
    Trichinella s.
    trichinosis s.
    tularemia s.
    varicella-zoster virus s.
    viral s.
Seromycin
    S. Pulvules
seronegative
seropedicae
    Herbaspirillum s.
seropositive
    gG-2 s.
seropositivity
    hepatitis B, C s.
    LANA s.
seroprevalence
seropurulent
    s. exudate
serosa
Sero STAT
serostatus
Serostim
    S. Injection
serotonin-reuptake inhibitor

serotype
    s. typhi
serotyping
serous
    s. tuberculosis
serovar (sv.)
serovar-specific epitope
serpens
    Aquaspirillum s.
Serpens flexibilis (b)
serpent ulcer of cornea
serpiginous
    s. keratitis
serpigo
Serpulina (b)
    S. alvinipulli
    S. hyodysenteriae
    S. innocens
    S. intermedia
    S. murdochii
    S. pilosicoli
Serra do Navio virus (SDNV)
serrata
    Linguatula s.
Serratia (b)
    S. entomophila
    S. ficaria
    S. fonticola
    S. grimesii
    S. liquefaciens
    S. marcescens
    S. marinorubra
    S. odorifera
    S. plymuthica
    S. proteamaculans subsp.
      proteamaculans
    S. proteamaculans subsp. *quinovora*
    S. rubidaea
Serratieae
serratus
    Aedes s.
sertraline
serum, pl. **sera**
    s. agar
    s. agglutinin
    s. alanine aminotransferase
    s. albumin
    s. alkaline phosphatase
    s. alpha-fetoprotein (AFP)
    s. ALT
    s. antibacterial activity
    s. antideoxyribonuclease-B titer
    s. antimicrobial activity test
    s. antinuclear antibody
    antirabies s. (ARS)
    s. aspartate aminotransferase
    s. aspartate transaminase
    s. bacterial inhibitory level

s. bactericidal dilution method
s. bactericidal test
s. beta-carotene level
s. chemistry
s. creatinine
s. creatinine concentration
s. cryptococcal antigen
s. cryptococcal antigen serology
s. electrolyte
s. endostatin level
equine antirabies s.
s. erythropoietin level
s. FTA-ABS
s. globulin
s. glutamate oxaloacetate
  transaminase
s. hepatitis
s. hormone binding globulin
  (SHBG)
human measles immune s.
human scarlet fever immune s.
s. IFA test
immune s.
s. immunoglobulin
s. inhibitory activity
s. inhibitory titer
s. lethal activity
neonatal s.
s. neopterin concentration
s. opacity factor
s. osmolality
s. p24 HIV-1 antigen assay
s. prolactin concentration
s. resistance factor
s. retinol level
s. sickness
s. T
s. T concentration
s. testosterone
s. testosterone level
s. TIBC
s. total bilirubin level
s. total testosterone
s. *Toxoplasma gondii* antibody titer
s. triglyceride
serum-casein-glucose-yeast extract
  medium (SCGYEM)
serum-neutralizing antibody
service
United States Public Health S.
  (USPHS)
sessile

setae
Kitasatospora s.
Streptomyces s.
Setaria (p)
S. cervi
S. equina
setonii
Streptomyces s.
Setora nitens virus
Setosphaeria (f)
S. holmii
S. monoceras
S. pedicellata
S. turcica
setosus
Linognathus s.
Seuratiaceae
seven-day fever
seventh nerve palsy
scviche
sexalatus
Physocephalus s.
sex factor
sexual
s. assault treatment
s. debut
s. generation
s. onset
sexually
s. transmitted disease (STD)
s. transmitted infection (STI)
seymouri
Leptomonas s.
Sézary syndrome
S-fluorocytosine
SFNV
sandfly fever Naples virus
SFSV
sandfly fever Sicilian virus
SFV
Semliki Forest virus
SF virus
SGAV
Salanga virus
SgCV
saguaro cactus virus
SGV virus
SHAART
salvage highly active antiretroviral
  therapy
shake culture

S

NOTES

shakespearei
     Legionella s.
Shaklee Dandruff Control
Shamonda virus (SHAV)
shampoo
     A-200 S.
     Anti-Dandruff S.
     Avant Garde S.
     Dandruff Treatment S.
     Exsel S.
     gamma benzene hexachloride s.
     Keep Clear Anti-Dandruff S.
     Lice-Enz S.
     Nizoral A-D S.
     Pronto S.
     P&S S.
     Pyrinex Pediculicide S.
     Pyrinyl Plus S.
     R & C S.
     RID S.
     Selsun Blue S.
     Tisit S.
     Zincon S.
Shampooing Anti-Pelliculaire
Shanghai rheumatism
shank fever
shannoni
     Anopheles s.
shape
     Y s.
shaposhnikovii
     Ectothiorhodospira s.
Shark River virus (SRV)
sharpeae
     Lactobacillus s.
SHAS
     Supplement to HIV/AIDS Surveillance
SHAV
     Shamonda virus
shave biopsy
SHBG
     serum hormone binding globulin
SHEA
     Society for Healthcare Epidemiology of
       America
shearii
     Pseudallescheria s.
sheath
     microfilarial s.
Sheather sucrose-flotation technique
shedding
     herpes simplex viral s.
     HIV s.
     viral s.
sheep
     s. bot
     circling disease of s.

     s. pox virus subgroup
     s. rotavirus
sheeppox virus
shehatae
     Candida s.
     Candida s. var. *shehatae*
shellfish poisoning
shepherd crook configuration
shermanii
     Propionibacterium freudenreichii
       subsp. *s.*
Shewanella (b)
     S. algae
     S. amazonensis
     S. baltica
     S. benthica
     S. colwelliana
     S. frigidimarina
     S. gelidimarina
     S. hanedai
     S. japonica
     S. oneidensis
     S. pealeana
     S. putrefaciens
     S. violacea
     S. woodyi
shibatae
     Sulfolobus s.
shift
     antigenic s.
Shiga
     S. bacillus (*See Shigella*
       dysenteriae)
     S. toxin
     S. toxin-producing *Escherichia coli*
       (STEC)
Shiga-Kruse bacillus (*See* **Shigella**
dysenteriae)
Shiga-like toxin
Shigella (b)
     S. boydii
     S. diarrhea
     S. dysenteriae
     S. dysenteriae serotype 1
     S. flexneri
     S. infection
     S. sonnei
shigellae
shigelloides
     Plesiomonas s.
shiloi
     Streptococcus s.
     Vibrio s.
shimamushi disease
shimoidei
     Mycobacterium s.
shin
     saber s.

shinbone fever
shingles
    s. culture
shinshuensis
    Leifsonia s.
shiotae
    Isaria s.
    Tritirachium s.
ship fever
shipping fever
shock
    endotoxic s.
    hypovolemic s.
    septic s.
Shokwe virus (SHOV)
short
    s. chain
    s. incubation hepatitis
short-acting benzodiazepine
shoulder
    s. arthrogram
    Head & S.'s
SHOV
    Shokwe virus
showae
    Campylobacter s.
showdoensis
    Streptomyces s.
showy flamecap mushroom
shriftii
    Selenihalanaerobacter s.
Shuni virus (SHUV)
shunt
    cerebrospinal fluid s.
    complex ventricular s.
    s. culture
    lumboperitoneal s.
    Quinton-Scribner external
      arteriovenous s.
    Scribner and Thomas s.
    ventricular s.
    ventriculoatrial s.
    ventriculoperitoneal s.
SHUV
    Shuni virus
SIADH
    syndrome of inappropriate antidiuretic
      hormone secretion
    syndrome of inappropriate secretion of
      antidiuretic hormone
sialadenitis
sialic acid-containing oligosaccharide

sialidase
    s. production test
sialoprotein
    bone s.
sialyl-Tn (STn)
siamensis
    Asaia s.
Sia water test
sibericum
    Thialkalimicrobium s.
sibirica
    Kurthia s.
    Rickettsia s.
    Thiorhodospira s.
sibiricus
    Sandaracinobacter s.
sibonii
    Morganella morganii subsp. *s.*
sicca
    cholera s.
    Neisseria s.
    s. syndrome
siccus
siciliae
    Methanolobus s.
    Methanosarcina s.
sickener mushroom
sickle
    s. cell anemia
    s. cell disease
    s. form
sickness
    acute African sleeping s.
    African sleeping s.
    black s.
    chronic African sleeping s.
    East African sleeping s.
    Gambian sleeping s.
    motion s.
    Rhodesian sleeping s.
    serum s.
    sleeping s.
    spotted s.
    West African sleeping s.
SICU
    spinal intensive care unit
sicuani
    Simulium s.
siculi
    Thermococcus s.
SID
    selective intestinal decontamination

S

NOTES

siderocapsulatus
  Arthrobacter s.
siderophilic
siderophilus
  Thermoanaerobacter s.
siderophore
sierrensis
  Aedes s.
  Culicoides s.
sight
  gunbarrel s.
sight-threatening
Sigma virus
sigmoid colon
sigmoidoscopy
sign
  Brudzinski s.
  chandelier s.
  Faget s.
  Hutchinson s.
  Kerandel s.
  Kernig s.
  Nikolsky s.
  Pastia s.
  Romaña s.
  Romberg s.
  steeple s.
  water lily s.
  Winterbottom s.
signal
  s. lesion
  polyadenylation s.
  time to s.
signet ring
significance
  atypical squamous cells of
    uncertain s. (ASCUS)
  atypical squamous cells of
    undetermined s. (ASCUS)
  monoclonal gammopathy of
    undetermined s. (MUGS)
SIL
  squamous intraepithelial lesion
silaceus
  Chrysops s.
Silafed syrup
Silaminic Expectorant
Silapap
silastic catheter
Sildicon-E
Silfedrine
  Children's S.
Silicibacter (b)
  S. lacuscaerulensis
silicon
silicone-elastomer catheter
silicone oil injection
silicosis

Silphen DM
Siltussin
  S. DM
Siltussin-CF
SILV
  Silverwater virus
silvacetica
  Sporomusa s.
Silvadene
silvae
  Candida s.
silvanorum
  Candida s.
silvanus
  Meiothermus s.
  Thermus s.
silvatica
  Candida s.
silvaticum
  Mycobacterium avium subsp. s.
silver (Ag)
  Gomori methenamine s. (GMS)
  s. ions
  s. nitrate ($AgNO_3$)
  s. oxide/trichloroisocyanuric acid
  s. protein, mild
  s. stain
  s. sulfadiazine
  s. sulfadiazine cream
Silverwater virus (SILV)
silvestris
  Bacillus s.
silvicola
  Candida s.
silvicultrix
  Candida s.
sim 1–27
  simian adenovirus 1–27
simbae
  Mycoplasma s.
Simbu virus (SIMV)
simiae
  Fusobacterium s.
  Hepatocystis s.
  Herpesvirus s.
  Mycobacterium s.
simian
  s. adenovirus 1–27 (sim 1–27)
  s. enterovirus 1–18
  s. foamy virus
  s. hemorrhagic fever virus
  s. hepatitis A virus
  s. immunodeficiency virus (SIV)
  s. malaria
  s. sarcoma virus
  s. T-lymphotropic virus (STLV)
simicola
  Pneumonyssus s.

simii
>Arthroderma s.
>Pinoyella s.
>Trichophyton s.

similis
>Culex s.
>Vorticella s.

Simkania negevensis (b)
Simmons citrate medium
simondi
>Leucocytozoon s.

Simon focus
Simonsiella (b)
>S. crassa
>S. muelleri
>S. steedae

Simonsiellaceae
simple
>s. cystometrogram
>s. fission
>s. pulmonary eosinophilia

simplex
>Anisakis s.
>Arthrobacter s.
>Bacillus s.
>Desulfovibrio s.
>genital herpes s.
>herpes s. (HS)
>intraoral herpes s.
>mucocutaneous herpes s.
>Nocardioides s.
>Pimelobacter s.
>Psorergates s.

Simplexvirus (v)
simplicicolor
>Simulium s.

simplicissima
>Spicaria s.

Simplified Acute Physiology Score
simulans
>Corynebacterium s.
>Pulex s.
>Staphylococcus s.

Simuliidae
Simulium
>S. acarayense
>S. aestivum
>S. albicinctum
>S. albilineatum
>S. albopictum
>S. alirioi
>S. amazonicum

S. anamariae
S. anatinum
S. angrense
S. antillarum
S. antonii
S. antunesi
S. aranti
S. arcticum
S. argentatum
S. argus
S. aureum
S. auripellitum
S. auristriatum
S. baffinense
S. baiense
S. barbatipes
S. beaupertuyi
S. bicoloratum
S. bicorne
S. bivittatum
S. blancasi
S. bordui
S. botulibranchium
S. brachycladum
S. bracteatum
S. brevifurcatum
S. caledonense
S. canadense
S. canonicola
S. catarinense
S. cauchense
S. cerqueira
S. chalcocoma
S. clarkei
S. clavibranchium
S. congreenarum
S. conviti
S. corbis
S. cormonsi
S. costaricense
S. cotopaxi
S. craigi
S. croxtoni
S. cuneatum
S. decollectum
S. decorum
S. defoliarti
S. dinellii
S. diversibranchium
S. diversifurcatum
S. dixiense
S. downsi

S

NOTES

Simulium (continued)
- S. duplex
- S. dureti
- S. ecuadoriense
- S. emarginatum
- S. encisoi
- S. escomeli
- S. ethelae
- S. euryadminiculum
- S. excisum
- S. exiguum
- S. fibrinflatum
- S. flavifemur
- S. flavipictum
- S. flavopubescens
- S. fulvibnotum
- S. furculatum
- S. gabaldoni
- S. gaudeatum
- S. gaurani
- S. giganteum
- S. goeidi
- S. gouldingi
- S. grerreroi
- S. griseum
- S. guianense
- S. guttatum
- S. haematopotum
- S. haysi
- S. herreri
- S. hirtipupa
- S. hoffmanni
- S. hunteri
- S. ignacioi
- S. ignescens
- S. impar
- S. inaequale
- S. incertum
- S. incrustatum
- S. inexorabile
- S. innocens
- S. iracouboense
- S. itaunense
- S. jacumbae
- S. jaimeramirezi
- S. jenningsi
- S. johannseni
- S. jonesi
- S. jujuyense
- S. jundiaiense
- S. kabanayense
- S. lahillei
- S. lakei
- S. laneportoi
- S. lassmanni
- S. laticalx
- S. latidigitus
- S. latipes
- S. lewisi

- S. limbatum
- S. longistylatum
- S. luggeri
- S. lurybayae
- S. lutzianum
- S. machadoallisoni
- S. major
- S. malyschevi
- S. manicatum
- S. maroniense
- S. matteabranchia
- S. mbarigui
- S. mediovittatum
- S. meridionale
- S. meruoca
- S. metallicum
- S. mexicanum
- S. minus
- S. minusculum
- S. morae
- S. mutucuna
- S. nebulosum
- S. nigricoxum
- S. nogueirai
- S. notatum
- S. notiale
- S. nunestovari
- S. nyssa
- S. obesum
- S. ochraceum
- S. opalinifrons
- S. orbitale
- S. ortizi
- S. oveidoi
- S. oviedoi
- S. oyapockense
- S. paraguayense
- S. paranense
- S. parnassum
- S. paynei
- S. penobscotensis
- S. perflavum
- S. pertinax
- S. petersoni
- S. pictipes
- S. pifanoi
- S. pilosum
- S. pintoi
- S. piperi
- S. podosterni
- S. prodexargenteum
- S. pruinosum
- S. pseudoexiguum
- S. pugetense
- S. pulverulentum
- S. quadrifidum
- S. quadristrigatum
- S. quadrivittatum

S. quebecense
S. racenisi
S. rangeli
S. rivasi
S. rivuli
S. rorotaense
S. rubiginosum
S. rubrithorax
S. rubtzovi
S. rugglesi
S. samboni
S. sanguineum
S. schmidtmummi
S. scutistriatum
S. seriatum
S. sicuani
S. simplicicolor
S. slossonae
S. snowi
S. solarii
S. spadicidorsum
S. spinibranchium
S. spinifer
S. strigatum
S. strigidorsum
S. striginotum
S. suarezi
S. subclavibranchium
S. subnigrum
S. subpallidum
S. tallaferroae
S. tarsale
S. tarsatum
S. taxodium
S. tescorum
S. townsendi
S. transiens
S. travassosi
S. trivittatum
S. truncata
S. tuberosum
S. underhilli
S. urubambanum
S. varians
S. venator
S. venustum
S. verecundum
S. vernum
S. versicolor
S. violacescens
S. virgatum
S. virus

S. vittatum
S. wuayaraka
S. wyomingense
S. yacuchuspi
SIMV
    Simbu virus
simvastatin
Sinarest 12 Hour Nasal solution
Sindbis
    S. fever
    S. virus (SINV)
    S. virus subtype Babanki
    S. virus subtype Kyzylagach
    S. virus subtype Ockelbo
    S. virus subtype Whataroa
sindenensis
    Streptomyces s.
Sine-Aid IB
sinense
    Methanocorpusculum s.
sinensis
    Bullera s.
    Clonorchis s.
sinensium
    Schistosoma s.
Sinex
    S. Long-Acting
    Vicks S.
singaporensis
    Actinopolymorpha s.
    Desulforhopalus s.
single
    s. nucleocapsid virus
    s. nucleopolyhedrovirus (SNPV)
    s. vial fixative
single-agent chemotherapy
single-host
    s.-h. pathogen
    s.-h. virus
single-lumen catheter
single-photon
    s.-p. emission computed
    tomography (SPECT)
    s.-p. emission tomography (SPECT)
single-shelled particle
single-strand conformation polymorphism (SSCP)
singulare
    Corynebacterium s.
Sin Nombre virus
sinoatrial node
sinonasal

S

NOTES

sinopulmonary mucosa
Sinorhizobium (b)
    S. arboris
    S. fredii
    S. kostiense
    S. medicae
    S. meliloti
    S. saheli
    S. terangae
    S. xinjiangense
sinuatum
    Entoloma s.
Sinubid
Sinufed Timecelles
Sinumist-SR Capsulets
sinuosum
    Aquaspirillum s.
    Lyticum s.
Sinupan
sinus
    s. empyema
    s. histiocytosis
    Motrin IB S.
    paranasal s.
    Plus S.
    subcutaneous s.
    s. tachycardia
    s. tract
sinusarabici
    Flexistipes s.
sinusitis
    acute s.
    Chlamydia pneumoniae s.
    chronic paranasal s.
    community-acquired s.
    maxillary s.
sinusoid
Sinutab SA
SINV
    Sindbis virus
sioyaensis
    Streptomyces s.
Siphona irritans (p)
Siphonaptera
Siphoviridae
siraeum
    Eubacterium s.
siralis
    Bacillus s.
siro
    Tyrophagus s.
Sirolpidiaceae
Sirop
    S. DM
    S. Expectorant
SIRS
    systemic inflammatory response
    syndrome

sisomicin
    1-*N*-ethyl s.
Sisomycin
SISPA
    sequence-independent single primer
    amplification
sitafloxacin
site
    sanctuary s.
site-specific
sitiens
    Culicoides s.
sitophila
    Chrysonilia s.
    Neurospora s.
situ
    in s.
sitz bath
SIV
    simian immunodeficiency virus
    vif-deleted SIV
sivashensis
    Orenia s.
Sixgun City virus (SCV)
SJAV
    Sandjimba virus
sjoestedi
    Hirudo s.
Sjögren syndrome
SJV
    San Juan virus
SK1 virus
skeletal
    s. muscle biopsy
    s. tuberculosis
skeleton
Skene
    S. duct
    S. gland
Skermanella parooensis (b)
Skermania piniformis (b)
skin
    s. antisepsis
    s. botfly
    s. culture for HSV
    s. degerming
    s. infection
    leopard s.
    lizard s.
    Oxy-5 Advanced Formula for
    Sensitive S.
    Oxy-10 Advanced Formula for
    Sensitive S.
    s. scraping
    s. snip
    s. test
    s. test antigen
    s. testing

s. test for penicillin allergy
s. test reactivity
s. viral culture
viral entry barrier s.
skinneri
    Cryptococcus s.
skip metastasis
skirrowii
    Arcobacter s.
skrjabini
    Paragonimus s.
    Thelazia s.
skull
    Madura s.
    s. tuberculosis
skunkpox virus
S/L
    A-Spas S/L
Slackia (b)
    S. exigua
    S. heliotrinreducens
slackii
    Actinomyces s.
slant culture
slapped cheek
slapped-cheek disease
slapping gait
SLE
    St. Louis encephalitis
    systemic lupus erythematosus
sleeping sickness
sleeved phlebotomy needle
SLEV
    St. Louis encephalitis virus
slide
    s. coagulase test
    Kodachrome s.
Slidex
    S. Staph
    S. Staph test
    S. Strep
slim disease
slip
    pH s.
slithyformis
    Runella s.
slit lamp
Slo-bid
slope culture
Slo-Phyllin
    S.-P. GG

slossonae
    Simulium s.
slot-blot assay
sloughing
slovaca
    Rickettsia s.
slow
    s. fever
    s. urease
    s. virus disease
SLR factor
S/LS
    S. EIA
    S. EIA testing
sludge
    activated s.
slug
    veronicellid s.
slurry
SM-1 virus
small
    s. DNA tumor virus
    s. noncleaved cell
    s. noncleaved cell lymphoma
    (SNC)
    s. round structured virus (SRSV)
    s. round virus (SRV)
smallpox
    hemorrhagic s.
    s. vaccine
smaragdinae
    Spirochaeta s.
SMB virus
smear
    acid-fast s.
    bacterial s.
    cervical *Trichomonas* s.
    cervicovaginal s.
    Chlamydia s.
    conjunctival s.
    corneal s.
    s. culture
    eye s.
    fecal s.
    fungus s.
    Giemsa-stained s.
    Legionella pneumophila s.
    malaria s.
    Papanicolaou s.
    peripheral s.
    suspension s.
    s. technique

S

NOTES

smear *(continued)*
>thick peripheral blood s.
>thin peripheral blood s.
>*Trichomonas* Pap s.
>Tzanck s.
>urethral *Trichomonas* s.
>vaginal s.
>vaginal *Trichomonas* s.

smegmatis
>*Mycobacterium* s.

Smithella propionica (b)
smithi
>*Leucocytozoon* s.

smithia
>*Aeromonas salmonicida* subsp. *s.*

smithii
>*Bacillus* s.
>*Methanobrevibacter* s.
>*Wyeomyia* s.

smoldering infection
smooth
>s. colony
>s. leprosy
>s. muscle antibody

smoothcap mushroom
SMP2 virus
smudge cell
smut
>corn s.

SMV
>Sena Madureira virus

SMX
>sulfamethoxazole

SMX-TMP
>sulfamethoxazole and trimethoprim

snail
>s. fever

snakehead rhabdovirus
SNAP
>Score for Neonatal Acute Physiology

Snaplets-EX
Snaplets-FR Granules
snare
>diathermy s.
>polypectomy s.

SNC
>small noncleaved cell lymphoma

SNC lymphoma
SNDV-like viruses (v)
snip
>skin s.

Sno-Strip
Snow
>S. Mountain agent
>S. Mountain virus

snowi
>*Culicoides* s.
>*Simulium* s.

snowshoe hare virus (SSHV)
SNPV
>single nucleopolyhedrovirus
>>*Trichoplusia ni* SNPV (TnSNPV)

soap
>s. bubble appearance
>Mazon Medicated S.

Sobemovirus (v)
sobria
>*Aeromonas* s.

sobrinus
>*Streptococcus* s.

sociabilis
>*Methanothermus* s.

Society
>Canadian Infectious Disease S.
>S. for Healthcare Epidemiology of America (SHEA)
>S. for Hospital Epidemiology of America

socranskii
>*Treponema socranskii* subsp. *s.*

Sodalis glossinidius (b)
sodium
>aminosalicylate s.
>ampicillin s.
>Ampicin S.
>s. bicarbonate
>s. bisulfite
>carbenicillin indanyl s.
>carboxymethylcellulose s.
>cefazolin s.
>cefmetazole s.
>cefonicid s.
>cefoperazone s.
>cefotaxime s.
>cefoxitin s.
>ceftizoxime s.
>ceftriaxone s.
>cefuroxime s.
>cephalothin s.
>cephapirin s.
>s. chloride tolerance test
>cloxacillin s.
>dantrolene s.
>DHPG s.
>s. dichloroisocyanurate
>diclazuril s.
>dicloxacillin s.
>s. dodecyl sulfate
>s. dodecyl sulfate-polyacrylamide gel electrophoresis (SDS-PAGE)
>GCV s.
>s. hippurate hydrolysis
>s. hydroxide

s. hydroxide digestion method
s. hypochlorite
s. hypochlorite solution
indanyl s.
s. iodate
methicillin s.
nafcillin s.
oxacillin s.
s. P.A.S.
piperacillin and tazobactam s.
s. polyanetholesulfonate (SPS)
s. polyanethol sulfonate
s. salicylate
stibogluconate s.
s. stibogluconate
S. Sulamyd
S. Sulamyd Ophthalmic
sulfacetamide s.
s. sulfacetamide
s. tetradecyl sulfate
s. thiosulfate
sodoku
sodomense
    Halobacterium s.
    Halorubrobacterium s.
    Halorubrum s.
    Rhodospirillum s.
sodomensis
    Rhodovibrio s.
soehngenii
    Methanothrix s.
soft
    s. chancre
    s. palate
    s. tick
    s. tissue infection
    s. tissue limb sarcoma
    s. tissue scan
soil
    s. ameba
    night s.
soil-borne spore
soiling
    polymicrobial s.
sokosho
Sokuluk virus (SOKV)
SOKV
    Sokuluk virus
solanacearum
    Burkholderia s.
    Pseudomonas s.
    Ralstonia s.

solani
    Candida s.
solar fever
solarii
    Simulium s.
Soldado virus (SOLV)
sole
solenamine
Solenopotes capillatus (p)
Solenopsis
    S. geminata
    S. invicta
    S. richteri
solfataricus
    Sulfolobus s.
Solganal
solitarius
    Enterococcus s.
solium
    Taenia s.
    taeniasis s.
sollicitans
    Aedes s.
Solobacterium moorei (b)
Solu-Cortef
Solugel
Solu-Medrol Injection
Solurex L.A.
Soluspan
    Celestone S.
solution
    Afrin Nasal s.
    AK-Spore Ophthalmic S.
    Allerest 12 Hour Nasal s.
    aqueous s.
    calcofluor white s.
    chlorhexidine diacetate aqueous s.
    chlorocresol aqueous s.
    Chlorphed-LA Nasal s.
    Clinda-Derm Topical s.
    C/T/S Topical s.
    Dey-Drop Ophthalmic s.
    dithiothreitol s.
    Dobell and O'Connor s.
    Dristan Long Lasting Nasal s.
    DuoFilm s.
    Duration Nasal s.
    enteral nutrition s. (ENS)
    Freezone s.
    Fungoid AF Topical s.
    isotonic s.
    KOH s.

S

NOTES

solution *(continued)*
    Lock s.
    Lotrimin AF s.
    Lugol s.
    Neosporin Ophthalmic s.
    Neo-Synephrine 12 Hour Nasal s.
    NTZ Long Acting Nasal s.
    nystatin s.
    Ocutricin Ophthalmic s.
    oral rehydration s. (ORS)
    piperazine s.
    potassium dichromate s.
    povidone-iodine aqueous s.
    Schaudinn fixative s.
    Sclavo-PPD s.
    Sinarest 12 Hour Nasal s.
    sodium hypochlorite s.
    SPG buffer s.
    starch-based electrolyte s.
    strong iodine s.
    sucrose-phosphate-glutamic acid
     buffer s.
    TOBI Inhalation s.
    tosylchloramide aqueous s.
    trifluridine s.
    Twice-A-Day Nasal s.
    Verukan s.
    virucidal s.
    4-Way Long Acting Nasal s.
Soluver
    S. Plus
SOLV
    Soldado virus
solventivorans
    Paracoccus s.
solvifaciens
    Streptomyces griseus subsp. *s.*
somaliensis
    Streptomyces s.
somatic
    s. agglutinin
    s. cell
    s. nucleus
    s. O antigen
    s. teniasis
somatosensory evoked potential (SSEP)
somatostatin
somatrem
somatropin
somfuk
sommermanae
    Culicoides s.
somnilux
    Entomoplasma s.
    Mycoplasma s.
somnolence
somnolent
Somophyllin

sonicated larva
sonicating
sonication
    vortex ± s.
sonnei
    Shigella s.
sonography
sonorensis
    Candida s.
Sopamycetin
sophiae-reginae
    Candida s.-r.
Sorangium schroeteri
sorbitol fermentation test
sorbophila
    Candida s.
sorbosa
    Candida s.
sorbose fermentation test
sorboxylosa
    Candida s.
Sordaria (f)
    S. fimicola
    S. macrospora
Sordariaceae
Sordariales
sordellii
    Clostridium s.
sordidellus
    Culicoides s.
sore
    cold s.
    fever s.
    oriental s.
    tropical s.
    water s.
sorediatum
    Polyangium s.
sorghina
    Phoma s.
sorivudine
sorokiniana
    Drechslera s.
Sororoca virus (SORV)
sorrel webcap mushroom
SORV
    Sororoca virus
soudanense
    Trichophyton s.
sounds
    absent bowel s.
    hypoactive bowel s.
source of carbon
sourekii
    Facklamia s.
South
    S. African tick-bite fever
    S. American blastomycosis

S. American trypanosomiasis
S. River virus
Southampton virus
Southern
S. blot
S. blot analysis
S. blot hybridization
sowda
soybean
s. oil
SP
Cordran S.
S. virus
SP10 virus
SP15 virus
SP3 virus
SP50 virus
SP8 virus
space
basal subarachnoid s.
lateral pharyngeal s. (LPS)
Virchow-Robin s.
space-occupying lesion
spadicidorsum
Simulium s.
spadix
Actinomadura s.
spandovensis
Candida s.
Spanish
S. fly
S. influenza
SPAr-2317 virus
sparfloxacin
sparganoma
sparganosis
ocular s.
sparganum
sparrowpox virus
sparsogenes
Streptomyces s.
sparsum
Streptoverticillium cinnamoneum
subsp. *s.*
sparsus
Streptomyces cinnamoneus subsp. *s.*
spasm
epidemic transient diaphragmatic s.
Spasmolin
spasticity
spathiger
Nematodirus s.

Spathulosporaceae
Spathulosporales
spear
Weck-cel ophthalmic surgical s.
specialist
disease intervention s. (DIS)
speciation
species
specific
s. active immunity
s. epithet
s. hemolysin
s. immune globulin (human)
s. immunotherapy
s. parasite
s. passive immunity
s. pathogen
s. urethritis
specificity
T-ccll s.
specimen
clean-catch urine s.
endocervical s.
first-catch urine s.
formalin-fixed stool s.
midvoid urine s.
needle biopsy s.
open-wedge biopsy s.
tampon s.
SPECT
single-photon emission computed
tomography
single-photon emission tomography
Spec-T
spectabilis
Gymnopilus s.
Streptomyces s.
Spectam
Spectazole
S. Topical
spectinomycin
spectra (*pl. of* spectrum)
Spectro
S. Gram
S. Tar
Spectrobid
S. tablet
spectrometry
gas chromatography/mass s.
(GC/MS)
gas isotope ratio mass s. (GIRMS)
mass s.

NOTES

S

spectroscopy
fluorescence s.
proton magnetic resonance s.
spectrum, pl. **spectra, spectrums**
speculum, pl. **specula**
Spegazzinia (f)
spegazzinii
Haemagogus s.
speleomycini
Streptomyces s.
Spelotrema nicolli (p)
spencerii
Aedes s.
spermatophilum
Mycoplasma s.
spermatozoa
spermine
Spermophilus
Spermospora columbianus (f)
Spersanicol
SPG
sucrose-phosphate-glutamic acid
SPG buffer solution
Sphaera (f)
Sphaerella (f)
Sphaeria (f)
sphaerica
Nigrospora s.
Planomonospora s.
sphaericus
Bacillus s.
Gluconobacter oxydans subsp. s.
Sphaerioidaceae
Sphaerobacter thermophilus (b)
Sphaerobolaceae
sphaeroides
Rhodobacter s.
Rhodopseudomonas s.
Sporomusa s.
Sphaeropsis subglobosa (f)
sphaerospermum
Cladosporium s.
Sphaerotilus natans (b)
sphagni
Mycobacterium s.
sphagnumensis
Culicoides s.
sphenoides
Amoebotaenia s.
Clostridium s.
spherical
spherocytosis
hereditary s.
spheroid colony
spheroides
Streptomyces s.
Spheroides maculatus
spheroplast

spherospermia
spherule
coccidioidal s.
Spherulin
sphincter
sphincterotomy
endoscopic s.
Sphingobacterium (b)
S. antarcticum
S. faecium
S. heparinum
S. mizutae
S. multivorum
S. piscium
S. spiritivorum
S. thalpophilum
Sphingobium (b)
S. chlorophenolicum
S. herbicidovorans
S. yanoikuyae
Sphingomonas (b)
S. adhaesiva
S. alaskensis
S. aquatilis
S. aromaticivorans
S. asaccharolytica
S. capsulata
S. chlorophenolica
S. chungbukensis
S. cloacae
S. echinoides
S. herbicidovorans
S. koreensis
S. macrogoltabidus
S. mali
S. natatoria
S. parapaucimobilis
S. paucimobilis
S. pituitosa
S. pruni
S. rosa
S. roseiflava
S. sanguinis
S. stygia
S. subarctica
S. suberifaciens
S. subterranea
S. taejonensis
S. terrae
S. trueperi
S. ursincola
S. wittichii
S. xenophaga
S. yanoikuyae
Sphingopyxis (b)
S. macrogoltabida
S. terrae
Spicaria simplicissima (f)

spicifer
spicifera
    Bipolaris s.
spiciferus
    Cochliobolus s.
spicule
    bone s.
spider
    s. angioma
    black widow s.
    brown recluse s.
    fiddleback s.
    hobo s.
    s. nevus
    vascular s.
    violin s.
spike
    fever s.
spiked condyloma
Spilopsyllus cuniculi (p)
spinal
    s. compressive lesion
    s. epidural abscess
    s. fluid analysis
    s. fluid VDRL
    s. intensive care unit (SICU)
    s. intramedullary cysticercosis
    s. tap
spin amplification
spindale
    Schistosoma s.
spindle cell
spine
    posterior superior iliac s. (PSIS)
spinibranchium
    Simulium s.
spinifer
    Simulium s.
spinifera
    Exophiala s.
spiniger
    Heterodoxus s.
spinigera
    Haemaphysalis s.
spinigerum
    Gnathostoma s.
spinipalpis
    Ixodes s.
spinosa
    Absidia s.
    Pseudomonas s.

    Pseudonocardia s.
    Saccharopolyspora s.
spinosporotrichia
    Saccharopolyspora s.
spinosum
    Acremonium s.
    Verrucomicrobium s.
spinosus
    Aspergillus s.
    Culicoides s.
spinoverrucosus
    Streptomyces s.
spiracle
spiracularis
    Megaselia s.
spiral
    Curschmann s.
    s. gradient endpoint method
    s. hypha
spirale
    Elytrosporangium s.
spiralis
    Actinomadura s.
    Microtetraspora s.
    Nonomuraea s.
    Streptomyces s.
    Trichinella s.
spiramycin
spirilla
spirillar
Spirilliplanes yamanashiensis (b)
Spirillospora (b)
    S. albida
    S. rubra
spirillum
    s. fever
    Obermeier s.
    Vincent s.
Spirillum volutans (b)
spiritensis
    Aquabacter s.
    Legionella s.
spiritivorum
    Flavobacterium s.
    Sphingobacterium s.
Spirocerca lupi (p)
Spirocercidae
Spirocerdinae
Spirochaeta (b)
    S. africana
    S. alkalica
    S. asiatica

S

NOTES

Spirochaeta (continued)
S. *aurantia* subsp. *aurantia*
S. *aurantia* subsp. *stricta*
S. *caldaria*
S. *halophila*
S. *isovalerica*
S. *litoralis*
S. *plicatilis*
S. *smaragdinae*
S. *stenostrepta*
S. *thermophila*
S. *zuelzerae*
Spirochaetaceae
Spirochaetales
spirochetal
s. infection
s. meningitis
spirochetal bacterium
spirochetal infection
spirochete
s. infection
spirochetemia
spirochetosis
intestinal s.
spirochetotic
spiroforme
Clostridium s.
Spirometra (p)
S. *erinaceieuropaei*
S. *mansoni*
S. *mansonoides*
spirometry
Spiromicrovirus (v)
Spiroplasma (b)
S. *alleghenense*
S. *apis*
S. *cantharicola*
S. *chinense*
S. *chrysopicola*
S. *citri*
S. *clarkii*
S. *corruscae*
S. *culicicola*
S. *diabroticae*
S. *diminutum*
S. *floricola*
S. *gladiatoris*
S. *helicoides*
S. *insolitum*
S. *ixodetis*
S. *kunkelii*
S. *lampyridicola*
S. *leptinotarsae*
S. *lineolae*
S. *litorale*
S. *melliferum*
S. *mirum*
S. *monobiae*

S. *montanense*
S. *phoeniceum*
S. *platyhelix*
S. *poulsonii*
S. *sabaudiense*
S. *syrphidicola*
S. *tabanidicola*
S. *taiwanense*
S. *turonicum*
S. *velocicrescens*
Spiroplasmataceae
Spirosomaceae
Spirosoma linguale (b)
Spirotrichea
Spirotrichum (f)
spiroverticillatus
Streptomyces s.
spirula
Onicola s.
Spirurida
Spirurina
spiruroid
s. larva migrans
Spiruroidea
spitsbergensis
Streptomyces s.
spizizenii
Bacillus subtilis subsp. s.
splanchnicus
Bacteroides s.
spleen cell culture
splendens
Eutrombicula s.
splendida
Beneckea s.
Splendidofilariinae
splendidus
Vibrio s.
Splendore-Hoeppli phenomenon
splenectomized
splenectomy
splenectomy-related sepsis
splenic gram
splenomegaly
Egyptian s.
hyperreactive s.
tropical s.
splinter hemorrhage
splinting
SPN
pneumolysin
SPN immunoblotting
Spondweni virus (SPOV)
spondylitis
ankylosing s.
tuberculous s.
spondyloarthropathy

sponge
> contraceptive s.
> Weck-cel s.

spongiform degeneration

spontaneous
> s. agglutination
> s. bacterial peritonitis (SBP)
> s. growth hormone level
> s. peritonitis
> s. rupture of membranes

sporadic

sporadin

sporangiophore

sporangium

Sporanox

spore
> airborne s.
> black s.
> soil-borne s.
> terminal s.

Sporendonema (f)

Sporichthya (b)
> S. brevicatena
> S. polymorpha

sporicidal

sporicide

Sporidesmlum (f)

sporidia (*pl. of* sporidium)

Sporidiaceae

Sporidiales

Sporidiobolus (f)
> S. johnsonli
> S. salmonicolor
> S. veronae

sporidium, pl. **sporidia**

sporium
> Methylosinus s.

Sporobacterium olearium (b)

Sporobacter termitidis (b)

sporoblast

Sporobolomyces (f)
> S. holsaticus
> S. odorus
> S. salmonicolor

Sporobolomycetacea

Sporobolomycetales

sporocidal

sporocinereus
> Streptomyces s.

sporoclivatus
> Streptomyces s.

Sporocybe (f)

sporocyst

Sporocytophaga (b)
> S. myxococcoides

sporodochium

sporogenes
> Clostridium s.

sporogenesis

sporogenous

sporogeny

sporogony

Sporohalobacter (b)
> S. lortetii
> S. marismortui

Sporolactobacillus (b)
> S. inulinus
> S. kofuensis
> S. lactosus
> S. nakayamae subsp. nakayamae
> S. nakayamae subsp. racemicus
> S. terrae

Sporomusa (b)
> S. acidovorans
> S. malonica
> S. ovata
> S. paucivorans
> S. silvacetica
> S. sphaeroides
> S. termitida

sporont

sporophore

sporoplasm

spororaveus
> Streptomyces s.

Sporosarcina (b)
> S. aquimarina
> S. globispora
> S. halophila
> S. pasteurii
> S. psychrophila
> S. ureae

sporosphaeroides
> Clostridium s.

sporotheca

sporothermodurans
> Bacillus s.

Sporothrix (f)
> S. antibody
> S. cyanescens
> S. schenckii

Sporotomaculum (b)
> S. hydroxybenzoicum

S

NOTES

sporotrichioides
    Fusarium s.
sporotrichoid leishmaniasis
sporotrichosis
    cutaneous s.
    disseminated s.
    extracutaneous s.
    lymphocutaneous s.
    multifocal extracutaneous s.
    osteoarticular s.
    plaque s.
    pulmonary s.
    s. serology
sporotrichositic chancre
Sporotrichum pruinosum (f)
sporoverrucosus
    Streptomyces s.
sporozoan
Sporozoasida
Sporozoea
sporozoite
sporozoon
sporular
sporulate
sporulated
sporulation
sporule
spot
    Biot s.
    café-au-lait s.
    depigmented s.
    Forscheimer s.
    Horder s.
    Koplik s.
    rose s.
    Roth s.
spotted
    s. fever
    s. sickness
SPOV
    Spondweni virus
SPP1 virus
spray
    CaldeCort Anti-Itch Topical S.
    ethyl chloride vinyl s.
    Ony-Clear S.
spread
    fecal-oral s.
    hematogenous s.
    horizontal s.
    olfactory s.
sprenti
    Dipetalonema s.
    Lagochilascaris s.
spring
    s. beauty latent virus
    s. viremia virus

Sprinkle
    Deconsal S.
    Humibid S.
sprue
    tropical s.
SPS
    sodium polyanetholesulfonate
spumans
    Mycoplasma s.
Spumavirus (v)
spumavirus
    human s.
spumicola
    Friedmanniella s.
spumosa
    Heterakis s.
spumosum
    Polyangium s.
spurious
    s. infection
    s. parasite
sputa (*pl. of* sputum)
sputi
    Gordonia s.
    Rhodococcus s.
sputigena
    Capnocytophaga s.
    Selenomonas s.
Sputolysin
sputorum
    Campylobacter sputorum subsp. *s.*
    Pandoraea s.
sputum, pl. **sputa**
    currant jelly s.
    s. fungus culture
    mucopurulent s.
    Papanicolaou stain of s.
    rusty s.
SPV
    San Perlita virus
SpV4-type phage
SPV4 virus
SPβ virus
SPy-2 virus
SQC
    semiquantitative culture
squama, squame
squamifemur
    Anopheles s.
squamiger
    Aedes s.
squamocolumnar
    s. epithelial cell
    s. junction
squamous
    s. cell
    s. cell cancer (SCC)
    s. cell carcinoma

s. epithelialization
s. epithelium
s. intraepithelial lesion (SIL)
s. metaplasia

squirrel
s. fibroma virus
s. monkey retrovirus
s. plague conjunctivitis

SQV
saquinavir

SQV-SGC

SR
Deconamine SR
Respaire-120 SR
Respaire-60 SR

3SR
self-sustaining sequence replication

Sr
Congess Sr

SRAV
Saraca virus

SRC Expectorant

SREV
Saumarez Reef virus

Sripur virus (SRIV)

SRIV
Sripur virus

srivastavai
Schistotaenia s

SRSV
small round structured virus

SRV
Shark River virus
small round virus

SSA
streptococcal superantigen

SSCP
single-strand conformation polymorphism

SSD
S. AF
S. Cream

ssDNA
isometric phage with s.

SSDP
sequence-specific DNA primer

SSEP
somatosensory evoked potential

SSHV
snowshoe hare virus

SSI
surgical site infection

SSKI
saturated solution of potassium iodide
supersaturated potassium iodide

SSPE
subacute sclerosing panencephalitis

ssRNA phage virus

SSSS
staphylococcal scalded skin syndrome

SST virus

SSV1-type phage virus

SSV1 virus

St.
St. Abbs Head virus
St. Joseph Cough Suppressant
St. Louis encephalitis (SLE)
St. Louis encephalitis virus (SLEV)
St. Louis equine encephalitis

St-1 virus

STA
standard tube agglutination test

stab culture

stabilis
Burkholderia s.

staccato cough

stachybotryotoxicosis

Stachybotrys (f)
S. chartarum
S. echinata

Stachylidium (f)

stadtmanae
Methanosphaera s.

Staf-Sistem 18-R test

stage
Ann Arbor s.
catarrhal s.
chancre s.
s. C HIV disease
convalescent s.
Dukes C colorectal carcinoma s.
exoerythrocytic s.
hemolymphatic s.
imperfect s.
incubative s.
latent s.
parasitemia s.
paroxysmal s.
perfect s.
prodromal s.
Tanner s.
Tanner s. I–V
trypanosome s.
UICC s.

S

NOTES

stage *(continued)*
    Union Internationale Contre La
      Cancer s.
staggers
staghorn calculus
stain
    acid-fast s.
    acridine orange s.
    AO s.
    auramine fluorochrome s.
    auramine O s.
    auramine-phenol s.
    auramine-rhodamine acid-fast s.
    azure II s.
    basic fuchsin s.
    bone marrow iron s.
    bovine rotavirus s.
    Brown-Brenn s.
    Brown & Hopps Gram s.
    calcofluor white s.
    carbol fuchsin s.
    chromotrope s.
    cold s.
    Congo red s.
    Coomassie blue s.
    cotton blue s.
    Cresylecht violet s.
    Cryptococcus s.
    Diene s.
    Dieterle s.
    Diff-Quik s.
    endocervical Gram s.
    fecal leukocyte s.
    flagellar s.
    fluorochrome s.
    Giemsa and Wilder reticulum s.
    Gimenez s.
    GMS s.
       Gomori methenamine silver stain
    Gomori methenamine s.
    Gomori methenamine silver s.
     (GMS stain, GMS)
    Gram s.
    Gram-chromotrope s.
    Gram-Weigert s.
    Grocott methenamine-silver s.
    Grocott modified silver s.
    Hansel s.
    H&E s.
    hematoxylin and eosin s.
    hot s.
    IF s.
    immunocytochemical s.
    immunofluorescence s.
    immunoperoxidase s.
    inclusion body s.
    India ink s.
    iodine s.

    iron s.
    iron-hematoxylin s.
    Kinyoun acid-fast s.
    Kinyoun carbol-fuchsin s.
    KOH s.
    Kokoskin s.
    lactophenol aniline blue s.
    Legionella DFA s.
    Leifson flagellar s.
    Leishman s.
    Loeffler methylene blue s.
    MacCallum-Goodpasture s.
    Macchiavellos s.
    Masson s.
    Masson-Fontana silver s.
    Mayer mucicarmine s.
    mepacrine s.
    methenamine silver s. (GMS)
    methylene blue s.
    modified Kinyoun acid-fast s.
    modified trichrome s.
    mucicarmine s.
    Nair buffered methylene blue s.
    overnight Giemsa s.
    Pap s.
    PAS s.
    periodic acid-Schiff s. (PAS)
    peroxidase-antiperoxidase
     immunocytochemical s.
    polyacrylamide gel electrophoresis
     with silver s. (PAGE-SS)
    potassium hydroxide s.
    rhodamine s.
    Romanovsky s.
    Ryan s.
    safranin s.
    Semichon acid carmine s.
    silver s.
    Steiner-Steiner s.
    toluidine blue O s.
    trichrome s.
    Warthin-Starry s.
    Wayson s.
    Weber modified trichrome s.
    Wheatley trichrome s.
    Wright s.
    Wright-Giemsa s.
    Ziehl-Neelsen acid-fast s.
staining
    DFA s.
    direct fluorescent antibody s.
    fluorescent actin s. (FAS)
    fluorochrome chitin s.
    immunohistochemical s.
    MicroTrak direct fluorescent
     antibody s.
    monoclonal antibody s.

rose bengal s.
trypan blue s.
Staleya guttiformus (b)
staleyi
    Pirella s.
    Pirellula s.
Stamey test
Stamnosoma
standard
    National Committee on Clinical
      Laboratory S.'s (NCCLS)
    S.'s for Pediatric Immunization
    s. precaution
    s. tube agglutination test (STA)
stanieri
    Pseudomonas s.
Staph
    RapiDEC S.
    S. Rapid test
    Slidex S.
StaphASE test
StaphAurex test
Staphcillin
Staphylatex test
staphylococcal
    s. abscess
    s. bacteremia
    s. coagglutination
    coagulase-negative s.
    s. endocarditis
    s. enterotoxin
    s. foodborne illness
    s. food poisoning
    s. infection
    s. intoxication
    s. pneumonia
    s. protein A COA
    s. protein A coagglutination
    s. scalded skin syndrome (SSSS)
    s. scarlet fever
    s. toxic shock syndrome
staphylococci (*pl. of* staphylococcus)
staphylococcic
staphylococcosis
Staphylococcus (b)
    S. arlettae
    S. aureus
    S. aureus subsp. *anaerobius*
    S. aureus subsp. *aureus*
    S. auricularis
    S. capitis subsp. *capitis*
    S. capitis subsp. *ureolyticus*

S. caprae
S. carnosus subsp. *carnosus*
S. carnosus subsp. *utilis*
S. caseolyticus
S. chromogenes
S. cohnii subsp. *cohnii*
S. cohnii subsp. *urealyticum*
S. condimenti
S. delphini
S. epidermidis
S. equorum
S. felis
S. fleurettii
S. food poisoning
S. gallinarum
S. haemolyticus
S. hominis subsp. *hominis*
S. hominis subsp. *novobiosepticus*
S. hyicus
S. hyicus subsp. *chromogenes*
S. intermedius
S. kloosii
S. lentus
S. lugdunensis
S. lutrae
S. muscae
S. pasteuri
S. piscifermentans
S. pulvereri
S. saccharolyticus
S. saprophyticus subsp. *bovis*
S. saprophyticus subsp.
  saprophyticus
S. schleiferi subsp. *coagulans*
S. schleiferi subsp. *schleiferi*
S. sciuri subsp. *carnaticus*
S. sciuri subsp. *lentus*
S. sciuri subsp. *rodentium*
S. sciuri subsp. *sciuri*
S. simulans
S. species coagulase-negative
S. succinus
S. vitulinus
S. warneri
S. xylosus
staphylococcus, pl. **staphylococci**
    s. antitoxin
    coagulase-negative s. (CNS, CONS)
    enterotoxigenic s.
staphyloenterotoxemia
staphyloenterotoxicosis
Staphyloslide

NOTES

Staphylothermus (b)
    S. hellenicus
    S. marinus
Staph-Zym test
Stappia (b)
    S. aggregata
    S. stellulata
starch
    s. hydrolysis test
    rice s.
starch-based electrolyte solution
Starkeya novella (b)
starkeyi
    Lipomyces s.
    Schizoblastosporion s.
Starkeyomyces (f)
starlingpox virus
starrii
    Bacteriovorax s.
    Bdellovibrio s.
stasis dermatitis
STAT
    Sero S.
state
    hypercoagulable s.
    imperfect s.
    perfect s.
Staticin
    O-V S.
    S. Topical
statin
stationary phase
stationis
    Brevibacterium s.
status epilepticus
staurosporea
    Saccharothrix aerocolonigenes
      subsp. s.
stavudine (d4T)
stay
    length of s. (LOS)
S-T Cort Topical
STD
    sexually transmitted disease
stearate
    erythromycin s.
stearothermophilus
    Bacillus s.
    Geobacillus s.
steatohepatitis
steatorrhea
steatosis
steatozoon
STEC
    Shiga toxin-producing *Escherichia coli*
steedae
    Simonsiella s.
steeple sign

steigerwaltii
    Legionella s.
Steiner-Steiner stain
steini
    Gregarina s.
Stella (b)
    S. humosa
    S. vacuolata
Stellantchasmus falcatus (p)
stellata
    Candida s.
    Hemispora s.
    Sagittula s.
    Seliberia s.
stellate
    s. abscess
    s. keratic
stellatoidea
    Procandida s.
stellifer
    Culicoides s.
stelliscabiei
    Streptomyces s.
stellulata
    Stappia s.
stellulatum
    Agrobacterium s.
stem
    s. cell
    s. cell rescue
    s. cell transplantation
    MicroScan Negative COMBO type
      5 system s.
    replicator system s.
Stemetil
Stemex
Stemonitales
stemonitis
    Doratomyces s.
Stemonitis flavogenita (f)
stemphylioides
    Alternaria s.
Stemphylium macrosporoideum (f)
stemphyloides
Stenella araguata (f)
stenocephala
    Uncinaria s.
stenosis, pl. stenoses
    anal s.
    aortic s.
    mitral s.
    urethral s.
    vaginal s.
stenostrepta
    Spirochaeta s.
Stenotrophomonas (b)
    S. africana

S. maltophilia
S. nitritireducens
stenoxenous
stenoxous parasite
Stensen duct
Stephanoascus ciferii (f)
Stephanofilaria stilesi (p)
Stephanosporium (f)
Stephanurus dentatus (p)
stercoralis
    Strongyloides s.
stercoraria
    Vitreoscilla s.
stercorarium
    Clostridium stercorarium subsp. *s.*
stercoris
    Bacteroides s.
    Collinsella s.
stereotaxic
sterigma
Sterigmatocystis (f) (*See* **Aspergillus**)
Sterigmatomyces (f)
    S. elviae
sterile
    s. abscess
    s. cyst
    s. granuloma
    s. urine culture
sterilization
    gas plasma s.
sternal osteomyelitis
sternoclavicular joint
sternotomy
steroid
    anabolic s.
    s. nasal inhaler
steroidogenesis
sterol
stethorae
    Rickettsiella s.
stetteri
    Thermococcus s.
Stetteria hydrogenophila (b)
Stevens-Johnson syndrome
stewartii
    Erwinia s.
    Pantoea stewartii subsp. *s.*
STI
    sexually transmitted infection
Stibiobacter senarmontii (b)

stibogluconate
    sodium s.
    s. sodium
stick
    heel s.
sticklandii
    Clostridium s.
sticticus
    Aedes s.
Stictidaceae
stiedai
    Eimeria s.
Stieva-A
    S.-A. Forte
stigma, pl. **stigmata**
stigmal plate
Stigmatella (b)
    S. aurantiaca
    S. erecta
Stilbellaceae
Stilbellales
Stilbospora (f)
stilbospora
    Taeniolella s.
Stilbosporaceae
stilesi
    Stephanofilaria s.
stillbirth
stilobezzioides
    Culicoides s.
Stilphostrol
stimulans
    Aedes s.
stimulant
    appetite s.
sting
stinging caterpillar
stipitatum
    Myxotrichum s.
stipitatus
    Myxococcus s.
stipitis
    Pichia s.
stippling
    basophilic s.
stirrer
    magnetic s.
St. John wort
STLV
    simian T-lymphotropic virus
STM
    streptomycin

S

NOTES

STMV
Santarem virus
STn
sialyl-Tn
STn-KLH cancer vaccine
stock
s. culture
s. strain
stockdaleae
Epidermophyton s.
stokesii
Leucosporidium s.
stolon
stolonifer
Rhizopus s.
stolpii
Bacteriovorax s.
Bdellovibrio s.
stoma
stomatis
Pasteurella s.
stomatitis
aphthous s.
bovine papular s. (BPSV)
Candida-associated denture s.
gonococcal s.
necrotizing s.
s. papulosa virus
Stomatococcus (b)
S. mucilaginosus
S. mucilaginosus sepsis
stomodeal
stomodeum
Stomoxyidae
Stomoxys calcitras (p)
stone
calcium carbonate s.
calcium phosphate s.
magnesium ammonium phosphate s.
struvite s.
triple phosphate s.
urinary s.
stonei
Culicoides s.
stool
s. adenovirus culture
s. for cryptosporidium
diarrheic s.
s. echovirus culture
s. enterovirus culture
Giardia O-positive s.
Giardia P-positive s.
s. poliovirus culture
s. viral culture
stopcock
strabismus
straight leg raising

strain
auxotrophic s.
carrier s.
EHEC O157:H7 Sakai s.
Haemophilus influenzae serotype
c s.
HFR s.
s. HM175 virus
hypothetical mean s. (HMS)
live vaccine s. (LVS)
lysogenic s.
mumps virus vaccine Jeryl Lynn s.
neotype s.
nitrate-negative s.
pathogenic s.
poliovirus type 2 Lansing s.
prototrophic s.
pseudolysogenic s.
recombinant s.
rheumatogenic streptococcal s.
stock s.
toxigenic s.
type s.
type b encapsulated s.
Vibrio cholerae O139 s.
VTEC 0111 s.
wild-type s.
zidovudine-resistant HIV-1 s.
strain-gauge plethysmography
straminea
Pseudomonas s.
stramineus
Streptomyces s.
strand displacement amplification (SDA)
stranskae
Planctomyces s.
strasburgensis
Pichia s.
Stratford virus (STRV)
stratification
stratifying
stratum corneum
strawberry tongue
straw itch
streak culture
streaming movement
streamlining antibiotic therapy
Strength
Allerest Maximum S.
Anbesol Maximum S.
Clearasil Maximum S.
Clocort Maximum S.
Orajel Maximum S.
Theraflu Non-Drowsy Formula
Maximum S.
Tylenol Flu Maximum S.
STREP
API Rapid S.

strep
    s. gangrene
    s. myositis
    Q Test S.
    s. screen
    Slidex S.
    s. throat screening culture
    S. TSS
streptavidin
Streptimonospora salina (b)
Streptoalloteichus hindustanus (b)
streptobacillary
Streptobacillus (b)
    S. moniliformis
streptocerca
    Agamofilaria s.
    Dipetalonema s.
    Mansonella s.
streptocerciasis
Streptococcaceae
streptococcal
    s. antibody titer
    s. balanoposthitis
    s. endocarditis
    s. gangrene
    s. impetigo
    s. M antigen
    s. pharyngitis
    s. pharyngotonsillitis
    s. pneumonia
    s. protein preabsorbing antigen
    s. pyrogenic exotoxin
    s. sore throat
    s. superantigen (SSA)
    s. toxic shock syndrome (Strep
      TSS, STSS)
streptococci (*pl. of* streptococcus)
streptococcic
streptococcosis
Streptococcus (b)
    S. acidominimus
    S. adjacens
    S. agalactiae
    S. alactolyticus
    S. anginosus
    S. australis
    S. bovis
    S. bovis endocarditis
    S. canis
    S. caprinus
    S. casseliflavus
    S. cecorum

S. constellatus subsp. *constellatus*
S. constellatus subsp. *pharyngis*
S. cremoris
S. criceti
S. cristatus
S. defectivus
S. didelphis
S. difficilis
S. downei
S. durans
S. dysgalactiae subsp. *dysgalactiae*
S. dysgalactiae subsp. *equisimilis*
S. equi subsp. *equi*
S. equinus
S. equi subsp. *zooepidemicus*
S. faecalis
S. faecium
S. ferus
S. gallinarum
S. gallolyticus
S. garvieae
S. gordonii
group A *S.* (GAS)
S. hansenii
S. hyointestinalis
S. hyovaginalis
S. infantarius subsp. *coli*
S. infantarius subsp. *infantarius*
S. infantis
S. infection
S. iniae
S. intermedius
S. intestinalis
S. lactis
S. lactis subsp. *cremoris*
S. lactis subsp. *diacetilactis*
S. macacae
S. macedonicus
S. M antigen
S. mitis
S. mitis bacteremia
S. morbillorum
S. mutans
S. oralis
S. orisratti
S. ovis
S. parasanguis
S. parauberis
S. parvulus
S. peroris
S. phocae
S. plantarum

S

NOTES

Streptococcus (continued)
   S. pleomorphus
   S. pluranimalium
   S. pneumoniae
   S. pneumoniae vaccine
   S. porcinus
   S. pyogenes
   pyogenic beta-hemolytic *S.*
   S. raffinolactis
   S. ratti
   S. saccharolyticus
   S. salivarius
   S. salivarius subsp. *thermophilus*
   S. sanguinis
   S. shiloi
   S. sobrinus
   S. suis
   S. thermophilus
   S. thoraltensis
   S. uberis
   S. urinalis
   S. vestibularis
   S. waius
streptococcus, pl. **streptococci**
   alpha hemolytic s.
   beta hemolytic s.
   gamma hemolytic s.
   group A beta-hemolytic s.
   group B s. (GBS)
   hemolytic streptococci
   Lancefield group D streptococci
   mutans streptococci
   nonhemolytic s.
   nutritionally variant s. (NVS)
   viridans s.
streptogramin
streptolysin O, S
Streptomonospora salina (b)
Streptomyces (f)
   S. abikoensis
   S. aburaviensis
   S. achromogenes subsp.
    achromogenes
   S. achromogenes subsp. *rubradiris*
   S. acidiscabies
   S. acrimycini
   S. aculeolatus
   S. aerocolonigenes
   S. afghaniensis
   S. alanosinicus
   S. albaduncus
   S. albiaxialis
   S. albidochromogenes
   S. albidoflavus
   S. albireticuli
   S. albofaciens
   S. alboflavus
   S. albogriseolus

S. albolongus
S. alboniger
S. albospinus
S. albosporeus
S. albosporeus subsp. *albosporeus*
S. albosporeus subsp.
  labilomyceticus
S. alboverticillatus
S. albovinaceus
S. alboviridis
S. albulus
S. albus subsp. *albus*
S. albus subsp. *pathocidicus*
S. almquistii
S. althioticus
S. amakusaensis
S. aminophilus
S. anandii
S. anthocyanicus
S. antibioticus
S. antimycoticus
S. anulatus
S. arabicus
S. ardus
S. arenae
S. argenteolus
S. armeniacus
S. asterosporus
S. atratus
S. atroaurantiacus
S. atroolivaceus
S. atrovirens
S. aurantiacus
S. aurantiogriseus
S. aureocirculatus
S. aureofaciens
S. aureorectus
S. aureoversilis
S. aureoverticillatus
S. autotrophicus
S. avellaneus
S. avidinii
S. azaticus
S. azureus
S. baarnensis
S. bacillaris
S. badius
S. baldaccii
S. bambergiensis
S. bellus
S. bikiniensis
S. biverticillatus
S. blastmyceticus
S. bluensis
S. bobili
S. bottropensis
S. brasiliensis
S. bungoensis

S

S. cacaoi
S. cacaoi subsp. asoensis
S. cacaoi subsp. cacaoi
S. caelestis
S. caeruleus
S. caespitosus
S. californicus
S. calvus
S. canarius
S. candidus
S. canescens
S. caniferus
S. canus
S. capillispiralis
S. capoamus
S. carpaticus
S. carpinensis
S. catenulae
S. caviscabies
S. cavourensis
S. cavourensis subsp. cavourensis
S. cavourensis subsp.
 washingtonensis
S. cellostaticus
S. celluloflavus
S. cellulolyticus
S. cellulosae
S. champavatii
S. chartreusis
S. chattanoogensis
S. chibaensis
S. chresiomyceticus
S. chromofuscus
S. chryseus
S. chrysomallus
S. chrysomallus subsp. chrysomallus
S. chrysomallus subsp. fumigatus
S. cinereorectus
S. cinereoruber
S. cinereoruber subsp. cinereoruber
S. cinereoruber subsp.
 fructofermentans
S. cinereospinus
S. cinereus
S. cinerochromogenes
S. cinnabarinus
S. cinnamonensis
S. cinnamoneus subsp. albosporus
S. cinnamoneus subsp. azacoluta
S. cinnamoneus subsp. cinnamoneus
S. cinnamoneus subsp. lanosus
S. cinnamoneus subsp. sparsus

S. cirratus
S. ciscaucasicus
S. citreofluorescens
S. clavifer
S. clavuligerus
S. cochleatus
S. coelescens
S. coelicoflavus
S. coelicolor
S. coeruleoflavus
S. coeruleofuscus
S. coeruleoprunus
S. coeruleorubidus
S. coerulescens
S. collinus
S. colombiensis
S. corchorusii
S. costaricanus
S. cremeus
S. crystallinus
S. curacoi
S. cuspidosporus
S. cyaneofuscatus
S. cyaneus
S. cyanoalbus
S. cystargineus
S. daghestanicus
S. diastaticus
S. diastaticus subsp. ardesiacus
S. diastaticus subsp. diastaticus
S. diastatochromogenes
S. distallicus
S. djakartensis
S. durhamensis
S. echinatus
S. echinoruber
S. ederensis
S. ehimensis
S. ekimensis
S. endus
S. enissocaesilis
S. erumpens
S. erythraeus
S. erythrogriseus
S. eurocidicus
S. europaeiscabiei
S. eurythermus
S. exfoliatus
S. felleus
S. fervens
S. fervens subsp. fervens
S. fervens subsp. melrosporus

NOTES

Streptomyces (continued)
- S. *filamentosus*
- S. *filipinensis*
- S. *fimbriatus*
- S. *fimicarius*
- S. *finlayi*
- S. *flaveolus*
- S. *flaveus*
- S. *flavidofuscus*
- S. *flavidovirens*
- S. *flaviscleroticus*
- S. *flavofungini*
- S. *flavofuscus*
- S. *flavogriseus*
- S. *flavopersicus*
- S. *flavotricini*
- S. *flavovariabilis*
- S. *flavovirens*
- S. *flavoviridis*
- S. *flocculus*
- S. *floridae*
- S. *fluorescens*
- S. *fradiae*
- S. *fragilis*
- S. *fulvissimus*
- S. *fulvorobeus*
- S. *fumanus*
- S. *fumigatiscleroticus*
- S. *galbus*
- S. *galilaeus*
- S. *gancidicus*
- S. *gardneri*
- S. *gedaensis*
- S. *gelaticus*
- S. *geysiriensis*
- S. *ghanaensis*
- S. *gibsonii*
- S. *glaucescens*
- S. *glaucosporus*
- S. *glaucus*
- S. *globisporus*
- S. *globisporus* subsp. *caucasicus*
- S. *globisporus* subsp. *flavofuscus*
- S. *globisporus* subsp. *globisporus*
- S. *globosus*
- S. *glomeratus*
- S. *glomeroaurantiacus*
- S. *gobitricini*
- S. *goshikiensis*
- S. *gougerotii*
- S. *graminearus*
- S. *graminofaciens*
- S. *griseinus*
- S. *griseoaurantiacus*
- S. *griseobrunneus*
- S. *griseocarneus*
- S. *griseochromogenes*
- S. *griseoflavus*

- S. *griseofuscus*
- S. *griseoincarnatus*
- S. *griseoloalbus*
- S. *griseolosporeus*
- S. *griseolus*
- S. *griseoluteus*
- S. *griseomycini*
- S. *griseoplanus*
- S. *griseorubens*
- S. *griseoruber*
- S. *griseorubiginosus*
- S. *griseosporeus*
- S. *griseostramineus*
- S. *griseoverticillatus*
- S. *griseoviridis*
- S. *griseus* subsp. *alpha*
- S. *griseus* subsp. *cretosus*
- S. *griseus* subsp. *griseus*
- S. *griseus* subsp. *solvifaciens*
- S. *hachijoensis*
- S. *halstedii*
- S. *hawaiiensis*
- S. *heliomycini*
- S. *helvaticus*
- S. *herbaricolor*
- S. *hiroshimensis*
- S. *hirsutus*
- S. *horton*
- S. *humidus*
- S. *humiferus*
- S. *hydrogenans*
- S. *hygroscopicus* subsp. *angustmyceticus*
- S. *hygroscopicus* subsp. *decoyicus*
- S. *hygroscopicus* subsp. *glebosus*
- S. *hygroscopicus* subsp. *hygroscopicus*
- S. *hygroscopicus* subsp. *ossamyceticus*
- S. *iakyrus*
- S. *indiaensis*
- S. *indigoferus*
- S. *intermedius*
- S. *inusitatus*
- S. *ipomoeae*
- S. *janthinus*
- S. *kanamyceticus*
- S. *kashmirensis*
- S. *kasugaensis*
- S. *katrae*
- S. *kentuckensis*
- S. *kifunensis*
- S. *kishiwadensis*
- S. *kunmingensis*
- S. *kurssanovii*
- S. *labedae*
- S. *ladakanum*
- S. *lanatus*

S. *lateritius*
S. *laurentii*
S. *lavendofoliae*
S. *lavendulae* subsp. *grasserius*
S. *lavendulae* subsp. *lavendulae*
S. *lavenduligriseus*
S. *lavendulocolor*
S. *levis*
S. *libani* subsp. *libani*
S. *libani* subsp. *rufus*
S. *lienomycini*
S. *lilacinus*
S. *limosus*
S. *lincolnensis*
S. *lipmanii*
S. *litmocidini*
S. *lividans*
S. *lomondensis*
S. *longisporoflavus*
S. *longispororuber*
S. *longisporus*
S. *longwoodensis*
S. *lucensis*
S. *luridus*
S. *lusitanus*
S. *luteofluorescens*
S. *luteogriseus*
S. *luteosporeus*
S. *luteoverticillatus*
S. *lydicus*
S. *macrosporus*
S. *malachitofuscus*
S. *malachitospinus*
S. *malaysiensis*
S. *mashuensis*
S. *massasporeus*
S. *matensis*
S. *mauvecolor*
S. *mediocidicus*
S. *mediolani*
S. *megasporus*
S. *melanogenes*
S. *melanosporofaciens*
S. *michiganensis*
S. *microflavus*
S. *minutiscleroticus*
S. *mirabilis*
S. *misakiensis*
S. *misionensis*
S. *mobaraensis*
S. *monomycini*
S. *morookaense*

S. *morookaensis*
S. *murinus*
S. *mutabilis*
S. *mutomycini*
S. *naganishii*
S. *narbonensis*
S. *nashvillensis*
S. *netropsis*
S. *neyagawaensis*
S. *niger*
S. *nigrescens*
S. *nigrifaciens*
S. *nitrosporeus*
S. *niveoruber*
S. *niveus*
S. *noboritoensis*
S. *nodosus*
S. *nogalater*
S. *nojiriensis*
S. *noursei*
S. *novaecaesareae*
S. *ochraceiscleroticus*
S. *odorifer*
S. *olivaceiscleroticus*
S. *olivaceoviridis*
S. *olivaceus*
S. *olivochromogenes*
S. *olivomycini*
S. *olivoreticuli* subsp. *cellulophilus*
S. *olivoreticuli* subsp. *olivoreticuli*
S. *olivoverticillatus*
S. *olivoviridis*
S. *omiyaensis*
S. *orientalis*
S. *orinoci*
S. *pactum*
S. *paracochleatus*
S. *paradoxus*
S. *parvisporogenes*
S. *parvulus*
S. *parvus*
S. *pentaticus* subsp. *jenensis*
S. *peucetius*
S. *phaeochromogenes*
S. *phaeofaciens*
S. *phaeopurpureus*
S. *phaeoviridis*
S. *phosalacineus*
S. *pilosus*
S. *platensis*
S. *plicatus*
S. *pluricolorescens*

S

NOTES

Streptomyces (continued)
S. polychromogenes
S. poonensis
S. praecox
S. prasinopilosus
S. prasinosporus
S. prasinus
S. prunicolor
S. psammoticus
S. pseudoechinosporeus
S. pseudogriseolus
S. pseudovenezuelae
S. pulcher
S. pulveraceus
S. puniceus
S. purpeofuscus
S. purpurascens
S. purpureus
S. purpurogeneiscleroticus
S. racemochromogenes
S. rameus
S. ramulosus
S. rangoon
S. rangoonensis
S. recifensis
S. rectiverticillatus
S. rectiviolaceus
S. regensis
S. resistomycificus
S. reticuli
S. reticuliscabiei
S. rimosus subsp. *paromomycinus*
S. rimosus subsp. *rimosus*
S. rishiriensis
S. rochei
S. roseiscleroticus
S. roseodiastaticus
S. roseoflavus
S. roseofulvus
S. roseolilacinus
S. roseolus
S. roseosporus
S. roseoverticillatus
S. roseoviolaceus
S. roseoviridis
S. ruber
S. rubiginosohelvolus
S. rubiginosus
S. rubrireticuli
S. rubrochlorinus
S. rubrogriseus
S. rubroverticillatus
S. rutgersensis subsp. *castelarensis*
S. rutgersensis subsp. *rutgersensis*
S. salmonis
S. sampsonii
S. sannanensis
S. sapporonensis

S. scabiei
S. scabies
S. sclerotialus
S. seoulensis
S. septatus
S. setae
S. setonii
S. showdoensis
S. sindenensis
S. sioyaensis
S. somaliensis
S. sparsogenes
S. spectabilis
S. speleomycini
S. spheroides
S. spinoverrucosus
S. spiralis
S. spiroverticillatus
S. spitsbergensis
S. sporocinereus
S. sporoclivatus
S. spororaveus
S. sporoverrucosus
S. stelliscabiei
S. stramineus
S. subrutilus
S. sulfonofaciens
S. sulphureus
S. syringium
S. takataensis
S. tanashiensis
S. tauricus
S. tendae
S. tenebrarius
S. termitum
S. thermoalcalitolerans
S. thermoautotrophicus
S. thermocarboxydovorans
S. thermocarboxydus
S. thermocoprophilus
S. thermodiastaticus
S. thermoflavus
S. thermogriseus
S. thermolineatus
S. thermonitrificans
S. thermoviolaceus subsp. *apingens*
S. thermoviolaceus subsp. *thermoviolaceus*
S. thermovulgaris
S. thioluteus
S. torulosus
S. toxytricini
S. tricolor
S. tsukubaensis
S. tubercidicus
S. tuirus
S. turgidiscabies
S. umbrinus

S. *variabilis*
S. *variegatus*
S. *varsoviensis*
S. *vastus*
S. *venezuelae*
S. *verticillatus*
S. *vinaceus*
S. *vinaceusdrappus*
S. *violaceochromogenes*
S. *violaceolatus*
S. *violaceorectus*
S. *violaceoruber*
S. *violaceorubidus*
S. *violaceus*
S. *violaceusniger*
S. *violarus*
S. *violascens*
S. *violatus*
S. *violens*
S. *virans*
S. *virens*
S. *virginiae*
S. *viridiviolaceus*
S. *viridobrunneus*
S. *viridochromogenes*
S. *viridodiastaticus*
S. *viridoflavum*
S. *viridoflavus*
S. *viridosporus*
S. *vitaminophilus*
S. *waksmanii*
S. *wedmorensis*
S. *werraensis*
S. *willmorei*
S. *xanthochromogenes*
S. *xanthocidicus*
S. *xantholiticus*
S. *xanthophaeus*
S. *yerevanensis*
S. *yokosukanensis*
S. *zaomyceticus*
Streptomycetaceae
streptomycete
streptomycin (STM)
    s. sulfate
streptomycin-containing anti-TB regimen
Streptomycoides glaucoflava (b)
Streptosporangiaceae
Streptosporangium (b)
    S. *albidum*
    S. *album*
    S. *amethystogenes*

S. *amethystogenes* subsp.
    amethystogenes
S. *amethystogenes* subsp. *fukuiense*
S. *carneum*
S. *claviforme*
S. *corrugatum*
S. *fragile*
S. *indianense*
S. *longisporum*
S. *nondiastaticum*
S. *pseudovulgare*
S. *roseum*
S. *violaceochromogenes*
S. *viridialbum*
S. *viridogriseum* subsp. *kofuense*
S. *viridogriseum* subsp.
    viridogriseum
S. *vulgare*
streptothrichosis
streptotrichiasis
streptotrichosis
Streptoverticillium (b)
    S. *abikoense*
    S. *albireticuli*
    S. *alboverticillatum*
    S. *album*
    S. *ardum*
    S. *aureoversile*
    S. *baldaccii*
    S. *biverticillatum*
    S. *blastmyceticum*
    S. *cinnamoneum* subsp. *albosporum*
    S. *cinnamoneum* subsp.
        cinnamoneum
    S. *cinnamoneum* subsp. *lanosum*
    S. *cinnamoneum* subsp. *sparsum*
    S. *distallicum*
    S. *ehimense*
    S. *eurocidicum*
    S. *fervens* subsp. *fervens*
    S. *fervens* subsp. *melrosporus*
    S. *flavopersicum*
    S. *griseocarneum*
    S. *griseoverticillatum*
    S. *hachijoense*
    S. *hiroshimense*
    S. *kashmirense*
    S. *kentuckense*
    S. *kishiwadense*
    S. *ladakanum*
    S. *lavenduligriseum*
    S. *lilacinum*

S

NOTES

Streptoverticillium (continued)
    S. luteoverticillatum
    S. mashuense
    S. mobaraense
    S. morookaense
    S. netropsis
    S. olivomycini
    S. olivoreticuli subsp. *cellulophilum*
    S. olivoreticuli subsp. *olivoreticuli*
    S. olivoverticillatum
    S. orinoci
    S. parvisporogenes
    S. rectiverticillatum
    S. roseoverticillatum
    S. salmonis
    S. sapporonense
    S. septatum
    S. syringium
    S. thioluteum
    S. viridoflavum
Streptozyme
stress fracture
striata
    Dirofilaria s.
striatum
    Amblyomma s.
    Corynebacterium s.
stricta
    Spirochaeta aurantia subsp. *s.*
stricto
    Borrelia burgdorferi sensu s.
    Leptospira interrogans sensu s.
    sensu s.
strictum
    Acremonium s.
    Rhodovulum s.
stricture
    urethral s.
stridor
    inspiratory s.
strigatum
    Simulium s.
Strigeatida
Strigeoidea
strigidorsum
    Simulium s.
striginotum
    Simulium s.
strigiphila
    Tetrameres s.
string test
strobila
strobilinum
    Coniosporium s.
strobilocercus
strobiloid
stroke
    heat s.

    lacunar s.
    subcortical s.
stroma
    erythrocyte s.
stromal
    s. cell
Stromectol
strong iodine solution
strongyle
Strongylida
Strongylidae
strongylina
    Ascarops s.
Strongyloidea
Strongyloides (p)
    S. esophagitis
    S. fuelleborni
    S. ratti
    S. stercoralis
strongyloides
    Pelodera s.
strongyloidiasis
    zoonotic s.
Strongyloididae
strongyloidosis
strongylosis
Strongylus vulgaris (p)
Strophariaceae
strophulus candidus
strumarium
    Chaetomium s.
strumosum
    Corynosoma s.
struvite
    s. stone
STRV
    Stratford virus
strychnine antagonist assay
STS
    serologic test for syphilis
ST-segment
STSS
    streptococcal toxic shock syndrome
stuartii
    Providencia s.
Stuart medium
studeri
    Bertia s.
    Bertiella s.
study
    AIDS Link to Intravenous
      Experiences s.
    ALIVE s.
    CHORUS s.
    cytogenetics s.
    electrodiagnostic s.
    HER S.
    HIV Epidemiology Research S.

HIVNET s.
HIV Vaccine Efficacy Trials
  Network s.
immunofluorescent s.
immunoperoxidase s.
joint s.
S. on Efficacy of Nosocomial
  Infection Control (SENIC)
radiographic s.
Tuskegee Syphilis S.
Vaccine Preparedness S. (VPS)
VIRADAPT s.
viral s.
Women and Infants
  Transmission S. (WITS)
Women's Interagency HIV S.
  (WIHS)
stupor
sturni
  Mycoplasma s.
sturniae
  Gigantobilharzia s.
stutzeri
  Pseudomonas s.
Stutzeri group of pseudomonads
stye
stygia
  Sphingomonas s.
stygiae
  Novosphingobium s.
Stygiolobus azoricus (b)
sualvi
  Mycoplasma s.
suarezi
  Simulium s.
suarezii
  Sanguibacter s.
suaveolens
  Moniliella s.
subacute
  s. bacterial endocarditis
  s. cellulitis
  s. sclerosing panencephalitis (SSPE)
  s. spongiform encephalopathy
suballiacea
  Amanita s.
subarachnoid
  s. hemorrhage (SAH)
subarctica
  Sphingomonas s.
subarcticum
  Novosphingobium s.

subcellular
subclass
subclavian
  s. catheter
  s. vein
subclavibranchium
  Simulium s.
subclinical
  s. coccidioidomycosis
  s. infection
  s. leptospirosis
subconjunctival
  s. hemorrhage
subcorticalis
  Coniochaeta s.
subcortical stroke
subculture
subcutaneous
  s. cysticercosis
  s. emphysema
  s. fungal infection
  s. interleukin-2
  s. myiasis
  s. necrotizing infection
  s. nodule
  s. sinus
  s. tissue
subcuticularc
subdermata
  Dirofilaria s.
subdiaphragmatic abscess
subdolum
  Mycoplasma s.
subdural
  s. empyema
  s. hematoma
subependymal nodular gliosis
subepicardial
subepidermal abscess
subepithelial hemorrhage
suberifaciens
  Rhizomonas s.
  Sphingomonas s.
suberosis
subfamily
subflava
  Neisseria s.
subgenus
subglaciescola
  Halomonas s.
subglobosa
  Sphaeropsis s.

S

NOTES

subglottic
subgroup
  fowlpox virus s.
  myxoma virus s.
  orf virus s.
  reovirus virus s.
  sheep pox virus s.
  swinepox virus s.
  vaccinia virus s.
  Yaba/Tanapox virus s.
subhepatic abscess
subiculosus
  Hypomyces s.
subimmaculatus
  Culicoides s.
subitum
  exanthem s.
  roseola s.
subjective synonym
subkingdom
sublaevis
  Figulus s.
sublettei
  Culicoides s.
subluxation
submandibular
  s. lymphadenitis
submicron mask
subnanogram level
subnigrum
  Simulium s.
subochrae
  Culiseta s.
suborder
suboxydans
  Gluconobacter oxydans subsp. *s.*
subpallidum
  Simulium p.
subpellicular
  s. fibril
  s. microtubule
subpelliculosa
  Hansenula s.
  Pichia s.
subperiodic periodicity
subphrenic abscess
subphylum
subpopulation
subrostratus
  Felicola s.
subrutilus
  Streptomyces s.
subSaharan Africa
subsalicylate
  bismuth s. (BSS)
subsegmental atelectasis

subset
  CD8$^+$ cell s.
  T-cell s.
subspecialist
  medical s.
  surgical s.
substance
  aggregation s.
substernal chest pain
substrate
  PyR s.
Subtercola (b)
  S. boreus
  S. frigoramans
subterminale
  Clostridium s.
subterranea
  Geotoga s.
  Sphingomonas s.
  Thermotoga s.
subterraneae
  Novosphingobium s.
subterraneum
  Methanobacterium s.
subterraneus
  Geobacillus s.
  Hydrogenobacter s.
  Thermoanaerobacter s.
subtherapeutic
subtile
  Bifidobacterium s.
subtilis
  Bacillus subtilis subsp. *s.*
subtribe
subtype
  Russian spring-summer encephalitis (Eastern s.)
  Russian spring-summer encephalitis (Western s.)
  tick-borne encephalitis (Central European s.)
  tick-borne encephalitis (Eastern s.)
subtyping
  HPV viral s.
  RFLP-based s.
subungual
  s. abscess
  s. splinter hemorrhage
subunit vaccine
subvibrioides
  Brevundimonas s.
  Caulobacter s.
succinea
  Kineosporia s.
succinicans
  Cytophaga s.
  Flavobacterium s.

succiniciproducens
Anaerobiospirillum s.
Succiniclasticum ruminis (b)
succinifaciens
Treponema s.
Succinimonas amylolytica (b)
Succinispira mobilis (b)
Succinivibrio dextrinosolvens (b)
succinivorans
Schwartzia s.
succinogenes
Actinobacillus s.
Bacteroides s.
Fibrobacter succinogenes subsp. s.
Vibrio s.
Wolinella s.
succinoxidans
Desulfuromusa s.
succinus
Staphylococcus s.
succiphila
Candida s.
sucker
sucking louse
Sucralfate
sucralfate
Sucre
DM Sans S.
Sucrets Cough Calmers
sucrofermentans
Acetobacter xylinus subsp. s.
Gluconacetobacter xylinus subsp. s.
sucromutans
Syntrophococcus s.
sucrose
s. test
thiosulfate citrate bile salts s.
(TCBS)
sucrose-phosphate-glutamic
s.-p.-g. acid (SPG)
s.-p.-g. acid buffer solution
suctioning
endo/nasotracheal s.
Sudafed
S. Cold & Cough
S. Cold & Cough Liquid Caps
S. DM
S. Expectorant
S. 12 Hour
S. Plus tablet
S. Severe Cold

sudden
s. acquired deafness
s. infant death syndrome
Sudodrin
sudoriparous abscess
SUDS-1 assay
suebicus
Lactobacillus s.
suecica
Candida s.
Sufedrin
sufrartyfex
Paryphostomum s.
sugar
pectin s.
suid
s. herpesvirus
s. herpesvirus 2
suihominis
Sarcocystis s.
suillum
Dechlorosoma s.
suimastitidis
Actinomyces s.
Suipoxvirus (v)
suis
Actinobacillus s.
Actinobaculum s.
Actinomyces s.
Bacteroides s.
Balantidium s.
Bifidobacterium s.
Brucella s.
Chlamydia s.
Eperythrozoon s.
Eubacterium s.
Haematopinus s.
Iodamoeba s.
Schistosoma s.
Streptococcus s.
Trichuris s.
sukumoe
Promicromonospora s.
Sulamyd
Sodium S.
sulbactam
ampicillin and s.
s. and ampicillin
cefoperazone s.
sulci
Eubacterium s.
Fusobacterium s.

NOTES

sulconazole
Sulcrate
sulcus
    coronal s.
Sulf-10
    S. Ophthalmic
sulfa
    triple s.
sulfacetamide
    s. and phenylephrine
    s. and prednisolone
    sodium s.
    s. sodium
    s. sodium and fluorometholone
    sulfur and s.
Sulfacet-R Topical
sulfacytine
sulfadiazine
    silver s.
sulfadiazine-chlorhexidine
sulfadoxine
sulfadoxine-pyrimethamine
Sulfa-Gyn
Sulfair
sulfamethazine
sulfamethiazole phenazopyridine
sulfamethizole
Sulfamethoprim
sulfamethoxazole (SMX)
    s. and phenazopyridine
    s. and trimethoprim (SMX-TMP)
sulfamethoxazole-phenazopyrine
sulfamethoxazole/trimethoprim test (SXT test)
Sulfamylon
    S. Topical
sulfanilamide
sulfasalazine
sulfatase
    chondroitin s.
sulfate
    amikacin s.
    atropine s.
    Capastat S.
    capreomycin s.
    dehydroepiandrosterone s. (DHEAS)
    ferric ammonium s.
    hydroxychloroquine s.
    magnesium s.
    Mycifradin S.
    neomycin s.
    polymyxin B s.
    quinidine s.
    quinine s.
    sodium dodecyl s.
    sodium tetradecyl s.
    streptomycin s.

sulfathiazole
    sulfabenzamide, sulfacetamide, and s.
    sulfabenzamide, sulfacetamide, and s.
sulfation reagent
Sulfatrim
    S. DS
sulfa-trimethoprim
Sulfa-Trip
Sulfex
sulfexigens
    Desulfocapsa s.
sulfide
    hydrogen s.
    selenium s.
sulfidophila
    Rhodopseudomonas s.
sulfidophilum
    Heliobacterium s.
    Rhodovulum s.
sulfidophilus
    Rhodobacter s.
sulfidovorans
    Methylophaga s.
sulfidoxydans
    Pseudonocardia s.
sulfisoxazole
    s. acetyl
    erythromycin and s.
    s. and phenazopyridine
Sulfitobacter (b)
    S. brevis
    S. mediterraneus
    S. pontiacus
Sulfizole
Sulfobacillus (b)
    S. acidophilus
    S. disulfidooxidans
    S. thermosulfidooxidans
sulfodismutans
    Desulfovibrio s.
Sulfolobaceae
Sulfolobales
Sulfolobus (b)
    S. acidocaldarius
    S. brierleyi
    S. hakonensis
    S. metallicus
    S. shibatae
    S. solfataricus
    S. yangmingensis
sulfonamide
    long-acting s.
    multiple s.
sulfonate
    carbazochrome sodium s. (AC-17)

2-mercaptoethane s.
sodium polyanethol s.
Sulfone syndrome
sulfonofaciens
  Streptomyces s.
sulfonylurea
  s. agent
Sulfophobococcus zilligii (b)
sulfosalicylate
  meclocycline s.
sulfoviridis
  Blastochloris s.
  Rhodopseudomonas s.
sulfur
  s. granule
  s. and salicylic acid
  s. shelf fungus
  s. and sulfacetamide
sulfureus
  Arthrobacter s.
  Enterococcus s.
Sulfurisphaera ohwakuensis (b)
Sulfurococcus (b)
  S. mirabilis
  S. yellowstonensis
sulfurophilus
  Thermoanaerobacter s.
Sulfurospirillum (b)
  S. arcachonense
  S. arsenophilum
  S. barnesii
  S. deleyianum
sulfurreducens
  Geobacter s.
sulphafurazole
sulphurea
  Amycolatopsis s.
  Nocardia s.
sulphureus
  Laetiporus s.
  Streptomyces s.
Sulsal
Sultrin
sumatriptan
summa
  Pygidiopsis s.
Sumycin Oral
Sunday Canyon virus (SCAV)
sundsvallense
  Corynebacterium s.
Supasa

superantigen
  endogenous viral s.
  streptococcal s. (SSA)
superficial
  s. aspergillosis
  s. candidiasis
  s. infection
  s. transitional cell carcinoma of
    the bladder
supergroup
  Bunyamwera s.
superinfection
  bacterial s.
superior vena cava syndrome
supernatant
superoxide
superoxol test
superparasite
superparasitism
supersaturated potassium iodide (SSKI)
supplement
  antioxidant s.
  S. to HIV/AIDS Surveillance
    (SHAS)
  mycobacteria antibiotic s. (MAS)
support
  pressor s.
suppository
  AVC S.
  miconazole o.
Suppress
Suppressant
  St. Joseph Cough S.
suppression
  bone marrow s.
  marrow s.
  viral load s.
suppressive therapy
suppressor T cell
suppuration
  contiguous s.
suppurativa
  hidradenitis s. (HS)
  hydradenitis s.
suppurative
  s. granulomatous lymphadenitis
  s. mediastinitis
  s. myositis
  s. oral infection
  s. peripheral phlebitis
  s. thrombophlebitis
supraclavicular

S

NOTES

supraglottitis
suprapubic
    s. aspiration
    s. aspiration of urine
    s. catheterization
    s. tenderness
supratentorial
Suprax
suramin
surface
    s. antigen of hepatitis B virus (HBsAg)
    s. area to volume ratio (SA/V)
    s. protein antigen
surfactant
surgery
    biliary tract s.
    cold blade s.
    conservative s.
    demolitive s.
    neck s.
surgical
    s. ablation
    s. maggot
    s. site infection (SSI)
    s. subspecialist
    s. wound infection (SWI)
surgicenter
surrenal gland
surrogate marker
surveillance
    S. and Control of Pathogens of Epidemiologic Importance (SCOPE)
    immune s.
    National Nosocomial Infection S. (NNIS)
    Supplement to HIV/AIDS S. (SHAS)
survey
    point-prevalent s. (PPS)
susceptibility testing
susceptible
Susp
    Megacillin S.
suspended animation
suspension
    AK-Spore H.C. Ophthalmic S.
    amphotericin B oral s.
    atovaquone s.
    barium sulfate s.
    cefuroxime axetil s. (CAE)
    Children's Advil s.
    Children's Motrin s.
    Cortisporin Ophthalmic s.
    Cortisporin-TC Otic s.
    FML-S Ophthalmic s.
    Fucidin Oral s.

    Mepron s.
    oral s.
    Poly-Pred Ophthalmic s.
    Rynatuss Pediatric s.
    s. smear
    Terra-Cortril Ophthalmic s.
Sus-Phrine
sustained response
Sustaire
Sustiva
Sutterella wadsworthensis (b)
Suttonella indologenes (b)
suttonii
    Pseudomicrodochium s.
suum
    Ascaris s.
sv.
    serovar
SV1 virus
SV2 virus
SV5 virus
SV40 virus
SV41 virus
SVDV
    swine vesicular disease virus
Svedburg unit (S)
SVV
    Sal Vieja virus
swab
    anal sphincter s.
    calcium alginate s.
    cellophane tape s.
    cervicovaginal mucosal s.
    conjunctival s.
    cotton s.
    Culturette s.
    Dacron s.
    endocervical s.
    external genital s.
    eye s.
    gingival s.
    high vaginal s.
    nasal s.
    nasopharyngeal s.
    rayon s.
    rectal s.
    Scotch tape s.
    s. test
    throat s.
    urethral s.
    vaginal secretion s.
    Virocult s.
    wound s.
swallow
    barium s.
swamp
    s. fever
    s. itch

Swan-Ganz
S.-G. catheter
S.-G. monitoring
S.-G. tip culture
swan-neck catheter Missouri catheter
swarming
sweat
s. mushroom
night s.
Sween Cream
Sweet syndrome
Sweetwater Branch virus
swelling
Calabar s.
fugitive s.
SWI
surgical wound infection
Swim-Ear Otic
swimmer's
s. ear
s. itch
swimming
s. pool conjunctivitis
s. pool granuloma
swine
s. erysipelas
s. fever
s. influenza
s. influenza vaccine
s. vesicular disease virus (SVDV)
swineherd fever
swineherd's disease
swinepox
s. virus
s. virus subgroup
swollen
s. belly disease
s. belly syndrome
swynnertoni
Glossina s.
SXT test
sycosiform fungous infection
sycosis
s. barbae
tinea s.
Sydenham chorea
Sydowia polyspora
sydowii
Aspergillus s.
sylvatic
s. plague

sylviarum
Liponyssus s.
Ornithonyssus s.
Sylvius
aqueduct of S.
Symadine
Symbiobacterium thermophilum (b)
symbion
symbiont
symbiosis
symbiosum
Clostridium s.
symbiote
Symbiotes lectularius (b)
symbiotic
Symmers clay pipestem fibrosis
Symmetrel
S. syrup
symmetrical peripheral gangrene
symmetry
axis of s.
sympathetic
s. ganglion
symptom
B s.
constitutional s.
hemorrhagic fever with renal s.
(HFRS)
symptomatic
s. fever
s. urinary tract infection
symptomology
Synacol CF
Synacort Topical
Synagis
Synalar-HP Topical
Synalar Topical
synanamorph
synaptobrevin
synaptophysin
synaptotagmin
Syncephalastraceae
Syncephalastrum racemosum (f)
Synchytriaceae
Synchytrium endobioticum (f)
syncope
orthostatic s.
syncytial
s. virus
syncytium, pl. syncytia
s. induction
syncytium-inducing phenotype

S

NOTES

syndrome

acquired immune deficiency s.
(AIDS)
acquired immunodeficiency s.
(AIDS)
acute retroviral s. (ARS)
acute toxic s.
acute urethral s.
adult respiratory distress s. (ARDS)
AIDS wasting s. (AWS)
appendicitis-like s.
aseptic meningitis s.
autoimmune lymphoproliferative s.
(ALPS)
Bannwarth s.
Budd-Chiari s.
capillary leak s.
cellular immunity deficiency s.
cepacia s.
cerebellar s.
chancriform s.
Chédiak-Higashi s.
chronic appendiceal s.
chronic EBV s.
chronic fatigue s. (CFS)
Clostridium difficile sepsis s.
CMV mononucleosis s.
compartment s.
congenital rubella s.
conus medullaris s.
cord compression s.
Cushing s.
dengue hemorrhagic fever/shock s.
(DHF-DSS)
dengue shock s. (DSS)
Down s.
Eaton-Lambert myasthenic s.
enterocolitis s.
euthyroid s.
Fanconi s.
Fanconi-like s.
febrile fasciolitic eosinophilic s.
Fisher Guillain-Barré s.
Fitz-Hugh-Curtis s.
Gerstmann-Straüssler-Scheinker s.
Gilbert s.
glove-and-stocking s.
Goodpasture s.
gray-baby s.
green nail s.
GSS s.
Guillain-Barré s.
Hantavirus pulmonary s.
hantavirus pulmonary s. (HPS)
hemolytic uremic s. (HUS)
hemophagocytic s.
hemorrhagic fever renal s.

hemorrhagic fever with renal s.
(HFRS)
Henoch-Schönlein s.
heterophil-negative s.
HIV-associated lipodystrophy s.
HIV wasting s.
Hurler s.
idiopathic nephrotic s.
Ikari s.
s. of inappropriate antidiuretic
hormone secretion (SIADH)
s. of inappropriate secretion of
antidiuretic hormone (SIADH)
infectious mononucleosis-like s.
intraamniotic infection s. (IAIS)
iron overload s.
Job s.
Katayama s.
Kawasaki s.
Kikuchi s.
Landry-Guillain-Barré s.
Lemierre s.
lipodystrophy s.
Löffler s.
lumpy jaw s.
lymphoproliferative s.
malabsorption s.
Meig s.
menstrual toxic shock s. (MTSS)
Mikulicz s.
Miller-Fisher s.
monoclonal lymphoproliferative s.
mononucleosis s.
mononucleosis-like s.
multiple organ dysfunction s.
(MODS)
myelodysplastic s. (MDS)
myeloproliferative s.
myoclonic alien hand s.
Nakalanga s.
nephrotic s.
neuroleptic malignant s. (NMS)
nonmenstrual toxic shock s.
(NMTSS)
orbital apex s.
Parinaud oculoglandular s.
pertussis-like s.
Pfiesteria-associated s.
Picchini s.
polyclonal lymphoproliferative s.
polymyositis s.
postencephalitis s.
posterior fossa s.
postpolio s.
presumed ocular histoplasmosis s.
(POHS)
Ramsay Hunt s.
red man s. (RMS)

Reiter s.
Reye s.
scalded skin s.
sepsis s.
sepsis inflammatory s.
septic shock-like s.
Sézary s.
sicca s.
Sjögren s.
staphylococcal scalded skin s.
  (SSSS)
staphylococcal toxic shock s.
Stevens-Johnson s.
streptococcal toxic shock s. (Strep
  TSS, STSS)
sudden infant death s.
Sulfone s.
superior vena cava s.
Sweet s.
swollen belly s.
systemic inflammatory response s.
  (SIRS)
tingling throat s.
toxic shock s. (TSS, TSST)
toxic shock-like s. (TSLS)
trichuris dysentery s.
tropical splenomegaly s. (TSS)
urethral s.
uvcoencephalitis s.
uveomeningitic s.
vaginitis s.
vascular leak s. (VLS)
viral hemophagocytic s.
virus-associated hemophagocytic s.
Vogt-Koyanagi-Harada s.
wasting s.
Waterhouse-Friderichsen s.
Weil s.
Wernicke-Korsakoff s.
whooping cough s.
Wiskott-Aldrich s.
s. X
Zollinger-Ellison s.
synechia, pl. **synechiae**
Synemol Topical
Synercid
synergism
Synergistes jonesii (b)
synergistic
  s. cellulitis
  s. gangrene

progressive bacterial s.
s. therapy
synergy
Synflex
Syngamidae
Syngaminae
Syngamus trachea (p)
Syn-Minocycline
synnaedendra
  Saccharomycopsis s.
synnemataformans
  Nocardiopsis s.
synonym
  objective s.
  senior s.
  subjective s.
Synosternus pallidus
synoviae
  Mycoplasma s.
synovial
  s. biopsy
  s. cyst
  s. fluid
  s. fluid cytology
  s. glucose
synovitis
  filarial s.
  granulomatous s.
syntaxin
Synthesiomyia
  S. nudiseta
synthesis
  peptidoglycan s.
synthetase
  RNase L 2'-5' oligoadenylate s.
synthetic opioid
Syntrophobacter (b)
  S. fumaroxidans
  S. pfennigii
  S. wolinii
Syntrophobotulus glycolicus (b)
Syntrophococcus sucromutans (b)
Syntrophomonas (b)
  S. sapovorans
  S. wolfei subsp. *saponavida*
  S. wolfei subsp. *wolfei*
Syntrophospora bryantii (b)
Syntrophothermus lipocalidus (b)
Syntrophus (b)
  S. buswellii
  S. gentianae

S

NOTES

synxantha
 Pseudomonas s.
Syphacia (p)
 S. muris
 S. obvelata
syphilid
 pustular s.
syphilis
 active s.
 benign s.
 cardiovascular s.
 s. chancre
 congenital s.
 disseminated s.
 early latent s.
 EL s.
 endemic s.
 incubating s.
 late benign s.
 late latent s.
 latent s.
 LL s.
 meningovascular s.
 nonvenereal s.
 ocular s.
 primary s.
 s. screening test
 secondary s.
 serologic s.
 serologic test for s. (STS)
 s. serology
 tertiary s.
syphilitic
 s. arthritis
 s. chancre
 s. dactylitis
 s. endarteritis
 s. fever
 s. lesion
 s. otitis
 s. retinitis
 s. ulceration
Sypringospora uvae
Syracol-CF
syringae
 Nocardiopsis s.
 Pseudomonas s.
 Pseudomonas syringae subsp. *s.*
 Saccharothrix s.
syringium
 Streptomyces s.
 Streptoverticillium s.
syringoma
syringomyelia
Syringospora albicans (f)
Syrphidae
syrphidae
 Mesoplasma s.

syrphidicola
 Spiroplasma s.
Syrphus americanus
syrup
 Actagen S.
 Allerfrin S.
 Allerphed s.
 Ambenyl Cough s.
 Amgenal Cough s.
 Anamine s.
 Aprodine S.
 Benylin Cough s.
 Bromanyl Cough S.
 Bromotuss w/Codeine Cough s.
 Bydramine Cough s.
 Cough s.
 Decofed s.
 Deconamine s.
 S. DM
 DM Cough s.
 S. DM-D
 S. DM-E
 Extra Action Cough s.
 Hydramyn s.
 hydrocodone PA s.
 Laniazid s.
 Naldecon-EX Children's s.
 Pediatric Cough s.
 Phanatuss Cough s.
 Silafed s.
 Symmetrel s.
 Triaminicol Multi-Symptom Cold s.
 Triofed s.
 Triposed s.
 Tussar SF s.
 Vicks Children's Cough and
  Congestion s.
system
 ACTG staging s.
 AIDS Clinical Trials Group
  staging s.
 amplification refractory mutation s.
  (ARMS)
 Androderm Transdermal S.
 An-IDENT s.
 antigen-antibody s.
 API 20NE nonenteric
  identification s.
 API Rapid 20E S.
 BACTEC 9440/9120 Blood
  Culture S.
 BACTEC radiometric s.
 Bartlett grading s.
 Behavioral Risk Factor
  Surveillance S. (BRFSS)
 Bethesda classification s.
 Biolog Microplate Identification S.
 central nervous s. (CNS)

cytochrome s.
Difco Extra Sensing Power (ESP)
  Blood Culture S.
ecological s.
electron transport s.
GonoGen II antigen detection s.
immune s.
InPouch s.
Isolator s.
Lancefield classification s.
luciferase enzyme-based
  luminescence s.
Merifluor direct immunofluorescence
  detection s.
Microbial Identification S. (MIDI,
  MIS)
Micro Drop yeast identification s.
Micro-ID s.
MicroScan S.
mononuclear phagocyte s.
Multitest CMI s.
mycobacteria growth indicator
  tube s.
National Nosocomial Infections
  Surveillance S. (NNIS)
O.A.S.I.S. Blood Culture S.
Oxoid Signal S.
RapID ANA II S.
rapid broth s.
Rapid NF Plus s.
RapID NH s.
RapID onE s.
reticuloendothelial s. (RES)
Sceptor S.
Sensititre S.
Septi-Chek AFB s.
Septi-Chek Blood Culture S.
Testoderm Transdermal S.
tuberculosis of lacrimal s.
vital blood culture s.

Walkaway (W/A) Rapid Bacterial
  Identification S.
systematic bacteriology
systemic
  s. antipseudomonal
  s. autoimmune disease
  s. azole
  betamethasone (s.)
  s. candidiasis
  s. chemotherapy
  s. CMV infection
  s. cytotoxic chemotherapy
  dexamethasone (s.)
  s. dissemination
  erythromycin (s.)
  s. fat embolism
  s. febrile disease
  s. fungal infection
  hydrocortisone (s.)
  s. inflammatory response
  s. inflammatory response syndrome
    (SIRS)
  s. interferon-gamma
  s. interleukin
  s. lupus erythematosus (SLE)
  s. mycosis
  s. phaeohyphomycosis
  s. pneumocystosis
  prednisolone (s.)
  triamcinolone (s.)
systolic regurgitant murmur
syzygial
syzygii
    Pseudomonas s.
syzygium
syzygy
szegediense
    Methylocaldum s.
szulgai
    Mycobacterium s.

NOTES

S

T
>testosterone
>>T body
>>T zone

T-20

T21 virus

T4/T8 ratio

TA
>tube agglutination
>>TA test

T1-A
>*Gaeumannomyces graminis*
>virus T.-A. (GgV-T1-A)

TAA
>tumor-associated antigen

Tab
>Apo-Doxy T.'s
>Meda T.

tabacinasalis
>*Facklamia t.*

tabanid
>t. fly

Tabanidae

tabanidae
>*Mesoplasma t.*

tabanidicola
>*Spiroplasma t.*

tabaniformis
>*Glossina t.*

Tabanus (p)
>*T. atratus*
>*T. nigrovittatus*
>*T. punctifer*

taberi
>*Saccharopolyspora t.*
>*Saccharopolyspora hirsuta* subsp. *t.*

tabes dorsalis

Tablet

tablet
>Actagen T.
>Actifed Allergy T. (Day)
>Allercon t.
>Allerfrin T.
>Aprodine T.
>Benadryl Decongestant Allergy t.
>Brontex T.
>Cenafed Plus t.
>Chlor-Trimeton 4 Hour Relief t.
>clotrimazole vaginal t.
>Deconamine t.
>Decongestant T.'s
>Fedahist t.
>Fucidin t.
>Genac t.
>Headache T.'s

>Klerist-D t.
>Pseudo-Gest Plus t.
>Spectrobid t.
>Sudafed Plus t.
>triple sulfa t.
>Triposed t.

TAC
>transient aplastic crisis

Tac-3 Injection

Tac-40 Injection

Tacaiuma virus (TCMV)

Tacaribe virus (TCRV)

TACE

tache noire

tachinoides
>*Glossina t.*

tachycardia
>ventricular t.

tachypnea

tachyzoite
>t. form

tacrolimus

tadpole edema virus

taejonensis
>*Sphingomonas t.*

Taenia (p)
>*T. brauni*
>*T. crassiceps*
>*T. glomeratus*
>*T. hydatigena*
>*T. multiceps*
>*T. ovis*
>*T. pisiformis*
>*T. saginata*
>*T. serialis*
>*T. solium*

Taeniarhynchus (p)

taeniasis
>Asian t.
>t. saginata
>t. solium

taeniid

Taeniidae

taenioid

Taeniolella stilbospora (f)

taeniopus
>*Culex t.*

taeniorhynchus
>*Aedes t.*

taeniospiralis
>*Caedibacter t.*
>*Hydrogenophaga t.*
>*Pseudomonas t.*

taetrolens
>*Pseudomonas t.*

T

Tagamet
Tagamet-HB
tagetidis
    Xanthobacter t.
Taggert virus (TAGV)
TAGV
    Taggert virus
TAHV
    Tahyna virus
Tahyna virus (TAHV)
Taiassui virus
taichui
    Haplorchis t.
tail
    fermented beaver t.
    phage with contractile t.
    phage with long noncontractile t.
    phage with short t.
tailed phage virus
TAIV
    Tai virus
Tai virus (TAIV)
taiwanense
    Spiroplasma t.
taiwanensis
    Natrialba t.
takataensis
    Streptomyces t.
talaje
    Ornithodoros t.
Talaromyces (f)
talc
    zinc oxide, cod liver oil, and t.
tallaferroae
    Simulium t.
talpae
    Bartonella t.
    Capillaria t.
    Grahamella t.
Tamana bat virus
tamarii
    Aspergillus t.
tamarindii
    Procandida t.
Tamdy virus (TDYV)
Tamiami virus (TAMV)
Tamiflu
Tamm-Horsfall protein
tamponade
    cardiac t.
tampon specimen
TAMV
    Tamiami virus
tamworthensis
    Amaricoccus t.
Tanac
Tanapox virus

tanashiensis
    Streptomyces t.
Tanga virus (TANV)
tangerinus
    Saccharothrix t.
Tanjong Rabok virus (TRV)
Tanner
    T. stage
    T. stage I–V
tannerae
    Prevotella t.
tannophilus
    Pachysolen t.
Tantafed
Tantaphen
tanukii
    Borrelia t.
TANV
    Tanga virus
tanzawaensis
    Candida t.
Tao
tap
    ascites fluid t.
    CSF t.
    dry t.
    joint t.
    pleural fluid t.
    spinal t.
    traumatic t.
    t. water bacillus
tapae
    Candida t.
Tapanol
TAPC
    total anomalous pulmonary circulation
tape
    cellulose t.
tapeticola
    Halospirulina t.
tapetis
    Vibrio t.
tapeworm
    t. cestode
Taphrinaceae
Taphrinales
tar
    coal t.
    DHS T.
    T. Distillate
    T. Doak
    Spectro T.
tarantellae
    Eubacterium t.
tarantula
    American t.
    black t.

European t.
Peruvian t.
tarassovi
  Leptospira interrogans serovar t.
tarda
  Edwardsiella t.
Tardan
tardum
  Eubacterium t.
Targel
  T. SA
targeted immunotherapy
target lesion
Targocid
Targretin
Taro-Ampicillin Trihydrate
Taro-Cloxacillin
Taro-Desoximetasone
Taro-Sone
tarsale
  Simulium t.
tarsalis
  Culex t.
tarsatum
  Simulium t.
tartaricus
  Ilyobacter t.
task
  word fluency t.
tassiana
  Mycosphaerella t.
TAT
  tetanus antitoxin
  total abdominal fat
Tataguine virus (TATV)
Taterapox virus
Tat gene
tationis
  Methanofollis t.
  Methanogenium t.
Tatlockia (b)
  T. *maceachernii*
  T. *micdadei*
Tatumella ptyseos (b)
TATV
  Tataguine virus
Tau-cheed
Taunton
  T. agent
  T. virus
tau protein

tauricus
  Streptomyces t.
taurinensis
  Legionella t.
Ta₁ virus
taxa
taxane
taxodium
  Simulium t.
taxon
taxonomic
taxonomy
  numerical t.
taylorae
  Enterobacter t.
Taylorella (b)
  T. *asinigenitalis*
  T. *equigenitalis*
taylorii
  Bartonella t.
  Methanolobus t.
tazarotene
Tazicef
Tazidime
tazobactam
Tazocin
Tazorac
TB
  tuberculosis
    multidrug-resistant TB
TB-attributable mortality rate
TBE
  tick-borne encephalitis
TBEV
  tick-borne encephalitis virus
TBI
  total body irradiation
TBK
  total body potassium
TBTV
  Timboteua virus
TBW
  total body water
3TC
  2′,3′-dideoxy-3′thiacytidine
  lamivudine
  lamivudine triphosphate
    AZT + 3TC
TCA
  tissue culture assay
  tricyclic antidepressant

T

NOTES

TCBS
> thiosulfate citrate bile salts sucrose
> TCBS agar

T-cell
> T.-c. costimulation
> T.-c. determinant
> T.-c. gene therapy
> T.-c. homeostasis
> T.-c. infiltrate
> T.-c. lymphoma
> T.-c. lymphoma virus
> T.-c. memory
> T.-c. profile
> T.-c. receptor (TCR, TcR)
> T.-c. specificity
> T.-c. subset
> T.-c. tropism

T-cell-tropic (T-tropic)
> T.-c.-t. virus

TCM
> traditional Chinese medicine

TCMV
> Tacaiuma virus

TCN
> tetracycline

TCR
> T-cell receptor
>> antigen-specific TCR

TcR
> T-cell receptor

TCRV
> Tacaribe virus

TCT
> tracheal cytotoxin

TCV

tD
> tetanus and diphtheria

T/Derm
> Neutrogena T.

TDH
> thermostable direct hemolysin

TDLN
> tumor-draining lymph node

TDLNC
> tumor-draining lymph node cell

TDMV
> Tindholmur virus

TDYV
> Tamdy virus

TE
> *Toxoplasma* encephalitis

Tebrazid

techellsii
> *Candida* t.

technetium scan

technique
> agar gel diffusion t.
> Baermann fecal extraction t.
> cellophane thick smear t.
> chromotrope-2R modified trichrome staining t.
> cold-knife t.
> counterimmunoelectrophoresis t.
> enzyme-multiplied immunoassay t. (EMIT)
> fecoculture t.
> formalin-ether sedimentation t.
> formalin-ethyl acetate concentration t.
> formalin-ethyl acetate sedimentation t.
> hemoconcentration t.
> immunoelectrotransfer blot t.
> immunohistochemical probe t.
> immunoperoxidase t.
> indirect immunofluorescence t.
> induced sputum t.
> iron-hematoxylin-phosphotungstic acid t.
> isoelectric focusing t.
> isoenzyme t.
> Kato-Katz thick smear t.
> Kato thick smear t.
> Knott t.
> lysis centrifugation t.
> Mantoux t.
> McKee-Farrar t.
> Movat t.
> plaque neutralization t.
> QBC t.
> quantitative buffy coat t.
> restriction fragment length polymorphism t.
> RFLP t.
> sedimentation t.
> sedimentation/centrifugation t.
> semiquantitative culture t.
> Sheather sucrose-flotation t.
> in situ hybridization t.
> smear t.
> zinc sulfate flotation t.

technology
> in vivo expression t. (IVET)

Tectibacter vulgaris (b)

Tectiviridae

Tectivirus (v)

tectus
> *Bacteroides* t.

TEE
> total energy expenditure
> transesophageal echocardiograph
> transesophageal echocardiography

Teejel

Teething
> Babee T.
> Numzit T.

tegetincola
    Flavobacterium t.
Tegopen
Tegretol
Tegrin
Tegrin-HC Topical
tegument
tegumentaria
    leishmaniasis t.
Tehran virus (TEHV)
TEHV
    Tehran virus
teichoic
    t. acid
    t. acid antibody
teicoplanin
Teladar Topical
Teladorsagia davtiani (p)
telangiectasia
    hemorrhagic t.
telemorph
teleomorph
telithromycin
Tellina virus (TV)
Telluria (b)
    T. chitinolytica
    T. mixta
Telmatoscopus albipunctatus
Telok Forest virus (TFV)
Telosporea
Telosporidia
TEM
    transmission electron microscopy
temafloxacin
Tembe virus (TMEV)
Tembusu virus (TMUV)
temefos
Temovate
temperans
    Acidovorax t.
temperata
    Photorhabdus t.
temperature
    basal body t.
temperature-sensitive phenotype
temporal
    t. arteritis
    t. ora serrata
    t. temperature gradient gel
    electrophoresis (TTGE)
temporary parasite
temporomandibular joint arthrogram

Tempra
    T. Cold Care
tenacious
tenax
    Eristalis t.
    Thermoproteus t.
    Trichomonas t.
Tenchoff catheter
Tench reovirus
tendae
    Streptomyces t.
tenderness
    cervical motion t.
    rebound t.
    suprapubic t.
tendinitis, tendonitis
tendon-reflex relaxation
tenebrarius
    Streptomyces t.
tenebrosa
    Cuterebra t.
tenella
    Eimeria t.
    Isaria t.
    Sarcocystis t.
tenesmus
    t. leukocyte
tenia
teniacide
teniafuge
tenial
teniasis
    somatic t.
tenicide
teniform
tenifugal
tenifuge
tenioid
teniposide
tenofovir
    t. disoproxil fumarate
Ten-O-Six
tenosynovitis
    destructive t.
    tuberculous t.
Tensaw virus (TENV)
Tensilon
tenue
    Caryophanon t.
    Cylindrocarpon cylindroides var. *t.*
    Eubacterium t.
    Rhodospirillum t.

T

NOTES

537

tenuicollis
    Cysticercus t.
    Opisthorchis t.
tenuifolia
    Amanita t.
tenuis
    Candida t.
    Dirofilaria t.
    Glycomyces t.
    Nitrosospira t.
    Rhodocyclus t.
    Trichostrongylus t.
tenuissima
    Alternaria t.
tenuistylus
    Culicoides t.
Tenuivirus (v)
TENV
    Tensaw virus
tepidarius
    Porphyrobacter t.
    Thermithiobacillus t.
    Thiobacillus t.
Tepidimonas ignava (b)
tepidum
    Chlorobium t.
    Chromatium t.
    Thermochromatium t.
Tequin
Terak Ophthalmic Ointment
terangae
    Sinorhizobium t.
teratocarcinoma
teratogenesis
teratogenic
teratogenicity
Terazol
    T. Vaginal
terbinafine
    t. (oral)
    t. (topical)
terconazole
teres
    Drechslera t.
    Pelodera t.
terevasa
    Pilimelia t.
terfenadine
Terfziaceae
Termeil virus (TERV)
terminal
    t. hematuria
    t. ileitis
    t. illness
    t. spore
terminalis
    Acanthocephala t.

termitida
    Sporomusa t.
termitidis
    Bacteroides t.
    Clostridium t.
    Desulfovibrio t.
    Sebaldella t.
    Sporobacter t.
termitum
    Streptomyces t.
termone
Ternidens deminutus (p)
terpene
terpenica
    Thauera t.
terpenotabidum
    Corynebacterium t.
terpin
    t. hydrate
    t. hydrate and codeine
Terrabacter tumescens (b)
Terracoccus luteus (b)
Terra-Cortril Ophthalmic suspension
terrae
    Actinokineospora t.
    Aureobacterium t.
    Gordonia t.
    Janibacter t.
    Microbacterium t.
    Mycobacterium t.
    Rhodococcus t.
    Sphingomonas t.
    Sphingopyxis t.
    Sporolactobacillus t.
terraenovae
    Calliphora t.
terragena
    Demetria t.
terramebiasis
Terramycin
    T. I.M. Injection
    T. Oral
    T. w/Polymyxin B Ophthalmic
      Ointment
Terranova decipiens (p)
terrea
    Pantoea t.
terregens
    Arthrobacter t.
    Aureobacterium t.
    Microbacterium t.
terreneum
    Eupenicillium t.
terrenus
    Ureibacillus t.
terrestre
    Trichophyton t.

terrestris
  Hyphelia t.
  Lumbricus t.
terretris
  Thielavia t.
terreum
  Scolecobasidium t.
terreus
  Aspergillus t.
  Cryptococcus t.
terricola
  Acanthamoeba t.
  Methylarcula t.
  Rhabditis t.
terrigena
  Comamonas t.
  Rauoltella t.
territans
  Culex t.
Tersa-Tar
tertanae
tertian
  t. fever
  t. malaria
  t. parasite
tertiana
  Plasmodium malariae t.
tertiary
  t. disease
  t. neurosyphilis
  t. syphilis
tertium
  Clostridium t.
TERV
  Termeil virus
Tesamone Injection
tescorum
  Simulium t.
Tessalon Perles
Tessaracoccus bendigoensis (b)
tessellarius
  Clavibacter michiganensis subsp. *t.*
  Corynebacterium michiganense subsp. *t.*
test
  AccuProbe *Campylobacter* Culture Identification T.
  AccuProbe Culture Confirmation T.
  Accu-Staph t.
  acetamide utilization t.
  acetate utilization t.
  acetoin production t.

N-acetyl-ʟ-cysteine-sodium hydroxide t. (NALC test)
acidometric t.
acid phosphatase t.
Acridine-Orange Leukocyte Cytospin T.
ACTH t.
adonitol fermentation t.
agar diffusion t.
agar dilution t.
ALA porphyrin t.
alpha-galactosidase t.
amebiasis serological t.
Ames t.
amidon fermentation t.
amine t.
Amplicor *Chlamydia trachomatis* t.
Amplicor *Mycobacterium tuberculosis* t.
Amplified *Mycobacterium tuberculosis* Direct T.
ANA t.
anthraxin skin t.
antibiotic-associated colitis toxin t.
antibody t.
anti-LFLA t.
antitreponemal antibody t.
API Rapid Strep t.
API STAPH t.
API Staph-IDENT t.
arabinose fermentation t.
ᴅ-arabitol fermentation t.
arginine t.
arylsulfatase activity t.
autofluorescence t.
automated reagin t. (ART)
bacitracin susceptibility t.
Bactcard *Candida* t.
bacterial phagocytosis t.
Bactigen *Haemophilus influenzae* type B t.
battery of t.'s
Bauer-Kirby susceptibility t.
bentonite flocculation t. (BFT)
beta-*N*-acetylglucosaminidase production t.
beta-galactosidase t.
beta-lactamase production t.
bile solubility t.
biopsy urease t.
broth dilution t.
broth susceptibility t.

T

NOTES

test (*continued*)

    Brucella card t.
    ^{13}C-labeled urea breath t.
    ^{14}C-labeled urea breath t.
    Calmette t.
    CAMP t.
    Candida skin t.
    capillary indirect
      hemagglutination t.
    capillary precipitin t.
    carbenicillin t.
    carbohydrate base t.
    card agglutination trypanosomiasis t.
      (CATT)
    casein hydrolysis t.
    catalase t.
    cat scratch skin t.
    cellobiose fermentation t.
    cellulose acetate t.
    cephalosporin t.
    cercarial agglutination t.
    CF t.
    Christie, Atkins, and Munch-
      Petersen t.
    chromogenic cephalosporin t.
    chromogenic enzyme substrate t.
    circumoval precipitin t.
    citrate utilization t.
    Clearview *Chlamydia* t.
    CLO t.
    Clostridium difficile t. (CLOtest)
    clue cell t.
    CMV antigen t.
    coagglutination t.
    coagulase t.
    coccidioidin skin t.
    colistin susceptibility t.
    colonial morphology t.
    complement fixation t.
    control t.
    Coombs t.
    cutaneous tuberculin t.
    cystine-tellurite blood agar t.
    cytochrome oxidase t.
    decarboxylase t.
    delta-aminolevulinic acid
      porphyrin t.
    deoxyribonuclease t.
    desferrioxamine susceptibility t.
    dexamethasone suppression t.
    dextran-from-sucrose t.
    dilution susceptibility t.
    direct agglutination t.
    direct antiglobulin t.
    direct Coombs t.
    direct fluorescent antibody t.
      (DFA)
    Directigen Meningitis T.

    direct immunofluorescence t.
    direct shiga toxin t.
    direct spot indole t.
    disk diffusion susceptibility t.
    DNA detection t.
    DNA hybridization t.
    DNA probe t.
    dulcitol fermentation t.
    duodenal string t.
    E t.
    ELISA t.
    enterobiasis t.
    epsilometer t. (E-test)
    erythritol fermentation t.
    esculin hydrolysis t.
    exoantigen t.
    exoantigen extraction t.
    Fairley t.
    false-negative patch t.
    FAS t.
    fecal concentration t.
    fibrinolysis t.
    filter in situ hybridization t.
    flocculation t.
    fluorescent actin staining t.
    fluorescent-denitrification t.
    fluorescent treponemal antibody
      absorption t. (FTA-ABS, FTA-
      Abs)
    fluorescent treponemal antigen-
      absorption t.
    formol-gel t.
    Frei t.
    FTA-ABS t.
    fungal precipitin t.
    furazolidone disk t.
    GAS antigen t.
    Gehan t.
    gelatinase t.
    gelatin hydrolysis t.
    Gen-Probe Pace 2 *Chlamydia* t.
    germ tube t.
    gluconate fermentation t.
    glucose fermentation t.
    glycerol fermentation t.
    glycogen fermentation t.
    glycogen hydrolysis t.
    GonoGen I t.
    Group A Streptococcus Direct T.
      (GP-ST)
    group B *Streptococcus* antigen t.
    group D antigen t.
    growth inhibition t.
    HAD t.
      hemadsorption test
    HAI t.
      hemagglutination inhibition test
    hair-baiting t.

HCG t.
Helicobacter pylori culture and urease t.
Helicobacter pylori urea breath t.
hemadsorption t. (HAD test)
hemadsorption virus t.
hemadsorption virus t. type 1, 2
hemagglutination inhibition t. (HAI test)
HerpChek t.
heterophil antibody t.
High and Leifson t.
histoplasmin skin t.
Hivagen antibody t.
H_2S t.
human chorionic gonadotropin t.
hybridization t.
hydrogen sulfide triple sugar iron t.
ICON Strep A t.
IDCF t.
ID32 Staph strip t.
IDTP t.
IgM t.
IHA t.
immune fluorescent antibody t.
immunodiffusion complement-fixing t.
immunodiffusion tube precipitin t.
immunofluorescence antibody t.
indirect Coombs t.
indirect fluorescent antibody t. (IFAT)
indole production t.
indoxyl acetate hydrolysis t.
inositol fermentation t.
intradermal t.
inulin t.
iron uptake t.
MYO-isositol fermentation t.
Jordan tartrate t.
Kahn t.
kanamycin susceptibility t.
Kirby-Bauer disc diffusion t.
Kirby-Bauer susceptibility t.
Kline t.
KPG skin t.
Kruskal-Wallis t.
LA t.
lactose fermentation t.
LAP t.
    leucine aminopeptidase test

latex agglutination t.
Legionella antigen t.
leishmanin skin t.
lepromin skin t.
leucine aminopeptidase t. (LAP test)
leukocyte esterase t. (LET)
liver enzyme t.
liver function t.
lupus band t.
Lyme disease antibody t.
lysine decarboxylase t.
lysostaphin susceptibility t.
lysozyme t.
Machado-Guerreiro t.
macroscopic broth dilution t.
Macro-Vue RPR Card T.
malonate utilization t.
maltose fermentation t.
mannitol fermentation t.
D-mannitol fermentation t.
mannose fermentation t.
D-mannose fermentation t.
Mantel-Haenszel t.
Mazzotti t.
MD t.
melezitose fermentation t.
melibiose fermentation t.
Meritec GC t.
metabolic products t.
methyl red t
4-methylumbelliferyl-beta-D-glucoronidase t. (MUG)
4-methylumbelliferyl-beta-D-glucuronidase t.
MHA-TP t.
    microhemagglutination test for *Treponema pallidum*
microbial susceptibility t.
microdilution broth dilution t.
microdilution broth susceptibility t.
microdilution serum bactericidal t.
microimmunofluorescence t.
microscopic agglutination t. (MAT)
MicroTrak direct fluorescent-antibody t.
microtube dilution t.
milk proteolysis t.
minimum inhibitory concentration susceptibility t.
Minitek *Neisseria* t.
miracidial immobilization t.
miracidium-hatching t.

NOTES

test *(continued)*
modified oxidase t.
Moeller decarboxylation t.
mono t.
Monospot t.
Monosticon Dri-Dot t.
Montenegro skin t.
motility t.
mouse neutralization t.
mucate fermentation t.
mucin clot t.
MUG t.
Murex *Candida albicans* t.
Mycobacterium leprae-stimulated
  lymphocyte transformation t.
N-acetylglucosamine fermentation t.
Nagler t.
NALC t.
    N-acetyl-L-cysteine-sodium
      hydroxide test
nalidixic acid t.
NAP t.
Neisseria gonorrhoeae DNA
  detection t.
Neisseria-Kwik t.
Neufeld capsular t.
neutralization t.
niacin accumulation t.
nitrate disk t.
nitrate reduction t.
nitrite reduction t.
Nitrocefin disk t.
nontreponemal serologic t.
nontreponemal syphilis t.
novobiocin susceptibility t.
nucleic acid amplification t.
nucleic acid hybridization t.
NucliSens t.
occult blood t.
Optochin susceptibility t.
ornithine t.
oxidase t.
oxidative-fermentative t.
Padebact GC OMNI t.
passive hemagglutination t.
Paul-Bunnell t.
PCR amplification t.
penicillinase t.
penicillin disk t.
penicillin skin t.
penicilloyl polylysine skin t.
Phadebact coagglutination t.
Phadebact GC OMNI t.
Phadebact *Haemophilus* t.
Phadebact *Haemophilus influenzae*
  type b COA t.
phenylalanine deaminase t.
pigment production t.

Pneumocystis carinii t.
POCkit HSV-2 Rapid T.
polysaccharide synthesis t.
PPD t.
PPL skin t.
precipitin t.
Pre-pen skin t.
prick t.
probe t.
pulmonary function t. (PFT)
pyocyanin t.
pyoverdin t.
PYR t.
pyrazinamidase t.
pyrrolidonyl arylamidase t.
quellung t.
radioallergosorbent t. (RAST)
raffinose fermentation t.
rapid antigen-detection t. (RADT)
rapid carbohydrate degradation t.
rapid carbohydrate utilization t.
rapid dipstick t.
RapiDEC aurease t.
RapiDEC Staph t.
rapid fermentation t.
rapid latex agglutination t.
rapid plasma reagent t.
rapid plasma reagin t.
rapid plasma reagin circle card t.
  (RPR-CT)
rapid streptococcal antigen t.
reaginic t.
reagin screen t. (RST)
recombinant HIV-1 latex
  agglutination t.
Remel t.
reverse CAMP t.
L-rhamnose fermentation t.
ribose fermentation t.
RIM-*Neisseria* t.
rose bengal t.
RPR CARD t.
Sabin-Feldman dye t.
salicin fermentation t.
Salmonella O antigen t.
salt tolerance t.
Schilling t.
schistosome egg-hatching t.
Schlichter t.
Scotch tape t.
scratch t.
Serodia-Myco II t.
serologic t.
serum antimicrobial activity t.
serum bactericidal t.
serum IFA t.
sialidase production t.
Sia water t.

skin t.
slide coagulase t.
Slidex Staph t.
sodium chloride tolerance t.
sorbitol fermentation t.
sorbose fermentation t.
Staf-Sistem 18-R t.
Stamey t.
standard tube agglutination t.
  (STA)
StaphASE t.
StaphAurex t.
Staph Rapid t.
Staphylatex t.
Staph-Zym t.
starch hydrolysis t.
string t.
sucrose t.
sulfamethoxazole/trimethoprim t.
  (SXT test)
superoxol t.
swab t.
SXT t.
    sulfamethoxazole/trimethoprim test
syphilis screening t.
TA t.
D-tagatose fermentation t.
tetrazolium reduction t.
thermonuclease t.
thermostable endonuclease t.
thyroid function t. (TFT)
toluidine red unheated serum t.
  (TRUST)
tourniquet t.
ToxA t.
toxigenicity t.
Toxin A T.
TPI t.
treadmill stress t.
trehalose fermentation t.
treponemal syphilis t.
Treponema pallidum t.
Treponema pallidum
  hemagglutination t. (TPHA)
Treponema pallidum
  immobilization t.
Trichophyton skin t.
triphenyltetrazolium chloride t.
triple sugar iron t.
TSI t.
TTC t.
tube agglutination t.

tube coagulase t.
tuberculin t.
tuberculin skin t. (TST)
tuberculosis skin t.
turamose fermentation t.
Tween-80 hydrolysis t.
tyrosine hydrolysis t.
Tzanck t.
unheated serum reagin t. (USR
  test)
urea breath t. (UBT)
urea hydrolysis t.
urease activity t.
urine dipstick t.
urine leukocyte esterase t.
USR t.
    unheated serum reagin
    unheated serum reagin test
UV light t.
vancomycin t.
VDRL slide t.
Venereal Disease Research
  Laboratory t. (VDRL)
Veri-Staph t.
virus fluorescent antibody t.
Voges-Proskauer t.
Wassermann t.
Weil-Felix t.
Western blot t.
whiff t.
xanthine hydrolysis t.
xylan fermentation t.
xylitol fermentation t.
xylose fermentation t.
D-xylose fermentation t.
yellow pigment t.

testa
Testacealobosia
testaceum
    Aureobacterium t.
    Brevibacterium t.
    Curtobacterium t.
    Microbacterium t.
testicular
    t. atrophy
    t. tuberculosis
testing
    adrenocortical axis t.
    Amplicor t.
    anaerobic susceptibility t.
    antibiotic sensitivity t.
    antifungal susceptibility t.

NOTES

testing *(continued)*
  antimicrobial susceptibility t.
  antimycobacterial susceptibility t.
  auditory brain-stem response t.
  BodPod t.
  breath H$_2$ t.
  cefinase t.
  cephalosporinase production t.
  counseling and t. (C&T)
  cryptococcal antigen t.
  DTH t.
  fungal skin t.
  genotypic t.
  group A *Streptococcus* antigen t.
  Haemophilus influenzae
    susceptibility t.
  HC t.
      home collection testing
  HIV-1 drug resistance t.
  HIV-1 mutations t.
  home collection t. (HC testing)
  HSV antibody t.
  immune status t.
  intracutaneous tuberculin skin t.
  intradermal skin t.
  KOH t.
  Mantoux skin t.
  microdilution susceptibility t.
  molecular probe t.
  Neisseria gonorrhoeae
    susceptibility t.
  neuropsychologic t.
  Nitrocefin t.
  NucliSens t.
  penicillin allergy skin t.
  penicillinase-producing organisms
    susceptibility t.
  pH t.
  phenotypic t.
  potassium hydroxide t.
  proportional susceptibility t.
  RSV t.
  sensitive/less sensitive enzyme
    immunoassay t.
  serologic t.
  skin t.
  S/LS EIA t.
  susceptibility t.
  tuberculin skin t.
  urodynamic t.
  whiff t.
Testoderm
  T. Transdermal System
  T. TTS patch
Testopel Pellet
testosterone (T)
  aqueous t.
  t. cypionate

  t. enanthate
  free t.
  t. propionate
  t. replacement therapy
  serum t.
  serum total t.
  total t.
testosteroni
  Comamonas t.
  Pseudomonas t.
Test-PPD
  Sclavo T.-P.
Testudinaceae
testudinalis
  Culicoides t.
testudinis
  Mycoplasma t.
  Pasteurella t.
testudinoris
  Corynebacterium t.
tetani
  Clostridium t.
  Clostridium t., Harvard strain 401
tetanolysin
tetanomorphum
  Clostridium t.
tetanospasmin
tetanus
  t. antitoxin (TAT)
  cephalic t.
  cryptogenic t.
  diphtheria and t. (DT)
  t. and diphtheria (tD)
  diphtheria, pertussis and t. (DPT)
  t. and diphtheria toxoid
  generalized t.
  t. immune globulin (TIG)
  t. immune globulin (human)
  t. immunoglobulin (TIG)
  localized t.
  neonatal t.
  t. toxin
  t. toxoid plain
  t. vaccine
tetany
TETEV
  Tete virus
Tete virus (TETEV)
Tetracap Oral
tetrachloroethylene
tetracoccus
tetracycline (TCN)
  bismuth subsalicylate, metronidazole,
    and t.
  t. hydrochloride
tetracycline-resistant *Neisseria*
  gonorrhoeae **(TRNG)**
Tetracyn

tetradius
> *Anaerococcus* t.
> *Peptostreptococcus* t.

tetradon poisoning

tetraedrale
> *Angulomicrobium* t.

Tetragenococcus (b)
> T. halophilus
> T. muriaticus

tetragenus

Tetrahymena pyriformis

TetraImmune vaccine

1,4,5,6-tetrakisphosphate
> D-myoinositol -t.

tetramastigote

tetramera
> *Drechslera* t.

Tetrameres strigiphila (p)

tetramethylparaphenylene diamine

tetramethylphenylene diamine

tetramethylrhodamine isothionate (TMRI)

Tetramitus (p) (*See* **Chilomastix mesnili**)

Tetramune vaccine

tetraodonis
> *Alteromonas* t.
> *Pseudoalteromonas* t.
> *Pseudoalteromonas haloplanktis* subsp. *t.*

Tetraodontiformes

Tetrapetalonema (p)

tetraplegia

Tetraploa aristata (f)

tetraptera
> *Aspiculuris* t.

Tetrasphaera (b)
> T. australiensis
> T. japonica

tetrasporus
> *Lipomyces* t.

Tetratrichomonas
> T. didelphis
> T. ovis

tetrazolium reduction test

tetrazonus
> *Aspergillus* t.

tetrodonic acid

tetrodotoxin

Texacort Topical

texasensis
> *Saccharothrix* t.

TFAV
> Thiafora virus

TFT
> thyroid function test
> trifluorothymidine

TFV
> Telok Forest virus

TG
> *Toxoplasma gondii*

T/Gel
> Neutrogena T.

TGT
> transdermal glyceryl trinitrate

thailandense
> *Dactylosporangium* t.

thailandensis
> *Burkholderia* t.
> *Weissella* t.

thalassemia
> alpha-t.
> beta-t.
> heterozygous t.

thalassemic

thalassica
> *Methylophaga* t.

thalassium
> *Chloroherpeton* t.
> *Microbacterium* t.

Thalassomonas viridans (b)

thalidomide

thallic

thallium
> t. negative

thallium-201

thallium-avid

thallium-gallium scanning

thallophyte

thallus

Thalomid

thalpophilum
> *Flavobacterium* t.
> *Sphingobacterium* t.

thalpophilus
> *Thermoactinomyces* t.

Thamnidiaceae

Thauera (b)
> T. aromatica
> T. chlorobenzoica
> T. linaloolentis
> T. mechernichensis
> T. selenatis
> T. terpenica

T

NOTES

Thayer-Martin medium
theicola
    Xanthomonas t.
Theiler
    T. murine encephalomyelitis virus
    (TMEV)
theileri
    Borrelia t.
    Trypanosoma t.
Theileria (p)
Thelazia
    T. *californiensis*
    T. *callipaeda*
    T. *gulosa*
    T. *lacrymalis*
    T. *skrjabini*
thelaziasis
Thelaziidae
Thelaziinae
Thelazoidea
thelcter
    Aedes t.
Thelebolaceae
Thelephoraceae
T-helper
    T.-h. cell
    T.-h. lymphocyte
Theo-24
Theobid
theobromae
    Botryodiplodia t. (*See Lasiodiplodia*
    theobromae)
    Lasiodiplodia t.
Theochron
Theoclear-80
Theoclear L.A.
Theo-Dur
Theolair
theophylline
    t. and guaifenesin
theoretically
theory
    cellular immune t.
    immune t.
Theo-Sav
Theospan-SR
Theo-SR
Theostat-80
Theovent
Theo-X
TheraCys
Theraflu Non-Drowsy Formula
  Maximum Strength
therapeutic
    t. malaria
    t. paracentesis
Theraplex Z

therapy
    adoptive cellular t.
    antibacterial t.
    antifungal t.
    antimicrobial t.
    antineoplastic t.
    antioxidant t.
    antiprotease t.
    antiprotozoal t.
    antiretroviral triple combination t.
    antisense oligonucleotide viral t.
    antitoxoplasmosis t.
    antitrichomonal t.
    antituberculosis t.
    antitumor necrosis factor-based t.
    antiviral t.
    argon laser t.
    combination t.
    cytokine t.
    directly observed t. (DOT)
    dual nucleoside t.
    electron beam t.
    empiric t.
    epitope-specific t.
    graft suppression t.
    hematopoietic stem cell gene t.
    heterovaccine t.
    highly active antiretroviral t.
    (HAART)
    HIV t.
    hormonal t.
    hormonal replacement t. (HRT)
    HSC gene t.
    hydroxyurea salvage t.
    immune-modulating t.
    immunomodulating t.
    immunosuppressive t.
    immunotoxin t. (IT)
    infectious disease t.
    infusion t.
    interferon t.
    intralesional t.
    intravirion gene t.
    low-dose VV t.
    parenteral t.
    photodynamic t.
    potent antiretroviral t.
    quadruple t.
    rescue t.
    salvage t.
    salvage highly active
    antiretroviral t. (SHAART)
    sequential antibiotic t.
    streamlining antibiotic t.
    suppressive t.
    synergistic t.
    T-cell gene t.

testosterone replacement t.
triple drug t.
Thermacetogenium phaeum (b)
thermacidophilum
    Bifidobacterium t.
Thermaerobacter marianensis (b)
Thermanaerovibrio (b)
    T. acidaminovorans
    T. velox
thermarum
    Thermotoga t.
Thermazene
Thermicanus aegyptius (b)
Thermithiobacillus tepidarius (b)
thermoacetica
    Moorella t.
thermoaceticum
    Clostridium t.
thermoacetophila
    Methanosaeta t.
    Methanothrix t.
thermoacetoxidans
    Desulfotomaculum t.
Thermoactinomyces (b)
    T. candidus
    T. dichotomicus
    T. intermedius
    T. peptonophilus
    T. putidus
    T. sacchari
    T. thalpophilus
    T. vulgaris
Thermoactinomycetaceae
thermoaerophilus
    Aneurinibacillus t.
    Bacillus t.
thermoaggregans
    Methanobacterium t.
thermoalcaliphilum
    Clostridium t.
    Methanobacterium t.
thermoalcalitolerans
    Streptomyces t.
thermoamylovorans
    Bacillus t.
Thermoanaerobacter (b)
    T. acetoethylicus
    T. brockii subsp. *brockii*
    T. brockii subsp. *finnii*
    T. brockii subsp. *lactiethylicus*
    T. ethanolicus
    T. finnii

    T. italicus
    T. kivui
    T. mathranii
    T. siderophilus
    T. subterraneus
    T. sulfurophilus
    T. thermocopriae
    T. thermohydrosulfuricus
    T. wiegelii
    T. yonsiensis
Thermoanaerobacterium (b)
    T. aotearoense
    T. polysaccharolyticum
    T. saccharolyticum
    T. thermosaccharolyticum
    T. thermosulfurigenes
    T. xylanolyticum
    T. zeae
Thermoanaerobium (b)
    T. acetigenum
    T. brockii
Thermoascus aurantiacus (f)
thermoautotrophica
    Moorella t.
thermoautotrophicum
    Clostridium t.
    Methanobacterium t.
thermoautotrophicus
    Methanothermobacter t
    Streptomyces t.
Thermobacillus xylanilyticus (b)
Thermobacteroides (b)
    T. acetoethylicus
    T. leptospartum
    T. proteolyticus
thermobenzoicum
    Desulfotomaculum t.
Thermobifida (b)
    T. alba
    T. fusca
Thermobispora bispora (b)
Thermobrachium celere (b)
thermobutyricum
    Clostridium t.
thermocarboxydovorans
    Streptomyces t.
thermocarboxydus
    Streptomyces t.
thermocatenulatus
    Bacillus t.
    Geobacillus t.

T

NOTES

thermocellum
    Clostridium t.
Thermochromatium tepidum (b)
thermocisternum
    Desulfotomaculum t.
Thermocladium modestius (b)
thermocloacae
    Bacillus t.
Thermococcaceae
Thermococcales
Thermococcus (b)
    T. acidaminovorans
    T. aegaeus
    T. aggregans
    T. alcaliphilus
    T. barophilus
    T. celer
    T. chitonophagus
    T. fumicolans
    T. gorgonarius
    T. guaymasensis
    T. hydrothermalis
    T. pacificus
    T. peptonophilus
    T. profundus
    T. siculi
    T. stetteri
    T. waiotapuensis
    T. zilligii
thermocopriae
    Clostridium t.
    Thermoanaerobacter t.
thermocoprophilus
    Streptomyces t.
Thermocrinis ruber (b)
Thermocrispum (b)
    T. agreste
    T. municipale
thermodenitrificans
    Bacillus t.
    Geobacillus t.
Thermodesulfobacterium (b)
    T. commune
    T. hveragerdense
    T. mobile
Thermodesulforhabdus norvegica (b)
Thermodesulfovibrio (b)
    T. islandicus
    T. yellowstonii
thermodiastatica
    Microbispora t.
thermodiastaticus
    Streptomyces t.
thermoduric
thermoferrooxidans
    Leptospirillum t.
Thermofilum pendens (b)

thermoflava
    Amycolatopsis t.
thermoflavus
    Streptomyces t.
thermoflexum
    Methanobacterium t.
thermoformicicum
    Methanobacterium t.
thermoglucosidasius
    Bacillus t.
    Geobacillus t.
thermogriseus
    Streptomyces t.
Thermohalobacter berrensis (b)
thermohalophilum
    Dichotomicrobium t.
Thermohydrogenium kirishiense (b)
thermohydrosulfuricum
    Clostridium t.
thermohydrosulfuricus
    Thermoanaerobacter t.
thermolacticum
    Clostridium t.
    Clostridium stercorarium subsp. *t.*
Thermoleophilum (b)
    T. album
    T. minutum
thermoleovorans
    Bacillus t.
    Geobacillus t.
thermolineatus
    Streptomyces t.
thermolithotrophicus
    Methanococcus t.
thermolithotrophum
    Desulfurobacterium t.
thermoluteolus
    Hydrogenophilus t.
thermometry
    ear t.
Thermomicrobium (b)
    T. fosteri
    T. roseum
Thermomonospora (b)
    T. alba
    T. chromogena
    T. curvata
    T. formosensis
    T. fusca
    T. mesophila
    T. mesouviformis
Thermomonosporaceae
thermomutatus
    Aspergillus t.
Thermomyces lanuginosus (f)
Thermonema (b)
    T. lapsum
    T. rossianum

thermonitrificans
    Streptomyces t.
thermonuclease test
thermopalmarium
    Clostridium t.
thermopapyrolyticum
    Clostridium t.
thermophila
    Methanosarcina t.
    Methanothrix t.
    Myceliophthora t.
    Pseudonocardia t.
    Saccharopolyspora t.
    Spirochaeta t.
thermophile
thermophilic
thermophilica
thermophilicum
    Methanogenium t.
thermophilum
    Bifidobacterium t.
    Dictyoglomus t.
    Flavobacterium t.
    Methanobacterium t.
    Symbiobacterium t.
thermophilus
    Deferribacter t.
    Desulfovibrio t.
    Hydrogenobacter t.
    Methanoculleus t.
    Methylococcus t.
    Saccharococcus t.
    Sphaerobacter t.
    Streptococcus t.
    Streptococcus salivarius subsp. t.
    Thermus t.
thermophylic
Thermoplasma (b)
    T. acidophilum
    T. volcanium
thermoplasma
Thermoproteaceae
Thermoproteales
Thermoproteus (b)
    T. neutrophilus
    T. phage TTV 1–3 virus
    T. tenax
thermoresistibile
    Mycobacterium t.
thermorosea
    Microbispora t.

thermoruber
    Bacillus t.
    Brevibacillus t.
thermosaccharolyticum
    Clostridium t.
    Thermoanaerobacterium t.
thermosapovorans
    Desulfotomaculum t.
Thermosipho (b)
    T. africanus
    T. geolei
    T. japonicus
    T. melanesiensis
thermosphacta
    Brochothrix t.
Thermosphaera aggregans (b)
thermosphaericus
    Bacillus t.
    Ureibacillus t.
thermostabile
thermostable
    t. direct hemolysin (TDH)
    t. endonuclease test
thermosuccinogenes
    Clostridium t.
thermosulfata
    Thiomonas t.
thermosulfatus
    Thiobacillus t.
thermosulfidooxidans
    Sulfobacillus t.
thermosulfurigenes
    Thermoanaerobacterium t.
thermosulfurogenes
    Clostridium t.
Thermosyntropha lipolytica (h)
Thermoterrabacterium ferrireducens (b)
thermoterrenum
    Anaerobaculum t.
Thermothrix (b)
    T. azorensis
    T. thiopara
Thermotoga (b)
    T. elfii
    T. hypogea
    T. maritima
    T. neapolitana
    T. subterranea
    T. thermarum
thermotolerans
    Haloterrigena t.
    Kluyveromyces t.

T

NOTES

thermoviolaceus
    Streptomyces thermoviolaceus subsp.
      t.
thermovulgaris
    Streptomyces t.
Thermus (b)
    T. antranikianii
    T. aquaticus
    T. brockianus
    T. chliarophilus
    T. filiformis
    T. igniterrae
    T. oshimai
    T. ruber
    T. scotoductus
    T. silvanus
    T. thermophilus
Theroxide Wash
thetaiotaomicron
    Bacteroides t.
thiabendazole
thiacetazone
thiacytidine derivative
Thiafora virus (TFAV)
Thialkalicoccus limnaeus (b)
Thialkalimicrobium (b)
    T. aerophilum
    T. sibericum
Thialkalivibrio (b)
    T. denitrificans
    T. nitratis
    T. versutus
thiamazole
thiamine
thiaminolyticus
    Bacillus t.
    Paenibacillus t.
thiamphenicol
Thiara (p)
thiazolidinediones
thibaulti
    Aedes t.
thickening
    sausage-roll nerve t.
thick peripheral blood smear
Thielavia (f)
    T. heterothallica
    T. terretris
Thielaviopsis basicola
thienamycin
thienylalanine
Thimiri virus (THIV)
thin
    t. peripheral blood smear
thinking abnormality
thin-layer chromatography
ThinPrep
thioanomide

Thiobacillus (b)
    T. acidophilus
    T. albertis
    T. aquaesulis
    T. caldus
    T. concretivorus
    T. delicatus
    T. denitrificans
    T. ferrooxidans
    T. halophilus
    T. hydrothermalis
    T. intermedius
    T. neapolitanus
    T. novellus
    T. perometabolis
    T. rapidicrescens
    T. tepidarius
    T. thermosulfatus
    T. thiooxidans
    T. thioparus
    T. thyasiris
    T. versutus
thiobacteria
Thiobacterium bovistum (b)
Thiocapsa (b)
    T. halophila
    T. litoralis
    T. pendens
    T. pfennigii
    T. rosea
    T. roseopersicina
Thiococcus pfennigii (b)
thiocyanatum
    Methylobacterium t.
thiocyanatus
    Paracoccus t.
thiocycli
    Catenococcus t.
Thiocystis (b)
    T. gelatinosa
    T. minor
    T. violacea
    T. violascens
Thiodictyon (b)
    T. bacillosum
    T. elegans
Thioflavicoccus mobilis (b)
thiogenes
    Trichlorobacter t.
thioglycolate
Thiohalocapsa halophila (b)
thiol
Thiolamprovum pedioforme (b)
thioluteum
    Streptoverticillium t.
thioluteus
    Streptomyces t.

thiomalate
    gold sodium t.
Thiomargarita namibiensis (b)
Thiomicrospira (b)
    T. chilensis
    T. crunogena
    T. denitrificans
    T. frisia
    T. kuenenii
    T. pelophila
    T. thyasirae
Thiomonas (b)
    T. cuprina
    T. intermedia
    T. perometabolis
    T. thermosulfata
thiooxidans
    Acidithiobacillus t.
    Bosea t.
    Limnobacter t.
    Roseinatronobacter t.
    Thiobacillus t.
thiopara
    Thermothrix t.
thioparus
    Thiobacillus t.
Thiopedia rosea (b)
thiophila
    Desulfuromonas t.
Thioploca (b)
    T. araucae
    T. chileae
    T. ingrica
    T. schmidlei
Thiorhodaceae
Thiorhodococcus minor (b)
Thiorhodospira sibirica (b)
Thiorhodovibrio winogradskyi (b)
Thiosphaera pantotropha (b)
Thiospira winogradskyi (b)
Thiospirillum (b)
    T. jenense
thiosulfate
    t. citrate bile salts sucrose (TCBS)
    t. citrate bile salts sucrose agar
    sodium t.
thiosulfatigenes
    Desulfonispora t.
thiosulfatophilus
    Roseococcus t.
Thiosulfil

Thiothrix (b)
    T. defluvii
    T. eikelboomii
    T. fructosivorans
    T. nivea
    T. unzii
thiouracil
Thiovulum majus (b)
thiozymogenes
    Desulfocapsa t.
third-generation cephalosporin
THIV
    Thimiri virus
thivervalensis
    Pseudomonas t.
ThMoV
thoenii
    Propionibacterium t.
Thogotovirus (v)
Thogoto virus (THOV)
tholozani
    Ornithodoros t.
thomasi
    Acanthocephala t.
    Anopheles t.
thomasii
    Anaerobiospirillum t.
Thominx aerophilus (p)
thomssenii
    Corynebacterium t.
thonzonium
    neomycin, colistin, hydrocortisone,
    and t.
thoracentesis
    diagnostic t.
    t. fluid cytology
thoracic
    t. actinomycosis
    t. adenopathy
    t. gland
    t. manifestation
thoracostomy
thoraltensis
    Streptococcus t.
thornei
    Pasteuria t.
thorny-headed worm
Thosea
    T. asigna
    T. asigna virus
Thottapalayam virus (TPMV)

NOTES

THOV
Thogoto virus
Thraustochytriaceae
threadworm
three-day
t.-d. fever
t.-d. measles culture
three-in-one vaccine
three-phase bone scan
threonine kinase
thresher's lung
thriambus
Culex t.
thrill
hydatid t.
thrive
failure to t. (FTT)
throat
streptococcal sore t.
t. swab
t. viral culture
thrombi (*pl. of* thrombus)
thrombin
thrombocyte
thrombocythemia
essential t.
thrombocytopenia
atypical immune-mediated t.
HIV-related t.
immune t.
profound t.
thrombocytopenic purpura
thromboembolic disease
thrombohemorrhage
thrombopenia
thrombophlebitis
pelvic t.
septic nonsuppurative t.
septic pelvic t.
suppurative t.
thrombosis, pl. **thromboses**
cavernous sinus t.
deep vein t. (DVT)
internal carotid artery t.
mural t.
ovarian vein t.
puerperal ovarian vein t. (POVT)
septic t.
thrombospondin
thrombospondin-1 (TSP-1)
thrombospondin-related adhesive protein
thrombotic thrombocytopenic purpura (TTP)
thromboxane
thrombus, pl. **thrombi**
thrush
t. fungus
oral t.

thuringiensis
Bacillus t.
thyasirae
Thiomicrospira t.
thyasiris
Thiobacillus t.
thymidine
t. analog
t. kinase
Thymoctonan
thymopoiesis
thymosin alpha
thymosine-alpha$_1$
thymus
Thynnascaris (p)
Thyro-Block
thyroid function test (TFT)
thyroiditis
autoimmune t.
chagasic t.
Hashimoto t.
parasitic t.
thyroid-stimulating hormone (TSH)
thyroxine
L-thyroxine
thyrse
en t.
Thysanosoma actinoides (p)
Thysanotaenia congolensis (p)
tiabendazole
Tiacid
Tiamol
tianshanense
Mesorhizobium t.
Rhizobium t.
TIBC
total iron-binding capacity
serum TIBC
tibetense
Natronorubrum t.
tibia
proximal t.
saber t.
tibiamaculatus
Anopheles t.
Tibrogargan virus (TIBV)
TIBV
Tibrogargan virus
Ticar
ticarcillin
t. clavulanate
t. and clavulanate potassium
t. disodium
TICE BCG
tick
t. bite fever
hard t.
ixodid t.

Lone Star t.
pajaroello t.
t. paralysis
soft t.
t. toxicosis
t. typhus
tick-borne
t.-b. borreliosis
t.-b. encephalitis (TBE)
t.-b. encephalitis (Central European subtype)
t.-b. encephalitis (Eastern subtype)
t.-b. encephalitis virus (TBEV)
t.-b. relapsing fever
tide
alkaline t.
tidoxil
fozivudine t. (FZD)
tiedjei
Desulfomonile t.
TIG
tetanus immune globulin
tetanus immunoglobulin
Tigan
tigertop mushroom
tigre disease virus
TIL
tumor-infiltrating lymphocyte
tillae
Borrelia t.
Tilletiaceae
Tilligerry virus (TILV)
TILV
Tilligerry virus
Timboteua virus (TBTV)
Timbo virus (TIMV)
time
activated partial thromboplastin t. (aPTT)
dilute Russell viper venom t. (DRVVT)
prothrombin t. (PT)
prothrombin time and partial thromboplastin t. (PT/PTT)
t. to signal
Timecelles
Sinufed T.
time-dependent bactericidal activity
Timentin
timidum
Eubacterium t.
Mogibacterium t.

timonae
Massilia t.
timori
Brugia t.
timothy hay bacillus
TIMV
Timbo virus
Tinactin
T. for Jock Itch
Tinaroo virus (TINV)
tinctura
Fabry t.
tincture
Fungoid T.
t. of opium
Tindale agar
Tindallia magadiensis (b)
tindarius
Methanolobus t.
Tindholmur virus (TDMV)
T-inducer cell
tinea
t. barbae
t. capitis
t. circinata
t. corporis
t. cruris
t. faciei
t. favosa
t. glabrosa
t. imbricata
t. incognito
t. inguinalis
t. kerion
t. manus
t. manuum
t. nigra
t. nigra palmaris
t. pedis
t. sycosis
t. tonsurans
t. tropicalis
t. unguium
t. versicolor
Tine Test PPD
Ting
tingling throat syndrome
tinidazole
tinnitus
Tinted
Oxy-5 T.

T

NOTES

TINV
    Tinaroo virus
Tinver
tioconazole
Tipranavir
Tipula
    T. paludosa
Tipulidae
Tisit
    T. Blue Gel
    T. Liquid
    T. Shampoo
Tissierella (b)
    T. creatinini
    T. creatinophila
    T. praeacuta
tissoti
    Culicoides t.
tissue
    t. biopsy
    bronchus-associated lymphoid t.
    (BALT)
    core of t.
    t. culture assay (TCA)
    gut-associated lymphoid t. (GALT)
    t. imprint
    lymphoid t.
    mucosa-associated lymph t.
    (MALT)
    mucosa-associated lymphoid t.
    (MALT)
    t. schizont
    subcutaneous t.
titer
    antibody t.
    anti-DNase-B t.
    antistreptococcal DNase-B t.
    antistreptolysin O t.
    Aspergillus IgG t.
    Bordetella pertussis t.
    chickenpox t.
    cold agglutinin t.
    cold-reactive autoantibody t.
    Coxiella burnetii t.
    Coxsackie B_1 virus t.
    Coxsackie B_2 virus t.
    Coxsackie B_3 virus t.
    Coxsackie B_4 virus t.
    Coxsackie B_5 virus t.
    Coxsackie B_6 virus t.
    EBV t.
    encephalitis t.
    IFA t.
    IgG antibody t.
    IgM antibody t.
    Proteus OXK agglutinin t.
    RPR t.
    RSV t.

    serum antideoxyribonuclease-B t.
    serum inhibitory t.
    serum *Toxoplasma gondii*
      antibody t.
    streptococcal antibody t.
    TORCH t.
    toxoplasmosis t.
    VCA t.
    viral t.
    virus t.
    zoster t.
Ti-U-Lac HC
Tlacotalpan virus (TLNV)
T1-like viruses (v)
T4-like viruses (v)
T5-like viruses (v)
T7-like viruses (v)
TLNV
    Tlacotalpan virus
T lymphocyte-tropic
TMA
    transcription-mediated amplication
TMEV
    Tembe virus
    Theiler murine encephalomyelitis virus
TML
    typhimurium strain T.
TMP
    trimethoprim
TMP-SMX
    trimethoprim-sulfamethoxazole
TMP-SMZ
    trimethoprim-sulfamethoxazole
TMP/SMZ
TMRI
    tetramethylrhodamine isothionate
TMTX
    trimetrexate
TMUV
    Tembusu virus
T-mycoplasma
TNF
    tumor necrosis factor
TNF-a
    tumor necrosis factor-alpha
TNF-alpha
    tumor necrosis factor-alpha
TNM
    tumor-node-metastases
TnSNPV
    Trichoplusia ni SNPV
TOA
    tuboovarian abscess
toadstool poisoning
toast
    banana, white rice, apple, and
      white t. (BRAT)

banana, white rice, apple, and
   white t. diet
Tobamovirus (v)
TOBEC
   total body electrical conductivity
Tobia fever
TOBI Inhalation solution
TobraDex
   T. Ophthalmic
tobramycin
   t. and dexamethasone
   t. level
**tobramycin-impregnated polymethyl
   methacrylate spacer block**
Tobravirus (v)
Tobrex
   T. Ophthalmic
toe itch
tofu
Togaviridae
togoi
   Aedes t.
tokaiense
   Mycobacterium t.
Tokelau ringworm
tolaasii
   Pseudomonas t.
tolaasinivorans
   Mycetocola t.
tolbutamide
tolerance
   glucose t.
tolerans
   Hyphomicrobium facile subsp. *t.*
   Lactobacillus casei subsp. *t.*
   Lactobacillus paracasei subsp. *t.*
   Roseovarius t.
toletana
   Pichia t.
tolnaftate
tolosanus
   Parachordodes t.
toluclasticus
   Azoarcus t.
toluene
toluidine
   t. blue O stain
   t. red unheated serum test
   (TRUST)
tolulyticus
   Azoarcus t.
Tolumonas auensis (b)

toluolica
   Desulfobacula t.
Tolu-Sed DM
toluvora
   Azoarcus t.
Tolypocladium inflatum
tomato
   Macrosporium t.
Tombusvirus (v)
tomography
   computed t. (CT)
   computed transaxial t.
   positron emission t. (PET)
   single-photon emission t. (SPECT)
   single-photon emission computed t.
   (SPECT)
tompkinsii
   Leptosphaeria t.
Tomycine Ophthalmic
tongue
   posterior t.
   raspberry t.
   strawberry t.
tonkinense
   Cylindrocarpon t.
tonometer
tonsil
   Luschka t.
tonsillar
   t. biopsy
   t. crypt
   t. fossa
   t. pillar
   t. tissue
tonsillarum
   Erysipelothrix t.
tonsillitis
   necrotizing t.
tonsurans
   tinea t.
   Trichophyton t.
Topactin
tophaceous gout
Topica
   Polysporin T.
topical
   t. ablation
   Achromycin T.
   Aclovate T.
   Acticort T.
   Aeroseb-HC T.
   Akne-Mycin T.

T

NOTES

topical *(continued)*
Ala-Cort T.
Ala-Scalp T.
Alphatrex T.
Anusol HC-1 T.
Anusol HC-2.5% T.
Aristocort A T.
A/T/S T.
Baciguent T.
BactoShield T.
Betalene T.
betamethasone t.
Betatrex T.
Beta-Val T.
Borofax T.
CaldeCort T.
Caldesene T.
Carmol-HC T.
Cetacort T.
t. chlorhexidine gluconate
Cleocin T T.
Clinda-Derm T.
Cloderm T.
Corque T.
CortaGel T.
Cortaid Maximum Strength T.
Cortaid with Aloe T.
Cort-Dome T.
Cortef Feminine Itch T.
Cortizone-5 T.
Cortizone-10 T.
Cyclocort T.
Delcort T.
Del-Mycin T.
Delta-Tritex T.
Dermacort T.
Dermarest Dricort T.
Derma-Smoothe/FS T.
Dermolate T.
Dermtex HC with Aloe T.
DesOwen T.
dexamethasone t.
Diprolene AF T.
Diprosone T.
Dyna-Hex T.
Eldecort T.
Emgel T.
Eryderm T.
Erygel T.
Erymax T.
E-Solve-2 T.
ETS-2% T.
Eurax T.
Exelderm T.
Fluonid T.
Flurosyn T.
Flutex T.
fluticasone t.

FS Shampoo T.
Furacin t.
G-myticin T.
Gynecort T.
Hibiclens T.
Hibistat T.
Hi-Cor-1.0 T.
Hi-Cor-2.5 T.
Hycort t.
Hydrocort T.
hydrocortisone t.
Hydro-Tex T.
Hytone T.
t. imidazole
Kenalog T.
Kenonel T.
LactiCare-HC T.
Lanacort T.
Lida-Mantle HC T.
Locoid T.
Maxivate T.
Meclan T.
MetroGel T.
Micatin T.
t. microbicide
Monistat-Derm T.
Mycifradin Sulfate T.
Mycitracin T.
Mycogen II T.
Mycolog-II T.
Myconel T.
Mytrex F T.
NeoDecadron T.
Neomixin T.
N.G.T. T.
Novacet T.
Nutracort T.
t. nystatin
Orabase HCA T.
Ovide T.
Oxistat T.
Pedi-Pro T.
Penecort T.
Psorion T.
Retin-A Micro T.
Rogaine T.
Scalpicin T.
t. spastic paraparesis
Spectazole T.
Staticin T.
S-T Cort T.
Sulfacet-R T.
Sulfamylon T.
Synacort T.
Synalar T.
Synalar-HP T.
Synemol T.
Tegrin-HC T.

Teladar T.
terbinafine t.
Texacort T.
Topicycline T.
tretinoin t.
Triacet T.
triamcinolone t.
Tridesilon T.
t. trifluridine
Triple Antibiotic T.
Tri-Statin II T.
T-Stat T.
U-Cort T.
Valisone T.
Westcort T.
Topicort
Topicort-LP
Topicycline Topical
Topilene
Topisone
topoisomerase II inhibitor
Topsyn
TOPV
  trivalent poliovirus vaccine
Tor
  Vibrio cholerae O1 El T.
TORCH
  T. serology
  T. serology battery
  T. titer
tormentor
  Aedes t.
Tornalate
Toronto virus
Torovirus (v)
torovirus
torquens
  Lactobacillus coryniformis subsp. t.
torques
  Ruminococcus t.
torquis
  Psychroflexus t.
torrens
  Leptoconops t.
torresii
  Candida t.
torreyae
  Culicoides t.
torridus
  Culicoides t.
  Picrophilus t.
torticollis

tortilis
  Aedes t.
tortuosum
  Eubacterium t.
Torula (f)
  T. heteroderae
  T. humicola
Torulaspora
  T. hansenii
Torulomyces lagena (f)
Torulopsis (*See* **Candida**)
Torulospora (f)
torulosus
  Streptomyces t.
Toscana virus (TOSV)
Tospovirus (v)
TOSV
  Toscana virus
tosylchloramide aqueous solution
Totacillin
Totacillin-N
total
  t. abdominal fat (TAT)
  t. anomalous pulmonary circulation (TAPC)
  t. body electrical conductivity (TOBEC)
  t. body irradiation (TBI)
  t. body potassium (TBK)
  t. body water (TDW)
  t. energy expenditure (TEE)
  t. iron-binding capacity (TIBC)
  t. laryngectomy
  t. lymphocyte count
  t. parenteral nutrition (TPN)
  t. protein
  t. testosterone
Totivirus (v)
touch preparation
tourniquet test
Touro
  T. Ex
  T. LA
toweri
  Culex t.
townsendi
  Simulium t.
toxaphene
Toxascaris (p)
  T. leonina
ToxA test

T

NOTES

toxic
- t. cholangitis
- t. encephalopathy
- t. epidermal necrolysis
- t. epidermal neurolysis
- t. granulation
- t. hepatitis
- t. megacolon
- t. scarlet fever
- t. shock-like syndrome (TSLS)
- t. shock syndrome (TSS, TSST)
- t. shock syndrome toxin-1

toxicity
- calcium-mediated t.
- dose-limiting t. (DLT)
- hematologic t.
- immune-mediated t.
- liver t.
- mitochondrial t.
- nucleoside-associated mitochondrial t.

toxicogenic conjunctivitis

toxicology
- urine t.

toxicosis, pl. toxicoses
- tick t.

toxicus
- *Clavibacter t.*
- *Gambierdiscus t.*
- *Rathayibacter t.*

toxigenic
- t. bacterial infection
- t. strain

toxigenicity test

toxin
- adenylate cyclase t. (ACT)
- T. A Test
- bacterial t.
- beta t.
- botulinal t.
- T. CD enzyme immunoassay
- cholera t.
- clostridial t.
- dermonecrotic t. (DNT)
- diarrheal t.
- dinophysis t.
- diphtheria t.
- disulfiram-like t.
- edema t.
- emetic t.
- erythrogenic t.
- *Escherichia coli* shiga t.
- exfoliative t.
- heat-labile t.
- intracellular t.
- lethal t.
- pertussis t. (PT)
- Shiga t.

- Shiga-like t.
- tetanus t.
- zonula occludens t. (zot)

toxin-1
- toxic shock syndrome t.

toxin-induced diarrhea

toxin-mediated disease

toxinogenotyping

toxin-producing

Toxocara (p)
- *T. canis*
- *T. cati*
- *T. mystax*

toxocariasis

Toxocarinae

toxoid
- adsorbed tetanus t.
- diptheria t.
- fluid tetanus t.
- tetanus and diphtheria t.

toxoneme

Toxoplasma (p)
- *T.* antigen
- *T.* encephalitis (TE)
- *T. gondii* (TG)
- *T. gondii* encephalitis
- *T. gondii* encephalitis
- *T. gondii* meningoencephalitis
- *T.* infection
- *T.* serology

toxoplasma
- t. encephalitis

Toxoplasmatidae

toxoplasmic
- t. chorioretinitis
- t. encephalitis

toxoplasmosis
- acute acquired t.
- t. antibody
- brain t.
- cerebral t.
- congenital ocular t.
- ocular t.
- t. titer

Toxothrix trichogenes (b)

toxytricini
- *Streptomyces t.*

TP
- tube precipitin
- TP antibody

TPHA
- *Treponema pallidum* hemagglutination
- *Treponema pallidum* hemagglutination assay
- *Treponema pallidum* hemagglutination test
- TPHA Test Kit

T-Phyl

TPI
  Treponema pallidum immobilization
    TPI test
TPMV
  Thottapalayam virus
TPN
  total parenteral nutrition
T-prolymphocytic leukemia
Trabulsiella guamensis (b)
trabulsii
  Koserella t.
trace positive
tracer
  radiolabeled t.
trachea
  Syngamus t.
tracheal
  t. aspirate
  t. colonization factor
  t. cryptosporidiosis
  t. cytotoxin (TCT)
tracheiphila
  Erwinia t.
tracheiphilum
tracheitis
  fulminant t.
tracheobronchial tree
tracheobronchitis
  acute febrile t.
  herpetic t.
Tracheophilus cucumerinum (p)
tracheotomy
Trachipleistophora (p)
  T. anthropophthera
  T. hominis
trachoma
  follicular t.
  t. and inclusion conjunctivitis
    (TRIC)
  t. inclusion conjunctivitis
  ocular t.
  t. virus
trachomatis
  C complex strain of *Chlamydia t.*
  Chlamydia t. (CT)
trachomatous
  t. conjunctivitis
trachuri
  Vibrio t.
tract
  biliary t.
  female genital t.

genitourinary t.
portal t.
respiratory t.
selective decontamination of the
  digestive t. (SDD)
sinus t.
uveal t.
tractellum
tractuosus
  Flexibacter t.
trade name
traditional Chinese medicine (TCM)
tranovarially
transactivation
transaminase
  alanine t.
  t. elevation
  hepatic t.
  serum aspartate t.
  serum glutamate oxaloacetate t.
transbronchial biopsy
transcript
  latency-associated t. (LAT)
transcriptase
  reverse t. (RT)
transcription-based amplification
transcription initiation codon
transcription-mediated amplification
  (TMA)
transdermal
  Alora T.
  Climara T.
  Esclim T.
  Estraderm T.
  t. glyceryl trinitrate (TGT)
  t. testosterone
  Vivelle T.
transducer-associated
transducer dome
transduction
  genetic t.
transesophageal
  t. echocardiograph (TEE)
  t. echocardiography (TEE)
transfection
transfer
  adenovirus-mediated gene t.
  cell t.
transferase
transferrin
transformant

T

NOTES

transformation
    cell t.
    t. zone (T zone)
transfusion
    cryoprecipitate t.
    exchange t.
    granulocyte t.
    t. hepatitis
    platelet t.
    red blood cell t.
transfusion-dependent anemia
transiens
    Simulium t.
transient
    t. aplastic anemia
    t. aplastic crisis (TAC)
    t. complete hematologic remission
    t. erythroblastopenia
    t. grade 2 granulocytopenia
    t. ischemic attack
    t. monocytopenia
    t. obstructive hydrocephalus
    t. pancytopenia
transjugular needle biopsy of the liver
translaryngeal aspiration
translation-competent genome
translucens
    Xanthomonas t.
transmissible
    t. mink encephalopathy
    t. neurodegenerative disease
    t. plasmid
transmission
    airborne t.
    t. electron microscopy (TEM)
    fecal t.
    mother-to-child t. (MTCT)
    mucocutaneous t.
    perinatal t.
    person-to-person t.
    transovarial t.
    transstadial t.
    vertical t.
transmural eosinophilic granuloma
transovarial
    t. transmission
transpeptidase
    gamma-glutamyl t. (gamma-GTP)
transpeptidation
transplacental
    t. transfer
transplacentally
transplant
    bone marrow t. (BMT)
    peripheral blood stem cell t.
Trans-Plantar Transdermal Patch
transplantation
    autologous stem cell t. (ASCT)

    bone marrow t. (BMT)
    European bone marrow t. (EBMT)
    heart t.
    hematopoietic stem cell t.
    pancreatic t.
    stem cell t.
transport
    electron t.
    t. host
    t. medium
transposable
    t. element
transposon
    conjugative t.
transstadial transmission
transtadially
transthoracic
    t. echocardiography
    t. pulmonary aspirate
transtracheal
    t. aspirate
    t. aspiration (TTA)
transudate
transudative ascites
transurethral prostate procedure (TURP)
transvaalensis
    Alkaliphilus t.
transvaginal
transvalensis
    Nocardia t.
transvector
transvenous
Trans-Ver-Sal Transdermal Patch
transverse myelitis
trapanicum
    Halobacterium t.
    Halorubrum t.
trauma
    abdominal t.
    corneal t.
traumatic
    t. herpes
    t. tap
travassosi
    Simulium t.
traveler's diarrhea
travisi
    Culicoides t.
trazodone
TRBV
    Tribec virus
treadmill stress test
treatment
    Anti-Acne Spot T.
    antibiotic t.
    azole t.
    Clear Pore T.

cytostatic t.
emetine t.
Head & Shoulders Intensive T.
t. modality
No-Name Dandruff T.
preventive t.
septicemia t.
sexual assault t.
Trecator-SC
tree
tracheobronchial t.
trehala
trehalophila
Pichia t.
trehalose
t. fermentation test
trehalosei
Nocardiopsis t.
trehalosi
Pasteurella t.
tremae
Pseudomonas t.
Trematoda
trematode
digenetic t.
trematum
Bordetella t.
Tremellaceae
Tremellales
tremens
delirium t
tremor
epidemic t.
optic atrophy t.
tremulousness
trench
t. fever
t. mouth
Trendar
Trental
Treponema (b)
T. amylovorum
T. brennaborense
T. bryantii
T. denticola
T. hyodysenteriae
T. innocens
T. lecithinolyticum
T. maltophilum
T. medium
T. minutum
T. pallidum

T. pallidum antigen
T. pallidum hemagglutination
(TPHA)
T. pallidum hemagglutination assay
(TPHA)
T. pallidum hemagglutination test
(TPHA)
T. pallidum immobilization (TPI)
T. pallidum immobilization test
T. pallidum subsp. pertenue
T. pallidum test
T. paraluiscuniculi
T. parvum
T. pectinovorum
T. pertenue
T. saccharophilum
T. socranskii subsp. buccale
T. socranskii subsp. paredis
T. socranskii subsp. socranskii
T. succinifaciens
treponemal
t. lysis
t. syphilis test
treponematosis
treponeme
treponemicidal
tretinoin
t. (topical)
trevisanii
Klebsiella t.
triacetin
Triacet Topical
triacetyloleandomycin
Triacin-C
triaconazole
triad
Charcot t.
Triaderm
trial
ALBI t.
field t.
HIV Network for Prevention T.'s
(HIVNET)
Triam-A Injection
Triamcine-A
Scheinpharm T.-A.
triamcinolone
t. (inhalation, oral)
nystatin and t.
t. (systemic)
t. (topical)
Triam Forte Injection

NOTES

Triaminic
    T. AM Decongestant Formula
    T. Cold & Fever
    T. Decongestant & Expectorant
    T. DM-D
    T. DM Daytime
    T. Long Lasting DM
Triaminicol Multi-Symptom Cold syrup
Triamonide Injection
triangularis
    Phaeotheca t.
triangulosporum
    Ophiostoma t.
triannulatus
    Anopheles t.
    Anopheles triannulatus t.
Triatoma (p)
    T. brasiliensis
    T. dimidiata
    T. infestans
    T. lethal paralysis virus
    T. recurva
    T. rubida
    T. rubida uhleri
    T. rubrofasciata
    T. sanguisuga
triatomid bug
Triatominae
triazolam
triazole
tribavirin
Tribec virus (TRBV)
Triblidiaceae
tribocorum
    Bartonella t.
TRIC
    trachoma and inclusion conjunctivitis
    TRIC agent
    TRIC agent culture
Tricercomonas
    T. intestinalis
Trichiales
trichina
Trichinella (p)
    T. britovi
    T. nativa
    T. nelsoni
    T. pseudospiralis
    T. serology
    T. spiralis
trichinelliasis
Trichinellidae
trichinellosis
trichiniasis
trichiniferous
trichinization
trichinoscope

trichinosis
    t. granuloma
    t. serology
trichinous
trichite
trichium
    Paramecium t.
trichiura
trichiuris
    Trichocephalus t.
trichloroacetic acid
Trichlorobacter thiogenes (b)
Trichobilharzia physellae (p)
Trichocephala
trichocephaliasis
Trichocephalus trichiuris (p)
Trichocladium asperum (f)
Trichococcus flocculiformis (b)
Trichocomaceae
Trichoconis padwickii (f)
trichocyst
Trichodectes canis (p)
Trichodectidae
Trichoderma (f)
    T. glaucum
    T. lignorum
    T. longibrachiatrum
    T. narcissi
    T. nigrescens
    T. truncorum
    T. viride
trichodes
    Lactobacillus t.
trichogenes
    Toxothrix t.
trichoides
    Oscillochloris t.
Tricholoma magnivelare (f)
Tricholomataceae
Trichomaris invadens (f)
Trichometasphaeria (f)
    T. fusispora
    T. turcica
trichomonacide
trichomonad
Trichomonadida
Trichomonadidae
trichomonal
    t. infection
    t. urethritis
    t. vulvovaginitis
Trichomonas (p)
    T. culture
    T. foetus
    T. medium Number 2
    T. Pap smear
    T. tenax
    T. urethritis

T. *vaginalis* (TV)
T. *vaginalis* culture
T. *vaginalis* wet preparation
trichomoniasis
vaginal t.
t. vaginitis
trichomycetosis
trichomycosis
t. axillaris
t. chromatica
t. nodosa
t. nodularis
t. palmellina
trichonocardiosis
t. axillaris
trichonodosis
trichophytic
trichophytid
trichophytin
Trichophyton (f)
T. *ajelloi*
T. *equinum* var. *autotrophicum*
T. *equinum* var. *quickeanum*
T. *gloriae*
T. *gourvilii*
T. *kanei*
T. *megninii*
T. *mentagrophytes*
T. *mentagrophytes* var. *goetzii*
T. *persicolor*
T *schoenleinii*
T. *simii*
T. skin test
T. *soudanense*
T. *terrestre*
T. *tonsurans*
T. *vanbreuseghemii*
T. *verrucosum*
T. *violaceum*
T. *yaoundei*
trichophytosis
t. barbae
t. capitis
t. corporis
t. cruris
t. unguium
Trichoplusia
T. *ni*
T. *ni* SNPV (TnSNPV)
Trichoptera
Trichopyton acuminatum
Trichosanthes cucumerina (p)

Trichosoma
trichosomatous
Trichosomoidiae
Trichosphaeriaceae
trichosporium
Methylosinus t.
Trichosporon (f)
T. *aneurinolyticum*
T. *appendiculare*
T. *asahii*
T. *asteroides*
T. *balzeri*
T. *beigelii*
T. *brasiliense*
T. *byrdii*
T. *capitatum*
T. *cerebriforme*
T. *coremiformis*
T. *cutaneum*
T. *dendriticum*
T. *faecale*
T. *giganteum*
T. *gracile*
T. *gracile*
T. *granulosum*
T. *hortai*
T. *humahuaquensis*
T. *infestans*
T. *inkin*
T. *jirovecii*
T. *klebahnii*
T. *krusei*
T. *lithogenes*
T. *matalense*
T. *minor*
T. *mucoides*
T. *ovale*
T. *ovoides*
T. *paraguay*
T. *pararugosum*
T. *pardi*
T. *penicillatum*
T. *piscium*
T. *proteolyticum*
T. *pullulans*
T. *ribeiroi*
T. *rotundatum*
T. *rugosum*
T. *uncinatum*
T. *venezuelunsis*
Trichosporonoides (f)
trichosporonosis

T

NOTES

trichosporosis
Trichostomatia
trichostrongyle
trichostrongyliasis
Trichostrongylidae
Trichostrongyloidea
trichostrongylosis
Trichostrongylus (p)
    T. axei
    T. brevis
    T. capricola
    T. colubriformis
    T. tenuis
trichothecenolyticum
    Aureobacterium t.
    Microbacterium t.
Trichothecium (f)
Trichovirus (v)
trichrome
    t. stain
trichuriasis
Trichurida
Trichuridae
trichuriid nematode
Trichuris (p)
    T. suis
    T. vulpis
trichuris
    t. dysentery syndrome
triclabendazole
Tri-Clear Expectorant
triclosan
tricolor
    Streptomyces t.
tricompartmental
Tricula
tricuspid
    t. valve
tricuspis
    Ollulanus t.
tricyclic antidepressant (TCA)
Tridesilon Topical
tridihexethyl
Trifed-C
triflorae
    Lasiodiplodia t.
trifluorothymidine (TFT)
    t. drops
trifluridine
    t. solution
    topical t.
trifolii
    Rhizobium t.
trifurcata
    Ostertagia t.
trigeminal
    t. dermatome

    t. nerve
    t. neuralgia
triglyceride
    long-chain t. (LCT)
    medium-chain t. (MCT)
    serum t.
trigonosporus
    Microascus t.
TriHIBit
trihydrate
    amoxicillin t.
    ampicillin t.
    Apo-Ampi T.
    Jaa Amp T.
    Nu-Ampi T.
    Taro-Ampicillin T.
Tri-Immunol
triiodothyronine
Trikacide
TRIKOF-D
Tri-Kort Injection
Trilisate
trilocalis
    Hysterolecitha t.
Trilog Injection
Trilone Injection
trima
trimastigote
trimethobenzamide
trimethoprim (TMP)
    t. and polymyxin B
    sulfamethoxazole and t. (SMX-
    TMP)
trimethoprim-dapsone
trimethoprim-induced hematotoxicity
trimethoprim-sulfamethoxazole (TMP-
    SMX, TMP-SMZ, TS)
trimethylsilyl derivative
trimetrexate (TMTX)
    t. glucuronate
Trimmatostroma betulinum
trimodality regimen
trimorphic
trimorphism
trimorphous
Trimox
Trimoxil
Trimpex
trinitrate
    transdermal glyceryl t. (TGT)
Triofed syrup
Tripedia
Tripedia/ActHIB
tripethoprim
Triphenyl Expectorant
triphenyltetrazolium
    t. chloride (TTC)
    t. chloride test

triphosphatase
  adenosine t. (ATPase)
  guanosine t.
triphosphate
  adenosine t. (ATP)
  azidothymidine t. (AZTTP)
  deoxyguanosine t. (dGTP)
  dideoxyadenosine t. (ddATP)
  guanosine t. (GTP)
triple
  T. Antibiotic Topical
  t. drug therapy
  t. phosphate
  t. phosphate stone
  t. quartan
  t. sugar iron (TSI)
  t. sugar iron agar
  t. sugar iron test
  t. sulfa
  t. sulfa tablet
  T. X Liquid
triple-lumen central venous catheter
triplex
  Mycobacterium t.
Triposed
  T. syrup
  T. tablet
Triprofed
triprolidinc
  t. and pseudoephedrine
  t., pseudoephedrine, and codeine
trisaccharide
  3-deoxy-D-manno-octulosonic acid t.
trisalicylate
  choline magnesium t.
trisdine
triseriatus
  Aedes t.
trismus
trisodium phosphonoformate
Trisoject Injection
Tri-Statin II Topical
tristriatulus
  Culicoides t.
Trisulfa
trisulfapyrimidine
Trisulfa-S
Tri-Tannate Plus
Tritec
tritici
  Clavibacter t.
  Corynebacterium t.

  Gaeumannomyces graminis var. *t.*
  Ochrobactrum t.
  Pyemotes t.
  Rathayibacter t.
Tritimovirus (v)
Tritin
  Dr Scholl's Maximum Strength T.
Tritirachium (f)
  T. brumptii
  T. musae
  T. oryzae
  T. purpureum
  T. roseum
  T. shiotae
Tritrichomonas foetus (p)
Trivagizole 3
trivalent poliovirus vaccine (TOPV)
triviale
  Mycobacterium t.
trivittatum
  Simulium t.
trivittatus
  Aedes t.
  t. virus (TVTV)
trivolus
  Echinostoma t.
TRNG
  tetracycline-resistant *Neisseria gonorrhoeae*
Trobicin
Trocal
trocar suprapubic cystostomy
trochanter
troche
  clotrimazole t.
  Mycelex T.
Troglotrema salmincola
Troglotrematata
Troglotrematidae
troglotrematoid
trogontum
  Helicobacter t.
troleandomycin
Trombetas virus
Trombicula (p)
  T. alfreddugesi
  T. autumnalis
trombiculiasis
trombiculid
Trombiculidae
Trombidiformes
Trombidiidae

T

NOTES

Trombidioidea
tromethamine
    fosfomycin t.
    lodoxamide t.
Tropheryma whippelii (b)
trophic nucleus
trophoblastic metazoa
trophochromatin
trophochromidia
trophonucleus
trophozoite
    biflagellated t.
    Giardia t.
tropica
    acrodermatitis vesiculosa t.
    Leishmania t.
    myositis purulenta t.
    Nocardiopsis t.
tropical
    t. anemia
    t. measles
    t. medicine
    t. myositis
    t. pulmonary eosinophilia
    t. pyomyositis
    t. sore
    t. spastic paraparesis
    t. spastic paresis/HTLV-1-associated myelopathy (TSP/HAM)
    t. splenomegaly
    t. splenomegaly syndrome (TSS)
    t. sprue
    t. typhus
    t. ulcer
tropicalis
    Acetobacter t.
    Blomia t.
    Candida t.
    tinea t.
tropici
    Rhizobium t.
tropicum
    Chrysosporium t.
    granuloma t.
    granuloma inguinale t.
tropism
    cell t.
    macrophage t.
    T-cell t.
Trosyd
trota
    Aeromonas t.
trough blood level
TRoV
trovafloxacin
Trovan
Trubanaman virus (TRUV)

true
    t. hyperthermia
    t. hypha
trueperi
    Halobacillus t.
    Rhodospira t.
    Sphingomonas t.
truncal
    t. fat
    t. obesity
truncal-to-appendicular
truncata
    Simulium t.
truncatum
    Pseudamphistomum t.
truncatus
    Bulinus t.
truncorum
    Trichoderma t.
Truphylline
TRUST
    toluidine red unheated serum test
TRUV
    Trubanaman virus
Truxcillin
TRV
    Tanjong Rabok virus
trypan blue staining
trypanicidal
trypanicide
trypanid
trypanocidal
trypanocide
Trypanoplasma
Trypanosoma (p)
    T. avium
    T. brucei
    T. brucei brucei
    T. brucei gambiense
    T. brucei rhodesiense
    T. congolense
    T. cruzi
    T. cruzi meningoencephalitis
    T. cruzi parasitemia
    T. equinum
    T. equiperdum
    T. evansi
    T. gondii
    T. lewisi
    T. rangeli
    T. theileri
    T. vivax
trypanosomal
    t. chancre
    t. parasite
trypanosomatid
Trypanosomatidae
Trypanosomatina

trypanosome
    t. stage
trypanosomiasis
    acute t.
    African t.
    American t.
    Chagas t.
    chronic t.
    East African t.
    Gambian t.
    t. peripheral blood preparation
    Rhodesian t.
    South American t.
    West African t.
trypanosomic
trypanosomicide
trypanosomid
tryparsamide
Tryparsone
trypomastigote
    CSF t.
trypticase soy agar
tryptophan broth
Trysul
TS
    trimethoprim-sulfamethoxazole
tsetse
    t. fly
TSH
    thyroid-stimulating hormone
tshawytschae
    Scolecobasidium t.
TSI
    triple sugar iron
        TSI agar
        TSI test
TSLS
    toxic shock-like syndrome
TSP-1
    thrombospondin-1
TSP/HAM
    tropical spastic paresis/HTLV-1-
      associated myelopathy
TSS
    toxic shock syndrome
    tropical splenomegaly syndrome
      Strep TSS
        streptococcal toxic shock syndrome
TSST
    toxic shock syndrome
TST
    tuberculin skin test

T-Stat Topical
T-strain
    Mycoplasma T.-s.
tsuchiyae
    Candida t.
Tsukamurella (b)
    T. inchonensis
    T. paurometabola
    T. pulmonis
    T. tyrosinosolvens
    T. wratislaviensis
tsukubaensis
    Streptomyces t.
tsunoense
    Catellatospora t.
Tsuruse virus (TSUV)
tsutsugamushi
    t. disease
    t. fever
    Orientia t.
    Rickettsia t.
TSUV
    Tsuruse virus
TTA
    transtracheal aspiration
TTC
    triphenyltetrazolium chloride
      TTC test
TTE
    two-dimensional transthoracic
    echocardiography
TTGE
    temporal temperature gradient gel
    electrophoresis
TTP
    thrombotic thrombocytopenic purpura
T-tropic
    T-cell-tropic
    T-tropic virus
TTV
    TT virus
TTV1
    T. virus
    T. virus group
T1–T6 virus
T6–T20 virus
TT virus (TTV)
TU
    tuberculin unit
TUAV
    Turuna virus

T

NOTES

tubaeforme
  Ancylostoma t.
tubal
  t. factor infertility
  t. ligation
Tubasal
tube
  t. agglutination (TA)
  t. agglutination test
  blood lysis t.
  t. coagulase test
  t. diffusion
  fallopian t.
  t. feeding
  germ t.
  microhematocrit capillary t.
  Miescher t.
  mycobacteria growth indicator t.
    (MGIT)
  nasogastric t.
  NG t.
  PEG t.
  percutaneous endoluminal
    gastrostomy t.
  t. placement
  t. precipitin (TP)
  t. precipitin antibody
  QBC malaria t.
  quantitative buffy coat malaria t.
  roll t.
Tuberaceae
tubercidicus
  Streptomyces t.
tubercle
  t. bacillus
Tuberculariaceae
Tuberculariales
tuberculatus
  Haematopinus t.
tuberculid
  papulonecrotic t.
tuberculin
  Koch t.
  t. skin test (TST)
  t. skin testing
  t. test
  t. unit (TU)
**5 tuberculin unit strength purified
  protein derivative (PPD)**
tuberculocidal
tuberculoid
  borderline t. (BT)
  t. leprosy
tuberculoma
tuberculosis (TB)
  abdominal t.
  adult t.

aerosol transmission of
  Mycobacterium t.
anal t.
areactive t.
articular t.
bone and joint t.
t. of the brain
calvarial t.
cavitary t.
central nervous system t.
chronic hematogenous t.
chronic pulmonary t.
congenital t.
conjunctival t.
cryptic miliary t.
cutaneous t.
t. cutis
dermal t.
drug-resistant t.
endobronchial t.
endometrial t.
epididymal t.
extrapulmonary t.
t. of eyelid
fallopian tube t.
genitourinary t.
head and neck t.
hepatobiliary t.
HIV-associated t.
ileocecal t.
intestinal t.
t. of jejunum
t. of lacrimal system
laryngeal t.
lymphatic t.
mandibular t.
MDR t.
t. meningitis
miliary t.
multiple-drug resistant t. (MDRTB)
musculoskeletal t.
mycobacteria other than
  Mycobacterium t. (MOTT)
Mycobacterium t. (MTB)
Mycobacterium tuberculosis subsp. t.
neonatal t.
ocular t.
oral cavity t.
orbital t.
orificial t.
osteoarticular t.
ovarian t.
pancreatic t.
parotid gland t.
penile t.
pericardial t.
peripheral osteoarticular t.
pituitary t.

pleural t.
primary t.
pulmonary t.
reactivated t.
renal t.
t. of the retina
salivary gland t.
serous t.
skeletal t.
t. skin test
skull t.
testicular t.
urethral t.
vaginal t.
vertebral t.
vulvovaginal t.
warty t.
W strain of *Mycobacterium t.*

tuberculostearic acid
tuberculous

t. abscess
t. adenoiditis
t. arthritis
t. ascites
t. blepharitis
t. chancre
t. colitis
t. dactylitis
t. empyema
t. enteritis
t. gingivitis
t. gumma
t. iritis
t. lymphadenitis
t. meningitis
t. osteomyelitis
t. otitis media
t. pericarditis
t. peritonitis
t. pleurisy
t. polyserositis
t. spondylitis
t. tenosynovitis

tubericola
Lasiodiplodia t.
tuberosity
ischial t.
tuberosum
Simulium t.
Tubersol
Tubeufiaceae

tubiashi
Acanthamoeba t.
tubiashii
Vibrio t.
Tubifera ferruginosa (f)
tubingensis
Aspergillus t.
tuboovarian abscess (TOA)
tubular
t. cell
t. interstitial nephritis
tubule
malpighian t.
tubulointerstitial
t. lesion
t. nephritis
tubuloreticular
tucsonensis
Legionella t.
Tucunduba virus
tuggertensis
Leptopsylla algira t.
tuirus
Streptomyces t.
tularemia
glandular t.
oculoglandular t.
oropharyngeal t.
pharyngeal t.
pneumonic t.
t. serology
typhoidal t.
ulceroglandular t.
t. vaccine
tularemic conjunctivitis
tularensis
Francisella tularensis subsp. *t.*
Francisella tularensis biogroup *t.*
tulasnei
Mycosphaerella t.
Tulasnellaceae
Tulasnellales
Tulostomataceae
Tulostomatales
tumbu
t. dermal myiasis
t. fly
tumefaciens
Agrobacterium t.
tumescens
Arthrobacter t.

T

NOTES

tumescens (continued)
>> Pimelobacter t.
>> Terrabacter t.

tumor
>> t. antigen
>> t. burden
>> Buschke-Löwenstein t.
>> t. challenge
>> episialin t.
>> mucosa-associated lymphoid t.
>> (MALToma)
>> t. necrosis factor (TNF)
>> t. necrosis factor-alpha (TNF-a,
>> TNF-alpha)
>> t. regression
>> t. vaccine
>> vanishing t.
>> t. virus
>> Wilms t.

tumor-associated
>> t.-a. antigen (TAA)
>> t.-a. glycoprotein-72

tumor-draining
>> t.-d. lymph node (TDLN)
>> t.-d. lymph node cell (TDLNC)

tumor-infiltrating
>> t.-i. leukocyte
>> t.-i. lymphocyte (TIL)

tumor-lysis syndrome
tumor-node-metastases (TNM)
TuMV
tundrae
>> Acetobacterium t.

***Tunga penetrans* (p)**
tungiasis
Tungidae
tunicata
>> Pseudoalteromonas t.

tunica vaginalis
tunnel
>> t. disease
>> t. infection

tunneled catheter
tupaiae
>> Brugia t.

***Tupaia* virus**
turamose fermentation test
turbata
>> Cellulomonas t.
>> Oerskovia t.

Turbatrix aceti
Turbellaria
turbidity
turbinate
turbot reovirus
turcica
>> Drechslera t.

>> Setosphaeria t.
>> Trichometasphaeria t.

turcicum
turdi
>> Borrelia t.

turgida
>> Lagochilascaris t.

turgidiscabies
>> Streptomyces t.

turgidum
>> Dictyoglomus t.
>> Gnathostoma t.

turicata
>> Ornithodoros t.

turicatae
>> Borrelia t.

***Turicella otitidis* (b)**
turicensis
>> Actinomyces t.

turkestanica
>> Orientobilharzia t.

turkey
>> t. coronavirus
>> t. rhinotracheitis virus

turkeypox virus
Turkish massage of Weinstein
turkmeniaca
>> Actinomadura t.
>> Microtetraspora t.
>> Nonomuraea t.

turkmenica
>> Haloterrigena t.

turkmenicus
>> Halococcus t.

Turlock virus (TURV)
turonicum
>> Spiroplasma t.

TURP
>> transurethral prostate procedure

Turuna virus (TUAV)
TURV
>> Turlock virus

tusciae
>> Bacillus t.
>> Mycobacterium t.

Tusibron
Tusibron-DM
Tuskegee Syphilis Study
Tuss
>> HycoClear T.

Tussafed Drops
Tussafin Expectorant
Tuss-Allergine Modified T.D. Capsule
Tussar SF syrup
Tuss-DM
Tussigon
Tussionex
Tussi-Organidin DM NR

Tuss-LA
Tussodan DM
Tussogest Extended Release Capsule
TV
    Tellina virus
    Trichomonas vaginalis
        TV culture
TVTV
    trivittatus virus
TVX virus
TWAR
    Chlamydia T.
T-wave
Tween
    human blood bilayer T. (HBT)
Tween-80 hydrolysis test
Twice-A-Day Nasal solution
twitching
    myoclonic t.
two-dimensional transthoracic
  echocardiography (TTE)
Twort-d'Herelle phenomenon
Twort virus
TY1-S-33 medium
Ty21a typhoid vaccine
tykaremia
Tylenchida
Tylenchidae
Tylenchinae
Tylenol
    T. Cold Medication (Daytime)
    T. Cold No Drowsiness
    T. Cough
    T. Cough with Decongestant
    T. Flu Maximum Strength
Tymovirus (v)
tympanic
    t. membrane
    t. membrane aspirate
tympanocentesis
tympanometry
tympanostomy tube insertion
TYMV
Ty-Pap
type
    t. A, B, C, D satellite virus
    t. A viral hepatitis
    t. b conjugate vaccine
    t. b encapsulated strain
    t. culture
    t. F virus
    t. II mixed cryoglobulinemia

    nomenclatural t.
    t. strain
typeable
typhi
    Rickettsia t.
    Salmonella t.
    serotype t.
typhimurium
    Salmonella t.
    t. strain GM3
    t. strain TML
Typhim Vi
typhinia
typhlitis
Typhlocoelum cucumerinum (p)
typhoid
    abdominal t.
    t. bacillus
    t. cholera
    t. fever
    fowl t.
    Malaysian t.
    t. vaccine
typhoidal
    t. listeremia
    t. tularemia
typhus
    endemic t.
    epidemic t.
    flea-borne t.
    louse-borne t.
    mite t.
    North Asian tick t.
    Queensland tick t.
    recrudescent louse-borne t.
    scrub t.
    tick t.
    tropical t.
typing
    bacteriophage t.
    electrophoretic protein t.
    epidemiologic t.
    HLA t.
    molecular t.
    multilocus sequence t. (MLST)
    Opa t.
    phage t.
    radiorespirometry t.
    serologic t. (SERO)
    verocytotoxin t.
tyrobutyricum
    Clostridium t.

T

NOTES

Tyrodone Liquid
tyrofermentans
    Brachybacterium t.
Tyroglyphoidea
Tyroglyphus longior (p)
Tyrophagidae
Tyrophagus
    T. farinae
    T. putrescentiae
    T. siro
tyrosinase
tyrosine hydrolysis test
tyrosinosolvens
    Tsukamurella t.

tyrrhenii
    Microtetraspora t.
TYSGM-9 medium
Tyuleniy virus (TYUV)
TYUV
    Tyuleniy virus
Tyzzeria (p)
Tzanck
    T. preparation
    T. smear
    T. test

U3 virus
UAA
UAD Otic
Uasin Gishu disease virus
uberis
    Streptococcus u.
ubiquitin
ubiquitous
    u. saprophytic mold
ubonensis
    Burkholderia u.
UBT
    urea breath test
U-Cort Topical
uda
    Cellulomonas u.
UFISH
    ultrasensitive fluorescence in situ
    hybridization
Ugandan eye worm
Uganda S virus (UGSV)
UGSV
    Uganda S virus
uhleri
    Triatoma rubida u.
UICC
    Union Internationale Contre La Cancer
    UICC classification
    UICC stage
ulcer
    Aden u.
    aphthous u.
    Bairnsdale u.
    burrowing u.
    Buruli u.
    chancroid u.
    chiclero u.
    corneal u.
    decubitus u.
    diphtheritic u.
    duodenal u.
    Gaboon u.
    genital aphthous u.
    herpetic u.
    HIV genital u.
    hypopyon u.
    idiopathic oral aphthous u.
    intraoral u.
    lingual u.
    Meleny u.
    Mooren corneal u.
    oriental u.
    peptic u.
    perforated duodenal u.
    pudendal u.

    tropical u.
    Zambesi u.
ulcerans
    Corynebacterium u.
    Fusobacterium u.
    Mycobacterium u.
ulcerating granuloma of pudenda
ulceration
    aphthous u.
    chancroidal u.
    esophageal u.
    genital u.
    herpetic u.
    mucosal u.
    neuropathic u.
    oral u.
    syphilitic u.
    vulvovaginal u.
ulcerative
    u. colitis
    u. disease
    u. disease rhabdovirus
    u. enteritis
    u. gingivostomatitis
    u. subcutaneous nodule
ulceroglandular
    u. disease
    u. tularemia
uli
    Lactobacillus u.
uliginosa
    Cellulophaga u.
    Cytophaga u.
    Zobellia u.
uliginosum
    Clostridium u.
    Flavobacterium u.
    Methanobacterium u.
Ulocladium chartarum (f)
ULR-LA
Ultra
    Grisactin U.
Ultracef
Ultracortenol
ultracytostome
ultrafiltrate
ultramicrosize
    griseofulvin u.
Ultramop
ultrasensitive
    u. fluorescence in situ hybridization
    (UFISH)
    u. quantitative PCR
    u. viral load assay
ultrasonography

U

ultrasound
  abdominal u.
  u. guidance
  kidney u.
  peripheral arteries and veins u.
  popliteal u.
  renal u.
  retroperitoneal u.
ultrasound-enhanced
  u.-e. latex agglutination
  u.-e. particle agglutination
Ultravate
ultraviolet (UV)
  u. germicidal irradiation (UVGI)
  u. irradiation
  u. light B therapy
ultunense
  Clostridium u.
ulvae
  Pseudoalteromonas u.
Umatilla virus (UMAV)
UMAV
  Umatilla virus
umbilical hernia
umbilicated papule
umbilication
umbilicus
Umbravirus (v)
Umbre virus (UMBV)
umbrina
  Actinomadura u.
  Hyphelia u.
umbrinus
  Streptomyces u.
UMBV
  Umbre virus
UMN
  upper motor neuron
  UMN disease
UNAIDS
  United Nations AIDS Control Program
unambiguous
unambiguously
unarmed rostellum
Unasyn
UNAV
  Una virus
Una virus (UNAV)
uncal herniation
Uncinaria (p)
  U. americana
  U. stenocephala
uncinariasis
Uncinariidae
uncinatum
  Arthroderma u.
  Trichosporon u.
Uncinocarpus (f)

uncircumcised
uncomplicated lupus
undecylenate
undecylenic acid and derivatives
underhilli
  Simulium u.
undicola
  Allorhizobium u.
  Rhizobium u.
undina
  Alteromonas u.
  Pseudoalteromonas u.
undosum
  Heliobacterium u.
undulant fever
undulata
  Holospora u.
undulate
undulating membrane
undulipodium
ungiari
  Gigantorhynchus u.
unguis
  Aspergillus u.
unguis-hominis
  Pyrenochaeta u.-h.
unguium
  tinea u.
  trichophytosis u.
unheated
  u. serum reagin (USR test)
  u. serum reagin test (USR test)
Uni-Ace
unicellular
unicolor
  Culicoides u.
unicompartmental
  double u.
Unicort
unidimensional echocardiogram
unidirectional
Uni-Dur
uniflagellate
uniforme
  Eubacterium u.
uniformis
  Bacteroides u.
  Nocardia u.
uniguttulata
uniguttulatum
  Filobasidium u.
uniguttulatus
  Cryptococcus u.
unilateral hyperlucent lung
unilocular hydatid cyst
unimicrobial bacteremia
uninhibited bladder

Union
U. Internationale Contre La Cancer (UICC)
U. Internationale Contre La Cancer classification
U. Internationale Contre La Cancer stage

Unipen
U. Injection
U. Oral

Uniphyl
Uni-Pro
unit
bone marrow transplant u. (BMTU)
colony forming u. (CFU)
ELISA u.
hemagglutinating u.
intensive care u. (ICU)
medical intensive care u. (MICU)
million u.'s (MU)
pediatric intensive care u. (PICU)
spinal intensive care u. (SICU)
Svedburg u. (S)
tuberculin u. (TU)

United
U. Nations AIDS Control Program (UNAIDS)
U. States Public Health Service (USPHS)

Uni-tussin
U.-t. DM

univariate
unknown origin
unpneumococcal
unsegmented
unsporulated
unstable
u. angina pectoris
u. bladder

unstained saline mount
untractable
unusual opportunistic infection
unzii
Thiothrix u.

uPA
urokinase plasminogen activator
up-gaze paresis
Upolu virus (UPOV)
UPOV
Upolu virus
upper
u. gastrointestinal endoscopy

u. motor neuron (UMN)
u. motor neuron disease
u. respiratory infection (URI)
u. respiratory tract infection
upsaliensis
Campylobacter u.
uptake
BrdU u.
iron u.
Uracel
uralensis
Calliphora u.
Uranotaenia sapphirina
Urasal
urate
ammonium u.
u. crystal
u. nephropathy
urativorans
Psychrobacter u.
uratoxydans
Arthrobacter u.
urban cutaneous leishmaniasis
urea
u. breath test (UBT)
u. and hydrocortisone
u. hydrolysis
u. hydrolysis test
u. nitrogen clearance
ureae
Actinobacillus u.
Pasteurella u.
Sporosarcina u.
ureafaciens
Arthrobacter u.
urealyticum
Corynebacterium u.
Staphylococcus cohnii subsp. *u.*
Ureaplasma u.
ureaphilum
Hyphomicrobium facile subsp. *u.*
Ureaplasma (b)
U. *canigenitalium*
U. *cati*
U. *diversum*
U. *felinum*
U. *gallorale*
U. *urealyticum*
U. *urealyticum* culture
ureaplasmal infection
urease
u. activity test

U

urease *(continued)*
    u. production
    slow u.
urease-positive bacteriuria
Uredinaceae
Uredinales
Urediniomycetes
uredovora
    Erwinia u.
Ureibacillus (b)
    U. terrenus
    U. thermosphaericus
ureidopenicillin
Uremol-HC
ureolytica
    Oligella u.
ureolyticus
    Bacteroides u.
    Staphylococcus capitis subsp. *u.*
urethral
    u. catheter
    u. *Chlamydia* culture
    u. chlamydial infection
    u. discharge
    u. enzyme immunoassay
    u. fistula
    u. stenosis
    u. stricture
    u. swab
    u. syndrome
    u. *Trichomonas* smear
    u. tuberculosis
urethralis
    Moraxella u.
    Oligella u.
urethritis
    chlamydial u.
    gonococcal u. (GCU)
    gonorrheal u.
    Neisseria gonorrhoeae u.
    nongonococcal u. (NGU)
    noninfectious u.
    specific u.
    trichomonal u.
    Trichomonas u.
    u. venerea
urethritis-cervicitis
urethropexy
    retropubic u.
urethroprostatitis
Urex
URI
    upper respiratory infection
uric
    u. acid
    u. acid crystal
Uridon Modified

urinae
    Aerococcus u.
urinaeequi
    Pediococcus u.
urinaehominis
    Aerococcus u.
urinalis
    Streptococcus u.
urinalysis
urinarius
    Bodo u.
urinary
    u. bilharziasis
    u. schistosomiasis
    u. stone
    u. tract candidiasis
    u. tract infection (UTI)
    u. tract infection prevention
urine
    u. bacterial screen
    u. bacteria screen
    u. cast
    catheterized u.
    clean-catch midstream u.
    u. crystal
    u. dipstick
    u. dipstick test
    first-void u. (FVU)
    u. fungus culture
    u. *Legionella* antigen
    u. leukocyte esterase
    u. leukocyte esterase test
    u. meter
    u. nitrite
    u. osmolality
    u. ova and parasites
    u. for parasites
    u. protein
    random u.
    u. sediment
    suprapubic aspiration of u.
    u. toxicology
    u. *Trichomonas* wet mount
uris
    Dirofilaria u.
Uriscreeen
Urised
Uri-Tet Oral
Uritin
Urobak
urobilinogen
urobilirubin
urodynamic testing
uroepithelial
uroepithelium
urogenital
    u. candidiasis
    u. schistosomiasis

urogenitalis
  Actinomyces u.
urography
urokinase plasminogen activator (uPA)
Urolene Blue
urolithiasis
Uromitexan
uromucoid
uropathogen
uropathogenic
uropathogenicity
Uroplus DS, SS
uroprotection
urosepsis
urosubulatus
  Globocephalus u.
urothelium
Urov disease
ursi
  Diphyllobothrium u.
ursincola
  Blastomonas u.
  Erythromonas u.
  Sphingomonas u.
ursodiol
urticaria
urticarial
  u. fever
urticarioides
uruhambanum
  Simulium u.
Urucuri virus (URUV)
uruguayensis
URUV
  Urucuri virus
usamii
user
  injecting drug u. (IDU)
  injection drug u. (IDU)
  intravenous drug u. (IVDU)
usingeri
  Culicoides u.
USPHS
  United States Public Health Service
USR test
Ustilaginaceae
Ustilaginales
Ustilaginomycetes
Ustilago (f)
  U. maydis
ustus
  Aspergillus u.

usual
  u. adult regimen
  u. discase
Usutu virus (USUV)
USUV
  Usutu virus
uta
utahensis
  Actinoplanes u.
  Culicoides u.
  Halorhabdus u.
uteri
  Phocoenobacter u.
utero
  in u.
uterobilateralis
  Paragonimus u.
UTI
  urinary tract infection
utilis
  Candida u.
  Staphylococcus carnosus subsp. u.
Utinga virus (UTIV)
UTIscreen
UTIV
  Utinga virus
Utive virus
utowana
  Culicoides u.
utricularis
  Badhamia u.
Uukuniemi virus (UUKV)
UUKV
  Uukuniemi virus
UV
  ultraviolet
    UV crosslinking
    UV light test
uvae
  Sypringospora u.
uvarum
  Saccharomyces u.
uveal tract
uveitis
  acanthamebic u.
  anterior u.
  granulomatous u.
  HTLV-1 u.
  HTLV-1-associated u.
uveoencephalitis syndrome
uveomeningitic syndrome
uveoparotid fever

U

NOTES

UVGI
   ultraviolet germicidal irradiation
Uvitex 2B

Uzbekistan hemorrhagic fever
uzenensis
   Geobacillus u.

V/517
    Escherichia coli strain V/517
vaccae
    Mycobacterium v.
vaccination
    anticytokine v.
vaccine
    acellular v.
    acellular pertussis v.
    anthrax v.
    antipertussis acellular v.
    aqueous v.
    autogenous v.
    autologous tumor v.
    bacterial v.
    BCG v.
    v. body
    botulinum toxoid pentavalent v.
    cellular v.
    chickenpox v.
    cholera v.
    conjugate v.
    diphtheria v.
    diphtheria-tetanus-pertussis v.
    diphtheria, tetanus toxoids and
      whole-cell pertussis v. (DTP)
    DTP v.
    duck embryo origin v.
    encephalitis v.
    flu virus v.
    foot-and-mouth disease virus v.
    formalin-inactivated v.
    German measles v.
    g209-2M peptide v.
    Haemophilus b conjugate v.
    Haemophilus influenzae type b v.
    Haffkine v.
    HAVRIX v.
    HbOC v.
    heat-phenol inactivated v.
    hepatitis A v.
    hepatitis B v.
    HibTITER v.
    Hib-TT v.
    high-egg-passage v.
    HIV-1$_{IIIB}$ rgp160 polypeptide v.
    human diploid cell culture
      rabies v. (HDCV)
    human diploid cell rabies v.
      (HDCV)
    IIIB-Mel-J allogeneic tumor cell v.
    Imovax Rabies I.D. V.
    inactivated Japanese encephalitis
      virus v.
    inactivated poliomyelitis virus v.

    inactivated whole virus v.
    influenza virus v.
    IVP-Salk v.
    Japanese B encephalitis v.
    killed v. (KV)
    live attenuated virus v.
    live measles virus v.
    live mumps virus v.
    live oral polio v.
    live oral poliovirus v.
    live rubella virus v.
    low-egg-passage v.
    Lyme disease v.
    measles, mumps, rubella v.
    measles and rubella v.
    meningococcal v.
    MMR v.
    multivalent group B streptococcal
      polysaccharide-tetanus toxoid
      conjugate v.
    mumps v.
    Neisseria meningitidis v.
    OmniHIB v.
    OPV-Sabin v.
    oral attenuated poliomyelitis
      virus v.
    oral polio v. (OPV)
    oral poliovirus v. (OPV)
    PCEC rabies v.
    PedvaxHIB v.
    plague v.
    pneumococcal v.
    polio v. (IPV)
    polynucleotide v.
    polyvalent pneumococcal
      polysaccharide v.
    V. Preparedness Study (VPS)
    ProHIBIT v.
    PRP-D v.
    PRP-OMPC v.
    PRP-T v.
    Q fever v.
    rabies virus v.
    recombinant expressed v.
    rgp160 v.
    rhesus rotavirus-tetravalent v.
    RRV-TV v.
    rubella and measles v.
    Sabin v.
    Salk v.
    Schwarz v.
    smallpox v.
    STn-KLH cancer v.
    v. strain infection
    Streptococcus pneumoniae v.

V

vaccine *(continued)*
    subunit v.
    swine influenza v.
    tetanus v.
    TetraImmune v.
    Tetramune v.
    three-in-one v.
    trivalent poliovirus v. (TOPV)
    tularemia v.
    tumor v.
    Ty21a typhoid v.
    type b conjugate v.
    typhoid v.
    14-valent v.
    23-valent v.
    7-valent pneumococcal conjugate v.
    varicella virus v.
    varicella-zoster virus v.
    viral protein subunit v.
    virus-like particle v.
    VLP v.
    VZV v.
    whole-cell v.
    yellow fever v.
    zoster v.
    Zostrix v.
vaccine-related paralytic polio
vaccinia
    v. infection
    v. virus (VACV)
    v. virus subgroup
vaccinii
    Candida v.
    Nocardia v.
vaccinostercus
    Lactobacillus v.
vacuolar myelopathy
vacuolata
    Ectothiorhodospira v.
    Methanosarcina v.
    Polaromonas v.
    Stella v.
vacuolated
    v. prickle cell
vacuolation
    neuronal v.
vacuolatum
    Halorubrum v.
    Natronobacterium v.
vacuolatus
    Desulforhopalus v.
vacuole
    contractile v.
    glycogen v.
    parasitophorous v.
vacuolization
    cytoplasmic v.

VACV
    vaccinia virus
    recombinant VV
Vaejovidae, **Vejovidae**
Vaejovis, **Vejovis**
vaga
    Alteromonas v.
    Marinomonas v.
vagabond's disease
Vagifem
Vagilia
vaginae
    Atopobium v.
    Cylindrocarpon v.
vaginal
    v. candidiasis
    Cleocin V.
    v. cuff
    v. culture
    Dalacin V.
    v. discharge
    v. dryness
    v. flora
    v. flora score
    v. inflammation
    v. microbicide
    Monistat V.
    Ortho-Dienestrol V.
    v. pH
    v. pruritus
    v. secretion
    v. secretion swab
    v. smear
    v. stenosis
    Terazol V.
    v. *Trichomonas* smear
    v. trichomoniasis
    v. tuberculosis
    Vagistat-1 V.
    v. wet mount
vaginalis
    Anaerococcus v.
    Falcivibrio v.
    Gardnerella v.
    Haemophilus v.
    Lactobacillus v.
    Peptostreptococcus v.
    portio v.
    Trichomonas v. (TV)
    tunica v.
vaginitis
    amebic v.
    Candida v.
    Candida albicans v.
    Gardnerella v.
    infectious v.
    pinworm v.
    v. syndrome

trichomoniasis v.
 yeast v.
vaginosis
 bacterial v. (BV)
 nonspecific v.
Vaginulus plebeius
Vagistat-1 Vaginal
Vagitrol
Vagococcus (b)
 V. fessus
 V. fluvialis
 V. lutrae
 V. salmoninarum
vagotomy
vagrant's disease
vagum
 Oceanospirillum v.
Vahlkampfia (p)
 V. avara
 V. magna
 V. russelli
Vahlkampfiidae
valacyclovir HCl
valaisiana
 Borrelia v.
valderianum
 Phormidium v.
valdiviana
 Candida v.
valganciclovir
valida
 Candida v.
validus
 Bacillus v.
 Paenibacillus v.
Valisone Topical
valley fever
vallismortis
 Bacillus v.
 Haloarcula v.
 Halobacterium v.
 Salinivibrio costicola subsp. *v.*
valproic acid
Valsaceae
Valtrex
value
 hemoglobin A$_{2C}$ v.
 positive predictive v. (PPV)
 predictive v.
valve
 aortic v.
 Hancock porcine aortic v.

mitral v.
 posterior urethral v.
 tricuspid v.
valvular
valvulitis
 rheumatic v.
VAMC
 Veterans Administration Medical Center
vampire bat
Vampirolepis (p)
Vampirovibrio chlorellavorus (b)
VanB *Enterococcus faecium* (VBEF)
vanbreuseghemii
 Arthroderma v.
 Microsporum v.
 Trichophyton v.
Vancocin
 V. CP
 V. Injection
 V. Oral
Vancoled Injection
vancomycin
 v. level
 v. test
vancomycin-resistant
 v.-r. enterococcus (VRE)
 v.-r. *Enterococcus faecium* (VREF)
 v.-r. *Staphylococcus aureus* (VRSA)
Vancor
vancouverensis
 Pseudomonas v.
vanderwaltii
 Candida v.
vandii
 Burkholderia v.
vanillism
Vaniqa Cream
vanishing tumor
vanneervenii
 Prosthecobacter v.
vannielii
 Methanococcus v.
 Rhodomicrobium v.
Vanoxide
Vanoxide-HC
Vanrija
 V. humicola
Vansil
Vantin
Vaponefrin
vaporized hydrogen peroxide (VHP)

V

NOTES

Vaporole
Amyl Nitrate V.
VAQTA
vargasi
Anopheles v.
variabile
Corynebacterium v.
Hyphomicrobium v.
variabilis
Arthrobacter v.
Brevundimonas v.
Bullera v.
Caulobacter v.
Dermatocentor v.
Desulfosarcina v.
Halomonas v.
Halovibrio v.
Streptomyces v.
Xenopsylla v.
varians
Kocuria v.
Micrococcus v.
Simulium v.
variant
v. Creutzfeldt-Jakob disease (vCJD)
L-phase v.
v. surface glycoprotein (VSG)
v. surface glycoprotein gene
v. tuberculin reactivity
viral v.
variation
amino acid sequence v.
varicaedens
Caedibacter v.
variceal sclerotherapy
varicella
congenital v.
v. immune globulin (VZIG)
v. pneumonia
v. virus vaccine
v. virus vaccine, live
varicella-zoster
v.-z. immune globulin (VZIG)
v.-z. immunoglobulin (VZIG)
v.-z. infection
v.-z. prevention
v.-z. retinitis
v.-z. virus (VZV)
v.-z. virus 1
v.-z. virus culture
v.-z. virus infection
v.-z. virus retinal necrosis
v.-z. virus serology
v.-z. virus vaccine
varicelliform lesion
varicellosus
herpes zoster v.
Varicellovirus (v)

varices (*pl. of* varix)
Varicosavirus (v)
varicose eczema
variegata
Atherix v.
variegatum
Amblyomma v.
variegatus
Streptomyces v.
varigena
Mannheimia v.
variglandis
Austrobilharzia v.
Microbilharzia v.
variipennis
Culicoides v.
variola
v. virus
variotii
Paecilomyces v.
Variovorax paradoxus (b)
varipalpus
Aedes v.
varium
Anaeroplasma v.
Fusobacterium v.
Procerovum v.
varius
Paragordius v.
Varivax
varix, pl. varices
lymph varices
varsoviensis
Streptomyces v.
vartiovaarae
Candida v.
vascular
v. adhesion molecule-1 (VCAM-1)
v. endothelial growth factor/vascular
permeability factor (VEGF/VPF)
v. leak syndrome (VLS)
v. pannus
v. spider
vasculitic purpura
vasculitis
cerebral v.
cutaneous v.
eosinophilic v.
Henoch-Schönlein v.
necrotizing v.
vasculogenic
vasculopathy
Vaseline-paraffin mixture
vasicola
Xanthomonas v.
vasiformis
Saksenaea v.

vasinfecta
    Neocosmospora v.
vasoactive
    v. amine
Vasocidin Ophthalmic
vasodilatation, vasodilation
vasodilator
vasodilatory
Vasofrinic
vasopressor
vasorum
    Angiostrongylus v.
    vaso v.
Vasosulf Ophthalmic
vaso vasorum
Vaspar
vastator
    Dactylogyrus v.
vastus
    Streptomyces v.
VAT
    visceral abdominal fat
VAT:TAT ratio
VBEF
    VanB *Enterococcus faecium*
VCA
    viral capsid antigen
      VCA titer
VCAM-1
    vascular adhesion molecule-1
V-Cillin K
vCJD
    variant Creutzfeldt-Jakob disease
VD13 virus
V-Dec-M
VDRL
    Venereal Disease Research Laboratory
    Venereal Disease Research Laboratory
    test
      CSF VDRL
      VDRL slide test
      spinal fluid VDRL
vection
vector
    adenoviral v.
    anopheline v.
    arthropod v.
    biologic v.
    insect v.
    mechanical v.
vector-borne
vectorial

Vectrin
vecuronium
vedderi
    Bacillus v.
VEE
    Venezuelan equine encephalitis
Veetids
VEEV
    Venezuelan equine encephalitis virus
vegetation
    heart valve v.
VEGF/VPF
    vascular endothelial growth
    factor/vascular permeability factor
Veillonella (b)
    V. alcalescens
    V. alcalescens subsp. *alcalescens*
    V. alcalescens subsp. *criceti*
    V. alcalescens subsp. *dispar*
    V. alcalescens subsp. *ratti*
    V. atypica
    V. caviae
    V. criceti
    V. dispar
    V. parvula
    V. parvula subsp. *atypica*
    V. parvula subsp. *parvula*
    V. parvula subsp. *rodentium*
    V. ratti
    V. rodentium
Veillonellaceae
vein
    femoral v.
    internal jugular v.
    subclavian v.
Vejovidae (*var. of Vaejovidae*)
Vejovis (*var. of Vaejovis*)
veldkampii
    Rhodobacter v.
Veldona
Vellore virus (VELV)
velocicrescens
    Spiroplasma v.
Velosef
velox
    Thermanaerovibrio v.
VELV
    Vellore virus
velvet ant
Vena medinensis
venator
    Simulium v.

V

NOTES

veneficus
  Archaeoglobus v.
venerea
  lues v.
  urethritis v.
venereal
  V. Disease Research Laboratory
    (VDRL)
  V. Disease Research Laboratory
    test (VDRL)
  v. wart
venerealis
  Campylobacter fetus subsp. v.
venereum
  granuloma v.
  lymphogranuloma v. (LGV)
  malum v.
venetianus
  Pelobacter v.
venezuelae
  Beijerinckia derxii subsp. v.
  Streptomyces v.
Venezuelan
  V. equine encephalitis (VEE)
  V. equine encephalitis virus
    (VEEV)
  V. hemorrhagic fever
venezuelensis
  Borrelia v.
  Leishmania v.
  Ornithodoros v.
  Planomonospora v.
venezuelunsis
  Trichosporon v.
venipuncture
venoconstriction
Venoglobulin-I, -S
venom
  dilute Russell viper v. (DRVV)
venomegaly
venoocclusive disease
venous catheter culture
venous-irritating
Ventodisk
Ventolin
  V. Rotocaps
ventral gland
ventricle
  left v. (LV)
ventricosus
  Haemodipsus v.
  Pediculoides v.
ventricular
  v. apex
  v. arrhythmia
  v. empyema
  v. fibrillation

  v. shunt
  v. tachycardia
ventriculi
  Sarcina v.
ventriculitis
ventriculoatrial
  v. shunt
  v. shunt infection
ventriculoperitoneal shunt
ventriculostomy
ventriculus
ventriosum
  Eubacterium v.
ventrovittis
  Aedes v.
Venturiaceae
venulosum
  Oesophagostomum v.
venusta
  Deleya v.
  Halomonas v.
venustum
  Simulium v.
venustus
  Alcaligenes v.
  Culicoides v.
verecundum
  Mycoplasma v.
  Simulium v.
Vergogel Gel
Veriderm
  Medrol V.
veriformis
  Hartmannella v.
Veri-Staph test
Vermes
vermicidal
vermicide
vermicular
Vermicularia (f)
vermicularis
  Enterobius v.
  Oxyuris v.
vermicule
vermiculose
vermiculus
vermiform
vermiformis
  Eimeria v.
vermifugal
vermifuge
vermin
verminal
vermination
verminous
  v. abscess
  v. appendicitis
vermis

Vermizine
Vermox
verna
    Amanita v.
vernal
    v. conjunctivitis
    v. encephalitis
vernalis
    Cyclops v.
vernum
    Simulium v.
verocytotoxin
    Escherichia coli v.
    v. typing
verocytotoxin-producing *Escherichia coli*
  (VTEC)
veronae
    Kluyveromyces v.
    Sporidiobolus v.
Veronaea botryosa (f)
veronensis
    Amaricoccus v.
veronicellid slug
veronii
    Aeromonas v.
    Pseudomonas v.
veroralis
    Bacteroides v.
    Prevotella v.
verotoxin (VT)
Verpa bohemica (f)
Verrex-C&M
verruca, pl. **verrucae**
    v. acuminata
    v. peruana
    v. vulgaris
verrucaria
    Myrothecium v.
verruciformis
    epidermodysplasia v.
Verrucomicrobium spinosum (b)
verrucosa
    Phialophora v.
verrucose
Verrucosispora gifhornensis (b)
verrucosospora
    Actinomadura v.
verrucosum
    Trichophyton v.
verrucosus
    Ornithodoros v.
verrucous appearance

verruculosa
    Curvularia v.
verruculosum
    Penicillium v.
verruculosus
    Cochliobolus v.
verruga peruana
Versacaps
versatilis
    Candida v.
Versed
Versel
Versiclear
versicolor
    Aspergillus v.
    pityriasis v.
    Simulium v.
    tinea v.
versiforme
    Natrinema v.
versutus
    Paracoccus v.
    Thialkalivibrio v.
    Thiobacillus v.
vertebral
    v. body
    v. osteomyelitis
    v. tuberculosis
vertical transmission
verticillatus
    Streptomyces v.
Verticillium alboatrum (f)
vertigo
Verukan solution
vescum
    Mogibacterium v.
vesica
vesical
vesicatoria
    Lytta v.
    Xanthomonas v.
vesicle
    endocytic v.
    herpetic v.
    mucocutaneous v.
vesicopustular rash
vesicoureteral
vesicourethral reflux
vesicular
    v. eruption
    v. exanthem
    v. exanthema swine virus (VESV)

V

NOTES

vesicular *(continued)*
    v. fluid
    v. rash
    v. rickettsiosis
    v. stomatitis Alagoas virus (VSAV)
    v. stomatitis Indiana virus (VSIV)
    v. stomatitis New Jersey virus
      (VSNJV)
    v. stomatitis virus (VSV)
    v. stomatitis virus group
    v. viral infection
vesicularis
    Brevundimonas *v.*
    Pseudomonas *v.*
vesicularum
    Brachiola *v.*
vesiculation
    cytoplasmic v.
Vesiculovirus (v)
vespertillionis
    Argas *v.*
vestibular
vestibularis
    Streptococcus *v.*
Vestibuliferida
vestimenti
    pediculosis v.
vestitipennis
    Anopheles *v.*
VESV
    vesicular exanthema swine virus
veterana
    Nocardia *v.*
**Veterans Administration Medical Center
(VAMC)**
vexans
    Aedes *v.*
    Isaria *v.*
Vf12 virus
Vf33 virus
V factor
vHL
    von Hippel-Lindau
VHP
    vaporized hydrogen peroxide
VHSV
    viral hemorrhagic septicemia virus
Vi
    Vi antigen
    Typhim Vi
Vibramycin
    V. IV
Vibra-Tabs
Vibrio (b)
    V. aerogenes
    V. aestuarianus
    V. albensis
    V. alginolyticus

V. anguillarum
V. campbellii
V. carchariae
V. cholerae
V. cholerae gastroenteritis
V. cholerae-induced gastroenteritis
V. cholerae O139 Bengal
V. cholerae O1 biotype El Tor
    serotype Ogawa
V. cholerae O1 El Tor
V. cholerae O139 strain
V. cholerae serotype 01 *Hikojima*
V. cholerae serotype 01 Inaba
V. cholerae serotype O1 of El
    Tor biotype
V. cholerae serotype Ogawa
V. cincinnatiensis
V. costicola
V. cyclitrophicus
V. damsela
V. diabolicus
V. diazotrophicus
V. fischeri
V. fluvialis
V. furnissii
V. gazogenes
V. halioticoli
V. harveyi
V. hollisae
V. ichthyoenteri
V. iliopiscarius
V. lentus
V. logei
V. marinus
V. mediterranei
V. metschnikovii
V. mimicus
V. mytili
Nasik *V.*
V. natriegens
V. navarrensis
V. nereis
V. nigripulchritudo
non-cholera *V.* (NCV)
V. ordalii
V. orientalis
V. parahaemolyticus
V. parahaemolyticus-associated
    gastroenteritis
V. pectenicida
V. pelagius
V. penaeicida
V. proteolyticus
V. rumoiensis
V. salmonicida
V. scophthalmi
V. shiloi
V. splendidus

V. *succinogenes*
V. *tapetis*
V. *trachuri*
V. *tubiashii*
V. *viscosus*
V. *vulnificus*
V. *wodanis*
vibrio
El Tor *v.*
vibrioforme
Chlorobium v.
vibrioformis
Desulfobacter v.
Oxalobacter v.
vibrioides
Caulobacter v.
Propionispora v.
Vibrionaceae
vibriosis
vibriostatic agent O/129
vicina
Calliphora v.
Musca domestica v.
Vicks
V. Children's Cough and Congestion syrup
V. DayQuil Sinus Pressure & Congestion Relief
V. 44D Cough & Head Congestion
V. Formula 44
V. Formula 44 Pediatric Formula
V. 44 Non-Drowsy Cold & Cough Liqui-Caps
V. Pediatric Formula 44E
V. Sinex
vidarabine
v. ointment
video-assisted thoracoscopic
videomicroscope image analysis
Videx EC
vietnamiensis
Burkholderia v.
vif-deleted SIV
Vif gene
vigil
Wohlfahrtia v.
ViII virus
villitis
villorum
Enterococcus v.

villosipennis
Culicoides v.
villosum
Clostridium v.
villosus
Filifactor v.
villous polyp
villus
chorionic v.
v. epithelium
v. ischemia
villus-attached enterocyte
Vil virus
Vilyuisk
V. encephalomyelitis
V. human encephalomyelitis virus
V. virus
vinacea
Actinomadura v.
vinaceum
Dactylosporangium v.
vinaceus
Streptomyces v.
vinaceusdrappus
Streptomyces v.
vinblastine
Vincent
V. angina
V. bacillus
V. disease
V. infection
V. spirillum
V. white mycetoma
vincentii
Clostridium v.
Fusobacterium nucleatum subsp. *v.*
Vinces virus (VINV)
vincristine
vinegar eel
vinelandii
Azotobacter v.
Methylococcus v.
vini
Candida v.
Pichia v.
vinosum
Allochromatium v.
Chromatium v.
vinsonii
Bartonella vinsonii subsp. *v.*
Rochalimaea v.

V

NOTES

VINV
 Vinces virus
Vioform
violacea
 Lentzea v.
 Microellobosporia v.
 Saccharothrix v.
 Shewanella v.
 Thiocystis v.
violaceochromogenes
 Streptomyces v.
 Streptosporangium v.
violaceolatus
 Streptomyces v.
violaceorectus
 Streptomyces v.
violaceoruber
 Streptomyces v.
violaceorubidus
 Streptomyces v.
violaceous
 v. papule verrucous lesion
violacescens
 Simulium v.
violaceum
 Actinosporangium v.
 Chromobacterium v.
 Trichophyton v.
violaceus
 Parachordodes v.
 Streptomyces v.
violaceusniger
 Streptomyces v.
violarus
 Streptomyces v.
violascens
 Chromatium v.
 Streptomyces v.
 Thiocystis v.
violatus
 Streptomyces v.
violens
 Chainia v.
 Streptomyces v.
violet
 crystal v.
 v. crystal
 gentian v.
violin spider
viper
 v. retrovirus
 Russell v.
Vira-A
 V.-A. Ophthalmic
Viracept
VIRADAPT
 V. data
 V. study

viral
 v. agent
 v. antigen
 v. antigenemia
 v. aseptic meningitis
 v. burden
 v. capsid antigen (VCA)
 v. conjunctivitis
 v. culture
 v. direct detection by fluorescent
  antibody
 v. disease
 v. encephalitis
 v. encephalomyelitis
 v. endophthalmitis
 v. entry barrier skin
 v. enzyme
 v. exanthema
 v. gastroenteritis
 v. genome
 v. hemagglutinin
 v. hemophagocytic syndrome
 v. hemorrhagic fever
 v. hemorrhagic septicemia virus
  (VHSV)
 v. hepatitis
 v. immunization
 v. inclusion
 v. isolate
 v. isolation
 v. laryngitis
 v. load (VL)
 v. load quantification
 v. load rebound
 v. load suppression
 v. nucleic acid
 v. nucleotide sequence
 v. pathogenesis
 v. protein
 v. protein subunit vaccine
 v. replication
 v. respiratory infection
 v. rhinitis
 v. serology
 v. shedding
 v. study
 v. titer
 v. variant
Viramune
virans
 Streptomyces v.
Virazole
 V. Aerosol
Virchow-Robin space
viremia
 chronic v.
 high-titer v.
 HIV v.

low-titer v.
maternal v.
plasma v.
primary v.
secondary v.
virens
    Gliocladium v.
    Streptomyces v.
virescens
    Myxococcus v.
virgatum
    Simulium v.
Virgibacillus (b)
    V. pantothenticus
    V. proomii
virgin
    v. generation
    V. River virus (VRV)
virginiae
    Streptomyces v.
viridans
    Aerococcus v.
    v. hemolysis
    v. streptococcus
    Thalassomonas v.
viride
    Clostridium v.
    Trichoderma v.
viridescens
    Calliphora v.
    Eidamia v.
    Lactobacillus v.
    Weissella v.
viridialbum
    Streptosporangium v.
viridiflava
    Pseudomonas v.
viridilutea
    Actinomadura v.
    Excellospora v.
viridis
    Actinomadura v.
    Blastochloris v.
    Euglena v.
    Microbispora v.
    Microtetraspora v.
    Paecilomyces v.
    Rhodopseudomonas v.
    Saccharomonospora v.
viridiviolaceus
    Streptomyces v.

viridobrunneus
    Streptomyces v.
viridochromogenes
    Streptomyces v.
viridodiastaticus
    Streptomyces v.
viridoflavum
    Streptomyces v.
    Streptoverticillium v.
viridoflavus
    Streptomyces v.
viridogrisea
    Kutzneria v.
viridogriseum
    Streptosporangium viridogriseum
    subsp. *v.*
viridosporus
    Streptomyces v.
virion
    infectious v.
Virocult swab
viroid
virologic
    v. failure
    v. rebound
    v. response
virology
Viroptic
    V. Ophthalmic
virosa
    Amanita v.
    Weeksella v.
virucidal
    v. solution
virulence
virulent
    v. bubo
virus
    A v.
    A-4 v.
    A6 v.
    A19 v.
    A23 v.
    A25 v.
    AA-1 v.
    A5/A6 v.
    Abras v. (ABRV)
    Abu Hammad v. (AHV)
    Abu Mina v. (ABMV)
    AC-1 v.
    Acado v. (ACDV)
    Acara v. (ACAV)

V

NOTES

·

virus *(continued)*
Acherontia atropas v.
Acholeplasma phage L2 v.
Acholeplasma phage MV-L51 v.
A1-Dat v.
Adelaide River v. (ARV)
adenoassociated v. (AAV)
adenoassociated v. 1–5 (AAV 1–5)
AE-2 v.
Aeh-2 v.
African horse sickness v. (AHSV)
African horse sickness v. 1–9
  (AHSV 1–9)
African tick v.
Aguacate v. (AGUV)
AIDS-related v. (ARV)
Akabane v. (AKAV)
Alajuela v.
Alenquer v. (ALEV)
Alfuy v.
Almeirim v. (AMRV)
Almpiwar v. (ALMV)
Altamira v. (ALTV)
Alteromonas phage PM2 v.
ALV-related v.
Amapari v. (AMAV)
American eel v. (EVA)
Ananindeua v. (ANUV)
Andasibe v. (ANDV)
Anhanga v. (ANHV)
Anhembi v. (AMBV)
Anopheles A, B v.
AN25S-1 v.
Antequera v. (ANTV)
Antheraea eucalypti v.
anti-Epstein-Barr v.
anti-hepatitis E v. (anti-HEV)
AP50 v.
Apeu v. (APEUV)
aphid lethal paralysis v.
Aphthovirus A v.
Apoi v. (APOIV)
Ar-577 v.
Ar-578 v.
Aransas Bay v. (ABV)
Arbia v. (ARBV)
Arboledas v. (ADSV)
Argentine hemorrhagic fever v.
Arkonam v. (ARKV)
Aroa v. (AROAV)
Arp v.
Arracacha A v. (AVA)
Arracacha B v. (AVB)
Arracacha latent v.
Arracacha Y v.
arthropod-borne v.
Aruac v. (ARUV)
Arumowot v. (AMTV)

AS-1 v.
AU v.
Aura v. (AURAV)
Auzduk disease v.
AV-1 v.
Avalon v. (AVAV)
avian encephalomyelitis v.
avian erythroblastosis v.
avian infectious bronchitis v. (IBV)
avian infectious laryngotracheitis v.
avian influenza v.
avian leukosis v. (ALV)
avian lymphomatosis v.
avian myeloblastosis v.
avian paramyxovirus v. 1–9 (PMV
  1–9)
B v.
B6 v.
B7 v.
B12 v.
B19 v.
Babahoya v. (BABV)
Babanki v.
bacterial v.
Bagaza v. (BAGV)
Bahig v. (BAHV)
Bakau v. (BAKUV)
Baku v. (BAKUV)
Bam35 v.
Bandia v. (BDAV)
Bangoran v. (BGNV)
Bangui v. (BGIV)
Banna v. (BAV)
Banzi v. (BANV)
Barmah Forest v. (BFV)
Barranqueras v. (BQSV)
Barur v. (BARV)
Batai v. (BATV)
Batama v. (BMAV)
Batken v.
Bauline v. (BAUV)
Bayou v. (BAYV)
Bdellovibrio phage v.
BE/1 v.
BeAn 157575 v. (BeAnV-157575)
BeAr 328208 v. (BAV)
bebaru v. (BEBV)
Beijing v.
Belem v. (BLMV)
Belgrade v.
Belmont v. (BELV)
Belterra v. (BELTV)
Benevides v. (BENV)
Benfica v. (BENV)
Berne v. (BEV)
Berrimah v. (BRMV)
Bertioga v.
Bhanja v.

Bimbo v. (BBOV)
Bimiti v. (BIMV)
Birao v. (BIRV)
Bivens Arm v.
BJ5-T v.
BK v.
black beetle v. (BBV)
Black Creek Canal v. (BCCV)
BLE v.
B/LEE/40 v.
bluetongue v. 1–24 (BLUV 1–24,
  BTV 1–24)
B11-M15 v.
Bobaya v. (BOBV)
Bobia v. (BIAV)
Boletus v. X (BolVX)
Boraceia v. (BORV)
border disease v. (BDV)
Borna disease v. (BDV)
Bornholm disease v.
Botambi v. (BOTV)
Boteke v. (BTKV)
Bouboui v. (BOUV)
bovine AAV v. (BAAV)
bovine immunodeficiency v.
bovine leukemia v.
bovine respiratory syncytial v.
bovine viral diarrhea v. (BVDV)
Bozo v.
Breda v.
Bruconha v.
Buenaventura v. (DMV)
buffalopox v.
Buggy Creek v.
Bujaru v.
Bukalasa bat v.
Bunyamwera v. (BUNV)
Bunyip Creek v. (BCV)
Bushbush v. (BSBV)
Bussuquara v. (BSQV)
Buttonwillow v. (BUTV)
Bwamba v. (BWAV)
C-1 v.
C16 v.
Cabassou v.
Cache Valley v. (CVV)
Cacipacore v. (CPCV)
Caddo Canyon v.
Caimito v. (CAIV)
Calchaqui v. (CQIV)
California encephalitis v. (CEV)
Cananeia v. (CANV)

canarypox v.
Caninde v. (CNAV)
Cape Wrath v. (CWV)
Capim v. (CAPV)
caprine arthritis encephalitis v.
v. capsid
Carajas v.
Caraparu v. (CARV)
Carey Island v. (CIV)
Catu v. (CATUV)
CbaAr 426 v.
CEb v.
CELO v.
central European encephalitis v.
  (CEEV)
Cf v.
Cflt v.
C group v.
Chaco v. (CHOV)
Chagres v. (CHGV)
Chandipura v. (CHPV)
Changuinola v. (CGLV)
Charleville v. (CHVV)
Chenuda v. (CNUV)
chickenpox v.
chikungunya v. (CHIKV)
Chilibre v. (CHIV)
Chim v. (CHIMV)
Chobar Gorge v. (CGV)
c2-like v.'s
Clo Mor v. (CMV)
CM$_1$ v.
CoAr 1071 v.
CoAr 3624 v.
CoAr 3627 v.
coastal plains v. (CPV)
Cocal v.
coital exanthema v.
ColAn 57389 v.
Colorado tick fever v. (CTFV)
Columbia SK v.
common cold v.
Connecticut v. (CNTV)
contagious pustular stomatitis v.
Convict Creek 104 v.
Convict Creek 74 v.
CONX v.
Corfou v. (CFUV)
Corriparta v. (CORV)
coryza v.
Cotia v. (CPV)
Cowbone Ridge v. (CRV)

V

NOTES

virus *(continued)*

cowpox v.
Coxsackie v.
Cp-1 v.
Crimean-Congo hemorrhagic
  fever v.
croup-associated v.
CSIRO Village v. (CVGV)
CT4 v.
CVA 1 v.
CV-AL1A v.
CV-AL2A v.
CV-AL2C v.
CVB 1 v.
CV-BJ2C v.
CV-CA1A v.
CV-CA4A v.
CV-CA4B v.
CV-CA1D v.
CVG 1 v.
CV-IL2A v.
CV-IL3A v.
CV-IL2B v.
CV-IL3D v.
CV-IL5-2s1 v.
CVM 1 v.
CV-MA1D v.
CV-MA1E v.
CV-NC1A v.
CV-NC1B v.
CV-NC1C v.
CV-NC1D v.
CV-NE8A v.
CV-NE8D v.
CV-NY2A v.
CV-NY2B v.
CV-NYb1 v.
CV-NY2C v.
CV-NY3F v.
CV-NYs1 v.
CVR 1 v.
CV-SC1A v.
CV-SC1B v.
CV-SH6 v.
CV-XZ3A v.
CV-XZ4A v.
CV-XZ4C v.
CV-XZ5C v.
CV-XZ6E v.
cytolytic v.
cytoplasmic polyhedrosis v. (CPV)
D3 v.
dφ3 v.
dφ4 v.
dφ5 v.
Dabakala v.
D'Aguilar v. (DAGV)
Dakar bat v. (DBV)

DakArK 7292 v.
Darna trima v.
dDVI v.
dengue v. 1–4 (DENV 1–4)
Dera Ghazi Khan v. (DGKV)
Desert Shield v.
v. detection
Dhori v.
Diplocarpon rosae v. (DrV)
direct detection of v.
direct fluorescent antibody test
  for v.
disseminated herpes simplex v.
  type 2
distemper v.
DNA tumor v.
Douglas v. (DOUV)
Drosophila A v. (DAV)
Drosophila C v. (DCV)
Drosophila P v. (DPV)
Drosophila X v. (DXV)
dsDNA algal v.
duck hepatitis B v. (DHBV)
duck influenza v.
duck plague v.
Dugbe v. (DUGV)
Duvenhage v.
E v.
eastern equine encephalitis v.
  (EEEV)
Ebola v. (EBOV)
Ebola-like v.'s
Ec9 v.
ECHO v.
ectromelia v.
Edge Hill v. (EHV)
EEE v.
EgAn 1825-61 v.
Egtved v.
El Moro Canyon v.
Embu v.
EMC v.
emerging v.
encephalitis v.
v. encephalomyelitis
encephalomyocarditis v. (EMCV)
endogenous latent v.
Enseada v. (ENSV)
Entebbe bat v. (ENTV)
enteric v.
enteropathogenic v.
epidemic gastroenteritis v.
epidemic keratoconjunctivitis v.
epidemic myalgia v.
epidemic parotitis v.
epidemic pleurodynia v.
epizootic hemorrhagic disease v.
  1–8 (EHDV)

Epstein-Barr v. (EBV)
equine abortion v. (EAV)
Eret-147 v.
Erve v.
Escherichia-7-11 v.
Estero Real v. (ERV)
Eubenangee v. (EUBV)
European eel v.
Everglades v. (EVEV)
Eyach v. (EYAV)
F116 v.
FA v.
Facey's Paddock v. (FPV)
Farallon v. (FARV)
FC3-9 v.
feline immunodeficiency v. (FIV)
feline infectious peritonitis v.
  (FIPV)
feline panleukopenia v. (FPLV,
  FPV)
fer-de-lance v.
F1, F2 v.
FH5 v.
Fiji disease v. (FDV)
filamentous phage v.
Flanders v. (FLAV)
Flexal v. (FLEV)
flock house v.
v. fluorescent antibody test
foamy v.
Fomede v. (FOMV)
foot-and-mouth disease v.
Forecariah v. (FORV)
Fort Morgan v. (FMV)
Fort Sherman v. (FSV)
fowlpox v.
Fraser Point v.
fri v.
Frijoles v. (FRIV)
Fukuoka v.
G v.
G4 v.
G6 v.
G13 v.
G14 v.
GA v.
GA-1 v.
Gabek Forest v. (GFV)
Gadget's Gully v. (GGYV)
GAL v.
Gamboa v. (GAMV)
Gan Gan v. (GGV)

garland chrysanthemum
  temperate v.
gastroenteritis v. type A, B
GB v. (GBV)
genital herpes simplex v.
German measles v.
Germiston v. (GERV)
Getah v. (GETV)
Gibbon ape leukemia v.
goatpox v.
golden shiner v. (GSV)
Gomoka v. (GOMV)
Gomphrena v.
Gordil v. (GORV)
Gossas v. (GOSV)
Grand Arbaud v. (GAV)
Gray Lodge v. (GLOV)
Great Island v. (GIV)
Great Saltee v.
group A, B, C, D, E, F v.
Guajara v. (GJAV)
Guama v. (GMAV)
Guanarito v.
Guaratuba v.
Guaroa v. (GROV)
Gumbo Limbo v. (GLV)
Gurupi v. (GURV)
GU71U-344 v.
GU71U-350 v.
gypsy moth v.
H-1 v.
HA1 v.
HA2 v.
Hantaan v. (HTNV)
Hantaan-like v.
hare fibroma v.
Hart Park v. (HPV)
Hawaii v.
Hazara v. (HAZV)
HB v.
Helenium S v.
Helenium Y v.
helper v.
hemadsorbing v.
Hendra v.
Hendra-like v.
hepatitis v.
hepatitis A v. (HAV)
hepatitis B v. (HBV)
hepatitis C v. (HCV)
hepatitis D v. (HDV)
hepatitis delta v. (HDV)

V

NOTES

virus *(continued)*

hepatitis E v. (HEV)
hepatitis G v. (HGV)
hepatopancreatic parvo-like v.
herpes simplex v. (HSV)
herpes simplex v. 1 (HSV-1)
herpes simplex v. 2 (HSV-2)
herpesvirus ateles v.
herpes zoster v.
Highlands J v. (HJV)
H-19J v.
H1N1 v.
HN131 v.
HN199 v.
HN295 v.
HN59 v.
hog cholera v.
horse papilloma v.
HR v.
Huacho v. (HUAV)
Hughes v. (HUGV)
human foamy v.
human hepatitis A v. (HHAV)
human immunodeficiency v. (HIV)
human immunodeficiency v. 1, 2
  (HIV-1, HIV-2)
human immunodeficiency v.-type 1
  (HIV-1)
human immunodeficiency v.-type 2
  (HIV-2)
human orf v.
human papilloma v.
human respiratory syncytial v.
  (HRSV)
human T-cell leukemia v.
human T-cell leukemia v. I
human T-cell leukemia v. II
human T cell lymphotrophic v.
human T cell lymphotrophic v.
  type II
human T-cell lymphotropic v.
  (HTLV)
human T-cell lymphotropic v. I
  (HTLV-I)
human T-cell lymphotropic v. II
  (HTLV-II)
human T-lymphotrophic v. type 2
  (HTLV-II)
human T-lymphotrophic
  virus/lymphadenopathy
  associated v. (HTLV-III/LAV)
human T-lymphotropic v. (HTLV-1)
human T-lymphotropic v. 1
  (HTLV-1)
human T-lymphotropic v. 2
  (HTLV-2)
human T-lymphotropic v. type 3
Humpty Doo v. (HDoov)

hv v.
hw v.
I v.
I3 v.
I$_2$-2 v.
Iaco v. (IACOV)
I-alpha v.
Ibaraki v. (IBAV)
Icoaraci v. (ICOV)
icosahedral v.
Ictalurid herpes-like v.'s
Ieri v. (IERIV)
Ife v. (IFEV)
If1, If2 v.
Ilesha v. (ILEV)
Ilheus v. (ILHV)
inclusion conjunctivitis v.
infectious bursal disease v. (IBDV)
infectious hematopoietic necrosis v.
  (IHNV)
infectious pancreatic necrosis v.
  (IPNV)
influenza v.
influenza A v.
influenza B v.
influenza v. type A, B
Ingwavuma v. (INGV)
Inini v. (INIV)
Inkoo v. (INKV)
Ippy v. (IPPYV)
IPy-1 v.
Irituia v. (IRIV)
Isfahan v. (ISFV)
Isla Vista v.
Issyk-Kul v. (ISKV)
Itaituba v. (ITAV)
Itaporanga v. (ITPV)
Itaqui v. (ITQV)
Itimirim v. (ITIV)
Itupiranga v. (ITUV)
IV v.
Jacareacanga v. (JACV)
Jamanxi v. (JAMV)
Jamestown Canyon v. (JCV)
Japanaut v. (JAPV)
Japanese B encephalitis v.
Japanese encephalitis v. (JEV)
Jari v. (JARIV)
Jersey v.
JH v.
JKT-6423 v.
JKT-6969 v.
JKT-7041 v.
JKT-7075 v.
Joa v.
Joinjakaka v. (JOIV)
Juan Diaz v. (JDV)
Jugra v. (JUGV)

juncopox v.
Junin v. (JUNV)
Jurona v. (JURV)
Jutiapa v. (JUTV)
K v.
K19 v.
Kachemak Bay v.
Kadam v. (KADV)
Kaeng Khoi v. (KKV)
Kaikalur v. (KAIV)
Kairi v. (KRIV)
Kaisodi v. (KSOV)
Kamese v. (KAMV)
Kammavanpettai v. (KMPV)
Kannamangalam v. (KANV)
Kao Shuan v. (KSV)
Karimabad v.
Karshi v. (KSIV)
Kasba v. (KASV)
Kasokero v.
Kemerovo v. (KEMV)
Kern Canyon v. (KCV)
Ketapang v. (KETV)
Keuraliba v. (KEUV)
Keystone v. (KEYV)
Kf1 v.
Khasan v.
Kimberley v. (KIMV)
Kismayo v. (KISV)
Klamath v. (KLAV)
Kokobern v. (KOKV)
Kolongo v. (KOLV)
Koongol v. (KOOV)
Korean hemorrhagic fever v.
Kotonkan v. (KOTV)
Koutango v. (KOUV)
Kowanyama v. (KOWV)
KSY1 v.
Kunjin v. (KUNV)
Kwatta v. (KWAV)
Kyasanur Forest disease v.
Kyzylagach v. (KYZV)
L3 v.
La Crosse v. (LACV)
lactate dehydrogenase elevating v.
  (LDV)
lactic dehydrogenase v. (LDHV)
Lagos bat v. (LBV)
La Joya v. (LJV)
Lake Clarendon v. (LCV)
Landjia v. (LJAV)
Langat v. (LGTV)

Langur v.
Lanjan v.
La-Piedad-Michoacan-Mexico v.
Las Maloyas v.
Lassa v. (LASV)
Latino v. (LATV)
Lato river v.
LCM v.
Leanyer v.
Lebombo v. (LEBV)
Le Dantec v. (LDV)
Lednice v. (LEDV)
λ-*like* v.'s
φ29-*like* v.'s
Lipovnik v. (LIPV)
Llano Seco v. (LLSV)
Lokern v. (LOKV)
Lone Star v. (LSV)
Lordsdale v.
louping ill v. (LIV)
LPP-1 v.
LT v.
Lu-III v.
Lukuni v. (LUKV)
Lymantria ninayi v.
lymphadenopathy-associated v.
  (LAV)
lymphocytic choriomeningitis v.
  (LCMV)
lymphogranuloma venereum v.
lytic v.
M v.
M6 v.
M12 v.
M13 v.
M14 v.
M20 v.
M_1 v.
Macaua v. (MCAV)
Machupo v. (MACV)
macrophage-tropic v.
Madrid v. (MADV)
Maguari v. (MAGV)
Mahogany Hammock v. (MHV)
Main Drain v. (MDV)
Malakal v. (MALV)
mal de Rio Cuarto v.
Malpais Spring v.
Manawa v. (MWAV)
Manawatu v.
Mapputta v. (MAPV)
Maprik v. (MPKV)

NOTES

V

595

virus *(continued)*

Mapuera v. (MPRV)
Maraba v.
Marburg v. (MARV, MBGV)
Marburg-like v.'s
Marco v. (MCOV)
Marek's disease-like v.'s
Marituba v. (MTBV)
marmosetpox v.
Marrakai v. (MARV)
Mason-Pfizer monkey v.
Matruh v. (MTRV)
Matucare v. (MATV)
Mayaro v. (MAYV)
Mboke v.
Meaban v. (MEAV)
measles v.
Melao v. (MELV)
Mermet v. (MERV)
Mexico v.
mibuna temperate v.
Middelburg v.
milker's nodule v.
Minatitlan v. (MNTV)
Minnal v. (MINV)
Mirim v. (MIRV)
Mitchell River v. (MRV)
MM v.
Mn936-77 v.
Mobala v. (MOBV)
Modoc v.
Moju v. (MOJUV)
Mojui Dos Campos v. (MDCV)
Mokola v.
molluscum contagiosum v.
monkeypox v.
monocyte tropic v.
Mono Lake v. (MLV)
Montana myotis leukoencephalitis v.
  (MMLV)
Monte Dourado v. (MDOV)
Montgomery County v.
Mopeia v.
mor1 v.
Moriche v. (MORV)
Mosqueiro v. (MQOV)
Mossuril v. (MOSV)
Mount Elgon bat v. (MEBV)
mousepox v.
MP13 v.
MP15 v.
MpV v.
MS2 v.
MSP8 v.
MSV v.
MT v.
M-tropic v.
Mu v.

Mucambo v. (MUCV)
mucosal disease v.
Mudjinbarry v.
Muerto Canyon v.
Muir Springs v.
Mu-like v.'s
multidrug resistant v.
multimammate papilloma v.
multiple nucleocapsid v.
mumps v.
Munguba v. (MUDV, MUNV)
Murray Valley encephalitis v.
  (MVE, MVEV)
Murre v.
Murutucu v. (MURV)
MVG-51 v.
Mykines v. (MYKV)
myxoma v.
N1 v.
N4 v.
N5 v.
Nairobi sheep disease v. (NSDV)
Naranjal v. (NJLV)
Nasoule v. (NAS)
Navarro v. (NAVV)
Ndelle v. (NDEV)
Ndumu v. (NDUV)
Neckar river v. (NRV)
NE-8D v.
Nepuyo v. (NEPV)
Netivot v.
Newcastle disease v. (NDV)
New Minto v. (NMV)
New York v.
Ngaingan v. (NGAV)
Ngari v. (NRIV)
Nipah v.
Nique v. (NIQV)
Nkolbisson v. (NKOV)
NM1 v.
Nodamura v.
Nola v.
non-A, non-B hepatitis v.
noncytolytic v.
nonenteropathogenic v.
nonenveloped v.
nonlytic v.
Northway v. (NORV)
Norwalk v.
nt-1, -2 v.
Ntaya v. (NTAV)
nuclear polyhedrosis v.
Nugget v. (NUGV)
Nyando v. (NDOV)
O1 v.
O087 v.
o6 v.
Oak-Vale v.

Obodhiang v.
Oceanside v.
Ockelbo v.
Oc1r v.
Odrenisrou v. (ODRV)
Oita 296 v.
Okhotskiy v. (OKHV)
Okola v. (OKOV)
Olifantsvlei v. (OLIV)
Omo v. (OMOV)
Omsk hemorrhagic fever v.
  (OHFV)
O'nyong-nyong v. (ONNV)
orf v.
Oriboca v. (ORIV)
Oriximina v. (ORXV)
ornithosis v.
Oropouche v. (OROV)
orphan v.
Orungo v. (ORUV)
Ossa v. (OSSAV)
Ouango v. (OUAV)
Oubi v. (OUBIV)
Ourem v.
ovine AAV v.
OXN-100P v.
OXN-52P v.
oyster v. (OV)
φH-like v.'s
P1 v.
P2 v.
P107 v.
P22 v.
P335 v.
P45 v.
PA-2 v.
P-a-1 v.
Pacora v. (PCAV)
Pacui v. (PACV)
Pahayokee v. (PAHV)
Palestina v. (PLSV)
Palyam v. (PALV)
Pangola stunt v.
parainfluenza v.
parainfluenza v. type 1–4
Paramushir v. (PMRV)
Paraná v. (PARV)
paravaccinia v.
Paroo River v. (PRV)
Parry Creek v.
v. particle
parvo-like v.

Pata v. (PATAV)
Pathum Thani v. (PTHV)
Patois v. (PATV)
PAV v.
PB-1 v.
PBCV-1 v.
PBP1 v.
PBS1 v.
PbV v.
PC84 v.
Pc-fV v.
PcV v.
PE1 v.
Peaton v.
penguinpox v.
Penicillium brevicompactum v.
  (PbV)
Penicillium chrysogenum v. (PcV)
Penicillium cyaneo-fulvum v. (Pc-
  fV)
Penicillium stoloniferum F v. (PsV-
  F)
Penicillium stoloniferum S v. (PsV-
  S)
Perinet v. (PERV)
peste-des-petits-ruminants v.
Pf1, Pf2, Pf3 v.
Phialophora radicicola 2 2 Λ v.
phlebotomus fever v.
Phnom Penh bat v. (PPBV)
Pichinde v. (PICV)
Picola v. (PIAV)
PIIBNV6 v.
PIIBNV6-C v.
Piry v. (PIRYV)
Pixuna v. (PIXV)
PL-1 v.
Playas v. (PLAV)
pleomorphic phage v.
P1-like v.'s (v)
P2-like v.'s (v)
P22-like v.'s (v)
poliomyelitis v.
Pongola v. (PGAV)
Ponteves v. (PTVV)
porcine hemagglutinating
  encephalomyelitis v.
porcine transmissible
  gastroenteritis v.
Porton v.
Powassan v. (POWV)
PP7 v.

V

NOTES

virus *(continued)*

PP8 v.
PR3 v.
PR4 v.
PR772 v.
Prague strain Rous sarcoma v. (PRSV)
Precarious Point v. (PPV)
Pretoria v. (PREV)
PR64FS v.
primate T-lymphotropic v. 1, 2, 3
progeny v.
Prospect Hill v. (PHV)
PRR1 v.
PS4 v.
PS8 v.
PS17 v.
pseudocowpox v.
Pseudomonas phage chi-6 v.
pseudorabies v.
psittacinepox v.
psittacosis v.
PST v.
PT11 v.
PTB v.
Puchong v. (PUCV)
Pueblo Viejo v.
Puffin Island v.
Punta Salinas v. (PSV)
Punta Toro v. (PTV)
Purus v. (PURV)
Puumala v. (PUUV)
Qβ v.
Qalyub v. (QYBV)
Queensland fruit fly v.
R v.
R5 v.
R17 v.
R23 v.
R34 v.
R_1 v.
R_2 v.
RA-1 v.
rabies v.
Radi v. (RADIV)
rat v. (RV)
Raza v.
Razdan v. (RAZV)
reassortant v.
recombinant vaccinia v.
Reed Ranch v.
Resistencia v. (RTAV)
respiratory v.
respiratory enteric orphan v.
respiratory infection v.
respiratory syncytial v. (RSV)
Restan v. (RESV)
reticuloendotheliosis v.

Rhizidiomyces v.
Rift Valley fever v. (RVFV)
rinderpest v.
Rio Bravo v. (RBV)
Rio Grande v. (RGV)
Rio Grande cichlid v.
Rio Segunda v.
RML-105355 v.
RMV v.
R1-Myb v.
RNA tumor v.
Rochambeau v. (RBUV)
Rocio v. (ROCV)
Ross River v. (RRV)
Rous sarcoma v.
Royal Farm v. (RFV)
RPV v.
RR66 v.
RT v.
rubella v.
Russian spring-summer encephalitis v. (RSSEV)
S-6 v.
S13 v.
SA10 v.
SA12 v.
Sabia v.
Sabo v. (SABOV)
Saboya v. (SABV)
sacbrood v.
Sagiyama v. (SAGV)
saguaro cactus v. (SgCV)
Saint-Floris v. (SAFV)
Sakhalin v. (SAKV)
Salanga v. (SGAV)
Salehabad v. (SALV)
Salmon River v.
Sal Vieja v. (SVV)
San Angelo v. (SAV)
sandfly fever v.
sandfly fever Naples v. (SFNV)
sandfly fever Sicilian v. (SFSV)
Sandjimba v. (SJAV)
Sango v. (SANV)
San Juan v. (SJV)
San Perlita v. (SPV)
Santarem v. (STMV)
Santa Rosa v. (SARV)
Santosai temperate v.
sapphire II v.
Sapporo v.
Sapporo-like v.'s
Saraca v. (SRAV)
Sathuperi v. (SATV)
Saturnia pavonia v.
Saumarez Reef v. (SREV)
sawgrass v. (SAWV)
SD1 v.

sd v.
sealpox v.
Seletar v. (SELV)
Semliki Forest v. (SFV)
Sena Madureira v. (SMV)
Sendai v.
Seoul v. (SEOV)
Sepik v. (SEPV)
Serra do Navio v. (SDNV)
Setora nitens v.
SF v.
SGV v.
Shamonda v. (SHAV)
Shark River v. (SRV)
sheeppox v.
Shokwe v. (SHOV)
Shuni v. (SHUV)
Sigma v.
Silverwater v. (SILV)
Simbu v. (SIMV)
simian foamy v.
simian hemorrhagic fever v.
simian hepatitis A v.
simian immunodeficiency v. (SIV)
simian sarcoma v.
simian T-lymphotropic v. (STLV)
Simulium v.
Sindbis v. (SINV)
single-host v.
single nucleocapsid v.
Sin Nombre v.
Sixgun City v. (SCV)
SK1 v.
skunkpox v.
S-2L v.
S-4L v.
SM-1 v.
small DNA tumor v.
small round v. (SRV)
small round structured v. (SRSV)
SMB v.
SMP2 v.
SNDV-like v.'s
Snow Mountain v.
snowshoe hare v. (SSHV)
Sokuluk v. (SOKV)
Soldado v. (SOLV)
Sororoca v. (SORV)
Southampton v.
South River v.
SP v.
SPβ v.

SP3 v.
SP8 v.
SP10 v.
SP15 v.
SP50 v.
SPAr-2317 v.
sparrowpox v.
Spondweni v. (SPOV)
SPP1 v.
spring beauty latent v.
spring viremia v.
SPV4 v.
SPy-2 v.
squirrel fibroma v.
Sripur v. (SRIV)
ssRNA phage v.
SST v.
SSV1 v.
SSV1-type phage v.
St-1 v.
St. Abbs Head v.
starlingpox v.
St. Louis encephalitis v. (SLEV)
stomatitis papulosa v.
strain HM175 v.
Stratford v. (STRV)
Sunday Canyon v. (SCAV)
surface antigen of hepatitis B v.
 (HBsAg)
SV1 v.
SV2 v.
SV5 v.
SV40 v.
SV41 v.
Sweetwater Branch v.
swinepox v.
swine vesicular disease v. (SVDV)
syncytial v.
T21 v.
Ta$_1$ v.
Tacaiuma v. (TCMV)
Tacaribe v. (TCRV)
tadpole edema v.
Taggert v. (TAGV)
Tahyna v. (TAHV)
Tai v. (TAIV)
Taiassui v.
tailed phage v.
Tamana bat v.
Tamdy v. (TDYV)
Tamiami v. (TAMV)
Tanapox v.

NOTES

V

virus *(continued)*

Tanga v. (TANV)
Tanjong Rabok v. (TRV)
Tataguine v. (TATV)
Taterapox v.
Taunton v.
T-cell lymphoma v.
T-cell-tropic v.
Tehran v. (TEHV)
Tellina v. (TV)
Telok Forest v. (TFV)
Tembe v. (TMEV)
Tembusu v. (TMUV)
Tensaw v. (TENV)
Termeil v. (TERV)
Tete v. (TETEV)
Theiler murine encephalomyelitis v.
  (TMEV)
Thermoproteus phage TTV 1–3 v.
Thiafora v. (TFAV)
Thimiri v. (THIV)
Thogoto v. (THOV)
Thosea asigna v.
Thottapalayam v. (TPMV)
Tibrogargan v. (TIBV)
tick-borne encephalitis v. (TBEV)
tigre disease v.
Tilligerry v. (TILV)
Timbo v. (TIMV)
Timboteua v. (TBTV)
Tinaroo v. (TINV)
Tindholmur v. (TDMV)
v. titer
Tlacotalpan v. (TLNV)
T1-like v.'s
T4-like v.'s
T5-like v.'s
T7-like v.'s
Toronto v.
Toscana v. (TOSV)
trachoma v.
Triatoma lethal paralysis v.
Tribec v. (TRBV)
trivittatus v. (TVTV)
Trombetas v.
Trubanaman v. (TRUV)
Tsuruse v. (TSUV)
TT v. (TTV)
T1–T6 v.
T6–T20 v.
T-tropic v.
TTV1 v.
Tucunduba v.
tumor v.
Tupaia v.
turkeypox v.
turkey rhinotracheitis v.
Turlock v. (TURV)

Turuna v. (TUAV)
TVX v.
Twort v.
type A, B, C, D satellite v.
type F v.
Tyuleniy v. (TYUV)
U3 v.
Uasin Gishu disease v.
Uganda S v. (UGSV)
Umatilla v. (UMAV)
Umbre v. (UMBV)
Una v. (UNAV)
Upolu v. (UPOV)
Urucuri v. (URUV)
Usutu v. (USUV)
Utinga v. (UTIV)
Utive v.
Uukuniemi v. (UUKV)
vaccinia v. (VACV)
varicella-zoster v. (VZV)
variola v.
VD13 v.
Vellore v. (VELV)
Venezuelan equine encephalitis v.
  (VEEV)
vesicular exanthema swine v.
  (VESV)
vesicular stomatitis v. (VSV)
vesicular stomatitis Alagoas v.
  (VSAV)
vesicular stomatitis Indiana v.
  (VSIV)
vesicular stomatitis New Jersey v.
  (VSNJV)
Vf12 v.
Vf33 v.
ViII v.
Vil v.
Vilyuisk v.
Vilyuisk human
  encephalomyelitis v.
Vinces v. (VINV)
viral hemorrhagic septicemia v.
  (VHSV)
Virgin River v. (VRV)
visna/maedi v.
volepox v.
VP1 v.
VP3 v.
VP5 v.
VP11 v.
v1, v2 v.
v4–v7 v.
W31 v.
WA/1 v.
Wad Medani v. (WMV)
Wallal v. (WALV)
Wanowrie v. (WANV)

Warrego v. (WARV)
Weldona v.
Wesselsbron v. (WESSV)
western equine encephalitis v.
  (WEE)
western equine encephalomyelitis v.
West Nile v.
West Nile encephalitis v. (WNV)
WF/1 v.
Whataroa v. (WHAV)
wild-type v.
Witwatersrand v. (WITV)
Wongal v. (WONV)
Wongorr v. (WGRV)
woolly monkey sarcoma v.
wound tumor v. (WTV)
WRSV v.
WT1 v.
WTV v.
WW/1 v.
Wyeomyia v. (WYOV)
X v.
X29 v.
v. X disease
Xf v.
Xf2 v.
Xiburema v. (XIBV)
Xingu v.
XP5 v.
y5 v.
Yaba 1, -7 v.
Yaba-like disease v.
Yaba monkey tumor v.
Yacaaba v. (YACV)
yam mosaic v. (YMV)
Yaquina Head v. (YHV)
Yuta v. (YATAV)
yellow fever v. (YFV)
YIV v.
Yogue v. (YOGV)
Yokose v.
Yug Bogdanovac v. (YBV)
Zaliv Terpeniya v. (ZTV)
Zegla v. (ZEGV)
ZG/1 v.
ZG/2 v.
ZG/3A v.
ZIK/1 v.
Zika v. (ZIKAV)
Zirqa v. (ZIRV)
ZJ/1 v.
ZJ/2 v.

ZL/3 v.
ZS/3 v.
virus-A
  GB v.-A.
virus-associated hemophagocytic
  syndrome
virus-B
  GB v.-B.
virus-C
  GB v.-C.
virus-cell infectious cycle
virus-host interaction
virus-induced immunopathy
virus-like
  v.-l. infectious agent (VLIA)
  v.-l. particle (VLP)
  v.-l. particle vaccine
virus-transformed cell
viscera (*pl. of* viscus)
visceral
  v. abdominal fat (VAT)
  v. abdominal fat to total
    abdominal fat ratio (VAT:TAT
    ratio)
  v. abscess
  v. gnathostomiasis
  v. Hodgkin disease
  v. larva migrans (VLM)
  v. leishmaniasis
  v. metastasis
viscerotropic *Leishmania tropica*
  infection
viscosa
  Moritella v.
viscosus
  Actinomyces v.
  Arthrobacter v.
  Vibrio v.
viscus, pl. **viscera**
vishniacii
  Cryptococcus v.
Visine
  V. L.R. Ophthalmic
  V. Workplace
vision
  cloudy v.
visna/maedi virus
Vistide
vistulensis
  Culicoides v.
visual
  v. acuity

NOTES

V

visual *(continued)*
    v. cortex
    v. field defect
visualization
viswanathii
    Candida v.
vitaeruminis
    Corynebacterium v.
vital blood culture system
vitamin
    v. A and vitamin D
    v. B_{12} malabsorption
vitaminophilum
    Actinosporangium v.
vitaminophilus
    Streptomyces v.
vitarumen
    Brevibacterium v.
viteae
    Acanthocheilonema v.
    Dipetalonema v.
Vitek
    V. Anaerobe Identification (ANI) card
    V. GPI card
    V. *Neisseria-Haemophilus* Identification Card
    V. NHI Card
vitellarium
vitelline reservoir
vitellinum
    Polyangium v.
vitiating
vitiligo
vitis
    Agrobacterium v.
    Rhizobium v.
Vitivirus (v)
Vitrasert
Vitravene
vitrectomy
    pars plana v.
vitreoretinal
Vitreoscilla (b)
    V. *beggiatoides*
    V. *filiformis*
    V. *stercoraria*
vitreous
    v. aspiration
    v. exudate
    v. haze
    v. hemorrhage
in vitro
Vitronectin R
Vittaforma (p)
    V. *corneae*
    V. *corneum*

vittatum
    Simulium v.
vittatus
    Aedes v.
vituli
    Acholeplasma v.
    Linognathus v.
vitulinus
    Lactobacillus v.
    Staphylococcus v.
vitulorum
    Neoascaris v.
vivax
    v. fever
    v. malaria
    Plasmodium v.
    Trypanosoma v.
Vivelle Transdermal
viverrini
    Opisthorchis v.
vivipara
    Probstymayria v.
viviparus
    Dictyocaulus v.
vivo
    in v.
Vivotif Berna
Vizellaceae
VK
    Apo-Pen VK
    Lanacillin VK
    pen VK
    Robicillin VK
VL
    viral load
VLIA
    virus-like infectious agent
VLM
    visceral larva migrans
VLP
    virus-like particle
    VLP vaccine
VLS
    vascular leak syndrome
vogeli
    Echinococcus v.
Vogesella indigofera (b)
Voges-Proskauer test
Vogt-Koyanagi-Harada syndrome
voice prosthesis
volantium
    Pasteurella v.
volar
volatile hydrazine
Volcaniella eurihalina (b)
volcanii
    Halobacterium v.
    Haloferax v.

volcanium
    Thermoplasma v.
vole
    field v.
volepox virus
Volhynia fever
Volmax
voltae
    Methanococcus v.
volume
    residual v.
volumetric flask
voluminous
volutans
    Spirillum v.
Volutella cinerescens (f)
volutin
    v. granule
Volvox
    V. carteri
    V. globactor
volvulosis
volvulus
    Onchocerca v.
vomiting
    epidemic v.
    grade 2 v.
vomitoria
    Calliphora v.
vomitus
von
    V. Economo encephalitis
    V. Economo encephalitis lethargica
    v. Hippel-Lindau (vHL)
    v. Willebrand disease
vordarabine
voriconazole
vortex, pl. **vortices**
    v. mixer
    v. ± sonication
    v. vein
vortexed
vortexing
Vorticella similis
vortices (*pl. of* vortex)
VoSol HC Otic
VP11 virus
VP1 virus
VP3 virus
VP5 virus
VPS
    Vaccine Preparedness Study

vpu
    v. gene
vpx-related gene
V/Q scan
VRE
    vancomycin-resistant enterococcus
VREF
    vancomycin-resistant *Enterococcus faecium*
VRSA
    vancomycin-resistant *Staphylococcus aureus*
VRV
    Virgin River virus
VSAV
    vesicular stomatitis Alagoas virus
VSG
    variant surface glycoprotein
    VSG gene
VSIV
    vesicular stomatitis Indiana virus
VSNJV
    vesicular stomatitis New Jersey virus
VSV
    vesicular stomatitis virus
VT
    verotoxin
VTEC
    verocytotoxin-producing *Escherichia coli*
    VTEC 0111 strain
vuloani
    Bacillus v.
    Methanolobus v.
vulcanius
    Methanococcus v.
vulgare
    Hyphomicrobium v.
    Ketogulonicigenium v.
    Streptosporangium v.
vulgaris
    acne v.
    Desulfovibrio vulgaris subsp. *v.*
    impetigo v.
    lupus v.
    Nitrobacter v.
    Proteus v.
    Strongylus v.
    Tectibacter v.
    Thermoactinomyces v.
    verruca v.
vulgatus
    Bacteroides v.

V

NOTES

vulneris
    Escherichia v.
vulnifica
    Beneckea v.
vulnificus
    Vibrio v.
vulpis
    Crenosoma v.
    Trichuris v.
vulva, gen. and pl. **vulvae**
    pruritus vulvae
vulval mucosa
vulvar
    v. pruritus
vulvovaginal
    v. candidiasis
    v. candidosis
    v. itching

v. tuberculosis
v. ulceration
vulvovaginitis
    Candida v.
    herpetic v.
    trichomonal v.
Vumon
V.V.S.
v1, v2 virus
v4–v7 virus
VZIG
    varicella immune globulin
    varicella-zoster immune globulin
    varicella-zoster immunoglobulin
VZV
    varicella-zoster virus
        VZV vaccine

W
   W. antigen
   W. strain of *Mycobacterium*
     tuberculosis
W31 virus
WA/1 virus
Waddlia chondrophila (b)
Wad Medani virus (WMV)
wadsworthensis
   Sutterella w.
wadsworthia
   Bilophila w.
wadsworthii
   Legionella w.
Waikavirus (v)
waiotapuensis
   Thermococcus w.
waist:hip ratio (WHR)
waius
   Streptococcus w.
Wakana disease
waksmanii
   Streptomyces w.
Waldenstrom macroglobulinemia
Waldermaria (f)
Walkaway (W/A) Rapid Bacterial
  Identification System
walkeri
   Anopheles w.
walking pneumonia
Wallal virus (WALV)
Wallemia sebi (f)
wallerian degeneration
waltersii
   Legionella w.
WALV
   Wallal virus
Wangiella dermatitidis (f)
Wanowrie virus (WANV)
WANV
   Wanowrie virus
warble
   w. botfly
   w. fly
   ox w.
Wardomyces inflatus (f)
Wardomycopsis (f)
Warfarin
warm agglutinin
warmboldiae
   Buttiauxella w.
warming
   global w.

warmingii
   Allochromatium w.
   Chromatium w.
warneri
   Staphylococcus w.
Warrego virus (WARV)
wart
   anogenital w.
   butcher's w.
   common w.
   filiform w.
   flat w.
   genital w.
   hyperproliferative w.
   intermediate w.
   juvenile w.
   mosaic w.
   Peruvian w.
   plane w.
   plantar w.
   W. Remover
   venereal w.
Wartec
Warthin-Starry stain
warty tuberculosis
WARV
   Warrego virus
wasabiae
   Erwinia carotovora subsp. *w.*
   Pectobacterium carotovorum subsp.
     w.
wash
   Benzac AC W.
   Benzac W W.
   Desquam-X W.
   Dryox W.
   Fostex 10% W.
   nasopharyngeal w.
   Oil-Free Acne W.
   Oxy 10 W.
   SAStid Plain Therapeutic Shampoo
     and Acne W.
   Theroxide W.
washing
   bronchial w.
   bronchoalveolar w.
washingtonensis
   Streptomyces cavourensis subsp. *w.*
Wassermann test
wasting
   w. disease
   fat w.
   peripheral fat w.
   w. syndrome

W

Watch
Oxy Night W.
water
deionized w.
distilled w.
extracellular w. (ECW)
intracellular w. (ICW)
w. itch
w. lily sign
w. sore
total body w. (TBW)
waterborne
Waterhouse-Friderichsen syndrome
watery diarrhea
watsoni
Watsonius w.
Watsonius watsoni (p)
wave
fluid w.
waxy cast
4-Way Long Acting Nasal solution
Wayson stain
waywayandensis
Lentzea w.
Saccharothrix w.
WB
Western blot
WB assay
WBC
white blood cell
WBH
whole-body hyperthermia
w/C
Aprodine w.
w/Codeine
Allerfrin w.
Bromphen DC w.
w/DM
Pherazine w.
weakness
proximal w.
weanling diarrhea
weaveri
Neisseria w.
Weber modified trichrome stain
Weck-cel
W.-c. ophthalmic surgical spear
W.-c. sponge
wedge resection
wedmorensis
Streptomyces w.
WEE
western equine encephalitis virus
Weeks bacillus (*See Haemophilus aegyptius*)
Weeksella (b)
W. virosa
W. zoohelcum

WEEV
Weichselbaum coccus (*See Neisseria meningitidis*)
Weigart focus
weight
extremely low birth w. (ELBW)
weihenstephanensis
Bacillus w.
Weil
W. disease
W. syndrome
Weil-Felix
W.-F. reaction
W.-F. test
weilii
Leptospira w.
Weinstein
Turkish massage of W.
weissei
Chromatium w.
Weissella (b)
W. confusa
W. halotolerans
W. hellenica
W. kandleri
W. minor
W. paramesenteroides
W. thailandensis
W. viridescens
Welch bacillus (*See Clostridium perfringens*)
Weldona virus
well-established
wellingtoni
Haemaphysalis w.
welshimeri
Listeria w.
wenyonii
Eperythrozoon w.
werkmanii
Citrobacter w.
werneckii
Hortaea w.
Pullularia w.
werneri
Culicoides w.
Wernicke disease
Wernicke-Korsakoff syndrome
werraensis
Streptomyces w.
Wesselsbron
W. fever
W. virus (WESSV)
WESSV
Wesselsbron virus
West
W. African fever
W. African sleeping sickness

W. African trypanosomiasis
W. Nile encephalitis virus (WNV)
W. Nile fever
W. Nile virus

Westcort Topical

westermani
Paragonimus w.

western
W. blot (WB)
W. blot assay
W. blot infection
W. blot test
w. equine encephalitis
w. equine encephalitis virus (WEE)
w. equine encephalomyelitis virus
W. immunoblot assay

wet
w. cutaneous leishmaniasis
w. gangrene
w. mount
w. mount preparation
w. prep

WF/1 virus
WGRV
Wongorr virus

Whataroa
Sindbis virus subtype W.
W. virus (WHAV)

Whatman No. 541 filter paper
WHAV
Whataroa virus

wheal
Wheatley trichrome stain
whiff
w. test
w. testing

whippelii
Tropheryma w.

Whipple disease
whipworm
white
w. blood cell (WBC)
calcofluor w.
w. mycetoma
w. piedra
w. piedra infection

whitei
Nosema w.

white-matter disease
Whitfield ointment

whitlow
herpes w.
herpetic w.

Whitmore bacillus
whittenburyi
Methylobacter w.
Methylococcus w.

whole-body
w.-b. bone scan
w.-b. hyperthermia (WBH)
w.-b. plethysmography

whole-brain radiation therapy
whole-cell
w.-c. pertussis
w.-c. vaccine

whooping
w. cough
w. cough syndrome

WHR
waist:hip ratio

Wickerhamiella (f)
wickerhamii
Candida w.
Hansenula w.
Prototheca w.

wick method
wide excision
wiegelii
Thermoanaerobacter w.

wieringae
Acetobacterium w.

Wigglesworthia glossinidia (b)
WIHS
Women's Interagency HIV Study

wikenii
Kluyveromyces w.

wild-type
w.-t. poliovirus
w.-t. strain
w.-t. virus

Willia (f) (*See* **Pichia**)
williamsae
Oceanospirillum maris subsp. w.

Williamsia murale (b)
Williopsis (f)
willmorei
Streptomyces w.

Wilms tumor
Wilson
W. disease
W. method

W

NOTES

wingei
  Hansenula w.
winogradskyi
  Nitrobacter w.
  Thiorhodovibrio w.
  Thiospira w.
Winpred
WinRho SD
winter
  w. diarrhea
  w. dysentery of cattle
Winterbottom sign
winthemi
  Margaropus w.
wirthi
  Culicoides w.
wisconsensis
  Moellerella w.
wisconsinensis
  Culicoides w.
Wiskott-Aldrich syndrome
witkop
WITS
  Women and Infants Transmission Study
wittichii
  Sphingomonas w.
WITV
  Witwatersrand virus
Witwatersrand virus (WITV)
WMV
  Wad Medani virus
WNV
  West Nile encephalitis virus
wodanis
  Vibrio w.
woesei
  Pyrococcus w.
Wohlfahrtia (p)
  W. magnifica
  W. opaca
  W. vigil
wohlfahrtiosis
Wolbachia (b)
  W. melophagi
  W. persica
  W. pipientis
wolbachii
  Leptospira w.
wolfei
  Methanobacterium w.
  Methanothermobacter w.
  Syntrophomonas wolfei subsp. *w.*
wolfii
  Mortierella w.
Wolinella (b)
  W. curva
  W. recta
  W. succinogenes

wolinii
  Syntrophobacter w.
wolinskyi
  Mycobacterium w.
Wollan agent
woluwensis
  Arthrobacter w.
Women
  W. and Infants Transmission Study
    (WITS)
  W. Interagency HIV Study (WIHS)
  Selsun Gold for W.
Wongal virus (WONV)
Wongorr virus (WGRV)
WONV
  Wongal virus
Woodburg bug
woodcutter's encephalitis
wooden tongue disease
woodii
  Acetobacterium w.
Wood lamp
woodsii
  Pseudomonas w.
woodyi
  Shewanella w.
woolly monkey sarcoma virus
woolsorter's
  w. disease
  w. pneumonia
word fluency task
worker
  health care w. (HCW)
  laboratory w. (LW)
Workplace
  Visine W.
worm
  w. abscess
  caddis w.
  cod w.
  eye w.
  fiery serpent w.
  giant kidney w.
  guinea w.
  herring w.
  heterophyid w.
  Manson eye w.
  meal w.
  Medina w.
  primary screw w.
  seal w.
  secondary screw w.
  thorny-headed w.
  Ugandan eye w.
worsleiensis
  Legionella w.
wound
  w. botulism

w. culture
w. dehiscence
w. fever
w. infection
w. myiasis
penetrating w.
saltwater-related w.
w. swab
w. tumor virus (WTV)
wratislaviensis
    Tsukamurella w.
Wright-Giemsa stain
Wright stain
wrist arthrogram
WRSV virus
WT1 virus
WTV
    wound tumor virus
    WTV virus
wuayaraka
    Simulium w.

Wuchereria (p)
    W. bancrofti
    W. kalimantani
    W. pacifica
wuchereriasis
wuyiensis
    Lasiohelea w.
WW/1 virus
Wyamycin S
Wycillin
Wyeomyia
    W. codiocampa
    W. moerbista
    W. occulta
    W. smithii
    W. virus (WYOV)
Wymox
wyomingense
    Simulium w.
WYOV
    Wyeomyia virus

NOTES

W

X

X factor
X virus
X29 virus
Xanax
xanthine hydrolysis test
xanthineolytica
Oerskovia x.
Xanthobacter (b)
X. agilis
X. autotrophicus
X. flavus
X. tagetidis
xanthochromogenes
Streptomyces x.
xanthocidicus
Streptomyces x.
xantholiticus
Streptomyces x.
Xanthomonas (b)
X. albilineans
X. ampelina
X. arboricola
X. axonopodis
X. bromi
X. campestris
X. cassavae
X. citri
X. codiaei
X. cucurbitae
X. cynarae
X. fragariae
X. hortorum
X. hyacinthi
X. maltophilia
X. melonis
X. oryzae
X. phaseoli
X. pisi
X. populi
X. saccari
X. theicola
X. translucens
X. vasicola
X. vesicatoria
xanthophaeus
Streptomyces x.
xanthum
Flavobacterium x.
xanthus
Myxococcus x.
xelajuensis
Anopheles x.
xenic culture
xenodiagnosis

xenograft
porcine x.
xenoparasite
xenophaga
Sphingomonas x.
xenopi
Mycobacterium x.
Xenopsylla (p)
X. cheopis
X. variabilis
Xenorhabdus (b)
X. beddingii
X. bovienii
X. japonica
X. luminescens
X. nematophila
X. nematophila subsp. beddingii
X. nematophila subsp. bovienii
X. nematophila subsp. poinarii
X. poinarii
xenozoonosis
Xerocomaceae
xeroderma
xerophthalmia
xerosis
Corynebacterium x.
xerostomia
xestobii
Candida x.
Xf2 virus
Xf virus
Xiburema virus (XIBV)
XIBV
Xiburema virus
Xingu virus
xinjiangense
Sinorhizobium x.
xinjiangensis
Actinobispora x.
Saccharomonospora x.
XL
Biaxin XL
X-linked
X-l. agammaglobulinemia
X-l. lymphoproliferative disease
XP
Cophene XP
XP5 virus
x-ray
x-r. crystallography
x-r. radiotherapy
X-Seb T
XT
Contuss XT
xylan fermentation test

X

xylanilyticus
> *Thermobacillus* x.

xylanolytica
> *Cytophaga* x.

xylanolyticum
> *Clostridium* x.
> *Thermoanaerobacterium* x.

xylanolyticus
> *Bacteroides* x.

xylanophilum
> *Eubacterium* x.

xylanophilus
> *Rubrobacter* x.

xylanovorans
> *Clostridium* x.

xylanus
> *Amphibacillus* x.

Xylaria (f)

Xylariaceae

Xylella fastidiosa (b)

xylene
> carbol x.

xyli
> *Clavibacter xyli* subsp. x.
> *Leifsonia xyli* subsp. x.

xylinum
> *Acetobacter aceti* subsp. x.

xylinus
> *Acetobacter xylinus* subsp. x.
> *Gluconacetobacter xylinus* subsp. x.

xylitol fermentation test

Xylocaine jelly

Xylohypha (f)

xylol

Xylophilus ampelinus (b)

xylosa
> *Pichia* x.

xylose fermentation test

D-xylose fermentation test

xylosoxidans
> *Achromobacter* x.
> *Achromobacter xylosoxidans* subsp. x.
> *Alcaligenes* x.

xylosus
> *Lactobacillus* x.
> *Staphylococcus* x.

Yaba
    Y. monkey tumor virus
Yaba-like disease virus
Yaba/Tanapox virus subgroup
Yaba-1, -7 virus
yabuuchiae
    Flavobacterium y.
Yacaaba virus (YACV)
yacuchuspi
    Simulium y.
YACV
    Yacaaba virus
yamanashiensis
    Lactobacillus y.
    Spirilliplanes y.
yam mosaic virus (YMV)
yanglingense
    Rhizobium y.
yangmingensis
    Sulfolobus y.
Yangtze
    Y. river edema
    Y. Valley fever
yanoikuyae
    Sphingobium y.
    Sphingomonas y.
yaoundei
    Trichophyton y
Yaquina Head virus (YHV)
Yarrowia (f)
    Y. lipolytica
yarrowii
    Cryptococcus y.
yasguri
    Cheyletiella y.
Yatapoxvirus (v)
YATAV
    Yata virus
Yata virus (YATAV)
yaw
    Bosch y.
    bush y.
    forest y.
    mother y.
yayanosii
    Moritella y.
YBV
    Yug Bogdanovac virus
yeast
    y. extract agar
    y. fungus
    y. infection
    y. vaginitis
yeastlike fungus

yeatsii
    Mycoplasma y.
yellow
    y. exudate
    y. fever (YF)
    y. fever vaccine
    y. fever virus (YFV)
    y. pigment test
yellowstonensis
    Sulfurococcus y.
yellowstonii
    Thermodesulfovibrio y.
yerevanensis
    Streptomyces y.
Yersinia (b)
    Y. aldovae
    Y. arthritis
    Y. bercovieri
    Y. enterocolitica biogroup 3A
    Y. enterocolitica biogroup 3B
    Y. enterocolitica biotype 1
    Y. enterocolitica biotype 1,
        serotype O:5
    Y. enterocolitica biovar 1
    Y. enterocolitica subsp.
        enterocolitica
    Y. enterocolitica subsp. *pulearctica*
    Y. frederiksenii
    Y. intermedia
    Y. kristensenii
    Y. mollaretii
    Y. pestis
    Y. philomiragia
    Y. pseudotuberculosis
    Y. pseudotuberculosis agglutinin
    Y. rohdei
    Y. ruckeri
yersiniosis
    pseudotubercular y.
yessotoxin
YF
    yellow fever
YFV
    yellow fever virus
YF-VAX
YHV
    Yaquina Head virus
YIV
    YIV virus
YMV
    yam mosaic virus
Yodoxin
Yogue virus (YOGV)
YOGV
    Yogue virus

Y

613

Yokenella regensburgei (b)
yokogawai
    Metagonimus y.
Yokose virus
yokosukanensis
    Streptomyces y.
yonsiensis
    Thermoanaerobacter y.
youngae
    Citrobacter y.
Y shape
Yug Bogdanovac virus (YBV)

yukonensis
    Culicoides y.
yumaensis
    Actinomadura y.
yunnanensis
    Actinobispora y.
yurii
    Eubacterium yurii subsp. *y.*
y5 virus

Zagam
zalcitabine (ddC)
Zaliv Terpeniya virus (ZTV)
Zambesi ulcer
zammitii
    Aedes *z.*
zanamivir
Zantac
    Z. 75
zaomyceticus
    Streptomyces *z.*
Zartan
zatmanii
    Methylobacterium *z.*
Zavarzinia (b)
    Z. compransoris
zavarzinii
    Hyphomicrobium *z.*
zeae
    Gibberella *z.*
    Lactobacillus *z.*
    Thermoanaerobacterium *z.*
Zcasorb-AF
    Z.-AF Powder
zebrae
    Habronema *z.*
Zefazone
Zegla virus (ZEGV)
ZEGV
    Zegla virus
Zeiss
    gland of Z.
Zephrex
    Z. LA
Zerit
Zetar
Zevalin
zeylanica
    Haemadipsa *z.*
zeylanoides
    Candida *z.*
ZG/1 virus
ZG/2 virus
ZG/3A virus
zhilinae
    Methanohalophilus *z.*
Ziagen
zidovudine (ZDV, ZVD)
    z. elixir
    z. and lamivudine
zidovudine-induced myelotoxicity
zidovudine-resistant HIV-1 strain
Ziehl-Neelsen acid-fast stain
Ziemann dots
ZIK/1 virus

Zika
    Z. fever
    Z. virus (ZIKAV)
ZIKAV
    Zika virus
zilligii
    Sulfophobococcus *z.*
    Thermococcus *z.*
Zinacef
    Z. Injection
Zinaderm
zinc
    DHS Z.
    z. oxide
    z. oxide, cod liver oil, and talc
    pyrithione z.
    z. sulfate douche
    z. sulfate flotation centrifugation
    z. sulfate flotation concentration
    z. sulfate flotation technique
Zincoderm
Zincofax
Zincon Shampoo
Zino
    Scholl Z.
ziracin
Zirqa virus (ZIRV)
ZIRV
    Zirqa virus
Zithromax
ZJ/1 virus
ZJ/2 virus
ZL/3 virus
ZNP Bar
zoa (*pl. of* zoon)
Zobellia (b)
    Z. galactanivorans
    Z. uliginosa
zobellii
    Idiomarina *z.*
    Metschnikowia *z.*
zoite
Zolicef
Zollinger-Ellison syndrome
zolpidem
Zonalon Topical Cream
zone
    T z.
        transformation zone
    transformation z. (T zone)
zonula occludens toxin (zot)
zooanthroponosis
zooepidemicus
    Streptococcus equi subsp. *z.*
zooglea

Z

zoogleiformans
> *Capsularis* z.

zoogleoformans
> *Bacteroides* z.
> *Prevotella* z.

Zoogloea (b)
> Z. *ramigera*
> Z. *resiniphila*

zoogloeoides
> *Duganella* z.

zoohelcum
> *Bergeyella* z.
> *Weeksella* z.

zooid
Zoomastigina
Zoomastigophorea
Zoomastigota
Zoon
> balanitis of Z.

zoon, pl. **zoa**
zoonosis
> direct z.

zoonotic
> z. cutaneous leishmaniasis
> z. disease
> z. listerial infection
> z. strongyloidiasis

Zoopagaceae
Zoopagales
zooparasite
zoophilic
zoophyte
zoosophus
> *Aedes* z.

Zopfia (f)
zopfii
> *Kurthia* z.
> *Prototheca* z.
> *Rhodococcus* z.

ZORprin
zoster
> acute herpes z.
> herpes z.
> z. immune globulin
> z. meningoencephalitis
> multidermatomeric herpes z.
> ocular z.
> ophthalmic z.
> z. ophthalmicus
> z. sine herpete
> z. titer
> z. vaccine

zosterae
> *Desulfovibrio* z.

zosteriform eruption
Zostrix
> Z. vaccine

Zostrix-HP
Zosyn
zot
> zonula occludens toxin

Zovirax
ZP 11
ZS/3 virus
ZTV
> Zaliv Terpeniya virus

Zubrod performance scale
zuelzerae
> *Spirochaeta* z.

ZVD
> zidovudine

Zygoascus (f)
Zygofabospora (f)
Zygohansenula (f)
zygoma, pl. **zygomata, zygomas**
zygomatic
Zygomycetes
zygomycosis
Zygomycotina
Zygopichia (f)
Zygorenospora (f)
Zygosaccharomyces (f)
zygosperm
zygospore
Zygosporium mansonii (f)
zygotoblast
zygotomere
Zygowillia (f)
Zygowilliopsis californicus
Zymobacter palmae (b)
Zymodebaryomyces (f)
zymodeme
Zymomonas (b)
> Z. *mobilis* subsp. *mobilis*
> Z. *mobilis* subsp. *pomaceae*

Zymonema (f)
Zymophilus (b)
> Z. *paucivorans*
> Z. *raffinosivorans*

Zymopichia (f)
zymotic papilloma
Zyvox

Appendix 1
Anatomical Illustrations

Bacteria

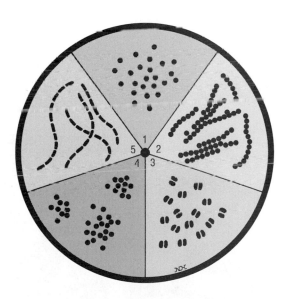

Figure 1. Bacteria. (1) cocci. (2) streptococci. (3) diplococci. (4) staphylococci. (5) bacilli.

Appendix 1

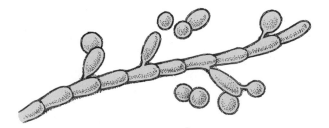

Figure 2.   Yeast: *Candida albicans.*

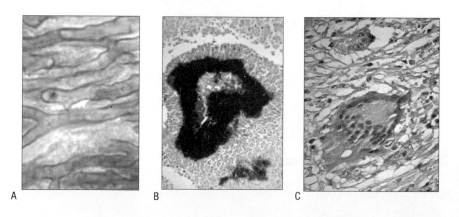

A   B   C

Figure 3.   Fungi. (A) *Aspergillus* hyphae: in tissue (periodic acid-Schiff stain). (B) mycetoma granule: in tissue (Brown and Brenn stain). (C) histoplasmosis: multinucleated giant cell in lung. These images, courtesy of Bennett J, PhD. for *Stedman's Medical Dictionary, 27th Edition,* Baltimore, Lippincott Williams & Wilkins, 2000, p. C7, appear here with permission and courtesy of Lippincott Williams & Wilkins.

Fungus

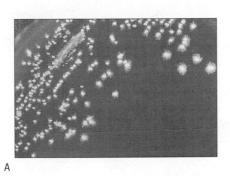

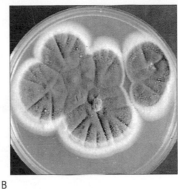

A   B

Figure 4. Fungi. (A) *Candida albicans* showing foot-like extensions of the colonies on the surface of 5% sheep blood agar. (B) *Alternaria* after 6 days' growth. These images, from Koneman EW, Allen SD, Janda WM, Schrechenberger PC & Winn WC, Jr., *Color Atlas and Textbook of Diagnostic Microbiology, 5th Edition*, Philadelphia, Lippincott, 1997, appear here with permission and courtesy of Lippincott Williams & Wilkins.

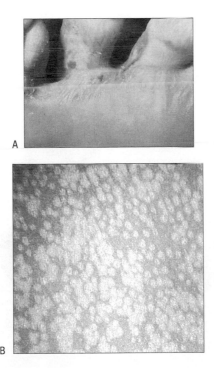

Figure 5. Fungal diseases. (A) tinea pedis: interdigital infection with *Trichophyton mentagrophytes*. (B) tinea versicolor: close-up view of hypopigmented macules on the back. These images, from Sanders CV, Nesbitt LT, Jr., *The Skin and Infection: A Color Atlas and Text*, Baltimore, Williams & Wilkins, 1995, appear here with permission and courtesy of Lippincott Williams & Wilkins.

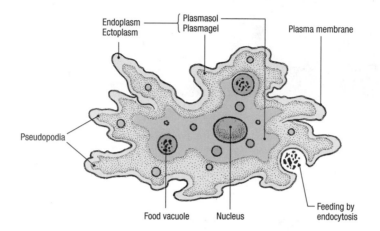

Endoplasm
Ectoplasm
Plasmasol
Plasmagel
Plasma membrane
Pseudopodia
Food vacuole
Nucleus
Feeding by
endocytosis

Figure 6.   Ameba: *Amoeba,* parasitic protozoon.

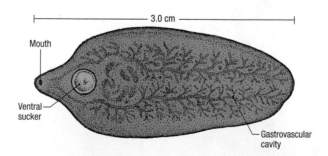

3.0 cm
Mouth
Ventral
sucker
Gastrovascular
cavity

Figure 7.   Trematode: *Fasciola hepatica,* liver fluke.

Parasite

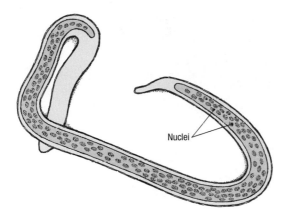

Figure 8. Filaria: microfilaria of *Wuchereria bancrofti.*

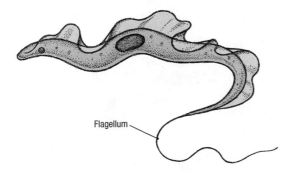

Figure 9. Flagellate: Mastigophora, subphylum of Protozoa.

Parasite

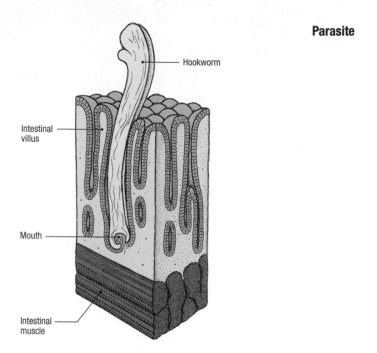

Figure 10. Nematode: *Necator americanus,* New World hookworm.

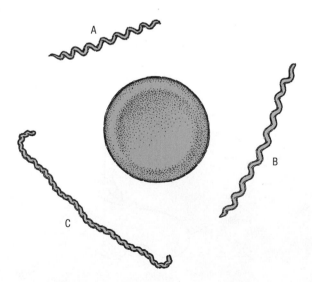

Figure 11. Spirochetes (parasitic bacteria shown for size comparison with red blood cell). (A) *Treponema.* (B) *Borrelia.* (C) *Leptospira.*

Parasite

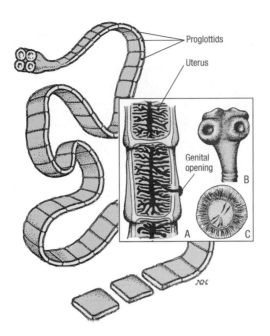

Figure 12. Beef tapeworm: *Taenia saginata.* (A) Body segment showing reproductive organs (×1.7). (B) Scolex (×12). (C) Egg (×550).

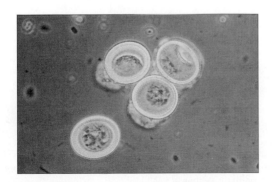

Figure 13. *Taenia:* Phase-contrast microscopy of four eggs. This image, from Sun T, *Parasitic Disorders, 2nd Edition,* Baltimore, Williams & Wilkins, 1998, Fig. 7.8, appears here with permission and courtesy of Lippincott Williams & Wilkins.

Parasite

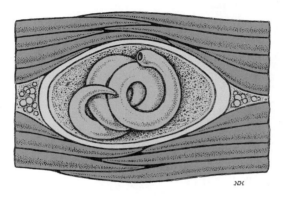

Figure 14. Nematode: *Trichinella spiralis,* pork worm, cause of trichinosis; larva encysted in human muscle.

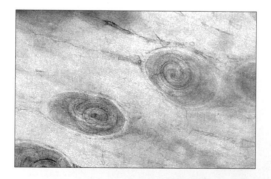

Figure 15. *Trichinella*: coiled larvae in laboratory mouse, unstained (×160). This image, from Sun T, *Parasitic Disorders, 2nd Edition,* Baltimore, Williams & Wilkins, 1998, fig. 23.7, appears here with permission and courtesy of Lippincott Williams & Wilkins.

Parasite

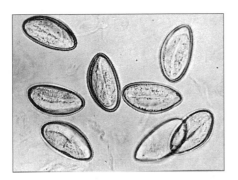

Figure 16. Nematodes: *Enterobius vermicularis*, pinworm ova; transparent tape preparation. This image, from Koneman EW, Allen SD, Janda WM, Schrechenberger PC & Winn WC, Jr., *Color Atlas and Textbook of Diagnostic Microbiology, 5th Edition*, Philadelphia, Lippincott, 1997, fig. 20.3G, appears here with permission and courtesy of Lippincott Williams & Wilkins.

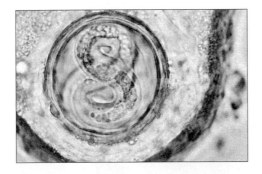

Figure 17. Nematode: *Ascaris lumbricoides*; egg containing larvae. This image, from Koneman EW, Allen SD, Janda WM, Schrechenberger PC & Winn WC, Jr., *Color Atlas and Textbook of Diagnostic Microbiology, 5th Edition*, Philadelphia, Lippincott, 1997, fig. 20.3C, appears here with permission and courtesy of Lippincott Williams & Wilkins.

Appendix 1

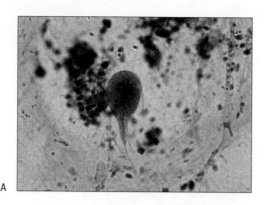

A

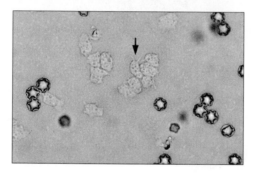

B

Figure 18. Trophozoites. (A) *Giarda lamblia*: trophozoite, trichrome stain (×400). (B) *Acanthamoeba*: trophozoites (arrow) and cysts, trypan blue (×40). These images, from Sun T, *Parasitic Disorders, 2nd Edition,* Baltimore, Williams & Wilkins, 1998, figs. 7.8 & 10.2, appear here with permission and courtesy of Lippincott Williams & Wilkins.

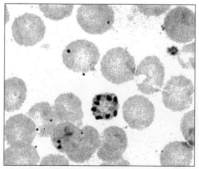

Figure 19. Protozoa: *Plasmodium malariae*; schizont with fewer than 13 segments in erythrocyte. This image, from Koneman EW, Allen SD, Janda WM, Schrechenberger PC & Winn WC, Jr., *Color Atlas and Textbook of Diagnostic Microbiology, 5th Edition,* Philadelphia, Lippincott, 1997, fig. 20.6P, appears here with permission and courtesy of Lippincott Williams & Wilkins.

Parasite

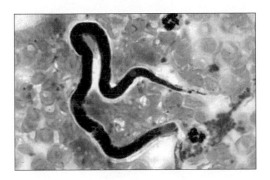

Figure 20.   Filaria: *Brugia malayi*; microfilaria (×300). This image, from Sun T, *Parasitic Disorders, 2nd Edition,* Baltimore, Williams & Wilkins, 1998, fig. 37.3, appears here with permission and courtesy of Lippincott Williams & Wilkins.

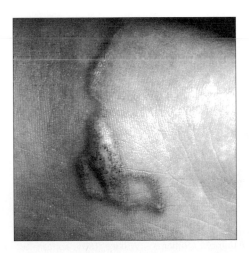

Figure 21.   Nematode: *Ancylostoma brazillense* or *A. canium* larvae, cutaneous larva migrans; serpiginous track with bulla formation on sole of foot. This image, from Sanders CV, Nesbitt LT, Jr., *The Skin and Infection: A Color Atlas and Text,* Baltimore, Williams & Wilkins, 1995, fig. 18.3, appears here with permission and courtesy of Lippincott Williams & Wilkins.

Parasite

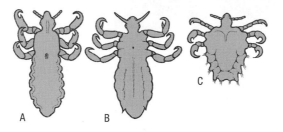

Figure 22. Common lice of humans. (A) Head louse (*Pediculus humanus* var *capitis*). (B) Body louse (*Pediculus* var *humanus corporis*). (C) Pubic louse (*Pthirus pubis*).

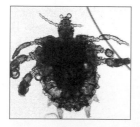

Figure 23. *Pthirus pubis* (adult female). This image, from Sanders CV, Nesbitt LT, Jr., *The Skin and Infection: A Color Atlas and Text,* Baltimore, Williams & Wilkins, 1995, appears here with permission and courtesy of Lippincott Williams & Wilkins.

Parasite

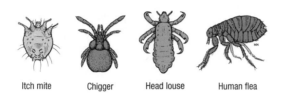

Itch mite　　Chigger　　Head louse　　Human flea

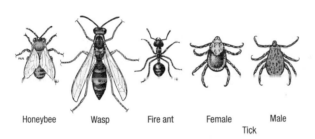

Honeybee　　Wasp　　Fire ant　　Female　　Male

Tick

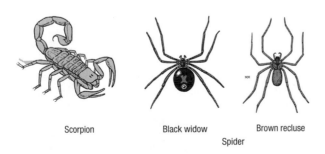

Scorpion　　Black widow　　Brown recluse

Spider

Figure 24. Biting and stinging insects and arachnids (insects shown are not drawn to scale). Nondangerous (top). Potentially dangerous (middle). Life-threatening (bottom).

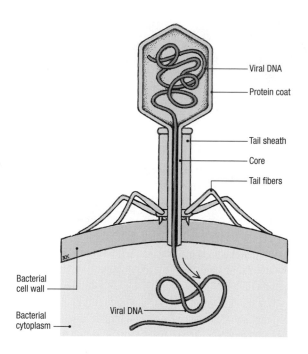

Figure 25. Bacteriophage virus.

Dermatology

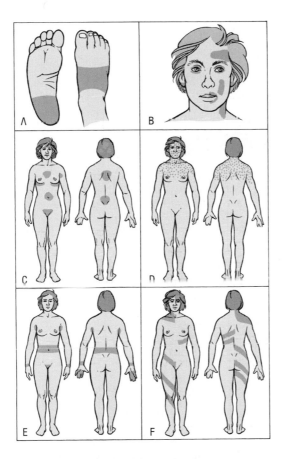

Figure 26. Anatomic distribution of common skin disorders. (A) Contact dermatitis (shoes). (B) Contact dermatitis (cosmetics, perfumes, and earrings). (C) Seborrheic dermatitis. (D) Acne. (E) Scabies. (F) Herpes zoster (shingles). This image, created by Mikki Senkarik, for Smeltzer SC & Bare BG, *Brunner & Suddarth's Textbook of Medical Surgical-Nursing, 8th Edition,* Philadelphia, JB Lippincott Company, 1996, fig. 53–5, appears here with permission and courtesy of Lippincott Williams & Wilkins.

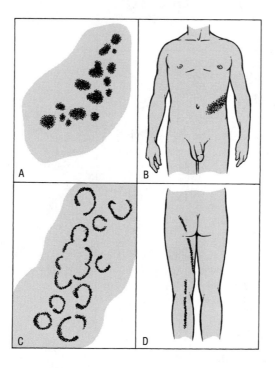

Figure 27. Different configurations of skin lesions. (A) Grouped. (B) Zosteroid. (C) Anular (circular) and arcuate (arc). (D) Linear. This image, created by Mikki Senkarik, for Pilliteri A, PhD, RN,RNP, *Maternal & Child Health Nursing: Care of the Childbearing and Childrearing Family, 3rd Edition,* Philadelphia, Lippincott Williams & Wilkins, 1998, fig. 21–12, appears here with permission and courtesy of Lippincott Williams & Wilkins.

Appendix 2
Poisonous and Hazardous Organisms

DEADLY, NEUROTOXIC, HALLUCINOGENIC, POISONOUS MUSHROOMS

Genus/Species	Common Name
Agaricus meleagris	grayscale
Amanita muscaria	fly agaric
Amanita pantherina	panthercap
Amanita phalloides	deathcap
Amanita verna	fools' mushroom
Boletus piperatus	pepper bolete
Boletus subvelutipes	red-mouth bolete
Chlorophyllum molybdites	green gill
Clitocybe dealbata	sweat mushroom
Conocybe filaris	deadly conocybe
Coprinus atramentarius	inky cap
Corinarius gentilis	goldband webcap
Entoloma lividum	gray pinkgill, lead poisoner
Entoloma strictior	straight-stalk pinkgill
Galerina autumnalis	autumn skullcap
Gymnophilus spectabilis	showy flamecap, big laughing mushroom
Gyromitra esculenta	false morel
Gyromitra infula	hooded false morel
Hebeloma crustuliniforme	poison pie
Hebeloma mesophaeum	dark disk
Inocybe fastigiata	conic fiberhead
Inocybe geophylla	earthblade fiberhead
Inocybe lanuginosa	fluff fiberhead
Lactarius piperatus	pepper cap
Lactarius representaneus	shaggy bear
Lactarius scrobiculatus	spotstalk
Lactarius torminosus	powderpuff milkcap
Lactarius uvidus	damp milkcap
Panaeolus campnaulatus	bell mottlegill
Paxillus involutus	naked brimcap
Psilocybe cubensis	bluestain smoothcap
Russula emetica	sickener
Russula fragilis	fragile brittlegill

RATTLESNAKES AND OTHER VENOMOUS ANIMALS

Genus/Species	Common Name
Blarina brevicauda	shorttail shrew
Crotalus adamanteus	eastern diamondback rattlesnake
Crotalus atrox	western diamondback rattlesnake
Crotalus cerastes cerastes	Mojave desert sidewinder
Crotalus cerastes cercobombus	Sonoran sidewinder
Crotalus cerastes laterorepens	Colorado desert sidewinder
Crotalus horridus	timber rattlesnake, canebrake rattler
Crotalus lepidus klauberi	banded rock rattlesnake
Crotalus lepidus lepidus	mottled rock rattlesnake
Crotalus mitchelii pyrrhus	southwestern speckled rattlesnake
Crotalus mitchelii stephensi	panamint rattlesnake
Crotalus pricei pricei	western twin-spotted rattlesnake
Crotalus ruber	red diamond rattlesnake
Crotalus scutulatus	Mojave rattlesnake
Crotalus tigris	tiger rattlesnake
Crotalus viridis abyssus	Grand Canyon rattlesnake
Crotalus viridis cerberus	Arizona black rattlesnake
Crotalus viridis concolor	midget faded rattlesnake
Crotalus viridis helleri	southern Pacific rattlesnake
Crotalus viridis hutosus	Great Basin rattlesnake
Crotalus viridis nuntius	Hopi rattlesnake
Crotalus viridis oreganus	northern Pacific rattlesnake
Crotalus viridis viridis	prairie rattlesnake
Crotalus willardi obscurus	New Mexico ridgenose rattlesnake
Crotalus willardi willardi	Arizona ridgenose rattlesnake
Heloderma suspectum cinctum	banded gila monster
Heloderma suspectum suspectum	reticulate gila monster
Sistrurus catenatus catenatus	eastern Massasauga (rattlesnake)
Sistrurus catenatus edwardsii	desert Massasauga (rattlesnake)
Sistrurus catenatus tergeminus	western Massasauga (rattlesnake)
Sistrurus miliarius barbouri	dusk pygmy rattlesnake
Sistrurus miliarius miliarius	Carolina pygmy rattlesnake
Sistrurus miliarius streckeri	western pygmy rattlesnake

COPPERHEAD SNAKES

Genus/Species	Common Name
Agkistrodon contortrix contortrix	southern copperhead
Agkistrodon contortrix laticinctus	broad-banded copperhead
Agkistrodon contortrix mokasen	northern copperhead
Agkistrodon contortrix phaeogaster	osage copperhead
Agkistrodon contortrix pictigaster	trans-Pecos copperhead

CORAL SNAKES AND KINGSNAKES

Genus/Species	Common Name
Lampropeltis triangulum	scarlet kingsnake
Micruroides euryxanthus euryoxanthus	Arizona coral snake
Micrurus fulvius	eastern coral snake
Micrurus fulvius tener	Texas coral snake

COTTONMOUTH SNAKES

Genus/Species	Common Name
Agkistrodon piscivorus conanti	Florida cottonmouth
Agkistrodon piscivorus leucostoma	western cottonmouth
Agkistrodon piscivorus piscivorus	eastern cottonmouth

REAR-FANGED SNAKES

Genus/Species	Common Name
Trimorphodon biscutatus lambda	Sonoran lyre snake
Trimorphodon biscutatus vandeburghi	California lyre snake
Trimorphodon biscutatus vilkinsonii	Texas lyre snake

SPIDERS, CENTIPEDES, SCORPIONS

Genus/Species	Common Name
centipedes	Phylum Chilopoda
Cheiracanthium mildei	yellow sac spider
Hadrurus spp.	scorpion
Latrodectus mactans	black widow spider
Loxosceles reclusa	brown recluse spider

STINGING INSECTS

Genus/Species	Common Name
Apis mellifera	honeybee
Bombas spp.	bumblebee
Polistes spp.	paper wasp
Vespula maculata	bald-faced hornet
Vespula spp.	yellowjacket

STINGING INSECTS, BLISTER BEETLES

Genus/Species	Common Name
Automeris io	Io moth caterpillar
blister beetle (300 species)	Family Meloidae
Dasymutilla magnifica	velvet ant (wingless female wasp)
Sibine stimulea	saddleback caterpillar

Simplified Virus Categories

Abbreviations and Conventions

-dae ending	**family name**
-nae ending	**subfamily**
-virus ending	**genus**
ds	**double stranded**
ss	**single stranded**
RT	**reverse transcriptase, reverse transcribing**
DNA	**deoxyribonucleic acid**
RNA	**ribonucleic acid**
(−)	**negative**
(+)	**positive**

FAMILIES AND GENERA OF VIRUSES INFECTING VERTEBRATES

dsDNA VIRUSES
Adenoviridae
Asfarviridae
Herpesviridae
Iridoviridae
   Ranavirus
   Lymphocytocystvirus
Papillomaviridae
Polyomaviridae
Poxviridae
   Chordopoxvirinae

ssDNA VIRUSES
Circoviridae
Parvoviridae
   Parvovirinae

dsDNA (RT) VIRUSES
Hepadnaviridae

dsRNA VIRUSES
Birnaviridae
   Aquabirnavirus
   Avibirnavirus
Reoviridae
   Orthoreovirus

Orbivirus
Coltivirus
Rotavirus
Aquareovirus

ssRNA (−)VIRUSES

Arenaviridae
Bornaviridae
Bunyaviridae
  Bunyavirus
  Hantavirus
  Nairovirus
  Phlebovirus
Filoviridae
Orthomyxoviridae
Paramyxoviridae
Rhabdoviridae
  Lyssavirus
  Vesiculovirus
  Ephemerovirus
  Novirhabdovirus
  Deltavirus

ssRNA (+) VIRUSES

Arteriviridae
Astroviridae
Calciviridae
Coronaviridae
Flaviviridae
HEV-like viruses
Nodaviridae
  Betanodavirus
Picornaviridae
Togaviridae

ssRNA (RT) VIRUSES

Retroviridae

FAMILIES OF VIRUSES INFECTING ALGAE, FUNGI, YEAST, AND PROTOZOA

dsDNA VIRUSES

Phycodnaviridae
  Rhizidiovirus

dsRNA VIRUSES
Hypoviridae
Partitiviridae
  Partitivirus
  Chrysovirus
Totiviridae

ssRNA (RT) VIRUSES
Metaviridae
  Metavirus
Pseudoviridae

ssRNA VIRUSES
Barnaviridae
Narnaviridae

FAMILIES AND GENERA OF VIRUSES INFECTING INVERTEBRATES

dsDNA VIRUSES
Ascoviridae
Baculoviridae
Iridoviridae
  Iridovirus
  Chloriridovirus
Polydnaviridae
  Ichnovirus
  Brachoviurs
Poxviridae
  Entomopoxvirinae

dsRNA VIRUSES
Birnaviridae
  Entomobirnavirus
Reoviridae
  Cypovirus

ssRNA (−) VIRUSES
Bunyaviridae
Rhabdoviridae

ssRNA (+) VIRUSES
CrPV-like
Flaviviridae
Nodaviridae

Picornaviridae
Teteraviridae
Togaviridae

ssRNA (RT) VIRUSES
Metaviridae
   Errantivirus

FAMILIES AND GENERA of VIRUSES INFECTING BACTERIA

dsDNA VIRUSES
Corticoviridae
Fuselloviridae
Lipothrixviridae
Myoviridae elongated head
Myoviridae isometric head
Plasmaviridae
Podoviridae
   SNDV-like viruses
Siphoviridae
Tectiviridae

dsRNA VIRUSES
Cystoviridae

ssDNA VIRUSES
Inoviridae
   Plectovirus
   Inovirus
Microviridae

ssRNA VIRUSES
Leviviridae

Sample Reports

COCCIDIOIDOMYCOSIS: ASSESSMENT

REASON FOR CONSULTATION: Rule out coccidioidomycosis.

HISTORY OF PRESENT ILLNESS: The patient is a 67-year-old Hispanic female seen in infectious disease consultation at the request of her primary care physician to evaluate for the possibility of pneumonia. Chart, labs, and chest x-rays were examined. She is intubated and poorly responsive and her family is not available. Therefore the available information is gathered from the chart, noting that she has a history of end-stage renal disease on hemodialysis. She also has history of hypertension and hyper-lipidemia. Reportedly she is allergic to morphine and cephalosporins, but details are not known. She was brought to this hospital due to unstable angina previously. A cardiac catheterization was launched, finding severe triple-vessel coronary artery disease and she was taken to the operating room where coronary artery bypass grafting x 4 with the left internal mammary to the left anterior descending was performed. Postoperatively the patient has had a very rocky course. She was noted to have seizures and had to be reintubated by the Emergency Room physician. She then developed a right-sided hemi-paresis. The CT scan was not impressive but the impression is that she has had a cere-brovascular accident (CVA). She remains on the ventilator, has been running low-grade temperatures, and her sputum is growing yeast. Her white blood count this morning is 15,800.

REVIEW OF SYSTEMS: Review of systems could not be obtained as the patient is on a ventilator and poorly responsive. According to her nurse, she has been suc-tioned of large amounts of tracheal secretions, which today are beige and yesterday were yellow. She has not had any diarrhea.

PAST MEDICAL/SOCIAL HISTORY: Further details are not available.

PHYSICAL EXAMINATION: GENERAL APPEARANCE: Shows an elderly Hispanic female who represents her age and appears acutely and chronically ill. She is small, thin, and frail. VITAL SIGNS: Temperature is 100.1, heart rate is around 100, blood pressure is 110/70, respiratory rate 20 per minute while on the ventilator, and she is having oxygen saturations of 100%. HEENT: Her pupils are small and she has some corneal rings. She has no conjunctival petechiae and no scleral icterus. Nasogastric and endotracheal tubes are in place. NECK: Supple. CHEST: The midsternal incision looks clean, and in the right subclavian area she has a Cordis with a thickened insertion site with no diastolic sounds or friction rubs. LUNGS: Show decreased breath sounds in the bases, but I could not hear any crackles. ABDOMEN: Does not seem to have any scars or distention. Bowel sounds are hypoactive but present. I could not feel liver or spleen, and there is no tenderness or guarding. LOWER EXTREMITIES: Surgical incisions on the right lower extremity look clean. Pedal pulses are absent but she has no acute ischemic changes. Her extremities show marked muscle wasting, and she has no signs of peripheral embolization. UPPER EXTREMITIES: On the left forearm, she has well-healed scars and on the right arm she has an A-V fistula with a good thrill. NEUROLOGIC: She is unresponsive. She has a few purposeless movements of left-sided extremities. Her right side is paralyzed and she had some up-going toes.

X-RAY DATA: Chest x-rays were reviewed and show a geriatric chest with bibasilar atelectasis and/or effusion.

ASSESSMENT: Considering the patient's bronchorrhea and leukocytosis, she may indeed have tracheobronchitis of early pneumonia. In this setting, it should be a bacterial process, and since she is allergic to cephalosporins, I agree with keeping her on Levaquin. If she were to deteriorate, we will give her vancomycin plus an aminoglycoside and may consider adding an anaerobic coverage as well. With regard to the presence of yeast, that most likely reflects colonization of the airways. Because of where she lives, the patient may be at risk for coccidioidomycosis. Therefore we may consider starting fluconazole being aware that if she stays in intensive care for awhile and continues to require central lines and broad-spectrum antibiotics in the future, she will be at risk for systemic candidiasis.

ESCHERICHIA COLI: ASSESSMENT

REASON FOR CONSULTATION: Rule out Escherichia coli (E. coli).

HISTORY OF PRESENT ILLNESS: This 47-year-old black female physician is being evaluated because of Escherichia coli (E. coli) sepsis. Specifically, I was asked to address the possible etiology or source of the infection. At this point I have reviewed the medical records, spoken to doctor, and reviewed the history with the patient. The patient has really had a very difficult and stormy medical history since last fall. She apparently presented with pancreatitis and the acute onset of diabetes. At that point, she received appropriate and supportive care and survived this tragic illness.

She certainly had complications, which included pseudocyst, deep venous thrombosis (DVT) of the right lower extremity, acute tubular necrosis, and unfortunately ischemic compromise of both of her lower extremities, from the ankles to the feet. Subsequent to her surviving the acute illness they attempted to salvage both of her feet over the last 5 or 6 months. This has involved hyperbaric oxygen, meticulous surgical debridement and wound care, but ultimately when they repeated an MRI they found that she had basically compromised and dead bone. With that in mind, they decided to proceed with bilateral below-the-knee amputations (BKAs), which took place. She relates that basically 2 weeks before the surgical intervention she began to notice that the area of the feet began to look a little bit inflamed and so the patient did cultures of the open wounds. A number of organisms were recovered, and she empirically placed herself on ciprofloxacin.

The patient continued that medication for two weeks leading up to the surgery. At that point, her primary care doctor (PCP) did bilateral BKAs and then converted her to Levaquin, which the patient continued. She also had a Foley in place. She was then transferred to rehabilitation after the BKAs and was actually doing relatively well. The patient relates that she had a little dysuria, but certainly was not having fevers, chills, flank pain, nausea, or vomiting. She then relates that she began to feel worse. At that time, her PCP obtained urine and blood cultures. The urinalysis had 15 to 25 red cells and greater than 100 white cells along with bacteria. Ultimately, the blood cultures and the urine cultures grew E. coli with exactly the same susceptibility patterns. When her condition began to change, she added gentamicin to her Levaquin. She has continued on gentamicin until today. Two days after admission, the patient acutely deteriorated in rehabilitation, now having fevers, tachycardia, and a transient hypotension. She was therefore transferred to the ICU for supportive care. At that point, they changed her to Claforan plus gentamicin, which she continues through today. As I stated, the urine and the blood cultures have all grown E. coli. Based upon that finding, they obtained a CT scan of the abdomen.

On review, what you appreciate is that she does have, what looks like, an intraabdominal collection on the left side, most likely next to the colon. It is suggested that this may be an abscess evolving or arising from the colon. However, what is confusing is the fact that the patient has had previous CT scans, for which we have the report and they also had demonstrated this left-sided collection which was approximately 6 x 4 cm. At that point, they considered it may well be a pseudocyst given her history of pancreatitis and pseudocyst. They also considered the possibility of an organized hematoma. In essence, we believe that this is actually the same process that is defined on both CT scans.

Subsequent to her transfer to the ICU and resuscitation, the patient is doing dramatically better as of today. She relates that yesterday she had some fevers but none today. She is not having any progressive head and neck complaints. No pulmonary, cardiovascular, GI, or GU complaints. She certainly denies any dysuria, frequency, urgency, hematuria, nausea, or vomiting. With regard to her BKA sites, she relates those are clean and dry, without incident.

PAST MEDICAL HISTORY: Septic shock, diabetes, pancreatitis, pseudocyst, DVT, acute tubular necrosis, thyroid goiter, mitral valve prolapse, hypertension.

PAST SURGICAL HISTORY: Total abdominal hysterectomy, appendectomy, bilateral BKAs.

MEDICATIONS: Claforan and gentamicin.

ALLERGIES: Questionably to penicillin. She actually has taken it many times but she relates that a couple of days after a shot of penicillin she will notice that she gets some swelling of her tongue or a hand or a leg, and so it has been attributed to penicillin. Yet, please note she takes cephalosporins with no difficulty.

SOCIAL HISTORY: No smoking, no ethanol. Occupation is that of a physician.

PHYSICAL EXAMINATION: GENERAL APPEARANCE: A pleasant female who is lying in bed in absolutely no distress. She is afebrile. NECK: Supple with good range of motion. She does have a scar in the anterior neck which is well healed without any erythema, warmth, or tenderness. Examination is basically unrevealing. BACK: Benign with no costovertebral angle (CVA) tenderness. CHEST: Clear to auscultation and percussion. HEART: Regular rhythm, S1-S2 without a significant rub or murmur tonight. ABDOMEN: Bowel sounds present. Abdomen is soft, nontender. No guarding or rebound. No palpable masses in the left lower quadrant. GENITALIA: Normal female genitalia. RECTAL: Exam deferred. LOWER EXTREMITIES: The bilateral BKA sites are absolutely immaculate. They are clean and dry. There is no erythema, warmth, fluctuance or tenderness. Absolutely no drainage is appreciated. NEUROLOGIC: She is awake, alert and oriented x 3.

LABORATORY EXAMINATION: White count 10,500, H&H 10/31, platelets 539,000. Her chem-12 showed a BUN of 13, creatinine 1.3, total bilirubin 0.4, SGOT 40, SGPT 73, alkaline phosphatase 210. As I stated, urinalysis had 15–25 red cells, white cells were greater than 100, and positive bacteria. The blood cultures had E. coli sensitive to ampicillin, cephazolin, Rocephin, gentamicin, piperacillin and Septra. The urine had E. coli with the exact same susceptibilities.

ASSESSMENT: Escherichia coli pyelonephritis: At this point after review, I truly believe that her primary infection is arising from the kidneys. Please appreciate that the patient has had a very acute onset of a febrile illness which is very consistent with pyelonephritis. In addition, you have to believe that she had a very convincing urinalysis with gross pyuria. With that in mind, I certainly would continue your approach as though this were primary pyelonephritis. Please recognize that with severe pyelonephritis it takes, on average, three days for the patient to become afebrile. I think we can safely say that it was not until two days after admission that antibiotics were altered enough to truly have an impact on her infection. With that in mind, we are really only on day three. I would suggest, though, that we could certainly simplify antibiotics to just Ancef, given the susceptibility patterns. Over the course of the next one to two days, I would also think that we could move towards oral antibiotics if she continues to do well. With regard to the left lower quadrant collection, I certainly respect all of your concerns. However, if we were to suggest that this is truly a diverticular abscess or a residual infection from her previous episodes, then we would have to explain why it is that she has had absolutely no fevers, chills, or other systemic symptoms over the last two months. I fully respect that what may have happened is that her E. coli sepsis may secondarily feed this site if indeed it was a hematoma. For the moment, I would prefer not to proceed with aspiration but follow her clinical course. If over the next 48 hours, despite appropriate antibiotics, the patient continues to have fever then I agree we will have to aspirate to see if the site is secondarily infected. If, on the other hand, all symptoms resolve and she is afebrile with a normal white count I would leave that collection alone.

PLAN: Discontinue gentamicin, discontinue Claforan. Start Ancef 1 g IV q.8h. If the patient continues to have fever over the next 48 hours, then I would consider aspiration of the left lower quadrant collection. All of this has been reviewed with the patient and her PCP.

OSTEOMYELITIS AND STAPHYLOCOCCUS AUREUS INFECTION: ASSESSMENT

REASON FOR CONSULTATION: Rule out Staphylococcus aureus.

HISTORY OF PRESENT ILLNESS: The patient is a 43-year old male with a history of hypertension, diabetes mellitus, and peripheral neuropathy. He states that for several years he has had an ulcer on his right great toe that waxes and wanes and appeared to be healing but it has gotten worse recently. He has been seen by his PCP and has had x-rays that show extensive bone destruction. He was brought in for incision and drainage. The patient denies any unusual exposures to the foot. His foot has not come into contact with lake or river water; he has not injured it in the dirt; he has not been bitten or scratched by any animals. He was on oral antibiotics prior to coming in, but he does not recall the name of the medication. He has never had any problems like this that required hospitalization or surgery.

PAST MEDICAL HISTORY: Otherwise unremarkable.

MEDICATIONS: He was started last evening on vancomycin and Cipro.

ALLERGIES: He has no known antimicrobial allergies.

PHYSICAL EXAMINATION: Nontoxic-appearing adult Caucasian male in no acute distress. Alert and oriented. Temperature overnight was normal. Vital signs are stable. Sclerae are clear. He has no oral or pharyngeal lesions. Neck is supple. Lungs are clear to auscultation. Regular heart rate and rhythm. Abdomen is soft and non-tender with positive bowel sounds. The foot was covered by surgical dressing and so was not examined. There is no redness, streaks, or anything above the level of the dressing on the ankle. The other foot has no lesions on it.

LABORATORY STUDIES: White blood cell count was 3.9 with an unremarkable differential. Hematocrit 31.9, platelets 237,000. Sedimentation rate was 57. BUN 24 and creatinine 1.6. Cultures showed no growth thus far.

ASSESSMENT: Diabetic foot infection with associated osteomyelitis. I would worry about a polymicrobial infection to include gram-positive cocci including Staphylococcus aureus, gram-negative rods, and anaerobes.

RECOMMENDATIONS: We will cover with vancomycin and Zosyn pending the results of the final cultures. Incision and drainage as per primary care physician (PCP). Length of therapy will depend on possibility of infected bone still being left. I will follow the patient with you.

PNEUMOCYSTIS PNEUMONIA: ASSESSMENT

REASON FOR CONSULTATION: Rule out Pneumocystis pneumonia.

HISTORY OF PRESENT ILLNESS: This is a 53-year-old white gentleman I am asked to evaluate for what appears to be Pneumocystis pneumonia and a new diagnosis of AIDS. At this point, I have reviewed the medical records and spoken to both the patient and his adopted son.

The patient indicates that he thought he was in his usual state of health until about three weeks ago. During that time, he states he had been experiencing a progressive dry, nonproductive cough, shortness of breath, dyspnea on exertion and fevers. In addition, he has anorexia and approximately a 10-pound weight loss. Because of the progressive nature of his shortness of breath, and dyspnea on exertion, he presented to his primary care physician (PCP). At that point he was evaluated in the office and it was felt that he had an atypical infection. He was therefore given a 5-day course of Zithromax. Unfortunately, the patient did not show clinical improvement and reappeared four days later for reevaluation. At that point, his PCP obtained a chest x-ray which demonstrated bilateral interstitial infiltrates, and for that reason he was admitted. He was empirically placed on Levaquin and Rocephin and was seen by the specialist from pulmonary services. At that point, there were concerns about the possibility of HIV, and appropriate serology was obtained. Today the patient was informed that his HIV status was positive, and he was placed on Septra and steroids. In addition, he was continued with the Levaquin and Rocephin.

At this point, the patient's primary complaints relate to his extreme shortness of breath, dyspnea on exertion, dry and nonproductive cough. He is not aware of any new head and neck complaints, GI, or GU complaints. The patient is a homosexual and has had multiple partners. He had checked his HIV status many years ago but not recently. He really did not know the status of any of his partners. He states he has not been sexually active for about four years. At this point, he resides in his own apartment. His only animal contact is with cats. He does not hunt, fish, camp, hike or have any water exposures. He does not do any extensive gardening. He enjoys bowling. His travels in the past have included Vietnam in the 1970s, Brazil, and Australia, but nowhere in the Middle East, Egypt, or Africa. In the United States, he has been in central California, Texas, and New York, but not in the Mississippi Valley. With regard to tuberculosis (TB), he had never had an active disease, but he states his PPD was known to be positive for the last 20 years. He never recalled receiving INH prophylaxis. The other interesting aspect is that he is known to have both hepatitis B and C although he has never received any therapy for these infections. He denies any intravenous (IV) drug abuse. He denied any history of syphilis, gonorrhea or herpes. No previous hypertension, diabetes, cardiac, or kidney problems.

PAST MEDICAL HISTORY: Significant for hepatitis B and C, colonic polyps, and positive PPD.

PAST SURGICAL HISTORY: Significant for tonsillectomy, tympanoplasty, repair of the tendon on the right first toe.

MEDICATIONS: Include Levaquin, Rocephin, Septra, and steroids.

ALLERGIES: None.

SOCIAL HISTORY: Smoked 1 pack per day x 45 years. Ethanol discontinued in 1985. He is a manager for a computer company.

REVIEW OF SYSTEMS: As above.

PHYSICAL EXAMINATION: Reveals acutely ill gentleman lying in bed who is in mild respiratory distress as soon as he starts talking. Vital signs reveal that initially his temperature was as high as 103 degrees but today he is afebrile. Head was unrevealing. Eyes are benign. Sinuses are nontender. Oral cavity without significant thrush. Neck is supple with no significant adenopathy. Back is benign with no costovertebral angle (CVA) tenderness. Chest demonstrates bilateral dry rales heard throughout. No pleural rub is heard. His heart was tachycardic, S1-S2 without significant rub. He does have a flow murmur of about 2/6. Bowel sounds are present. Abdomen is soft and nontender. No guarding or rebound. Liver and spleen are not palpable. Normal male genitalia without a Foley. Rectal exam deferred. Extremities without any unusual rash, lesions, or joint effusions. Neurologically he is awake, alert, and oriented x 3.

LABORATORY DATA: Potassium 3.4, glucose 191, BUN 10, creatinine 0.7, albumin 2.5, total bilirubin 1.2. SGOT of 90, SGPT 51, LDH 300, alkaline phosphatase 65. His white blood count is 1600, H&H 12.7 and 36.6. Platelets 66,000. Differential shows 87 polys, 7 bands, 5 lymphs. Chest x-ray shows the diffuse interstitial changes consistent with *Pneumocystis* pneumonia. HIV is positive. Western blot pending.

ASSESSMENT: Rule out Pneumocystis pneumonia.

At this point, I certainly respect your concerns and believe that *Pneumocystis* is the leading diagnosis. The fact that he did not show any response to Zithromax speaks against the atypical pneumonia. As such, I think it is unlikely that you are dealing with Legionella, Mycoplasma, or psittacosis. In light of the fact that he is now HIV positive, the 3-week history of fever, shortness of breath, dyspnea on exertion, dry cough, elevated LDH, and chest x-ray findings are all consistent with Pneumocystis. With that in mind, I certainly agree with using Septra at 15 mg/kg per day. In addition, I agree with steroids to reduce the inflammatory component. I do believe that the dose of steroids can be reduced. Since I do not believe that we are dealing with a community-acquired pneumonia, I have discontinued the Levaquin and Rocephin. I did review with the patient and his son the nature of this infection, the magnitude of the illness, and the fact that mortality can reach 15% to 20% despite best efforts. In addition, Septra is not always well tolerated by patients, and it may lead to the formation of rashes or other complications. I would offer that if he does fail Septra that he would need bronchoscopy to actually confirm the etiology and rule out acquired immunodeficiency syndrome. In light of the fact that we are considering all of the above, we have to believe that we are going to document that he has acquired immunodeficiency syndrome. I expect that his CD4 count is less than 200. We will not entertain antivirals until he has completely recovered from his pneumonia. This can be reviewed with him as an outpatient. Hepatitis B and C per PCP.

PLAN: Discontinue Rocephin and Levaquin. Change the Septra to 320 mg of trimethoprim IV q.8h. Decrease Solu-Medrol to 40 mg IV q.8h. Get an a.m. lymphocyte enumeration panel. HIV viral load by PCR. RPR. Hepatitis A total antibody. If the patient were to fail Septra, then we would need bronchoscopy to establish a clear diagnosis.

STREPTOCOCCAL BACTEREMIA: ASSESSMENT

REASON FOR CONSULTATION: Rule out streptococcal bacteremia.

HISTORY OF PRESENT ILLNESS: The patient is a 78-year-old Hispanic male seen in infectious disease consultation at the request of his primary care physician (PCP) for evaluation of streptococcal bacteremia. The available chart was reviewed.

All records were not available. The patient was a fairly good historian, was interviewed and examined.

This pleasant gentleman states that he fell off a ladder, suffering an injury to his right foot. Eventually he required an amputation of the fifth toe which was done by a physician, and subsequently the patient went home and was doing quite well. Dressing changes were being done as the wound was kept open. He tells me that approximately 6 days ago, he fell again, twisting his right foot and reinjuring it. Therefore he was brought to the hospital. When he arrived to the hospital his temperature was 100.9 degrees, and blood cultures were obtained which subsequently grew group A beta-hemolytic organism as well as methicillin-sensitive Staphylococcus aureus. The patient has been kept on Rocephin. While on this, he became afebrile but yesterday spiked again to 100.6 degrees.

LABORATORY DATA: His white blood count has stayed in the 10,000 to 11,000 range, but he has had as many as 30% bands. Blood sugars have been mildly elevated, and his creatinine on admission was 4.0, and 2 days ago was down to 2.9.

REVIEW OF SYSTEMS: The patient has been aware of the fever, but he denies any chills or malaise. He denies any changes in visual acuity, denies any respiratory, gastrointestinal, or genitourinary symptoms.

PAST MEDICAL HISTORY: Pertinent for hypertension and diabetes which were diagnosed approximately 14 years ago.

MEDICATIONS: At the present time, he is on insulin, but at home he was on Glucophage, Actos, and he was also on Vasotec. He denies having any allergies.

SOCIAL HISTORY: He is from Mexico City but has been living in the United States for 30 years. He retired over 10 years ago after working in maintenance. He denies smoking or drinking.

PHYSICAL EXAMINATION: Shows a very pleasant gentleman who represents his age and does not look ill. His temperature recorded is 97.6, heart rate is in the 80s, blood pressure is 142/60, and he is breathing 20 times a minute. He is well developed and well hydrated. Conjunctivae are pale with no petechia or scleral icterus. Pupils are small, and retinas are not examined. His nose is clear. Heart sounds are of good quality, and he has a soft systolic and a moderate diastolic sound. His lungs are clear on auscultation. Abdomen is soft and nontender, and his liver is felt at 1 cm below the right costal margin. Genital and rectal examinations are not done. His right foot is moderately warm, red, and swollen. There is no tenderness. The wound on the lateral aspect of the foot is clean and the fifth toe is absent. He has pounding pedal and radial pulses. His digits show no signs of peripheral embolization. He lacks any stigmata of endocarditis, but for completeness we will get a 2-D echocardiogram.

RECOMMENDATIONS: It is unusual for a foot cellulitis to cause bacteremia. It is noted that his wound looks clean; therefore I am going to take the liberty of getting a 2-D echocardiogram to rule out a deep-seated infection that may require incision and drainage. The antibiotic of choice for group A streptococcus would be plain penicillin, but for convenience, we will go with Unasyn which would also cover the Staphylococcus aureus which grew from the wound.

Appendix 5
Common Terms by Assessment

Coccidioidomycosis Assessment

aminoglycoside
anaerobic
antibiotic
atelectasis
beige
bibasilar
broad-spectrum antibiotics
bronchorrhea
central line
cephalosporins
coccidioidomycosis
colonization
conjunctival petechiae
crackles
decreased breath sounds
diarrhea
diastolic
effusion
embolization
fluconazole
friction rub
hemodialysis
ischemic
leukocytosis
Levaquin
morphine
pedal pulses
pneumonia
scleral icterus
sputum
systemic candidiasis
tracheal secretions
tracheobronchitis
vancomycin
ventilator
white blood count
yeast
yellow

Escherichia coli Assessment

abscess
afebrile
ampicillin
Ancef
aspirate
auscultation
below knee amputation (BKA)
cephalosporin
costovertebral angle tenderness
   (CVA)
chills
ciprofloxacin
Claforan
debridement
diabetes
deep vein thrombosis (DVT)
dysuria
Escherichia coli (E. coli)
erythema
fever
fluctuance
Foley
gentamicin
hematuria
hyperbaric oxygen
immaculate
intensive care unit (ICU)
intraabdominal
ischemic
Levaquin
magnetic resonance imaging (MRI)
organized hematoma
pancreatitis
primary care physician (PCP)
penicillin
percussion
piperacillin
pseudocyst
pyelonephritis

pyuria
Rocephin
sepsis
septic shock
Septra
supportive care
surgical debridement
susceptible
tachycardia
transient hypotension
tubular necrosis
wound care

Osteomyelitis Assessment

anaerobe
antimicrobial allergy
auscultation
blood urea nitrogen (BUN)
ciprofloxacin (Cipro)
creatinine
culture
diabetes mellitus
diabetic foot infection
drainage
gram-negative rods
gram-positive cocci
hematocrit
hypertension
incision and drainage
infected bone
oral antibiotic
osteomyelitis
primary care physician (PCP)
peripheral neuropathy
pharyngeal lesion
platelet
polymicrobial infection
sclerae
sedimentation rate
Staphylococcus aureus
surgical dressing
ulcer
vancomycin

white blood cell count
Zosyn

Pneumocystis Pneumonia Assessment

acquired immunodeficiency syndrome (AIDS)
animal contact
anorexia
antivirals
atypical
bronchoscopy
CD4 count
community-acquired pneumonia
diffuse interstitial changes
dry nonproductive cough
dyspnea on exertion
elevated LDH
empirically
ethanol
Foley
gardening
gonorrhea
hepatitis B
hepatitis C
herpes
HIV status
homosexual
human immunodeficiency virus (HIV)
hypertension
infiltrates
interstitial infiltrate
isonicotinic acid hydrazide (INH)
IV drug abuse
lactic dehydrogenase (LDH)
Legionella
Levaquin
lymphocyte
multiple partners
murmur
Mycoplasma
nonproductive cough
pleural rub

pneumonia
polyps
positive PPD
primary care physician (PCP)
prophylaxis
psittacosis
pulmonary services
purified protein derivative (PPD)
rales
reevaluation
Rocephin
rapid plasma reagin (RPR)
Septra
serology
Solu-Medrol
syphilis
tendon
tonsillectomy
tuberculosis (TB)
tympanoplasty
Western blot
water exposure
Zithromax

Streptococcal Assessment
afebrile
amputation
antibiotic
auscultation
bacteremia
bands
cellulitis
chills

conjunctivae
creatinine
deep-seated infection
diastolic
digit
drainage
echocardiogram
embolization
endocarditis
Glucophage
group A beta-hemolytic organism
group A streptococcus
hypertension
icterus
incision and drainage
insulin
malaise
methicillin-sensitive Staphylococcus
  aureus
penicillin
peripheral embolization
petechia
pounding pulse
primary care physician (PCP)
reinjuring
Rocephin
scleral icterus
spiked
stigmata
streptococcal bacteremia
Unasyn
Vasotec
wound

Drugs by Indication

ACNE

Acne Products

Acetoxyl (Can)

Acnomel BP 5 (Can)

adapalene

Advanced Formula Oxy® Sensitive Gel [OTC]

Akne-Mycin® Topical

Ambi 10® [OTC]

A/T/S® Topical

Ben-Aqua® [OTC]

Benoxyl®

Benzac AC® Gel

Benzac AC® Wash

Benzac W® Gel

Benzac W® Wash

5-Benzagel®

10-Benzagel®

Benzagel (Can)

Benzamycin®

Benzashave® Cream

benzoyl peroxide

benzoyl peroxide and hydrocortisone

BlemErase® Lotion [OTC]

Brevoxyl® Gel

Clearasil® B.P. Plus (Can)

Clear By Design® Gel [OTC]

Clearasil® Maximum Strength [OTC]

Cleocin HCl® Oral

Cleocin Pediatric® Oral

Cleocin Phosphate® Injection

Cleocin T® Topical

Cleocin® Vaginal

Clinda-Derm® Topical

clindamycin

Dalacin® C (Can)

Dalacin T (Can)

Dalacin Vaginal (Can)

Del Aqua-5® Gel

Del Aqua-10® Gel

Del-Mycin® Topical

Dermacne (Can)

Dermoxyl (Can)

Desquam-E™ Gel

Desquam-X® Gel

Desquam-X® Wash

Differin®

Dryox® Gel [OTC]

Dryox® Wash [OTC]

Emgel™ Topical

Eryderm® Topical

Erygel® Topical

Erymax® Topical

erythromycin and benzoyl peroxide

erythromycin (ophthalmic/topical)

E-Solve-2® Topical

ETS-2%® Topical

Exact® Cream [OTC]

Fostex® 10% BPO Gel [OTC]

Fostex® 10% Wash [OTC]

Fostex® Bar [OTC]

H_2Oxyl (Can)

Ilotycin® Ophthalmic

Loroxide® [OTC]

Neutrogena® Acne Mask [OTC]

Neutrogena® On-The-Spot Acne Lotion (Can)

Oxy-5® Advanced Formula for Sensitive Skin [OTC]

Oxy 5 (Can)

Oxy-5® Tinted [OTC]

Oxy-10® Advanced Formula for Sensitive Skin [OTC]

Oxy 10® Wash [OTC]

Oxyderm (Can)

PanOxyl®-AQ

PanOxyl® Bar [OTC]

Perfectoderm® Gel [OTC]

Peroxin A5®

Peroxin A10®

Persa-Gel®
Solugel (Can)
Staticin® Topical
Theroxide® Wash [OTC]
T-Stat® Topical
Vanoxide® [OTC]
Vanoxide-HC®
Antibiotic, Topical
Apo®-Metronidazole (Can)
Meclan® Topical
meclocycline
Metrocream (Can)
MetroGel® Topical
metronidazole
Neo-Metric (Can)
NidaGel (Can)
Noritate (Can)
Novo-Nidazol (Can)
Trikacide (Can)
Antiseborrheic Agent, Topical
Anti-Acne Formula for Men (Can)
Aveeno® Cleansing Bar [OTC]
Fostex® [OTC]
Meted (Can)
Night Cast R (Can)
Novacet® Topical
Pernox® [OTC]
SAStid® Plain Therapeutic Shampoo
and Acne Wash [OTC]
Sebulex (Can)
Sulfacet-R® Topical
sulfur and salicylic acid
sulfur and sulfacetamide
Sulsal (Can)
Keratolytic Agent
Acnex (Can)
Acnomel Acne Mask (Can)
Anti-Acne Control Formula
(Can)
Anti-Acne Spot Treatment (Can)
Blemish Control (Can)
Callus Salve (Can)

Clean & Clear Deep Cleaning
Astringent (Can)
Clean & Clear Invisible Clearasil
Clearstick (Can)
Clearasil® Pads (Can)
Clear Away® Disc [OTC]
Clear Pore Treatment (Can)
Compound W (Can)
Compound W Plus (Can)
Duoforte (Can)
Fostex® Medicated Cleansing (Can)
Freezone® Solution [OTC]
Gordofilm® Liquid
Ionil (Can)
Keralyt (Can)
Mediplast® Plaster [OTC]
Mosco (Can)
Mudd Acne (Can)
Neutrogena® Healthy Scalp Anti-
Dandruff (Can)
Nova Perfecting Lotion (Can)
Occlusal (Can)
Occlusal®-HP Liquid
Off-Ezy® (Can)
Oil-Free Acne Wash (Can)
Oxy Control (Can)
Oxy Deep Pore (Can)
Oxy Medicated Pads (Can)
Oxy Night Watch (Can)
Oxy Power Pads (Can)
Panscol® Lotion [OTC]
Panscol® Ointment [OTC]
PediaPatch Transdermal Patch
[OTC]
Propa PH (Can)
P&S® Shampoo [OTC]
Salac (Can)
Salacid® Ointment
Sal-Acid® Plaster
salicylic acid
Salseb (Can)
Scholl 2-Drop Corn Remedy (Can)

Scholl Corn, Callus Plaster
   Preparation (Can)
Scholl Corn Salve (Can)
Scholl Wart Remover (Can)
Scholl Zino (Can)
Sebcur (Can)
Soluver (Can)
tazarotene
Tazorac®
Ten-O-Six (Can)
Trans-Plantar® Transdermal Patch
   [OTC]
Trans-Ver-Sal® Transdermal Patch
   [OTC]
Vergogel® Gel [OTC]
Verukan® Solution
Wart Remover (Can)
X-Seb® (Can)
Retinoic Acid Derivative
   Accutane®
   Avita®
   isotretinoin
   Isotrex® (Can)
   Renova®
   Retin-A™ Micro Topical
   Retin-A™ Topical
   Retisol-A® (Can)
   Stieva-A® (Can)
   Stieva-A® Forte (Can)
   tretinoin (topical)
Tetracycline Derivative
   Achromycin® Ophthalmic
   Achromycin® Topical
   Achromycin V (Can)
   Apo®-Minocycline (Can)
   Apo®-Tetra (Can)
   Declomycin®
   demeclocycline
   Dynacin® Oral
   Minocin®
   Minocin® IV Injection
   minocycline

Nor-tet® Oral
Novo-Tetra (Can)
Nu-Tetra (Can)
Panmycin® Oral
Robitet® Oral
Sumycin® Oral
Syn-Minocycline (Can)
Tetracap® Oral
tetracycline
Tetracyn (Can)
Topicycline® Topical
Vectrin®
Topical Skin Product
   azelaic acid
   Azelex®

ACQUIRED IMMUNODEFICIENCY SYNDROME (AIDS)

Antiviral Agent
   abacavir
   adefovir
   Agenerase™
   amprenavir
   Apo®-Zidovudine (Can)
   Combivir™
   Crixivan®
   delavirdine
   didanosine
   efavirenz
   Epivir®
   Epivir®-HBV™
   Fortovase®
   Heptovir® (Can)
   Hivid®
   indinavir
   Invirase®
   Kaletra™
   lamivudine
   lopinavir and ritonavir
   nelfinavir
   nevirapine

Norvir®
Novo-AZT (Can)
Preveon®
Rescriptor®
Retrovir®
ritonavir
saquinavir
stavudine
Sustiva™
3TC® (Can)
Videx®
Viracept®
Viramune®
zalcitabine
Zerit®
zidovudine
zidovudine and lamivudine
Ziagen™

ALOPECIA
Antiandrogen
    finasteride
    Proscar®
Progestin
    hydroxyprogesterone caproate
    Hylutin®
    Hyprogest® 250
Topical
    Apo®-Gain (Can)
    minoxidil
    Minoxigaine® (Can)
    Rogaine® Topical

ALPHA 1-ANTITRYPSIN DEFICIENCY (CONGENITAL)
Antitrypsin Deficiency Agent
    alpha 1-proteinase inhibitor
    Prolastin®

AMEBIASIS
Amebicide
    Apo®-Metronidazole (Can)
    Diodoquin® (Can)

Flagyl® Oral
Humatin®
iodoquinol
Metrocream (Can)
MetroGel® Topical
MetroGel®-Vaginal
Metro I.V.® Injection
metronidazole
Neo-Metric (Can)
NidaGel (Can)
Noritate (Can)
Novo-Nidazol (Can)
paromomycin
Protostat® Oral
Trikacide (Can)
Yodoxin®
Aminoquinoline (Antimalarial)
    Aralen® Phosphate
    chloroquine phosphate

ANTHRAX
Vaccine
    anthrax vaccine, adsorbed
    Biothrax®

ASCARIASIS
Anthelmintic
    albendazole
    Albenza®

ASPERGILLOSIS
Antifungal Agent
    Abelcet™
    Amphotec®
    amphotericin B cholesteryl sulfate
        complex
    amphotericin B (conventional)
    amphotericin B lipid complex
    Ancobon®
    Ancotil® (Can)
    flucytosine
    Fungizone®
Antifungal Agent, Systemic
    AmBisome®
    amphotericin B liposomal

ATHLETE'S FOOT (SEE TINEA)

BACTERIAL ENDOCARDITIS (PROPHYLAXIS)

Aminoglycoside (Antibiotic)
  Alcomicin (Can)
  Cidomycin (Can)
  Diogent (Can)
  Garamycin®
  Garatec (Can)
  Genoptic®
  Gentacidin®
  Gent-AK®
  gentamicin
  Gentrasul®
  G-myticin®
  Jenamicin®
  Ocugram (Can)
  RO-Gentycin (Can)
Antibiotic, Miscellaneous
  Cleocin HCl® Oral
  Cleocin Pediatric® Oral
  Cleocin Phosphate® Injection
  Cleocin T® Topical
  Cleocin® Vaginal
  Clinda-Derm® Topical
  clindamycin
  Dalacin® C (Can)
  Dalacin T (Can)
  Dalacin Vaginal (Can)
  Lyphocin® Injection
  Vancocin® CP (Can)
  Vancocin® Injection
  Vancocin® Oral
  Vancoled® Injection
  vancomycin
Cephalosporin (First Generation)
  Apo®-Cephalex (Can)
  Biocef®
  cefadroxil
  Cefanex®

  cephalexin
  Ceporex (Can)
  Duricef®
  Keflex®
  Keftab®
  Novo-Lexin (Can)
  Nu-Cephalex (Can)
  Zartan®
Macrolide (Antibiotic)
  azithromycin
  Biaxin®
  Biaxin® XL
  clarithromycin
  Zithromax™
Penicillin
  amoxicillin
  Amoxil®
  ampicillin
  Ampicin (Can)
  Ampicin® Sodium (Can)
  Ampilean (Can)
  Apo®-Amoxi (Can)
  Apo®-Ampi (Can)
  Apo®-Pen VK (Can)
  Gen-Amoxicillin (Can)
  Jaa Amp® (Can)
  Marcillin®
  Nadopen-V® (Can)
  Novamoxin® (Can)
  Novo-Pen-VK® (Can)
  Nu-Amoxi (Can)
  Nu-Ampi (Can)
  Nu-Pen-VK (Can)
  Omnipen®
  Omnipen®-N
  penicillin V potassium
  Principen®
  Pro-Amox® (Can)
  Totacillin®
  Trimox®
  Truxcillin®
  Veetids®
  Wymox®

BERYLLIOSIS (SEE RESPIRATORY DISORDERS)

BITES (SNAKE)
Antivenin
  antivenin (Crotalidae) polyvalent
  antivenin (Micrurus fulvius)

BITES (SPIDER)
Antivenin
  antivenin (Latrodectus mactans)
Electrolyte Supplement, Oral
  calcium gluconate
  H-F Antidote (Can)
  Kalcinate®
Skeletal Muscle Relaxant
  methocarbamol
  Robaxin®

BLASTOMYCOSIS
Antifungal Agent
  itraconazole
  ketoconazole
  Nizoral®
  Nizoral® A-D Shampoo [OTC]
  Novo-Ketoconazole (Can)
  Nu-Ketocon (Can)
  Sporanox®

BLEPHARITIS
Antifungal Agent
  Natacyn®
  natamycin

BRONCHITIS
Adrenergic Agonist Agent
  Adrenalin® Chloride
  Airet®
  albuterol
  Apo®-Salvent (Can)
  Arm-a-Med® Isoetharine
  Arm-a-Med® Isoproterenol
  Asmavent (Can)
  AsthmaHaler® Mist [OTC]
  AsthmaNefrin® [OTC]

  Beta-2®
  bitolterol
  Bronitin® Mist [OTC]
  Bronkaid® Mist [OTC]
  Bronkometer®
  Bronkosol®
  Dey-Dose® Isoproterenol
  Dey-Lute® Isoetharine
  Dysne-Inhal (Can)
  ephedrine
  Epi EZ (Can)
  Epifrin®
  epinephrine
  EpiPen®
  EpiPen® Jr
  Glaucon®
  isoetharine
  isoproterenol
  Isuprel®
  Kondon's Nasal® [OTC]
  Medihaler-Epi (Can)
  Medihaler-Iso®
  microNefrin® [OTC]
  Novo-Salmol (Can)
  Pretz-D® [OTC]
  Primatene® Mist [OTC]
  Proventil®
  Proventil® HFA
  Sabulin® (Can)
  Sus-Phrine®
  Tornalate®
  Vaponefrin® [OTC]
  Ventodisk (Can)
  Ventolin®
  Ventolin® Rotocaps®
  Volmax (Can)
Antibiotic, Quinolone
  Avelox™
  moxifloxacin
  trovafloxacin
  Trovan®
Cephalosporin (Third Generation)
  cefdinir

Omnicef®
Mucolytic Agent
  acetylcysteine
  Airbron (Can)
  Mucomyst®
  Mucosil™
  Parvolex (Can)
Theophylline Derivative
  Acet-Am (Can)
  Acet-Am Expectorant (Can)
  Aerolate III®
  Aerolate JR®
  Aerolate SR®
  aminophylline
  Apo®-Theo (Can)
  Apo®-Theo LA (Can)
  Aquaphyllin®
  Asmalix®
  Bronchial®
  Choledyl (Can)
  Corophyllin (Can)
  Dilor®
  dyphylline
  Elixomin®
  Elixophyllin®
  Glycerol-T®
  Lufyllin®
  Novo-Triphyl (Can)
  oxtriphylline
  Palaron (Can)
  Phyllocontin®
  Pulmophylline (Can)
  Quibron®
  Quibron®-T/SR
  Respbid®
  Rouphylline (Can)
  Slo-bid™
  Slo-Phyllin®
  Slo-Phyllin® GG
  Somophyllin (Can)
  Sustaire®
  Theo-24®
  Theobid®

Theochron®
Theoclear-80®
Theoclear® L.A.
Theo-Dur®
Theolair™
theophylline
theophylline and guaifenesin
Theo-Sav®
Theospan®-SR
Theo-S® (Can)
Theostat-80®
Theovent®
Theo-X®
T-Phyl®
Truphylline®
Uni-Dur®
Uniphyl®

BRUCELLOSIS
Antibiotic, Aminoglycoside
  streptomycin

BULLOUS SKIN DISEASE
Antibacterial, Topical
  Dermazin® (Can)
  Flamazine® (Can)
  Silvadene®
  silver sulfadiazine
  SSD® AF
  SSD® Cream
  Thermazene®
Gold Compound
  Aurolate®
  aurothioglucose
  gold sodium thiomalate
  Myochrysine (Can)
  Solganal®
Immunosuppressant Agent
  azathioprine
  Imuran®

CANDIDIASIS
Antifungal Agent
  Abelcet™

Absorbine® Antifungal [OTC]
Absorbine® Antifungal Foot Powder
  [OTC]
Absorbine® Jock Itch [OTC]
Absorbine Jr.® Antifungal [OTC]
Aftate® [OTC]
Amphotec®
amphotericin B cholesteryl sulfate
  complex
amphotericin B (conventional)
amphotericin B lipid complex
Ancobon®
Ancotil® (Can)
Apo®-Fluconazole (Can)
AVC™ Cream
AVC™ Suppository
Breezee® Mist Antifungal [OTC]
butoconazole
Candistatin (Can)
Canesten (Can)
ciclopirox
Clotrimaderm (Can)
clotrimazole
Desenex® [OTC]
Diflucan®
econazole
Ecostatin® (Can)
Exelderm® Topical
Femizol-M® [OTC]
fluconazole
flucytosine
Fungizone®
Fungoid® Creme
Fungoid® Solution
Fungoid® Tincture
Genaspor® [OTC]
Gynazole• 1®
Gynecure (Can)
Gyne-Lotrimin® [OTC]
Gyne-Lotrimin® 3 [OTC]
Gyno-Trosyd (Can)
itraconazole
ketoconazole

Lamisil® Cream
Loprox®
Lotrimin®
Lotrimin® AF Cream [OTC]
Lotrimin® AF Lotion [OTC]
Lotrimin® AF Powder [OTC]
Lotrimin® AF Solution [OTC]
Lotrimin® AF Spray Liquid [OTC]
Lotrimin® AF Spray Powder [OTC]
Maximum Strength Desenex®
  Antifungal Cream [OTC]
Mestatin® (Can)
Micatin® Topical [OTC]
miconazole
Mitrazol® [OTC]
Monazole-7® (Can)
Monistat-Derm™ Topical
Monistat i.v.™ Injection
Monistat™ Vaginal
Mycelex®
Mycelex®-7
Mycelex®-G
Myclo-Derm (Can)
Myclo-Gyne (Can)
Mycostatin®
M-Zole® 7 Dual Pack [OTC]
Nadostine® (Can)
naftifine
Naftin®
Neo-Zol (Can)
Nilstat®
Nizoral®
Nizoral® A-D Shampoo [OTC]
Novo-Ketoconazole (Can)
NP-27® [OTC]
Nu-Ketocon (Can)
Nyaderm (Can)
nystatin
Nystat-Rx®
Nystex®
Ony-Clear® Spray
O-V Staticin®
oxiconazole

Oxistat® Topical
Pedi-Dri® Topical Powder
Pitrex (Can)
PMS-Nystatin (Can)
Prescription Strength Desenex®
  [OTC]
Scholl Athlete's Foot Preparations
  (Can)
Spectazole™
Sporanox®
sulconazole
sulfanilamide
Terazol® Vaginal
terbinafine (topical)
terconazole
Tinactin® [OTC]
tioconazole
tolnaftate
Tritin (Can)
Trivagizole 3™ [OTC]
Trosyd (Can)
Vagistat®-1 Vaginal [OTC]
Vagitrol®
Zeasorb-AF® [OTC]
Zeasorb-AF® Powder [OTC]
Antifungal Agent, Systemic
  AmBisome®
  amphotericin B liposomal
Antifungal/Corticosteroid
  Mycogen II Topical
  Mycolog®-II Topical
  Myconel® Topical
  Myco-Triacet® II
  Mytrex® F Topical
  N.G.T.® Topical
  nystatin and triamcinolone
  Tri-Statin® II Topical

CANKER SORE
Anti-infective Agent, Oral
  carbamide peroxide
  Gly-Oxide® Oral [OTC]
  Orajel® Perioseptic® [OTC]

Proxigel® Oral [OTC]
Anti-inflammatory Agent, Locally
  Applied
  amlexanox
  Aphthasol™
Local Anesthetic
  Americaine® [OTC]
  Anbesol® [OTC]
  Anbesol Baby (Can)
  Anbesol® Maximum Strength
    [OTC]
  Babee® Teething® [OTC]
  Baby Liquid (Can)
  Baby Nighttime (Can)
  Baby Orajel (Can)
  benzocaine
  Benzocol® [OTC]
  Benzodent® [OTC]
  Cylex® [OTC]
  Maximum Strength Anbesol® [OTC]
  Maximum Strength Orajel® [OTC]
  Numzitdent® [OTC]
  Numzit Teething® [OTC]
  Orabase®-B [OTC]
  Orabase®-O [OTC]
  Orajel® Maximum Strength [OTC]
  Orasept® [OTC]
  Orasol® [OTC]
  Spec-T® [OTC]
  Tanac® [OTC]
Protectant, Topical
  gelatin, pectin, and methylcellulose
  Orabase® Plain [OTC]

CHOLERA
Vaccine, Inactivated Bacteria
  cholera vaccine

CHROMOBLASTOMYCOSIS
Antifungal Agent
  ketoconazole
  Nizoral®
  Novo-Ketoconazole (Can)
  Nu-Ketocon (Can)

COCCIDIOIDOMYCOSIS
Antifungal Agent
ketoconazole
Nizoral®
Novo-Ketoconazole (Can)
Nu-Ketocon (Can)

COLD SORE
Antiviral Agent
Denavir™
penciclovir

CONDYLOMA ACUMINATA
Immune Response Modifier
Aldara™
imiquimod

CONDYLOMA ACUMINATUM
Antiviral Agent
interferon alfa-2b and ribavirin
combination pack
Rebetron™
Biological Response Modulator
Alferon® N
interferon alfa-2a
interferon alfa-2b
interferon alfa-2b and ribavirin
combination pack
interferon alfa-n3
Intron® A
Rebetron™
Roferon-A®
Keratolytic Agent
Condyline (Can)
Condylox®
Pod-Ben-25®
Podocon-25™
Podofilm® (Can)
podofilox
Podofin®
podophyllin and salicylic acid
podophyllum resin

Verrex-C&M®
Wartec (Can)

CONJUNCTIVITIS (BACTERIAL)
Antibiotic, Ophthalmic
Levaquin™
levofloxacin
Quixin™ Ophthalmic

CONJUNCTIVITIS (VIRAL)
Antiviral Agent
trifluridine
Viroptic® Ophthalmic

COUGH
Antihistamine
Allerdryl® (Can)
Allergy Elixir (Can)
Benylin® Cough Syrup [OTC]
Bydramine® Cough Syrup [OTC]
Diphen® Cough [OTC]
diphenhydramine
Hydramyn® Syrup [OTC]
Antihistamine/Antitussive
Ambenyl® Cough Syrup
Amgenal® Cough Syrup
Bromanyl® Cough Syrup
bromodiphenhydramine and codeine
Bromotuss® w/Codeine Cough Syrup
hydrocodone and chlorpheniramine
Phenameth® DM
Phenergan® With Codeine
Phenergan® With Dextromethorphan
Pherazine® w/DM
Pherazine® With Codeine
promethazine and codeine
promethazine and dextromethorphan
Prothazine-DC®
Tussionex®
Antihistamine/Decongestant/Antitussive
Actagen-C®
Allerfrin® w/Codeine
Aprodine® w/C

Bromanate® DC
Bromphen® DC w/Codeine
brompheniramine,
   phenylpropanolamine, and codeine
carbinoxamine, pseudoephedrine, and
   dextromethorphan
Carbodec DM®
Cardec DM®
Cerose-DM® [OTC]
chlorpheniramine, ephedrine,
   phenylephrine, and carbetapentane
chlorpheniramine, phenylephrine,
   and codeine
chlorpheniramine, phenylephrine,
   and dextromethorphan
chlorpheniramine,
   phenylpropanolamine, and
   dextromethorphan
chlorpheniramine, pseudoephedrine,
   and codeine
CoActifed (Can)
Codehist® DH
Cotridin (Can)
Cotrifed (Can)
Decohistine® DH
Dihistine® DH
Dimetane®-DC
hydrocodone, phenylephrine,
   pyrilamine, phenindamine,
   chlorpheniramine, and ammonium
   chloride
Myphetane DC®
Ornade-DM (Can)
Pediacof®
Pedituss®
Phenergan® VC With Codeine
Pherazine® VC w/ Codeine
Poly-Histine CS®
promethazine, phenylephrine, and
   codeine
Promethist® With Codeine
Prometh® VC With Codeine
Pseudo-Car® DM

P-V-Tussin®
Rentamine®
Rondamine-DM® Drops
Rondec®-DM
Ryna-C® Liquid
Rynatuss® Pediatric Suspension
Triacin-C®
Triaminicol® Multi-Symptom Cold
   Syrup [OTC]
Trifed-C®
triprolidine, pseudoephedrine, and
   codeine
Tri-Tannate Plus®
Tussafed® Drops
Antihistamine/Decongestant
   Combination
Allerest® Maximum Strength [OTC]
Anamine® Syrup [OTC]
Anaplex® Liquid [OTC]
Benylin® Cold (Can)
caramiphen and
   phenylpropanolamine
Chlorafed® Liquid [OTC]
chlorpheniramine and
   pseudoephedrine
Chlor-Trimeton® 4 Hour Relief
   Tablet [OTC]
Chlor-Tripolon Decongestant (Can)
Co-Pyronil® 2 Pulvules® [OTC]
Deconamine® SR
Deconamine® Syrup [OTC]
Deconamine® Tablet [OTC]
Fedahist® Tablet [OTC]
Hayfebrol® Liquid [OTC]
Klerist-D® Tablet [OTC]
Ordrine AT® Extended Release
   Capsule
Pseudo-Gest Plus® Tablet [OTC]
Rescaps-D® S.R. Capsule
Rhinosyn® Liquid [OTC]
Rhinosyn-PD® Liquid [OTC]
Ryna® Liquid [OTC]
Sudafed® Plus Tablet [OTC]

Tuss-Allergine® Modified T.D.
Capsule
Tussogest® Extended Release
Capsule
Vasofrinic (Can)
Antitussive
adextromethorphan
Balminil DM® (Can)
Benylin DM® [OTC]
Benylin® Pediatric [OTC]
benzonatate
Broncho-Grippol-DM (Can)
Bronchopan DM (Can)
Buckley's DM (Can)
Calmylin #1 (Can)
Centratuss DM (Can)
Children's Hold® [OTC]
codeine
Codeine Contin® (Can)
Contac Coughcaps (Can)
Cough Suppressant Syrup DM (Can)
Creo-Terpin® [OTC]
Delsym® [OTC]
DM Cough Syrup (Can)
DM Sans Sucre (Can)
Drixoral® Cough Liquid Caps [OTC]
Hold® DM [OTC]
Hycodan®
Hycomine® Compound
hydrocodone and homatropine
hydrocodone, chlorpheniramine,
phenylephrine, acetaminophen, and
caffeine
Hydromet®
Koffex DM (Can)
Linctus Codeine Blac (Can)
Neo-DM (Can)
Oncet®
Ornex-DM (Can)
Pertussin® CS [OTC]
Pertussin® ES [OTC]
Pharmilin-DM (Can)
Pharminil DM (Can)

Robidex (Can)
Robitussin® Cough Calmers [OTC]
Robitussin® Pediatric [OTC]
Scot-Tussin DM® Cough Chasers
[OTC]
Sedatuss DM (Can)
Silphen DM® [OTC]
Sirop DM (Can)
St. Joseph® Cough Suppressant
[OTC]
Sucrets® Cough Calmers [OTC]
Suppress® [OTC]
Syrup DM (Can)
Tessalon® (Can)
Tessalon® Perles
Triaminic DM (Can)
Triaminic Long Lasting DM (Can)
Trocal® [OTC]
Tussigon®
Vicks® Children's Cough Syrup
(Can)
Vicks Formula 44® [OTC]
Vicks Formula 44® Pediatric Formula
[OTC]
Antitussive/Analgesic
acetaminophen and
dextromethorphan
Bayer® Select® Chest Cold Caplets
[OTC]
Drixoral® Cough & Sore Throat
Liquid Caps [OTC]
Tylenol Cough (Can)
Antitussive/Decongestant
Balminil DM D (Can)
Benylin DM-D (Can)
Buckley's DM Decongestant (Can)
Calmylin #2 (Can)
Calmylin Pediatric (Can)
Centratuss DM-D (Can)
Children's Benylin DM-D (Can)
Codamine®
Codamine® Pediatric
Cough Syrup DM Decongestant (Can)

Cough Syrup DM Decongestant for
  Children (Can)
Demdec (Can)
DM Plus Decongestant (Can)
Drixoral® Cough & Congestion
  Liquid Caps [OTC]
Hycomine®
Hycomine® Pediatric
hydrocodone and
  phenylpropanolamine
Hydrocodone PA® Syrup
Koffex DM-D (Can)
Novahistex DM (Can)
Novahistine DM (Can)
Pediatric Cough Syrup (Can)
Personnelle DM (Can)
pseudoephedrine and
  dextromethorphan
Robitussin Pediatric Cough & Cold
  (Can)
Sudafed DM (Can)
Syrup DM-D (Can)
Triaminic DM-D (Can)
Tussodan DM (Can)
Vicks® 44D Cough & Head
  Congestion
Vicks® 44 Non-Drowsy Cold &
  Cough Liqui-Caps [OTC]
Vicks Children's Cough and
  Congestion Syrup (Can)
Antitussive/Decongestant/Expectorant
  Anatuss® [OTC]
Benylin® Codeine (Can)
Calmylin Codeine D-E (Can)
Codafed® Expectorant
Cophene XP®
CoSudafed Expectorant (Can)
Cough Syrup (Can)
Cycofed® Pediatric
Decohistine® Expectorant
Deproist® Expectorant With Codeine
Detussin® Expectorant
Dihistine® Expectorant

Dorcol® DM (Can)
guaifenesin, phenylpropanolamine,
  and dextromethorphan
guaifenesin, pseudoephedrine, and
  codeine
Guiatuss CF® [OTC]
Guiatuss DAC®
Guiatussin® DAC
Halotussin® DAC
hydrocodone, pseudoephedrine, and
  guaifenesin
Isoclor® Expectorant
Mytussin® DAC
Naldecon® DX Adult Liquid [OTC]
NF Cough Syrup with Codeine (Can)
Nucofed®
Nucofed® Pediatric Expectorant
Nucotuss®
Phenhist® Expectorant
Profen II DM®
Robafen® CF [OTC]
Robitussin-CF® [OTC]
Robitussin®-DAC
Ryna-CX®
Siltussin-CF® [OTC]
SRC® Expectorant
Triaminic DM Daytime (Can)
TRIKOF-D®
Tussafin® Expectorant
Tussar® SF Syrup
Antitussive/Expectorant
  Benylin® DM-E (Can)
Benylin® Expectorant [OTC]
Brontex® Liquid
Brontex® Tablet
Centratuss DM Expectorant (Can)
Cheracol®
Cheracol® D [OTC]
Clear Tussin® 30
Codiclear® DH
Contac® Cough Formula Liquid
  [OTC]
Cough Syrup DM-E (Can)

Cough Syrup DM Expectorant (Can)
Cough Syrup with Guaifenesin (Can)
Diabetic Tussin DM® [OTC]
DM E Suppressant Expectorant (Can)
DM Plus Expectorant (Can)
Extra Action Cough Syrup [OTC]
Fenesin™ DM
Genatuss DM® [OTC]
Glycotuss-dM® [OTC]
guaifenesin and codeine
guaifenesin and dextromethorphan
Guaifenex® DM
Guaituss AC®
GuiaCough® [OTC]
Guiatuss-DM® [OTC]
Guiatussin® With Codeine
Halotussin® DM [OTC]
Humibid® DM [OTC]
HycoClear Tuss®
Hycotuss® Expectorant Liquid
hydrocodone and guaifenesin
Iobid DM®
Kolephrin® GG/DM [OTC]
Kwelcof®
Monafed® DM
Muco-Fen-DM®
Mytussin® AC
Mytussin® DM [OTC]
Naldecon® Senior DX [OTC]
Phanatuss® Cough Syrup [OTC]
Pharmitussin DM (Can)
Phenadex® Senior [OTC]
Respa®-DM
Rhinosyn-DMX® [OTC]
Robafen® AC
Robafen DM® [OTC]
Robitussin® A-C
Robitussin®-DM [OTC]
Safe Tussin® 30 [OTC]
Scot-Tussin® Senior Clear [OTC]
Siltussin DM® [OTC]
Synacol® CF [OTC]
Syracol-CF® [OTC]

Syrup DM-E (Can)
terpin hydrate and codeine
Tolu-Sed® DM [OTC]
Tusibron-DM® [OTC]
Tuss-DM® [OTC]
Tussi-Organidin® DM NR
Tussi-Organidin® NR
Uni-tussin® DM [OTC]
Vicks® 44E [OTC]
Vicks® Pediatric Formula 44E
    [OTC]
Cold Preparation
    acetaminophen, dextromethorphan,
        and pseudoephedrine
    Alka-Seltzer® Plus Flu & Body
        Aches Non-Drowsy Liqui-Gels®
        [OTC]
    Anatuss® DM [OTC]
    Calmylin #3 (Can)
    Cold Medication Daytime Relief
        (Can)
    Cold Medication D (Can)
    Comtrex® Maximum Strength Non-
        Drowsy [OTC]
    Cough Syrup DM-D-E (Can)
    Cough Syrup DM Decongestant
        Expectorant (Can)
    Dayquil (Can)
    Dimacol® Caplets [OTC]
    DM Plus Decongestant Expectorant
        (Can)
    guaifenesin, pseudoephedrine, and
        dextromethorphan
    Histenol Cold (Can)
    Maxifed® DM
    Neo Citran Daycaps (Can)
    Novahistex DM Expectorant (Can)
    Novahistine DM Expectorant (Can)
    Personnelle Contre le Rhume (Can)
    Rhinosyn-X® Liquid [OTC]
    Robitussin Cough & Cold (Can)
    Ru-Tuss® Expectorant [OTC]
    Sudafed Cold & Cough (Can)

Sudafed® Cold & Cough Liquid Caps [OTC]
Sudafed® Severe Cold [OTC]
Tempra Cold Care (Can)
Theraflu® Non-Drowsy Formula Maximum Strength [OTC]
Triaminic Cold & Fever (Can)
Tylenol Cold Medication (Daytime) (Can)
Tylenol® Cold No Drowsiness [OTC]
Tylenol Cough with Decongestant (Can)
Tylenol® Flu Maximum Strength [OTC]
Cough and Cold Combination
  Detussin® Liquid
  Entuss-D® LIquid
  Histinex® D Liquid
  Histussin D® Liquid
  hydrocodone and pseudoephedrine
  Tyrodone® Liquid
Expectorant
  Anti-Tuss® Expectorant [OTC]
  Balminil® Expectorant (Can)
  Benylin-E (Can)
  Breonesin® [OTC]
  Calmylin Expectorant (Can)
  Diabetic Tussin® EX [OTC]
  Duratuss-G®
  Fenesin™
  Gee Gee® [OTC]
  Genatuss® [OTC]
  Glyate® [OTC]
  Glycotuss® [OTC]
  Glytuss® [OTC]
  guaifenesin
  Guaifenex® LA
  GuiaCough® Expectorant [OTC]
  Guiatuss® [OTC]
  Halotussin® [OTC]
  Humibid® L.A.
  Humibid® Sprinkle
  Hytuss® [OTC]

  Hytuss-2X® [OTC]
  Koffex Expectorant (Can)
  Liquibid®
  Medi-Tuss® [OTC]
  Monafed®
  Muco-Fen-LA®
  Mytussin® [OTC]
  Naldecon® Senior EX [OTC]
  Organidin® NR
  Pneumomist®
  Respa-GF®
  Resyl (Can)
  Robitussin® [OTC]
  Scot-Tussin® [OTC]
  Siltussin® [OTC]
  Sinumist®-SR Capsulets®
  Sirop Expectorant (Can)
  terpin hydrate
  Touro Ex®
  Tusibron® [OTC]
  Uni-tussin® [OTC]

CYCLOSERINE POISONING
Vitamin, Water Soluble
  B6–250 (Can)
  Hexa-Betalin (Can)
  Nestrex®
  pyridoxine

CYSTITIS (HEMORRHAGIC)
Antidote
  mesna
  Mesnex™
  Uromitexan (Can)

CYTOMEGALOVIRUS
Antiviral Agent
  cidofovir
  Cytovene®
  foscarnet
  Foscavir®
  ganciclovir
  Vistide®

Vitrasert®
Antiviral Agent, Ophthalmic
  fomivirsen
  Vitravene™
Immune Globulin
  CytoGam™
  cytomegalovirus immune globulin
    (intravenous-human)
  Gamimune® N
  Gammagard® S/D
  Gammar®-P I.V.
  immune globulin (intravenous)
  Polygam® S/D
  Sandoglobulin®
  Venoglobulin®-I
  Venoglobulin®-S

DANDRUFF

Antiseborrheic Agent, Topical
  Anti-Acne Formula for Men (Can)
  Anti-Dandruff Shampoo (Can)
  AquaTar® [OTC]
  Avant Garde Shampoo (Can)
  Aveeno® Cleansing Bar [OTC]
  Balnetar® [OTC]
  Capitrol®
  chloroxine
  coal tar
  coal tar and salicylic acid
  coal tar, lanolin, and mineral oil
  Dandruff Treatment Shampoo (Can)
  Dan-Gard (Can)
  Denorex® [OTC]
  DHS® Tar [OTC]
  DHS Zinc® [OTC]
  Doak-Oil (Can)
  Duplex® T [OTC]
  Estar® [OTC]
  Exsel® Shampoo
  Fostex® [OTC]
  Fototar® [OTC]
  Hair and Scalp (Can)
  Head & Shoulders® [OTC]

Ionil-T (Can)
Ionil-T Plus (Can)
Keep Clear Anti-Dandruff Shampoo
  (Can)
Lander Dandruff Control (Can)
Mazon Medicated Soap (Can)
Metasep® [OTC]
Meted (Can)
Neutrogena® T/Derm
Neutrogena T/Gel (Can)
Night Cast R (Can)
No-Name Dandruff Treatment (Can)
Out of Africa (Can)
parachlorometaxylenol
Pentrax® [OTC]
Pernox® [OTC]
Pert Plus (Can)
Polytar® [OTC]
psoriGel® [OTC]
P & S Plus (Can)
pyrithione zinc
SAStid® Plain Therapeutic Shampoo
  and Acne Wash [OTC]
Satinique Anti-Dandruff (Can)
Sebcur/T (Can)
Sebulex (Can)
Sebulon (Can)
selenium sulfide
Selsun Blue® Shampoo [OTC]
Selsun® Shampoo
Shaklee Dandruff Control (Can)
Shampooing Anti-Pelliculaire (Can)
Spectro Tar (Can)
sulfur and salicylic acid
Sulsal (Can)
Tardan (Can)
Tar Distillate (Can)
Tar Doak (Can)
Targel (Can)
Targel SA (Can)
Tegrin (Can)
Tersa-Tar (Can)
T/Gel® [OTC]

Theraplex Z® [OTC]
Versel (Can)
X-seb® T [OTC]
Zetar® [OTC]
Zincon® Shampoo [OTC]
ZNP® Bar [OTC]
ZP 11 (Can)

DERMATOLOGIC DISORDERS

Adrenal Corticosteroid
  Acthar®
  Actharn (Can)
  Adlone® Injection
  Aeroseb-Dex®
  Ak-Tate (Can)
  Amcort® Injection
  A-methaPred® Injection
  Apo®-Prednisone (Can)
  Aristocort® Forte Injection
  Aristocort® Intralesional Injection
  Aristocort® Oral
  Aristospan® Intra-articular Injection
  Aristospan® Intralesional Injection
  Atolone® Oral
  Balpred (Can)
  betamethasone (systemic)
  Celestone® Oral
  Celcstone® Phosphate Injection
  Celestone® Soluspan®
  Cel-U-Jec® Injection
  Colocort™
  Cortef®
  corticotropin
  cortisone acetate
  Cortone® Acetate
  Decadron® Injection
  Decadron®-LA
  Decadron® Oral
  Decadron® Phosphate
  Decaject®
  Decaject-LA®
  Delta-Cortef® Oral

Deltasone®
depMedalone® Injection
Depoject® Injection
Depo-Medrol® Injection
Depopred® Injection
dexamethasone (systemic)
dexamethasone (topical)
Dexasone®
Dexasone® L.A.
Dexone®
Dexone® LA
Diopred (Can)
D-Med® Injection
Duralone® Injection
Haldrone®
Hexadrol®
H.P. Acthar® Gel
hydrocortisone (systemic)
Hydrocortone® Acetate
Inflamase (Can)
Jaa-Prednisone® (Can)
Kenacort® Oral
Kenaject® Injection
Kenalog® Injection
Key-Pred® Injection
Key-Pred-SP® Injection
Liquid Pred®
Medralone® Injection
Medrol® Oral
Medrol Veriderm (Can)
methylprednisolone
Meticorten®
M-Prednisol® Injection
Novo-Prednisolone (Can)
Orasone®
paramethasone acetate
Pediapred® Oral
PMS-Dexamethasone (Can)
Prednicen-M®
prednisolone (systemic)
Prednisol® TBA Injection
prednisone
Prelone® Oral

RO-Predphate (Can)
Scheinpharm Triamcine-A (Can)
Solu-Cortef®
Solu-Medrol® Injection
Solurex L.A.®
Stemex®
Tac™-3 Injection
Tac™-40 Injection
Triam-A® Injection
triamcinolone (systemic)
Triam Forte® Injection
Triamonide® Injection
Tri-Kort® Injection
Trilog® Injection
Trilone® Injection
Trisoject® Injection
Ultracortenol (Can)
Winpred (Can)

DERMATOMYCOSIS

Antifungal Agent
  Absorbine® Antifungal Foot Powder
    [OTC]
  Breezee® Mist Antifungal [OTC]
  Femizol-M® [OTC]
  Fulvicin (Can)
  Fulvicin® P/G
  Fulvicin-U/F®
  Fungoid® Creme
  Fungoid® Tincture
  Grifulvin® V
  Grisactin®
  Grisactin® Ultra
  griseofulvin
  Grisovin®-FP (Can)
  Gris-PEG®
  ketoconazole
  Lotrimin® AF Powder [OTC]
  Lotrimin® AF Spray Liquid [OTC]
  Lotrimin® AF Spray Powder [OTC]
  Maximum Strength Desenex®
    Antifungal Cream [OTC]
  Micatin® Topical [OTC]

miconazole
Mitrazol® [OTC]
Monazole-7® (Can)
Monistat-Derm™ Topical
Monistat i.v.™ Injection
Monistat™ Vaginal
M-Zole® 7 Dual Pack [OTC]
naftifine
Naftin®
Nizoral®
Nizoral® A-D Shampoo [OTC]
Novo-Ketoconazole (Can)
Nu-Ketocon (Can)
Ony-Clear® Spray
oxiconazole
Oxistat® Topical
Prescription Strength Desenex®
  [OTC]
Zeasorb-AF® Powder [OTC]

DERMATOSIS

Anesthetic/Corticosteroid
  Lida-Mantle HC® Topical
  lidocaine and hydrocortisone
Corticosteroid, Topical
  Aclovate® Topical
  Acticort® Topical
  Aeroseb-HC® Topical
  Ala-Cort® Topical
  Ala-Scalp® Topical
  alclometasone
  Alocort (Can)
  Alphatrex® Topical
  amcinonide
  Anusol® HC-1 Topical [OTC]
  Anusol® HC-2.5% Topical [OTC]
  Aquacort® (Can)
  Aristocort® A Topical
  Aristocort® Topical
  Bactine® Hydrocortisone [OTC]
  Barriere-HC (Can)
  Beben (Can)
  Betacort (Can)

Betaderm (Can)
Betagel (Can)
Betalene® Topical
betamethasone (topical)
Betatrex® Topical
Beta-Val® Topical
Betnesol® (Can)
Betnovate (Can)
CaldeCort® Anti-Itch Topical Spray
CaldeCort® Topical [OTC]
Carmol-HC® Topical
Celestoderm (Can)
Cetacort® Topical
clobetasol
Clocort® Maximum Strength [OTC]
clocortolone
Cloderm® Topical
Cordran®
Cordran® SP
Cormax® Ointment
Cortacet (Can)
CortaGel® Topical [OTC]
Cortaid® Maximum Strength Topical
   [OTC]
Cortaid® with Aloe Topical [OTC]
Cortate (Can)
Cort-Dome® Topical
Cortef® Feminine Itch Topical
Cortizone®-5 Topical [OTC]
Cortizone®-10 Topical [OTC]
Cortoderm (Can)
Cutivate™
Cyclocort® Topical
Delcort® Topical
Delta-Tritex® Topical
Dermacort® Topical
Dermaflex HC (Can)
Dermarest Dricort® Topical
Derma-Smoothe/FS® Topical
Dermasone (Can)
Dermatop®
Dermolate® Topical [OTC]
Dermovate (Can)

Dermtex® HC with Aloe Topical
   [OTC]
Desocort (Can)
desonide
DesOwen® Topical
desoximetasone
diflorasone
Diprolene® AF Topical
Diprolene® Glycol (Can)
Diprolene® Topical
Diprosone (Can)
Diprosone® Topical
Drenison (Can)
Ectosone (Can)
Eldecort® Topical
Elocom® (Can)
Elocon®
Emo-Cort (Can)
Florone®
Florone E®
fluocinolone
fluocinonide
Fluoderm (Can)
Fluonid® Topical
flurandrenolide
Flurosyn® Topical
Flutex® Topical
fluticasone (topical)
Flutone (Can)
FS Shampoo® Topical
Gynecort® Topical [OTC]
halcinonide
halobetasol
Halog®
Halog®-E
Hi-Cor-1.0® Topical
Hi-Cor-2.5® Topical
Hycort
Hycort® Topical
Hyderm (Can)
hydrocortisone (topical)
Hydrocort® Topical
Hydrosone (Can)

Hydro-Tex® Topical [OTC]
Hytone® Topical
Kenalog® Topical
Kenonel® Topical
LactiCare-HC® Topical
Lanacort® Topical [OTC]
Lidemol (Can)
Lidex®
Lidex-E®
Locoid® Topical
Lyderm (Can)
Maxiflor®
Maxivate® Topical
mometasone furoate
Nasonex®
Novobetamet (Can)
Nutracort® Topical
Orabase® HCA Topical
Penecort® Topical
prednicarbate
Prevex B (Can)
Prevex HC (Can)
Psorcon™
Psorion® Topical
Rholosone (Can)
Rhoprolene (Can)
Rhoprosone (Can)
Rivasone (Can)
Sarna HC (Can)
Scalpicin® Topical
Sential (Can)
S-T Cort® Topical
Synacort® Topical
Synalar-HP® Topical
Synalar® Topical
Synemol® Topical
Taro-Desoximetasone (Can)
Taro-Sone (Can)
Tegrin®-HC Topical [OTC]
Teladar® Topical
Temovate®
Texacort® Topical
Tiamol (Can)

Ti-U-Lac HC (Can)
Topactin (Can)
Topicort®
Topicort®-LP
Topilene (Can)
Topisone (Can)
Topsyn (Can)
Triacet™ Topical
Triaderm (Can)
triamcinolone (topical)
Tridesilon® Topical
U-Cort™ Topical
Ultravate™
Unicort (Can)
urea and hydrocortisone
Uremol-HC (Can)
Valisone® Topical
Westcort® Topical

DIAPER RASH

Antifungal Agent
Caldesene® Topical [OTC]
Cruex (Can)
Fungoid® AF Topical Solution
[OTC]
Pedi-Pro Topical [OTC]
undecylenic acid and derivatives
Dietary Supplement
methionine
Pedameth®
Protectant, Topical
A and D™ Ointment [OTC]
Aquasol A & D (Can)
Desitin® [OTC]
Nutrol A D (Can)
vitamin A and vitamin D
zinc oxide, cod liver oil, and talc
Topical Skin Product
Babys Own Ointment (Can)
Diaparene® [OTC]
Diaper Rash (Can)
Herisan (Can)
Infazinc (Can)

methylbenzethonium chloride
Neoderm (Can)
Pate d'Unna (Can)
Perineal Skin Cleanser (Can)
Prevex Diaper Rash Cream (Can)
Puri-Clens™ [OTC]
Sween Cream® [OTC]
Zinaderm (Can)
Zincoderm (Can)
Zincofax (Can)
zinc oxide

DIARRHEA (BACTERIAL)
Aminoglycoside (Antibiotic)
Mycifradin® Sulfate
Myciguent (Can)
Neo-fradin®
neomycin
Neo-Tabs®

DIARRHEA (TRAVELERS)
Gastrointestinal Agent, Miscellaneous
Bismatrol® [OTC]
Bismed (Can)
bismuth subsalicylate
Bismylate (Can)
Pepto-Bismol® [OTC]

DIPHTHERIA
Antitoxin
diphtheria antitoxin

DIVERTICULITIS
Aminoglycoside (Antibiotic)
Alcomicin (Can)
Cidomycin (Can)
Diogent (Can)
Garamycin®
Garatec (Can)
Genoptic®
Gentacidin®
gentamicin
Gentrasul®
G-myticin®

Jenamicin®
Nebcin® Injection
Ocugram (Can)
PMS-Tobramycin (Can)
RO-Gentycin (Can)
tobramycin
Antibiotic, Miscellaneous
Apo®-Metronidazole (Can)
Azactam®
aztreonam
Cleocin HCl® Oral
Cleocin Pediatric® Oral
Cleocin Phosphate® Injection
Cleocin® Vaginal
Clinda-Derm® Topical
clindamycin
Dalacin® C (Can)
Dalacin T (Can)
Flagyl® Oral
Metro I.V.® Injection
metronidazole
Neo-Metric (Can)
NidaGel (Can)
Noritate (Can)
Novo-Nidazol (Can)
Protostat® Oral
Trikacide (Can)
Carbapenem (Antibiotic)
imipenem and cilastatin
Primaxin®
Cephalosporin (Second Generation)
cefmetazole
Cefotan®
cefotetan
cefoxitin
Mefoxin®
Zefazone®
Penicillin
ampicillin
ampicillin and sulbactam
Ampicin (Can)
Ampicin® Sodium (Can)
Ampilean (Can)

Apo®-Ampi (Can)
bacampicillin
Jaa Amp® (Can)
Marcillin®
Nu-Ampi (Can)
Omnipen®
Omnipen®-N
Penglobe (Can)
piperacillin and tazobactam sodium
Principen®
Spectrobid® Tablet
Tazocin (Can)
ticarcillin and clavulanate potassium
Timentin®
Totacillin®
Unasyn®
Zosyn™

DRACUNCULIASIS
Amebicide
Apo®-Metronidazole (Can)
Flagyl® Oral
Metro I.V.® Injection
metronidazole
Neo-Metric (Can)
NidaGel (Can)
Noritate (Can)
Novo-Nidazol (Can)
Protostat® Oral
Trikacide (Can)

ENCEPHALITIS (HERPESVIRUS)
Antiviral Agent
acyclovir
Avirax® (Can)
Zovirax®

ENDOCARDITIS TREATMENT
Aminoglycoside (Antibiotic)
Alcomicin (Can)
amikacin
Amikin®

Cidomycin (Can)
Diogent (Can)
Garamycin®
Garatec (Can)
Gentacidin®
Gent-AK®
gentamicin
Gentrasul®
G-myticin®
Jenamicin®
Nebcin® Injection
netilmicin
Netromycin®
Ocugram (Can)
PMS-Tobramycin (Can)
RO-Gentycin (Can)
tobramycin
Antibiotic, Miscellaneous
Lyphocin® Injection
Vancocin® CP (Can)
Vancocin® Injection
Vancocin® Oral
Vancoled® Injection
vancomycin
Antibiotic, Penicillin
pivampicillin (Canada only)
Pondocillin® (Can)
Antifungal Agent
amphotericin B (conventional)
Fungizone®
Cephalosporin (First Generation)
Ancef®
Cefadyl®
cefazolin
cephalothin
cephapirin
Ceporacin (Can)
Keflin (Can)
Kefzol®
Zolicef®
Penicillin
ampicillin
Ampicin (Can)

Ampicin® Sodium (Can)
Ampilean (Can)
Apo®-Ampi (Can)
Jaa Amp® (Can)
Marcillin®
nafcillin
Nallpen®
Nu-Ampi (Can)
Omnipen®
Omnipen®-N
oxacillin
penicillin G (parenteral/aqueous)
Pfizerpen®
Principen®
Totacillin®
Unipen® (Can)
Quinolone
　Ciloxan™ Ophthalmic
　Cipro®
　ciprofloxacin

EYE INFECTION
Antibiotic/Corticosteroid, Ophthalmic
　AK-Cide® Ophthalmic
　AK-Spore® H.C. Ophthalmic
　　Ointment
　AK-Spore® H.C. Ophthalmic
　　Suspension
　AK-Trol®
　bacitracin, neomycin, polymyxin B,
　　and hydrocortisone
　Blephamide® Ophthalmic
　Cetapred® Ophthalmic
　chloramphenicol and prednisolone
　chloramphenicol, polymyxin B, and
　　hydrocortisone
　Chloroptic-P® Ophthalmic
　Cortimyxin (Can)
　Cortisporin® Ophthalmic Ointment
　Cortisporin® Ophthalmic Suspension
　Dexacidin®
　Dexasporin®
　Dioptimyd (Can)

Dioptrol (Can)
Diospor HC (Can)
FML-S® Ophthalmic Suspension
Isopto® Cetapred® Ophthalmic
Maxitrol®
Metimyd® Ophthalmic
Neo-Cortef® Ophthalmic
NeoDecadron® Ophthalmic
Neo-Dexameth® Ophthalmic
neomycin and dexamethasone
neomycin and hydrocortisone
neomycin, polymyxin B, and
　dexamethasone
neomycin, polymyxin B, and
　hydrocortisone
neomycin, polymyxin B, and
　prednisolone
Neotricin HC® Ophthalmic Ointment
Ophthocort (Can)
oxytetracycline and hydrocortisone
Poly-Pred® Ophthalmic Suspension
Pred-G® Ophthalmic
prednisolone and gentamicin
sulfacetamide and prednisolone
sulfacetamide sodium and
　fluorometholone
Terra-Cortril® Ophthalmic
　Suspension
TobraDex® Ophthalmic
tobramycin and dexamethasone
Vasocidin® Ophthalmic
Antibiotic, Ophthalmic
　Achromycin® Ophthalmic
　Achromycin V (Can)
　AK-Chlor® Ophthalmic
　AK-Poly-Bac® Ophthalmic
　AK-Spore® Ophthalmic Ointment
　AK-Spore® Ophthalmic Solution
　AK-Sulf®
　AKTob® Ophthalmic
　AK-Tracin® Ophthalmic
　Alcomicin (Can)
　Antibiotic Ointment (Can)

Antibiotique Onguent (Can)
Apo®-Oflox (Can)
Apo®-Tetra (Can)
Bacimyxin (Can)
Bacitin (Can)
bacitracin
bacitracin and polymyxin B
bacitracin, neomycin, and
   polymyxin B
Balsulph (Can)
Betadine® First Aid Antibiotics +
   Moisturizer [OTC]
Bioderm® (Can)
Bleph®-10
Cetamide®
chloramphenicol
Chloroptic® Ophthalmic
Ciloxan™ Ophthalmic
Cipro®
ciprofloxacin
Diochloram (Can)
Diogent (Can)
Diosporin (Can)
Diosulf (Can)
erythromycin (ophthalmic/topical)
Fenicol (Can)
Floxin®
Garamycin®
Garatec (Can)
Genoptic®
Gentacidin®
Gent-AK®
gentamicin
Gentrasul®
G-myticin®
Ilotycin® Ophthalmic
Isopto® Cetamide® (Can)
I-Sulfacet®
Jenamicin®
Lanabiotic (Can)
Levaquin™
levofloxacin
Neo Bace (Can)

neomycin, polymyxin B, and
   gramicidin
Neosporin® Ophthalmic Ointment
Neosporin® Ophthalmic Solution
Neotopic (Can)
Novo-Chlorocap (Can)
Novo-Tetra (Can)
Nu-Tetra (Can)
Ocuflox™ Ophthalmic
Ocugram (Can)
ofloxacin
Ophthacet®
Ophtho-Chloram (Can)
Ophthochlor® Ophthalmic
Ophtho-Sulf (Can)
Optimyxin (Can)
Optimyxin Plus (Can)
oxytetracycline and polymyxin B
Panmycin® Oral
Pentamycetin® (Can)
PMS-Tobramycin (Can)
Polycidin (Can)
Polyderm (Can)
Polysporin® Ophthalmic
Polytopic (Can)
Polytracin (Can)
Polytrim® Ophthalmic
Quixin™ Ophthalmic
Robitet® Oral
RO-Gentycin (Can)
Sodium Sulamyd®
Sopamycetin (Can)
Spersanicol (Can)
Sulf-10®
sulfacetamide
sulfacetamide and phenylephrine
Sulfair®
Sulfex (Can)
Terak® Ophthalmic Ointment
Terramycin® Ophthalmic Ointment
Terramycin® w/Polymyxin B
   Ophthalmic Ointment
tetracycline

Tetracyn (Can)
tobramycin
Tobrex® Ophthalmic
Tomycine™ Ophthalmic (Can)
trimethoprim and polymyxin B
Vasosulf® Ophthalmic
Antibiotic, Topical
silver protein, mild

EYELID INFECTION
Antibiotic, Ophthalmic
mercuric oxide
Ocu-Merox®
Pharmaceutical Aid
boric acid
Borofax® Topical [OTC]
RO-Eyewash (Can)

FEVER
Antipyretic
Abenol® (Can)
Acephen® [OTC]
Aceta® [OTC]
Acetab (Can)
acetaminophen
Aches-N-Pain® [OTC]
Actiprofen® (Can)
Advil® [OTC]
A.F. Anacin® (Can)
222 AF (Can)
Aleve® [OTC]
Alsiphene (Can)
Amersol (Can)
Anacin® [OTC]
Anacin-3 (Can)
Anaprox®
Apacet® [OTC]
APF (Can)
Apo®-ASA (Can)
Apo®-Ibuprofen (Can)
Apo®-Napro-Na (Can)
Apo®-Naproxen (Can)
Argesic®-SA
Artha-G®

Arthrisin (Can)
Artria (Can)
Artritol (Can)
A.S.A. [OTC]
Asadrine (Can)
Asaphen (Can)
Ascriptin® [OTC]
Aspergum® [OTC]
aspirin
Aspirin Plus Stomach Guard (Can)
Atasol® (Can)
Bayer® Aspirin [OTC]
Bufferin® [OTC]
Cephanol (Can)
Children's Advil® Suspension
Children's Motrin® Suspension
[OTC]
Coryphen (Can)
Dapa® [OTC]
Dapacin® [OTC]
Disalcid®
Dodds (Can)
Dorcol® [OTC]
Easprin®
Ecotrin® [OTC]
Empirin® [OTC]
Entrophen® (Can)
Excedrin® IB [OTC]
Feverall™ [OTC]
Genapap® [OTC]
Genebs® [OTC]
Genpril® [OTC]
Halfprin® [OTC]
Haltran® [OTC]
Headache Tablets (Can)
Headarest (Can)
Ibuprin® [OTC]
ibuprofen
Ibuprohm® [OTC]
Ibu-Tab®
Junior Strength Motrin® [OTC]
Liquiprin® [OTC]
Mapap® [OTC]

Maranox® [OTC]
Marthritic®
Measurin® [OTC]
Meda-Cap® [OTC]
Meda® Tab [OTC]
Medipren® [OTC]
Menadol® [OTC]
Midol® IB [OTC]
Mono-Gesic®
Motrin®
Motrin® IB [OTC]
MSD® Enteric Coated ASA (Can)
Myapap® [OTC]
Naprelan®
Naprosyn®
naproxen
Naxen® (Can)
Neopap® [OTC]
Novasen (Can)
Novo-Gesic (Can)
Novo-Naprox (Can)
Novo-Profen® (Can)
Nu-Ibuprofen (Can)
Nu-Naprox (Can)
Nuprin® [OTC]
Pain Aid Free (Can)
Pamprin IB® [OTC]
Panadol® [OTC]
Pedia-Profen™
Pediatrix (Can)
Redutemp® [OTC]
Ridenol® [OTC]
Robigesic (Can)
Rounox (Can)
S-60 (Can)
Sal (Can)
Saleto-200® [OTC]
Saleto-400®
Salflex®
Salgesic®
Saliject (Can)
salsalate
Salsitab®

Silapap® [OTC]
Snaplets-FR® Granules [OTC]
sodium salicylate
Supasa (Can)
Synflex (Can)
Tantaphen® (Can)
Tapanol® [OTC]
Tempra® [OTC]
Trendar® [OTC]
Tylenol® [OTC]
Ty-Pap [OTC]
Uni-Ace® [OTC]
Uni-Pro® [OTC]
Uracel®
ZORprin®

FUNGUS (DIAGNOSTIC)
Diagnostic Agent
    Candida albicans (Monilia)
    coccidioidin skin test
    Dermatophytin®
    Dermatophytin-O
    Histolyn-CYL®
    histoplasmin
    Spherulin®
    Trichophyton skin test

GENITAL HERPES
Antiviral Agent
    famciclovir
    Famvir™
    valacyclovir
    Valtrex®

GENITAL WART
Immune Response Modifier
    Aldara™
    imiquimod

GIARDIASIS
Amebicide
    Apo®-Metronidazole (Can)
    Flagyl® Oral
    Humatin®
    Metro I.V.® Injection

metronidazole
Neo-Metric (Can)
NidaGel (Can)
Noritate (Can)
Novo-Nidazol (Can)
paromomycin
Protostat® Oral
Trikacide (Can)
Anthelmintic
albendazole
Albenza®
Antiprotozoal
furazolidone
Furoxone®

GINGIVITIS

Antibiotic, Oral Rinse
BactoShield® [OTC]
Baxedin (Can)
Betasept® [OTC]
chlorhexidine gluconate
Chlorhexseptic (Can)
Dyna-Hex® [OTC]
Hexifoam (Can)
Hibidil (Can)
Hibitane (Can)
Oro-Clense (Can)
Peridex®
Periochip®
PerioGard®
Rouhex-G (Can)
Spectro Gram (Can)

GONOCOCCAL OPHTHALMIA NEONATORUM

Topical Skin Product
Dey-Drop® Ophthalmic Solution
silver nitrate

GONORRHEA

Antibiotic, Macrolide
Rovamycine® (Can)
spiramycin (Canada only)

Antibiotic, Miscellaneous
spectinomycin
Trobicin®
Antibiotic, Quinolone
gatifloxacin
Tequin™
Cephalosporin (Second Generation)
cefoxitin
Ceftin® Oral
cefuroxime
Kefurox® Injection
Mefoxin®
Zinacef® Injection
Cephalosporin (Third Generation)
cefixime
ceftriaxone
Rocephin®
Suprax®
Quinolone
Apo®-Oflox (Can)
Ciloxan™ Ophthalmic
Cipro®
ciprofloxacin
Floxin®
Ocuflox™ Ophthalmic
ofloxacin
Tetracycline Derivative
Achromycin® Ophthalmic
Achromycin® Topical
Achromycin V (Can)
Apo®-Doxy Tabs (Can)
Apo®-Tetra (Can)
Bio-Tab®
Doryx®
Doxy-200®
Doxy-Caps®
Doxychel®
Doxycin (Can)
doxycycline
Doxy-Tabs®
Doxytec (Can)
Monodox®
Nor-tet® Oral

Novo-Doxylin (Can)
Novo-Tetra (Can)
Nu-Doxycycline (Can)
Nu-Tetra (Can)
Panmycin® Oral
Robitet® Oral
Sumycin® Oral
Tetracap® Oral
tetracycline
Tetracyn (Can)
Topicycline® Topical
Vibramycin®
Vibra-Tabs®

GRANULOMA (INGUINALE)

Antibiotic, Aminoglycoside
  streptomycin
Antitubercular Agent
  streptomycin

HAY FEVER

Adrenergic Agonist Agent
  Afrin® Children's Nose Drops [OTC]
  Afrin® Nasal Solution [OTC]
  Allerest® 12 Hour Nasal Solution
    [OTC]
  Chlorphed®-LA Nasal Solution
    [OTC]
  Dristan® Long Lasting Nasal
    Solution [OTC]
  Drixoral® (Can)
  Duramist Plus® [OTC]
  Duration® Nasal Solution [OTC]
  Nafrine (Can)
  Neo-Synephrine® 12 Hour Nasal
    Solution [OTC]
  Nostrilla® [OTC]
  NTZ® Long Acting Nasal Solution
    [OTC]
  OcuClear® Ophthalmic [OTC]
  oxymetazoline
  Sinarest® 12 Hour Nasal Solution
  Sinex® Long-Acting [OTC]
  Twice-A-Day® Nasal Solution [OTC]

Vicks® Sinex (Can)
Visine® L.®. Ophthalmic [OTC]
Visine® Workplace (Can)
4-Way® Long Acting Nasal Solution
  [OTC]
Antihistamine
  Allegra®
  fexofenadine
Antihistamine/Decongestant
  Combination
  acrivastine and pseudoephedrine
  Actagen® Syrup [OTC]
  Actagen® Tablet [OTC]
  Actifed 12 Hour (Can)
  Actifed (Can)
  Allercon® Tablet [OTC]
  Allerest® Maximum Strength [OTC]
  Allerfrin® Syrup [OTC]
  Allerfrin® Tablet [OTC]
  Allerphed® Syrup [OTC]
  Anamine® Syrup [OTC]
  Anaplex® Liquid [OTC]
  Aprodine® Syrup [OTC]
  Aprodine® Tablet [OTC]
  Benylin® Cold (Can)
  Cenafed® Plus Tablet [OTC]
  Chlorafed® Liquid [OTC]
  chlorpheniramine and
    pseudoephedrine
  Chlor-Trimeton® 4 Hour Relief
    Tablet [OTC]
  Chlor-Tripolon Decongestant (Can)
  Co-Pyronil® 2 Pulvules® [OTC]
  Deconamine® SR
  Deconamine® Syrup [OTC]
  Deconamine® Tablet [OTC]
  Fedahist® Tablet [OTC]
  Genac® Tablet [OTC]
  Hayfebrol® Liquid [OTC]
  Klerist-D® Tablet [OTC]
  Pseudo-Gest Plus® Tablet [OTC]
  Rhinosyn® Liquid [OTC]
  Rhinosyn-PD® Liquid [OTC]

Ryna® Liquid [OTC]
Semprex®-D
Silafed® Syrup [OTC]
Sudafed® Plus Tablet [OTC]
Triofed® Syrup [OTC]
Triposed® Syrup [OTC]
Triposed® Tablet [OTC]
Triprofed (Can)
triprolidine and pseudoephedrine
Vasofrinic (Can)

HELICOBACTER PYLORI
Antibiotic, Miscellaneous
  Apo®-Metronidazole (Can)
  Flagyl® Oral
  Metro I.V.® Injection
  metronidazole
  Neo-Metric (Can)
  NidaGel (Can)
  Noritate (Can)
  Novo-Nidazol (Can)
  Protostat® Oral
  Trikacide (Can)
Antidiarrheal
  bismuth subsalicylate, metronidazole,
    and tetracycline
  Helidac™
Gastrointestinal Agent, Gastric or
  Duodenal Ulcer Treatment
  ranitidine bismuth citrate
  Tritec®
Gastrointestinal Agent, Miscellaneous
  Bismatrol® [OTC]
  Bismed (Can)
  bismuth subsalicylate
  Bismylate (Can)
  Pepto-Bismol® [OTC]
Macrolide (Antibiotic)
  Biaxin®
  Biaxin® XL
  clarithromycin
Penicillin
  amoxicillin

Amoxil®
Apo®-Amoxi (Can)
Gen-Amoxicillin (Can)
Novamoxin® (Can)
Nu-Amoxi (Can)
Pro-Amox® (Can)
Trimox®
Wymox®
Tetracycline Derivative
  Achromycin V (Can)
  Apo®-Tetra (Can)
  Nor-tet® Oral
  Novo-Tetra (Can)
  Nu-Tetra (Can)
  Panmycin® Oral
  Robitet® Oral
  Sumycin® Oral
  Tetracap® Oral
  tetracycline
  Tetracyn (Can)

HEPATITIS A
Immune Globulin
  Gammabulin Immuno (Can)
  immune globulin (intramuscular)

HEPATITIS B
Antiviral Agent
  Epivir®
  Epivir®-HBV™
  Heptovir® (Can)
  interferon alfa-2b and ribavirin
  combination pack
  lamivudine
  Rebetron™
  3TC® (Can)
Biological Response Modulator
  interferon alfa-2b
  interferon alfa-2b and ribavirin
    combination pack
  Intron® A
  Rebetron™
Reverse Transcriptase Inhibitor
  adefovir

Preveon®

HEPATITIS C

Antiviral Agent
interferon alfa-2b and ribavirin
combination pack
Rebetron™
Biological Response Modulator
interferon alfa-2b
interferon alfa-2b and ribavirin
combination pack
Intron® A
Rebetron™
Interferon
Infergen®
interferon alfacon-1

HERPES SIMPLEX

Antiviral Agent
acyclovir
Avirax® (Can)
Cytovene®
famciclovir
Famvir™
foscarnet
Foscavir®
ganciclovir
trifluridine
vidarabine
Vira-A® Ophthalmic
Viroptic® Ophthalmic
Vitrasert®
Zovirax®

HERPES ZOSTER

Analgesic, Topical
Axsain (Can)
capsaicin
Capsin® [OTC]
Capzasin-P® [OTC]
Dolorac™ [OTC]
No Pain-HP® [OTC]
R-Gel® [OTC]
Zostrix® [OTC]

Zostrix®-HP [OTC]
Antiviral Agent
acyclovir
Avirax® (Can)
famciclovir
Famvir™
valacyclovir
Valtrex®
vidarabine
Vira-A® Ophthalmic
Zovirax®

HISTOPLASMOSIS

Antifungal Agent
amphotericin B (conventional)
Fungizone®
itraconazole
ketoconazole
Nizoral®
Novo-Ketoconazole (Can)
Nu-Ketocon (Can)
Sporanox®

HIV [SEE ACQUIRED IMMUNODEFICIENCY SYNDROME (AIDS)]

HOOKWORMS

Anthelmintic
albendazole
Albenza®
Antiminth® [OTC]
Combantrin (Can)
Jaa Pyral® (Can)
mebendazole
Pin-Rid® [OTC]
Pin-X® [OTC]
pyrantel pamoate
Reese's® Pinworm Medicine [OTC]
Vermox®

IMPETIGO

Antibiotic, Topical
bacitracin, neomycin, and polymyxin B

Bactroban®
Medi-Quick® Topical Ointment
    [OTC]
mupirocin
Mycitracin® Topical [OTC]
Neomixin® Topical
Neosporin® Topical Ointment [OTC]
Neotopic (Can)
Ocutricin® Topical Ointment
Septa® Topical Ointment [OTC]
Triple Antibiotic® Topical
Penicillin
Apo®-Pen VK (Can)
Ayercillin® (Can)
Crysticillin® A.S.
Nadopen-V® (Can)
Novo-Pen-VK® (Can)
Nu-Pen-VK (Can)
penicillin G procaine
penicillin V potassium
Truxcillin®
Veetids®
Wycillin®

INFLUENZA
Antiviral Agent
amantadine
Endantadine® (Can)
PMS-Amantadine (Can)
Symadine®
Symmetrel® Syrup
Antiviral Agent, Inhalation Therapy
Relenza®
zanamivir
Antiviral Agent, Oral
oseltamivir
Tamiflu™

INFLUENZA A
Antiviral Agent
amantadine
Endantadine® (Can)
Flumadine®
PMS-Amantadine (Can)

rimantadine
Symadine®
Symmetrel® Syrup

INFLUENZA VIRUS
Antiviral Agent
Flumadine®
rimantadine
Vaccine, Inactivated Virus
Fluogen®
Fluviral® (Can)
Fluzone®
influenza virus vaccine

KERATITIS (FUNGAL)
Antifungal Agent
Natacyn®
natamycin

KERATITIS (HERPES SIMPLEX)
Antiviral Agent
trifluridine
vidarabine
Vira-A® Ophthalmic
Viroptic® Ophthalmic

LEPROSY
Immunosuppressant Agent
Contergan®
Distaval®
Kevadon®
thalidomide
Thalomid®
Leprostatic Agent
clofazimine
Lamprene®
Sulfone
Avlosulfon®
dapsone

LICE
Scabicides/Pediculicides
A-200™ Shampoo [OTC]
Acticin® Cream

Barc™ Liquid [OTC]
Elimite™ Cream
End Lice® Liquid [OTC]
GBH (Can)
G-well®
Hexit® (Can)
Kwellada® (Can)
Lice-Enz® Shampoo [OTC]
lindane
malathion
Nix™ Creme Rinse
Ovide™ Topical
permethrin
PMS-Lindane (Can)
Prioderm (Can)
Pronto® Shampoo [OTC]
pyrethrins and piperonyl butoxide
Pyrinex® Pediculicide Shampoo [OTC]
Pyrinyl II® Liquid [OTC]
Pyrinyl Plus® Shampoo [OTC]
R & C® Shampoo [OTC]
RID® Mousse [OTC]
RID® Shampoo [OTC]
Tisit® Blue Gel [OTC]
Tisit® Liquid [OTC]
Tisit® Shampoo [OTC]
Triple X® Liquid [OTC]

LICHEN SIMPLEX CHRONICUS

Topical Skin Product
  doxepin
  Zonalon® Topical Cream

LYME DISEASE

Antibiotic, Penicillin
  pivampicillin (Canada only)
  Pondocillin® (Can)
Cephalosporin (Third Generation)
  ceftriaxone
  Rocephin®
Macrolide (Antibiotic)
  AK-Mycin®

Apo®-Erythro E-C (Can)
Diomycin (Can)
E.E.S.®
E-Mycin®
E-Mycin-E®
Erybid® (Can)
Eryc®
Ery-Tab®
Erythro-Base® (Can)
Erythrocin®
erythromycin (systemic)
Ilosone® Pulvules®
Ilotycin®
Novo-Rythro Encap (Can)
PCE®
PMS-Erythromycin (Can)
Wyamycin® S
Penicillin
  amoxicillin
  Amoxil®
  ampicillin
  Ampicin (Can)
  Ampicin® Sodium (Can)
  Ampilean (Can)
  Apo®-Amoxi (Can)
  Apo®-Ampi (Can)
  Apo®-Pen VK (Can)
  Gen-Amoxicillin (Can)
  Jaa Amp® (Can)
  Marcillin®
  Nadopen-V® (Can)
  Novamoxin® (Can)
  Novo-Pen-VK® (Can)
  Nu-Amoxi (Can)
  Nu-Ampi (Can)
  Nu-Pen-VK (Can)
  Omnipen®
  Omnipen®-N
  penicillin V potassium
  Principen®
  Pro-Amox® (Can)
  Totacillin®
  Trimox®

Truxcillin®
Veetids®
Wymox®
Tetracycline Derivative
Achromycin® Ophthalmic
Achromycin® Topical
Achromycin V (Can)
Apo®-Doxy Tabs (Can)
Apo®-Tetra (Can)
Bio-Tab®
Doryx®
Doxy-200®
Doxy-Caps®
Doxychel®
Doxycin (Can)
doxycycline
Doxy-Tabs®
Doxytec (Can)
Monodox®
Nor-tet® Oral
Novo-Doxylin (Can)
Novo-Tetra (Can)
Nu-Doxycycline (Can)
Nu-Tetra (Can)
Panmycin® Oral
Robitet® Oral
Sumycin® Oral
Tetracap® Oral
tetracycline
Tetracyn (Can)
Topicycline® Topical
Vibramycin®
Vibra-Tabs®
Vaccine
Lyme disease vaccine
LYMErix™

MALARIA

Aminoquinoline (Antimalarial)
Aralen® Phosphate
Aralen® Phosphate With Primaquine
Phosphate
chloroquine and primaquine

chloroquine phosphate
hydroxychloroquine
Plaquenil®
primaquine
Antimalarial Agent
atovaquone and proguanil
Formula Q®
Halfan®
halofantrine
Lariam®
Malarone™
mefloquine
quinine
Folic Acid Antagonist (Antimalarial)
Daraprim®
pyrimethamine
Sulfonamide
Coptin® (Can)
SSD (Can)
sulfadiazine
Tetracycline Derivative
Apo®-Doxy Tabs (Can)
Bio-Tab®
Doryx®
Doxy-200®
Doxy-Caps®
Doxychel®
Doxycin (Can)
doxycycline
Doxy-Tabs®
Doxytec (Can)
Monodox®
Novo-Doxylin (Can)
Nu-Doxycycline (Can)
Vibramycin®
Vibra-Tabs®

MEASLES (RUBELLA)

Vaccine, Live Virus
measles and rubella vaccines,
combined
MoRu-Viraten (Can)
M-R-VAX® II

A69

MEASLES (RUBEOLA)
Immune Globulin
  Gammabulin Immuno (Can)
  immune globulin (intramuscular)
Vaccine, Live Virus
  measles and rubella vaccines,
    combined
  MoRu-Viraten (Can)
  M-R-VAX® II

MENINGITIS (TUBERCULOUS)
Antibiotic, Aminoglycoside
  streptomycin

MOUTH INFECTION
Antifungal Agent, Topical
  Dequadin® (Can)
  dequalinium (Canada only)

MUMPS (DIAGNOSTIC)
Diagnostic Agent
  MSTA® Mumps
  mumps skin test antigen

MYCOBACTERIUM AVIUM-INTRACELLULARE
Antibiotic, Aminoglycoside
  streptomycin
Antibiotic, Miscellaneous
  Mycobutin®
  rifabutin
  Rifadin® Injection
  Rifadin® Oral
  rifampin
  Rimactane® Oral
  Rofact® (Can)
Antimycobacterial Agent
  ethambutol
  Etibi® (Can)
  Myambutol®
Antitubercular Agent
  streptomycin
Carbapenem (Antibiotic)

imipenem and cilastatin
  meropenem
  Merrem® I.V.
  Primaxin®
Leprostatic Agent
  clofazimine
  Lamprene®
Macrolide (Antibiotic)
  azithromycin
  Biaxin®
  Biaxin® XL
  clarithromycin
  Zithromax™
Quinolone
  Cipro®
  ciprofloxacin

MYCOSIS (FUNGOIDES)
Psoralen
  methoxsalen
  Oxsoralen (Can)
  Oxsoralen-Ultra®
  Ultramop (Can)

ONYCHOMYCOSIS
Antifungal Agent
  Fulvicin (Can)
  Fulvicin® P/G
  Fulvicin-U/F®
  Grifulvin® V
  Grisactin®
  Grisactin® Ultra
  griseofulvin
  Grisovin®-FP (Can)
  Gris-PEG®
  Lamisil® Oral
  terbinafine (oral)

OSTEOMYELITIS
Antibiotic, Miscellaneous
  Cleocin HCl® Oral
  Cleocin Pediatric® Oral
  Cleocin Phosphate® Injection
  Cleocin T® Topical

Cleocin® Vaginal
Clinda-Derm® Topical
clindamycin
Dalacin® C (Can)
Dalacin T (Can)
Dalacin Vaginal (Can)
Lyphocin® Injection
Vancocin® CP (Can)
Vancocin® Injection
Vancocin® Oral
Vancoled® Injection
vancomycin
Antifungal Agent, Systemic
  Fucidin® I.V. (Can)
  Fucidin® Oral Suspension (Can)
  Fucidin® Tablet (Can)
  fusidic acid (Canada only)
Carbapenem (Antibiotic)
  imipenem and cilastatin
  meropenem
  Merrem® I.V.
  Primaxin®
Cephalosporin (First Generation)
  Ancef®
  Cefadyl®
  cefazolin
  cephalothin
  cephapirin
  Ceporacin (Can)
  Keflin (Can)
  Kefzol®
  Zolicef®
Cephalosporin (Second Generation)
  cefmetazole
  cefonicid
  Cefotan®
  cefotetan
  cefoxitin
  Ceftin® Oral
  cefuroxime
  Kefurox® Injection
  Mefoxin®
  Monocid®

Zefazone®
Zinacef® Injection
Cephalosporin (Third Generation)
  Cefizox®
  Cefobid®
  cefoperazone
  cefotaxime
  ceftazidime
  ceftizoxime
  ceftriaxone
  Ceptaz™
  Claforan®
  Fortaz®
  Rocephin®
  Tazicef®
  Tazidime®
Penicillin
  ampicillin and sulbactam
  bacampicillin
  dicloxacillin
  Dycill®
  Dynapen®
  nafcillin
  Nallpen®
  oxacillin
  Pathocil®
  Penglobe (Can)
  Spectrobid® Tablet
  ticarcillin and clavulanate potassium
  Timentin®
  Unasyn®
  Unipen® (Can)
Quinolone
  Cipro®
  ciprofloxacin

OTITIS EXTERNA
Aminoglycoside (Antibiotic)
  Alcomicin (Can)
  amikacin
  Amikin®
  Cidomycin (Can)
  Diogent (Can)

Garamycin®
Garatec (Can)
Gentacidin®
Gent-AK®
gentamicin
Gentrasul®
G-myticin®
Jenamicin®
kanamycin
Kantrex®
Mycifradin® Sulfate
Myciguent (Can)
Nebcin® Injection
Neo-fradin®
neomycin
Neo-Tabs®
netilmicin
Netromycin®
Ocugram (Can)
PMS-Tobramycin (Can)
RO-Gentycin (Can)
tobramycin
Tobrex® Ophthalmic
Tomycine™ Ophthalmic (Can)
Antibacterial, Otic
  acetic acid
  VoSol® Otic
Antibiotic/Corticosteroid, Otic
  Acetasol® HC Otic
  acetic acid, propylene glycol
    diacetate, and hydrocortisone
  AK-Spore® H.C. Otic
  AntibiOtic® Otic
  ciprofloxacin and hydrocortisone
  Cipro® HC Otic
  colistin, neomycin, and
    hydrocortisone
  Coly-Mycin Otic (Can)
  Coly-Mycin® S Otic Drops
  Cortatrigen® Otic
  Cortimyxin (Can)
  Cortisporin® Otic
  Cortisporin-TC® Otic

Cortisporin®-TC Otic Suspension
Diospor HC (Can)
neomycin, colistin, hydrocortisone,
  and thonzonium
neomycin, polymyxin B, and
  hydrocortisone
Octicair® Otic
Otic-Care® Otic
Otobiotic® Otic
Otocort® Otic
Otosporin® Otic
Pediotic® Otic
polymyxin B and hydrocortisone
UAD Otic®
VoSol® HC Otic
Antibiotic, Otic
  chloramphenicol
  ofloxacin
Cephalosporin (Third Generation)
  ceftazidime
  Ceptaz™
  Fortaz®
  Tazicef®
  Tazidime®
Corticosteroid, Topical
  Aclovate® Topical
  Acticort® Topical
  Aeroseb-HC® Topical
  Ala-Cort® Topical
  Ala-Scalp® Topical
  alclometasone
  Alocort (Can)
  Alphatrex® Topical
  amcinonide
  Anusol® HC-1 Topical [OTC]
  Anusol® HC-2.5% Topical [OTC]
  Aquacort® (Can)
  Aristocort® A Topical
  Aristocort® Topical
  Bactine® Hydrocortisone [OTC]
  Barriere-HC (Can)
  Beben (Can)
  Betacort (Can)

Betaderm (Can)
Betagel (Can)
Betalene® Topical
betamethasone (topical)
Betatrex® Topical
Beta-Val® Topical
Betnesol® (Can)
Betnovate (Can)
CaldeCort® Anti-Itch Topical Spray
CaldeCort® Topical [OTC]
Carmol-HC® Topical
Celestoderm (Can)
Cetacort® Topical
clobetasol
Clocort® Maximum Strength [OTC]
clocortolone
Cloderm® Topical
Cordran®
Cordran® SP
Cormax® Ointment
Cortacet (Can)
CortaGel® Topical [OTC]
Cortaid® Maximum Strength Topical
  [OTC]
Cortaid® with Aloe Topical [OTC]
Cortate (Can)
Cort-Dome® Topical
Cortef® Feminine Itch Topical
Cortizone®-5 Topical [OTC]
Cortizone®-10 Topical [OTC]
Cortoderm (Can)
Cutivate™
Cyclocort® Topical
Delcort® Topical
Delta-Tritex® Topical
Dermacort® Topical
Dermaflex HC (Can)
Dermarest Dricort® Topical
Derma-Smoothe/FS® Topical
Dermasone (Can)
Dermatop®
Dermolate® Topical [OTC]
Dermovate (Can)

Dermtex® HC with Aloe Topical
  [OTC]
Desocort (Can)
desonide
DesOwen® Topical
desoximetasone
diflorasone
Diprolene® AF Topical
Diprolene® Glycol (Can)
Diprolene® Topical
Diprosone (Can)
Diprosonc® Topical
Drenison (Can)
Ectosone (Can)
Eldecort® Topical
Elocom® (Can)
Elocon®
Emo-Cort (Can)
Florone®
Florone E®
fluocinolone
fluocinonide
Fluoderm (Can)
Fluonid® Topical
flurandrenolide
Flurosyn® Topical
Flutex® Topical
fluticasone (topical)
Flutone (Can)
FS Shampoo® Topical
Gynecort® Topical [OTC]
halcinonide
halobetasol
Halog®
Halog®-E
Hi-Cor-1.0® Topical
Hi-Cor-2.5® Topical
Hycort
Hycort® Topical
Hyderm (Can)
hydrocortisone (topical)
Hydrocort® Topical
Hydrosone (Can)

Hydro-Tex® Topical [OTC]
Hytone® Topical
Kenalog® in Orabase®
Kenalog® Topical
Kenonel® Topical
LactiCare-HC® Topical
Lanacort® Topical [OTC]
Lidemol (Can)
Lidex®
Lidex-E®
Locoid® Topical
Lyderm (Can)
Maxiflor®
Maxivate® Topical
mometasone furoate
Nasonex®
Novobetamet (Can)
Nutracort® Topical
Orabase® HCA Topical
Penecort® Topical
prednicarbate
Prevex B (Can)
Prevex HC (Can)
Psorcon™
Psorion® Topical
Rholosone (Can)
Rhoprolene (Can)
Rhoprosone (Can)
Rivasone (Can)
Sarna HC (Can)
Scalpicin® Topical
Sential (Can)
S-T Cort® Topical
Synacort® Topical
Synalar-HP® Topical
Synalar® Topical
Synemol® Topical
Taro-Desoximetasone (Can)
Taro-Sone (Can)
Tegrin®-HC Topical [OTC]
Teladar® Topical
Temovate®
Texacort® Topical

Tiamol (Can)
Ti-U-Lac HC (Can)
Topactin (Can)
Topicort®
Topicort®-LP
Topilene (Can)
Topisone (Can)
Topsyn (Can)
Triacet™ Topical
Triaderm (Can)
triamcinolone (topical)
Tridesilon® Topical
U-Cort™ Topical
Ultravate™
Unicort (Can)
urea and hydrocortisone
Uremol-HC (Can)
Valisone® Topical
Westcort® Topical
Otic Agent, Analgesic
    Allergan® Ear Drops
    Antiben®
    antipyrine and benzocaine
    Auralgan®
    Aurodex®
    Auroto®
    Dolotic®
Otic Agent, Anti-infective
    aluminum acetate and acetic acid
    Cresylate®
    m-cresyl acetate
    Otic Domeboro®
Quinolone
    Cipro®
    ciprofloxacin
    lomefloxacin
    Maxaquin®
    nalidixic acid
    NegGram®

OTITIS MEDIA
Antibiotic, Carbacephem
    Lorabid™

loracarbef
Antibiotic, Miscellaneous
  Primsol®
  Proloprim®
  trimethoprim
  Trimpex®
Antibiotic, Otic
  Apo®-Oflox (Can)
  Floxin®
  ofloxacin
Antibiotic, Penicillin
  pivampicillin (Canada only)
  Pondocillin® (Can)
Cephalosporin (First Generation)
  Apo®-Cephalex (Can)
  Biocef®
  cefadroxil
  Cefanex®
  cephalexin
  Ceporex (Can)
  Duricef®
  Keflex®
  Keftab®
  Novo-Lexin (Can)
  Nu-Cephalex (Can)
  Zartan®
Cephalosporin (Second Generation)
  Apo®-Cefaclor (Can)
  Ceclor®
  Ceclor® CD
  cefaclor
  cefpodoxime
  cefprozil
  Ceftin® Oral
  cefuroxime
  Cefzil®
  Kefurox® Injection
  Novo-Cefaclor (Can)
  Vantin®
  Zinacef® Injection
Cephalosporin (Third Generation)
  Cedax®
  cefdinir

cefixime
ceftibuten
Omnicef®
Suprax®
Macrolide (Antibiotic)
  AK-Mycin®
  Apo®-Erythro E-C (Can)
  Diomycin (Can)
  E.E.S.®
  E-Mycin®
  E-Mycin-E®
  Erybid® (Can)
  Eryc®
  Ery-Tab®
  Erythro-Base® (Can)
  Erythrocin®
  erythromycin and sulfisoxazole
  erythromycin (systemic)
  Eryzole®
  Ilosone® Pulvules®
  Ilotycin®
  Novo-®ythro Encap (Can)
  PCE®
  Pediazole®
  PMS-Erythromycin (Can)
  Wyamycin® S
Otic Agent, Analgesic
  Allergan® Ear Drops
  Antiben®
  antipyrine and benzocaine
  Auralgan®
  Aurodex®
  Auroto®
  Dolotic®
Penicillin
  amoxicillin
  amoxicillin and clavulanate potassium
  Amoxil®
  ampicillin
  Ampicin (Can)
  Ampicin® Sodium (Can)
  Ampilean (Can)
  Apo®-Amoxi (Can)

Apo®-Ampi (Can)
Augmentin®
Clavulin® (Can)
Gen-Amoxicillin (Can)
Jaa Amp® (Can)
Marcillin®
Novamoxin® (Can)
Nu-Amoxi (Can)
Nu-Ampi (Can)
Omnipen®
Omnipen®-N
Principen®
Pro-Amox® (Can)
Totacillin®
Trimox®
Wymox®
Sulfonamide
  Apo®-Sulfamethoxazole (Can)
  Apo®-Sulfatrim (Can)
  Bactrim™
  Bactrim™ DS
  Cotrim®
  Cotrim® DS
  co-trimoxazole
  erythromycin and sulfisoxazole
  Eryzole®
  Gantrisin®
  Novo-Soxazole (Can)
  Novo-Trimel (Can)
  Nu-Cotrimox (Can)
  Pediazole®
  Protrin (Can)
  Roubac® (Can)
  Septra®
  Septra® DS
  Sulfamethoprim®
  sulfamethoxazole
  Sulfatrim®
  Sulfatrim® DS
  sulfisoxazole
  Sulfizole® (Can)
  Trisulfa® (Can)
  Trisulfa-S® (Can)

Uroplus® DS
Uroplus® SS
Tetracycline Derivative
  Achromycin V (Can)
  Apo®-Doxy Tabs (Can)
  Apo®-Minocycline (Can)
  Apo®-Tetra (Can)
  Bio-Tab®
  Doryx®
  Doxy-200®
  Doxy-Caps®
  Doxychel®
  Doxycin (Can)
  doxycycline
  Doxy-Tabs®
  Doxytec (Can)
  Dynacin® Oral
  Minocin®
  Minocin® IV Injection
  minocycline
  Monodox®
  Nor-tet® Oral
  Novo-Doxylin (Can)
  Novo-Tetra (Can)
  Nu-Doxycycline (Can)
  Nu-Tetra (Can)
  oxytetracycline
  Panmycin® Oral
  Robitet® Oral
  Sumycin® Oral
  Syn-Minocycline (Can)
  Terramycin® I.M. Injection
  Terramycin® Oral
  Tetracap® Oral
  tetracycline
  Tetracyn (Can)
  Vectrin®
  Vibramycin®
  Vibra-Tabs®

PARACOCCIDIOIDO-MYCOSIS

Antifungal Agent

ketoconazole
Nizoral®
Novo-Ketoconazole (Can)
Nu-Ketocon (Can)

PEPTIC ULCER
Antibiotic, Miscellaneous
  Apo®-Metronidazole (Can)
  Flagyl® Oral
  Metro I.V.® Injection
  metronidazole
  Neo-Metric (Can)
  NidaGel (Can)
  Noritate (Can)
  Novo-Nidazol (Can)
  Protostat® Oral
  Trikacide (Can)
Anticholinergic Agent
  Anaspaz®
  Apo®-Chlorax (Can)
  A-Spas® S/L
  atropine
  Banthine®
  Barbidonna®
  belladonna
  Bellatal®
  Cantil®
  clidinium and chlordiazepoxide
  Clindex®
  Corium® (Can)
  Cystospaz®
  Cystospaz-M®
  Donnamar®
  Donnatal®
  ED-SPAZ®
  Gastrosed™
  glycopyrrolate
  hyoscyamine
  hyoscyamine, atropine, scopolamine,
    and phenobarbital
  Hyosophen®
  Levbid®
  Levsin®

Levsinex®
Levsin/SL®
Librax®
mepenzolate
methantheline
methscopolamine
Pamine®
Pathilon®
Pro-Banthine®
ProChlorax (Can)
Propanthel (Can)
propantheline
Robinul®
Robinul® Forte
Spasmolin®
tridihexethyl
Antidiarrheal
  bismuth subsalicylate, metronidazole,
    and tetracycline
  Helidac™
Gastric Acid Secretion Inhibitor
  lansoprazole
  Losec® (Can)
  omeprazole
  Prevacid®
  Prilosec™
Gastrointestinal Agent, Gastric or
    Duodenal Ulcer Treatment
  Carafate®
  Novo-Sucralate (Can)
  PMS-Sucralfate (Can)
  sucralfate
  Sulcrate®
Gastrointestinal Agent, Miscellaneous
  Bismatrol® [OTC]
  Bismed (Can)
  bismuth subsalicylate
  Bismylate (Can)
  Pepto-Bismol® [OTC]
Histamine H_2 Antagonist
  Apo®-Cimetidine (Can)
  Apo®-Famotidine (Can)
  Apo®-Nizatidine (Can)

Apo®-®anitidine (Can)
Axid®
Axid® AR [OTC]
cimetidine
famotidine
Gaviscon Prevent (Can)
Maalox H2 Acid Controller (Can)
nizatidine
Novo-Cimetine (Can)
Novo-Famotidine (Can)
Novo-Ranidine (Can)
Nu-Cimet (Can)
Nu-Famotidine (Can)
Nu-Ranit (Can)
Pepcid®
Pepcid® AC Acid Controller [OTC]
Pepcid RPD®
Peptol® (Can)
ranitidine hydrochloride
Tagamet®
Tagamet-HB® [OTC]
Zantac®
Zantac® 75 [OTC]
Macrolide (Antibiotic)
  Biaxin®
  Biaxin® XL
  clarithromycin
Penicillin
  amoxicillin
  Amoxil®
  Apo®-Amoxi (Can)
  Gen-Amoxicillin (Can)
  Novamoxin® (Can)
  Nu-Amoxi (Can)
  Pro-Amox® (Can)
  Trimox®
  Wymox®

PHARYNGITIS

Antibiotic, Penicillin
  pivampicillin (Canada only)
  Pondocillin® (Can)
Cephalosporin (First Generation)

Apo®-Cephalex (Can)
Biocef®
cefadroxil
Cefanex®
cephalexin
Ceporex (Can)
Duricef®
Keflex®
Keftab®
Novo-Lexin (Can)
Nu-Cephalex (Can)
Zartan®
Cephalosporin (Second Generation)
  cefpodoxime
  cefprozil
  Ceftin® Oral
  cefuroxime
  Cefzil®
  Kefurox® Injection
  Vantin®
  Zinacef® Injection
Cephalosporin (Third Generation)
  Cedax®
  ceftibuten
Macrolide (Antibiotic)
  AK-Mycin®
  Apo®-Erythro E-C (Can)
  azithromycin
  Diomycin (Can)
  E.E.S.®
  E-Mycin®
  E-Mycin-E®
  Erybid® (Can)
  Eryc®
  Ery-Tab®
  Erythro-Base® (Can)
  Erythrocin®
  erythromycin (systemic)
  Ilosone® Pulvules®
  Ilotycin®
  Novo-Rythro Encap (Can)
  PCE®
  PMS-Erythromycin (Can)

Wyamycin® S
Zithromax™
Penicillin
  amoxicillin
  Amoxil®
  ampicillin
  Ampicin (Can)
  Ampicin® Sodium (Can)
  Ampilean (Can)
  Apo®-Amoxi (Can)
  Apo®-Ampi (Can)
  Apo®-Pen VK (Can)
  Ayercillin® (Can)
  Bicillin® C-R
  Bicillin® C-R 900/300
  Bicillin® L-A
  Crysticillin® A.S.
  Gen-Amoxicillin (Can)
  Jaa Amp® (Can)
  Marcillin®
  Megacillin (Can)
  Nadopen-V® (Can)
  Novamoxin® (Can)
  Novo-Pen-VK® (Can)
  Nu-Amoxi (Can)
  Nu-Ampi (Can)
  Nu-Pen-VK (Can)
  Omnipen®
  Omnipen®-N
  penicillin G benzathine
  penicillin G benzathine and procaine
    combined
  penicillin G procaine
  penicillin V potassium
  Permapen®
  Principen®
  Pro-Amox® (Can)
  Totacillin®
  Trimox®
  Truxcillin®
  Veetids®
  Wycillin®
  Wymox®

Tetracycline Derivative
  Achromycin® Ophthalmic
  Achromycin® Topical
  Achromycin V (Can)
  Apo®-Doxy Tabs (Can)
  Apo®-Minocycline (Can)
  Apo®-Tetra (Can)
  Bio-Tab®
  Doryx®
  Doxy-200®
  Doxy-Caps®
  Doxychel®
  Doxycin (Can)
  doxycycline
  Doxy-Tabs®
  Doxytec (Can)
  Dynacin® Oral
  Minocin®
  Minocin® IV Injection
  minocycline
  Monodox®
  Nor-tet® Oral
  Novo-Doxylin (Can)
  Novo-Tetra (Can)
  Nu-Doxycycline (Can)
  Nu-Tetra (Can)
  oxytetracycline
  Panmycin® Oral
  Robitet® Oral
  Sumycin® Oral
  Syn-Minocycline (Can)
  Terramycin® I.M. Injection
  Terramycin® Oral
  Tetracap® Oral
  tetracycline
  Tetracyn (Can)
  Topicycline® Topical
  Vectrin®
  Vibramycin®
  Vibra-Tabs®

PINWORMS
Anthelmintic

Antiminth® [OTC]
Combantrin (Can)
Jaa Pyral® (Can)
mebendazole
Pin-®id® [OTC]
Pin-X® [OTC]
pyrantel pamoate
Reese's® Pinworm Medicine [OTC]
Vermox®

PLAGUE
Antibiotic, Aminoglycoside
  streptomycin

PNEUMOCYSTIS CARINII
Miscellaneous
  atovaquone
  Mepron™
  Neutrexin®
  NebuPent™ Inhalation
  Pentacarinat® Injection
  Pentam-300® Injection
  pentamidine
  Pneumopent (Can)
  Primsol®
  Proloprim®
  trimethoprim
  trimetrexate glucuronate
  Trimpex®
Sulfonamide
  Apo®-Sulfatrim (Can)
  Bactrim™
  Bactrim™ DS
  Cotrim®
  Cotrim® DS
  co-trimoxazole
  Novo-Trimel (Can)
  Nu-Cotrimox (Can)
  Protrin (Can)
  Roubac® (Can)
  Septra®
  Septra® DS
  Sulfamethoprim®
  Sulfatrim®

Sulfatrim® DS
Trisulfa® (Can)
Trisulfa-S® (Can)
Uroplus® DS
Uroplus® SS
Sulfone
  Avlosulfon®
  dapsone

PNEUMONIA
Aminoglycoside (Antibiotic)
  Alcomicin (Can)
  amikacin
  Amikin®
  Cidomycin (Can)
  Diogent (Can)
  Garamycin®
  Garatec (Can)
  Gentacidin®
  Gent-AK®
  gentamicin
  Gentrasul®
  G-myticin®
  Jenamicin®
  Nebcin® Injection
  netilmicin
  Netromycin®
  Ocugram (Can)
  PMS-Tobramycin (Can)
  RO-Gentycin (Can)
  TOBI™ Inhalation Solution
  tobramycin
Antibiotic, Miscellaneous
  Azactam®
  aztreonam
  Cleocin HCl® Oral
  Cleocin Pediatric® Oral
  Cleocin Phosphate® Injection
  clindamycin
  Dalacin® C (Can)
  Dalacin T (Can)
  Dalacin Vaginal (Can)
  Lyphocin® Injection

Vancocin® CP (Can)
Vancocin® Injection
Vancocin® Oral
Vancoled® Injection
vancomycin
Antibiotic, Penicillin
  pivampicillin (Canada only)
  Pondocillin® (Can)
Antibiotic, Quinolone
  gatifloxacin
  Levaquin™
  levofloxacin
  Tequin™
Carbapenem (Antibiotic)
  imipenem and cilastatin
  meropenem
  Merrem® I.V.
  Primaxin®
Cephalosporin (First Generation)
  Ancef®
  Apo®-Cephalex (Can)
  Biocef®
  cefadroxil
  Cefadyl®
  Cefanex®
  cefazolin
  cephalexin
  cephalothin
  cephapirin
  cephradine
  Ceporacin (Can)
  Ceporex (Can)
  Duricef®
  Keflex®
  Keflin (Can)
  Keftab®
  Kefzol®
  Novo-Lexin (Can)
  Nu-Cephalex (Can)
  Velosef®
  Zartan®
  Zolicef®
Cephalosporin (Second Generation)

Cefotan®
cefotetan
cefoxitin
cefpodoxime
cefprozil
Ceftin® Oral
cefuroxime
Cefzil®
Kefurox® Injection
Mefoxin®
Vantin®
Zinacef® Injection
Cephalosporin (Third Generation)
  cefdinir
  cefixime
  Cefizox®
  Cefobid®
  cefoperazone
  cefotaxime
  ceftazidime
  ceftizoxime
  ceftriaxone
  Ceptaz™
  Claforan®
  Fortaz®
  Omnicef®
  Rocephin®
  Suprax®
  Tazicef®
  Tazidime®
Cephalosporin (Fourth Generation)
  cefepime
  Maxipime®
Macrolide (Antibiotic)
  AK-Mycin®
  Apo®-Erythro E-C (Can)
  azithromycin
  Biaxin®
  Biaxin® XL
  clarithromycin
  Diomycin (Can)
  dirithromycin
  Dynabac®

E.E.S.®
E-Mycin®
E-Mycin-E®
Erybid® (Can)
Eryc®
Ery-Tab®
Erythro-Base® (Can)
Erythrocin®
erythromycin (systemic)
Ilosone® Pulvules®
Ilotycin®
Novo-Rythro Encap (Can)
PCE®
PMS-Erythromycin (Can)
Wyamycin® S
Zithromax™
Penicillin
  amoxicillin
  amoxicillin and clavulanate potassium
  Amoxil®
  ampicillin
  ampicillin and sulbactam
  Ampicin (Can)
  Ampicin® Sodium (Can)
  Ampilean (Can)
  Apo®-Amoxi (Can)
  Apo®-Ampi (Can)
  Apo®-Cloxi (Can)
  Apo®-Pen VK (Can)
  Augmentin®
  Ayercillin® (Can)
  bacampicillin
  Bactopen (Can)
  Bicillin® C-R
  Bicillin® C-R 900/300
  Bicillin® L-A
  carbenicillin
  Clavulin® (Can)
  cloxacillin
  Cloxapen®
  Crysticillin® A.S.
  dicloxacillin
  Dycill®

Dynapen®
Gen-Amoxicillin (Can)
Geocillin®
Geopen® (Can)
Jaa Amp® (Can)
Marcillin®
Megacillin (Can)
Mezlin®
mezlocillin
Nadopen-V® (Can)
nafcillin
Nallpen®
Novamoxin® (Can)
Novo-Cloxin (Can)
Novo-Pen-VK® (Can)
Nu-Amoxi (Can)
Nu-Ampi (Can)
Nu-Cloxi (Can)
Nu-Pen-VK (Can)
Omnipen®
Omnipen®-N
Orbenin® (Can)
oxacillin
Pathocil®
Penglobe (Can)
penicillin G benzathine
penicillin G benzathine and procaine
  combined
penicillin G (parenteral/aqueous)
penicillin G procaine
penicillin V potassium
Permapen®
Pfizerpen®
piperacillin
piperacillin and tazobactam sodium
Pipracil®
Principen®
Pro-Amox® (Can)
Pyopen (Can)
Spectrobid® Tablet
Taro-Cloxacillin® (Can)
Tazocin (Can)
Tegopen (Can)

Ticar®
ticarcillin
ticarcillin and clavulanate potassium
Timentin®
Totacillin®
Trimox®
Truxcillin®
Unasyn®
Unipen® (Can)
Veetids®
Wycillin®
Wymox®
Zosyn™
Quinolone
  Apo®-Oflox (Can)
  Cipro®
  ciprofloxacin
  Floxin®
  lomefloxacin
  Maxaquin®
  ofloxacin
  sparfloxacin
  Zagam®
Sulfonamide
  Apo®-Sulfatrim (Can)
  Bactrim™
  Bactrim™ DS
  Cotrim®
  Cotrim® DS
  co-trimoxazole
  Novo-Trimel (Can)
  Nu-Cotrimox (Can)
  Protrin (Can)
  Roubac® (Can)
  Septra®
  Septra® DS
  Sulfamethoprim®
  Sulfatrim®
  Sulfatrim® DS
  Trisulfa® (Can)
  Trisulfa-S® (Can)
  Uroplus® DS
  Uroplus® SS

PNEUMONIA, COMMUNITY-ACQUIRED
Antibiotic, Quinolone
  Avelox™
  moxifloxacin

POISON IVY
Protectant, Topical
  bentoquatam
  IvyBlock®

POISON OAK
Protectant, Topical
  bentoquatam
  IvyBlock®

POISON SUMAC
Protectant, Topical
  bentoquatam
  IvyBlock®

PROTOZOAL INFECTIONS
Antiprotozoal
  Apo®-Metronidazole (Can)
  Flagyl® Oral
  furazolidone
  Furoxone®
  Metrocream (Can)
  MetroGel® Topical
  MetroGel®-Vaginal
  Metro I.V.® Injection
  metronidazole
  NebuPent™ Inhalation
  Neo-Metric (Can)
  NidaGel (Can)
  Noritate (Can)
  Novo-Nidazol (Can)
  Pentacarinat® Injection
  Pentam-300® Injection
  pentamidine
  Pneumopent (Can)
  Protostat® Oral
  Trikacide (Can)

PULMONARY TUBERCULOSIS
Antitubercular Agent
  Priftin®
  rifapentine

PYELONEPHRITIS
Antibiotic, Quinolone
  gatifloxacin
  Tequin™

RABIES
Serum
  antirabies serum (equine)

RAT-BITE FEVER
Antibiotic, Aminoglycoside
  streptomycin

RATTLESNAKE BITE
Antivenin
  antivenin (Crotalidae) polyvalent

RESPIRATORY DISORDERS
Adrenal Corticosteroid
  Acthar®
  Actharn (Can)
  Adlone® Injection
  Ak-Tate (Can)
  Amcort® Injection
  A-methaPred® Injection
  Apo®-Prednisone (Can)
  Aristocort® Forte Injection
  Aristocort® Intralesional Injection
  Aristocort® Oral
  Aristospan® Intra-articular Injection
  Aristospan® Intralesional Injection
  Atolone® Oral
  Azmacort™ Oral Inhaler
  Balpred (Can)
  betamethasone (systemic)
  Celestone® Oral
  Celestone® Phosphate Injection
  Celestone® Soluspan®

Cel-U-Jec® Injection
Cortef®
corticotropin
cortisone acetate
Cortone® Acetate
Decadron® Injection
Decadron®-LA
Decadron® Oral
Decaject®
Decaject-LA®
Delta-Cortef® Oral
Deltasone®
depMedalone® Injection
Depoject® Injection
Depo-Medrol® Injection
Depopred® Injection
Dexacort® Phosphate in Respihaler®
dexamethasone (oral inhalation)
dexamethasone (systemic)
Dexasone®
Dexasone® L.A.
Dexone®
Dexone® LA
Diopred (Can)
D-Med® Injection
Duralone® Injection
Haldrone®
Hexadrol®
H.P. Acthar® Gel
hydrocortisone (systemic)
Hydrocortone® Acetate
Inflamase (Can)
Jaa-Prednisone® (Can)
Kenacort® Oral
Kenaject® Injection
Kenalog® Injection
Key-Pred® Injection
Key-Pred-SP® Injection
Liquid Pred®
Medralone® Injection
Medrol® Oral
Medrol Veriderm (Can)
methylprednisolone

Meticorten®
M-Prednisol® Injection
Novo-Prednisolone (Can)
Orasone®
paramethasone acetate
Pediapred® Oral
PMS-Dexamethasone (Can)
Prednicen-M®
prednisolone (systemic)
Prednisol® TBA Injection
prednisone
Prelone® Oral
RO-Predphate (Can)
Scheinpharm Triamcine-A (Can)
Solu-Cortef®
Solu-Medrol® Injection
Solurex L.A.®
Stemex®
Tac™-3 Injection
Tac™-40 Injection
Triam-A® Injection
triamcinolone (inhalation, oral)
triamcinolone (systemic)
Triam Forte® Injection
Triamonide® Injection
Tri-Kort® Injection
Trilog® Injection
Trilone® Injection
Trisoject® Injection
Ultracortenol (Can)
Winpred (Can)

RESPIRATORY SYNCYTIAL VIRUS (RSV)

Monoclonal Antibody
palivizumab
Synagis®

RESPIRATORY TRACT INFECTION

Aminoglycoside (Antibiotic)
AKTob® Ophthalmic
Alcomicin (Can)

Cidomycin (Can)
Diogent (Can)
Garamycin®
Garatec (Can)
Genoptic®
Gentacidin®
Gent-AK®
gentamicin
Gentrasul®
G-myticin®
Jenamicin®
Nebcin® Injection
netilmicin
Netromycin®
Ocugram (Can)
PMS-Tobramycin (Can)
RO-Gentycin (Can)
TOBI™ Inhalation Solution
tobramycin
Tobrex® Ophthalmic
Tomycine™ Ophthalmic (Can)
Antibiotic, Carbacephem
Lorabid™
loracarbef
Antibiotic, Macrolide
Rovamycine® (Can)
spiramycin (Canada only)
Antibiotic, Miscellaneous
Azactam®
aztreonam
Cleocin HCl® Oral
Cleocin Pediatric® Oral
Cleocin Phosphate® Injection
Cleocin T® Topical
Cleocin® Vaginal
Clinda-Derm® Topical
clindamycin
Dalacin® C (Can)
Dalacin T (Can)
Dalacin Vaginal (Can)
Antibiotic, Penicillin
pivampicillin (Canada only)
Pondocillin® (Can)

Antibiotic, Quinolone
  gatifloxacin
  Levaquin™
  levofloxacin
  Quixin™ Ophthalmic
  Tequin™
Cephalosporin (First Generation)
  Ancef®
  Apo®-Cephalex (Can)
  Biocef®
  cefadroxil
  Cefadyl®
  Cefanex®
  cefazolin
  cephalexin
  cephalothin
  cephapirin
  cephradine
  Ceporacin (Can)
  Ceporex (Can)
  Duricef®
  Keflex®
  Keflin (Can)
  Keftab®
  Kefzol®
  Novo-Lexin (Can)
  Nu-Cephalex (Can)
  Velosef®
  Zartan®
  Zolicef®
Cephalosporin (Second Generation)
  Apo®-Cefaclor (Can)
  Ceclor®
  Ceclor® CD
  cefaclor
  cefamandole
  cefmetazole
  cefonicid
  Cefotan®
  cefotetan
  cefoxitin
  cefpodoxime
  cefprozil

Ceftin® Oral
cefuroxime
Cefzil®
Kefurox® Injection
Mandol®
Mefoxin®
Monocid®
Novo-Cefaclor (Can)
Vantin®
Zefazone®
Zinacef® Injection
Cephalosporin (Third Generation)
  Cedax®
  cefixime
  Cefizox®
  Cefobid®
  cefoperazone
  cefotaxime
  ceftazidime
  ceftibuten
  ceftizoxime
  ceftriaxone
  Ceptaz™
  Claforan®
  Fortaz®
  Rocephin®
  Suprax®
  Tazicef®
  Tazidime®
Cephalosporin (Fourth Generation)
  cefepime
  Maxipime®
Macrolide (Antibiotic)
  AK-Mycin®
  Apo®-Erythro E-C (Can)
  azithromycin
  Biaxin®
  Biaxin® XL
  clarithromycin
  Diomycin (Can)
  dirithromycin
  Dynabac®
  E.E.S.®

E-Mycin®
E-Mycin-E®
Erybid® (Can)
Eryc®
Ery-Tab®
Erythro-Base® (Can)
Erythrocin®
erythromycin and sulfisoxazole
erythromycin (systemic)
Eryzole®
Ilosone® Pulvules®
Ilotycin®
Novo-®ythro Encap (Can)
PCE®
Pediazole®
PMS-Erythromycin (Can)
Wyamycin® S
Zithromax™
Penicillin
  amoxicillin
  amoxicillin and clavulanate
    potassium
  Amoxil®
  ampicillin
  ampicillin and sulbactam
  Ampicin (Can)
  Ampicin® Sodium (Can)
  Ampilean (Can)
  Apo®-Amoxi (Can)
  Apo®-Ampi (Can)
  Apo®-Cloxi (Can)
  Apo®-Pen VK (Can)
  Augmentin®
  Ayercillin® (Can)
  bacampicillin
  Bactopen (Can)
  Bicillin® C-R
  Bicillin® C-R 900/300
  Bicillin® L-A
  carbenicillin
  Clavulin® (Can)
  cloxacillin
  Cloxapen®

Crysticillin® A.S.
dicloxacillin
Dycill®
Dynapen®
Gen-Amoxicillin (Can)
Geocillin®
Geopen® (Can)
Jaa Amp® (Can)
Marcillin®
Megacillin (Can)
Mezlin®
mezlocillin
Nadopen-V® (Can)
nafcillin
Nallpen®
Novamoxin® (Can)
Novo-Cloxin (Can)
Novo-Pen-VK® (Can)
Nu-Amoxi (Can)
Nu-Ampi (Can)
Nu-Cloxi (Can)
Nu-Pen-VK (Can)
Omnipen®
Omnipen®-N
Orbenin® (Can)
oxacillin
Pathocil®
Pcnglobe (Can)
penicillin G benzathine
penicillin G benzathine and procaine
  combined
penicillin G (parenteral/aqueous)
penicillin G procaine
penicillin V potassium
Permapen®
Pfizerpen®
piperacillin
piperacillin and tazobactam sodium
Pipracil®
Principen®
Pro-Amox® (Can)
Pyopen (Can)
Spectrobid® Tablet

Taro-Cloxacillin® (Can)
Tazocin (Can)
Tegopen (Can)
Ticar®
ticarcillin
ticarcillin and clavulanate potassium
Timentin®
Totacillin®
Trimox®
Truxcillin®
Unasyn®
Unipen® (Can)
Veetids®
Wycillin®
Wymox®
Zosyn™
Quinolone
  Apo®-Oflox (Can)
  Ciloxan™ Ophthalmic
  Cipro®
  ciprofloxacin
  Floxin®
  lomefloxacin
  Maxaquin®
  Ocuflox™ Ophthalmic
  ofloxacin
  sparfloxacin
  Zagam®
Sulfonamide
  erythromycin and sulfisoxazole
  Eryzole®
  Pediazole®

RHEUMATIC FEVER
Nonsteroidal Anti-inflammatory Drug
  (NSAID)
  Argesic®-SA
  Artha-G®
  Arthropan® [OTC]
  Back-Ese M (Can)
  choline magnesium trisalicylate
  choline salicylate
  Disalcid®

Doan's Backache Pills (Can)
Doan's®, Original [OTC]
Extra Strength Doan's® [OTC]
Herbogesic (Can)
Magan®
magnesium salicylate
Magsal®
Marthritic®
Mobidin®
Mono-Gesic®
Salflex®
Salgesic®
salsalate
Salsitab®
Teejel (Can)
Trilisate®
Penicillin
  Bicillin® C-R
  Bicillin® C-R 900/300
  penicillin G benzathine and procaine
    combined

ROUNDWORMS
Anthelmintic
  Antiminth® [OTC]
  Combantrin (Can)
  Jaa Pyral® (Can)
  mebendazole
  Pin-®id® [OTC]
  Pin-X® [OTC]
  pyrantel pamoate
  Reese's® Pinworm Medicine [OTC]
  Vermox®

SCABIES
Scabicides/Pediculicides
  A-200™ Shampoo [OTC]
  Acticin® Cream
  Barc™ Liquid [OTC]
  crotamiton
  Elimite™ Cream
  End Lice® Liquid [OTC]
  Eurax® Topical
  GBH (Can)

G-well®
Hexit® (Can)
Kwellada® (Can)
Lice-Enz® Shampoo [OTC]
lindane
Nix™ Creme Rinse
permethrin
PMS-Lindane (Can)
Pronto® Shampoo [OTC]
pyrethrins and piperonyl butoxide
Pyrinex® Pediculicide Shampoo
    [OTC]
Pyrinyl II® Liquid [OTC]
Pyrinyl Plus® Shampoo [OTC]
R & C® Shampoo [OTC]
RID® Mousse [OTC]
RID® Shampoo [OTC]
Tisit® Blue Gel [OTC]
Tisit® Liquid [OTC]
Tisit® Shampoo [OTC]
Triple X® Liquid [OTC]

SINUSITIS
Adrenergic Agonist Agent
    Actifed® Allergy Tablet (Day) [OTC]
    Afrinol® [OTC]
    Balminil® Decongestant (Can)
    Benylin Decongestant (Can)
    Cenafed® [OTC]
    Children's Silfedrine® [OTC]
    Congestac ND (Can)
    Congest Aid (Can)
    Congest-Eze (Can)
    Contac Cold Nondrowsy (Can)
    Decofed® Syrup [OTC]
    Decongestant Tablets (Can)
    Drixoral® Non-Drowsy [OTC]
    Durafedrin (Can)
    Efidac/24® [OTC]
    Eltor® (Can)
    Maxenal (Can)
    Nasal & Sinus Relief (Can)
    Neofed® [OTC]

Ornex Cold (Can)
Otrivin (Can)
PediaCare® Oral
Plus Sinus™ (Can)
PMS-Pseudoephedrine (Can)
pseudoephedrine
Pseudofrin (Can)
Robidrine® (Can)
Sudafed® [OTC]
Sudafed® 12 Hour [OTC]
Sudodrin (Can)
Sufedrin® [OTC]
Tantafed (Can)
Triaminic® AM Decongestant
    Formula [OTC]
Aminoglycoside (Antibiotic)
    Alcomicin (Can)
    Cidomycin (Can)
    Diogent (Can)
    Garamycin®
    Garatec (Can)
    Genoptic®
    Gentacidin®
    Gent-AK®
    gentamicin
    Gentrasul®
    G-myticin®
    Jenamicin®
    Ocugram (Can)
    RO-Gentycin (Can)
Antibiotic, Miscellaneous
    Cleocin HCl® Oral
    Cleocin Pediatric® Oral
    Cleocin Phosphate® Injection
    Cleocin T® Topical
    Cleocin® Vaginal
    Clinda-Derm® Topical
    clindamycin
    Dalacin® C (Can)
    Dalacin T (Can)
    Dalacin Vaginal (Can)
Antibiotic, Penicillin
    pivampicillin (Canada only)

Pondocillin® (Can)
Antibiotic, Quinolone
   Avelox™
   gatifloxacin
   Levaquin™
   levofloxacin
   moxifloxacin
   Quixin™ Ophthalmic
   Tequin™
Antihistamine/Decongestant/Analgesic
   phenyltoloxamine,
      phenylpropanolamine, and
      acetaminophen
   Sinubid®
   Sinutab® SA (Can)
Antihistamine/Decongestant
   Combination
   Actifed® Allergy Tablet (Night)
      [OTC]
   Banophen® Decongestant Capsule
      [OTC]
   Benadryl® Decongestant Allergy
      Tablet [OTC]
   Benylin® for Allergies (Can)
   diphenhydramine and
      pseudoephedrine
Cephalosporin (First Generation)
   Apo®-Cephalex (Can)
   Biocef®
   cefadroxil
   Cefanex®
   cephalexin
   cephradine
   Ceporex (Can)
   Duricef®
   Keflex®
   Keftab®
   Novo-Lexin (Can)
   Nu-Cephalex (Can)
   Velosef®
   Zartan®
Cephalosporin (Second Generation)
   Apo®-Cefaclor (Can)

Ceclor®
Ceclor® CD
cefaclor
cefpodoxime
cefprozil
Ceftin® Oral
cefuroxime
Cefzil®
Kefurox® Injection
Novo-Cefaclor (Can)
Vantin®
Zinacef® Injection
Cephalosporin (Third Generation)
   Cedax®
   cefdinir
   cefixime
   ceftibuten
   Omnicef®
   Suprax®
Cold Preparation
   Anatuss® DM [OTC]
   Calmylin #3 (Can)
   Cough Syrup DM-D-E (Can)
   Cough Syrup DM Decongestant
      Expectorant (Can)
   Deconsal® Sprinkle®
   Dimacol® Caplets [OTC]
   DM Plus Decongestant Expectorant
      (Can)
   Endal®
   guaifenesin and phenylephrine
   guaifenesin, pseudoephedrine, and
      dextromethorphan
   Maxifed® DM
   Novahistex DM Expectorant (Can)
   Novahistine DM Expectorant (Can)
   Rhinosyn-X® Liquid [OTC]
   Robitussin Cough & Cold (Can)
   Ru-Tuss® Expectorant [OTC]
   Sinupan®
   Sudafed® Cold & Cough Liquid Caps
      [OTC]
Decongestant/Analgesic

Advil® Cold & Sinus Caplets [OTC]
Dayquil Sinus with Pain Relief (Can)
Dimetapp® Sinus Caplets [OTC]
Dristan® Sinus Caplets [OTC]
Motrin® IB Sinus [OTC]
pseudoephedrine and ibuprofen
Sine-Aid® IB [OTC]
Expectorant/Decongestant
Ami-Tex LA®
Coldlac-LA®
Coldloc®
Conex® [OTC]
Congess® Jr
Congess® Sr
Congestac®
Contac Head & Chest Congestion
    (Can)
Contuss®
Contuss® XT
Deconsal® II
Defen®-LA
Dura Gest®
Dura-Vent®
Enomine®
Entex®
Entex® LA
Entex® PSE
Eudal-SR®
Fedahist® Expectorant [OTC]
Fedahist® Expectorant Pediatric
    [OTC]
Genagesic®
Genamin® Expectorant [OTC]
Glycofed®
Guaifed® [OTC]
Guaifed-PD®
guaifenesin and
    phenylpropanolamine
guaifenesin and pseudoephedrine
guaifenesin, phenylpropanolamine,
    and phenylephrine
Guaifenex®
Guaifenex® PPA 75

Guaifenex® PSE
GuaiMAX-D®
Guaipax®
Guaitab®
Guaivent®
Guai-Vent/PSE®
Guiatex®
Guiatuss PE® [OTC]
Halotussin® PE [OTC]
Maxifed®
Maxifed-G®
Myminic® Expectorant [OTC]
Naldecon-EX® Children's Syrup
    [OTC]
Nasabid™
Nolex® LA
Novahistex Expectorant (Can)
Partuss® LA
Phenylfenesin® L.A.
Profen II®
Profen LA®
Respa-1st®
Respaire®-60 SR
Respaire®-120 SR
Robitussin-PE® [OTC]
Robitussin® Severe Congestion
    Liqui-Gels [OTC]
Ru-Tuss® DE
Rymed®
Rymed-TR®
Silaminic® Expectorant [OTC]
Sildicon-E® [OTC]
Sinufed® Timecelles®
Snaplets-EX® [OTC]
Sudafed Expectorant (Can)
Touro LA®
Triaminic Decongestant &
    Expectorant (Can)
Triaminic® Expectorant [OTC]
Tri-Clear® Expectorant [OTC]
Triphenyl® Expectorant [OTC]
Tuss-LA®
ULR-LA®

V-Dec-M®
Versacaps®
Vicks® DayQuil® Sinus Pressure &
  Congestion Relief [OTC]
Zephrex®
Zephrex LA®
Macrolide (Antibiotic)
  AK-Mycin®
  Apo®-Erythro E-C (Can)
  Biaxin®
  Biaxin® XL
  clarithromycin
  Diomycin (Can)
  dirithromycin
  Dynabac®
  E.E.S.®
  E-Mycin®
  E-Mycin-E®
  Erybid® (Can)
  Eryc®
  Ery-Tab®
  Erythro-Base® (Can)
  Erythrocin®
  erythromycin (systemic)
  Ilosone® Pulvules®
  Ilotycin®
  Novo-Rythro Encap (Can)
  PCE®
  PMS-Erythromycin (Can)
  Wyamycin® S
Penicillin
  amoxicillin
  amoxicillin and clavulanate
    potassium
  Amoxil®
  ampicillin
  Ampicin (Can)
  Ampicin® Sodium (Can)
  Ampilean (Can)
  Apo®-Amoxi (Can)
  Apo®-Ampi (Can)
  Apo®-Cloxi (Can)
  Augmentin®

Bactopen (Can)
Clavulin® (Can)
cloxacillin
Cloxapen®
Gen-Amoxicillin (Can)
Jaa Amp® (Can)
Marcillin®
nafcillin
Nallpen®
Novamoxin® (Can)
Novo-Cloxin (Can)
Nu-Amoxi (Can)
Nu-Ampi (Can)
Nu-Cloxi (Can)
Omnipen®
Omnipen®-N
Orbenin® (Can)
oxacillin
Principen®
Pro-Amox® (Can)
Taro-Cloxacillin® (Can)
Tegopen (Can)
Totacillin®
Trimox®
Unipen® (Can)
Wymox®
Quinolone
  Apo®-Oflox (Can)
  Ciloxan™ Ophthalmic
  Cipro®
  ciprofloxacin
  Floxin®
  lomefloxacin
  Maxaquin®
  Ocuflox™ Ophthalmic
  ofloxacin
  sparfloxacin
  Zagam®
Sulfonamide
  Apo®-Sulfatrim (Can)
  Bactrim™
  Bactrim™ DS
  Cotrim®

Cotrim® DS
co-trimoxazole
Novo-Trimel (Can)
Nu-Cotrimox (Can)
Protrin (Can)
Roubac® (Can)
Septra®
Septra® DS
Sulfamethoprim®
Sulfatrim®
Sulfatrim® DS
Trisulfa® (Can)
Trisulfa-S® (Can)
Uroplus® DS
Uroplus® SS
Tetracycline Derivative
  Achromycin V (Can)
  Apo®-Doxy Tabs (Can)
  Apo®-Minocycline (Can)
  Apo®-Tetra (Can)
  Bio Tab®
  Doryx®
  Doxy-200™
  Doxy-Caps®
  Doxychel®
  Doxycin (Can)
  doxycycline
  Doxy-Tabs®
  Doxytec (Can)
  Dynacin® Oral
  Minocin®
  Minocin® IV Injection
  minocycline
  Monodox®
  Nor-tet® Oral
  Novo-Doxylin (Can)
  Novo-Tetra (Can)
  Nu-Doxycycline (Can)
  Nu-Tetra (Can)
  oxytetracycline
  Panmycin® Oral
  Robitet® Oral
  Sumycin® Oral

Syn-Minocycline (Can)
Terramycin® I.M. Injection
Terramycin® Oral
Tetracap® Oral
tetracycline
Tetracyn (Can)
Topicycline® Topical
Vectrin®
Vibramycin®
Vibra-Tabs®

SOFT TISSUE INFECTION
Aminoglycoside (Antibiotic)
  AKTob® Ophthalmic
  Alcomicin (Can)
  amikacin
  Amikin®
  Cidomycin (Can)
  Diogent (Can)
  Garamycin®
  Garatec (Can)
  Genoptic®
  Gentacidin®
  Gent-AK®
  gentamicin
  Gentrasul®
  G-myticin®
  Jenamicin®
  Nebcin® Injection
  netilmicin
  Netromycin®
  Ocugram (Can)
  PMS-Tobramycin (Can)
  RO-Gentycin (Can)
  tobramycin
Antibiotic, Carbacephem
  Lorabid™
  loracarbef
Antibiotic, Miscellaneous
  Cleocin HCl® Oral
  Cleocin Pediatric® Oral
  Cleocin Phosphate® Injection
  Cleocin T® Topical

Cleocin® Vaginal
Clinda-Derm® Topical
clindamycin
Dalacin® C (Can)
Dalacin T (Can)
Dalacin Vaginal (Can)
Lyphocin® Injection
Vancocin® CP (Can)
Vancocin® Injection
Vancocin® Oral
Vancoled® Injection
vancomycin
Antibiotic, Penicillin
  pivampicillin (Canada only)
  Pondocillin® (Can)
Antibiotic, Quinolone
  Levaquin™
  levofloxacin
  Quixin™ Ophthalmic
Antifungal Agent, Systemic
  Fucidin® I.V. (Can)
  Fucidin® Oral Suspension (Can)
  Fucidin® Tablet (Can)
  fusidic acid (Canada only)
Cephalosporin (First Generation)
  Ancef®
  Apo®-Cephalex (Can)
  Biocef®
  cefadroxil
  Cefadyl®
  Cefanex®
  cefazolin
  cephalexin
  cephalothin
  cephapirin
  cephradine
  Ceporacin (Can)
  Ceporex (Can)
  Duricef®
  Keflex®
  Keflin (Can)
  Keftab®
  Kefzol®

Novo-Lexin (Can)
Nu-Cephalex (Can)
Velosef®
Zartan®
Zolicef®
Cephalosporin (Second Generation)
  Apo®-Cefaclor (Can)
  Ceclor®
  Ceclor® CD
  cefaclor
  cefamandole
  cefmetazole
  cefonicid
  Cefotan®
  cefotetan
  cefoxitin
  cefpodoxime
  cefprozil
  Ceftin® Oral
  cefuroxime
  Cefzil®
  Kefurox® Injection
  Mandol®
  Mefoxin®
  Monocid®
  Novo-Cefaclor (Can)
  Vantin®
  Zefazone®
  Zinacef® Injection
Cephalosporin (Third Generation)
  Cedax®
  cefixime
  Cefizox®
  Cefobid®
  cefoperazone
  cefotaxime
  ceftazidime
  ceftibuten
  ceftizoxime
  ceftriaxone
  Ceptaz™
  Claforan®
  Fortaz®

Rocephin®
Suprax®
Tazicef®
Tazidime®
Cephalosporin (Fourth Generation)
  cefepime
  Maxipime®
Macrolide (Antibiotic)
  azithromycin
  dirithromycin
  Dynabac®
  Zithromax™
Penicillin
  amoxicillin
  amoxicillin and clavulanate
    potassium
  Amoxil®
  ampicillin
  ampicillin and sulbactam
  Ampicin (Can)
  Ampicin® Sodium (Can)
  Ampilean (Can)
  Apo®-Amoxi (Can)
  Apo®-Ampi (Can)
  Apo®-Cloxi (Can)
  Apo®-Pen VK (Can)
  Augmentin®
  Ayercillin® (Can)
  bacampicillin
  Bactopen (Can)
  Bicillin® C-R
  Bicillin® C-R 900/300
  Bicillin® L-A
  carbenicillin
  Clavulin® (Can)
  cloxacillin
  Cloxapen®
  Crysticillin® A.S.
  dicloxacillin
  Dycill®
  Dynapen®
  Gen-Amoxicillin (Can)
  Geocillin®

Geopen® (Can)
Jaa Amp® (Can)
Marcillin®
Megacillin (Can)
Mezlin®
mezlocillin
Nadopen-V® (Can)
nafcillin
Nallpen®
Novamoxin® (Can)
Novo-Cloxin (Can)
Novo-Pen-VK® (Can)
Nu-Amoxi (Can)
Nu-Ampi (Can)
Nu-Cloxi (Can)
Nu-Pen-VK (Can)
Omnipen®
Omnipen®-N
Orbenin® (Can)
oxacillin
Pathocil®
Penglobe (Can)
penicillin G benzathine
penicillin G benzathine and procaine
  combined
penicillin G (parenteral/aqueous)
penicillin G procaine
penicillin V potassium
Permapen®
Pfizerpen®
piperacillin
piperacillin and tazobactam sodium
Pipracil®
Principen®
Pro-Amox® (Can)
Pyopen (Can)
Spectrobid® Tablet
Taro-Cloxacillin® (Can)
Tazocin (Can)
Tegopen (Can)
Ticar®
ticarcillin
ticarcillin and clavulanate potassium

Timentin®
Totacillin®
Trimox®
Truxcillin®
Unasyn®
Unipen® (Can)
Veetids®
Wycillin®
Wymox®
Zosyn™
Quinolone
  Apo®-Oflox (Can)
  Cipro®
  ciprofloxacin
  Floxin®
  lomefloxacin
  Maxaquin®
  ofloxacin

SYPHILIS

Antibiotic, Miscellaneous
  chloramphenicol
  Chloromycetin® Injection
  Diochloram (Can)
  Fenicol (Can)
  Novo-Chlorocap (Can)
  Ophtho-Chloram (Can)
  Pentamycetin® (Can)
  Sopamycetin (Can)
  Spersanicol (Can)
Penicillin
  Ayercillin® (Can)
  Bicillin® L-A
  Crysticillin® A.S.
  Megacillin (Can)
  penicillin G benzathine
  penicillin G (parenteral/aqueous)
  penicillin G procaine
  Permapen®
  Pfizerpen®
  Wycillin®
Tetracycline Derivative
  Achromycin® Ophthalmic

Achromycin® Topical
Achromycin V (Can)
Apo®-Doxy Tabs (Can)
Apo®-Tetra (Can)
Bio-Tab®
Doryx®
Doxy-200®
Doxy-Caps®
Doxychel®
Doxycin (Can)
doxycycline
Doxy-Tabs®
Doxytec (Can)
Monodox®
Nor-tet® Oral
Novo-Doxylin (Can)
Novo-Tetra (Can)
Nu-Doxycycline (Can)
Nu-Tetra (Can)
Panmycin® Oral
Robitet® Oral
Sumycin® Oral
Tetracap® Oral
tetracycline
Tetracyn (Can)
Topicycline® Topical
Vibramycin®
Vibra-Tabs®

TAPEWORM INFESTATION
Amebicide
  Humatin®
  paromomycin
Anthelmintic
  Biltricide®
  praziquantel

TETANUS
Antibiotic, Miscellaneous
  Apo®-Metronidazole (Can)
  Flagyl® Oral
  Metro I.V.® Injection
  metronidazole
  Neo-Metric (Can)

NidaGel (Can)
Noritate (Can)
Novo-Nidazol (Can)
Protostat® Oral
Trikacide (Can)
Immune Globulin
  tetanus immune globulin (human)

TETANUS (PROPHYLAXIS)
Antitoxin
  tetanus antitoxin

THREADWORM (NONDISSEMINATED INTESTINAL)
Antibiotic, Miscellaneous
  ivermectin
  Stromectol®

TINEA
Antifungal Agent
  Absorbine® Antifungal [OTC]
  Absorbine® Antifungal Foot Powder [OTC]
  Absorbine® Jock Itch [OTC]
  Absorbine Jr.® Antifungal [OTC]
  Aftate® [OTC]
  benzoic acid and salicylic acid
  Breezee® Mist Antifungal [OTC]
  butenafine
  Caldesene® Topical [OTC]
  Canesten (Can)
  carbol-fuchsin solution
  ciclopirox
  clioquinol
  Clotrimaderm (Can)
  clotrimazole
  Cruex (Can)
  Desenex® [OTC]
  econazole
  Ecostatin® (Can)
  Exelderm® Topical
  Femizol-M® [OTC]
  Fulvicin (Can)

Fulvicin® P/G
Fulvicin-U/F®
Fungoid® AF Topical Solution [OTC]
Fungoid® Creme
Fungoid® Solution
Fungoid® Tincture
Genaspor® [OTC]
Grifulvin® V
Grisactin®
Grisactin® Ultra
griseofulvin
Grisovin®-FP (Can)
Gris-PEG®
Gyne-Lotrimin® [OTC]
Gyne-Lotrimin® 3 [OTC]
haloprogin
Halotex®
ketoconazole
Lamisil® Cream
Loprox®
Lotrimin®
Lotrimin® AF Cream [OTC]
Lotrimin® AF Lotion [OTC]
Lotrimin® AF Powder [OTC]
Lotrimin® AF Solution [OTC]
Lotrimin® AF Spray Liquid [OTC]
Lotrimin® AF Spray Powder [OTC]
Maximum Strength Desenex® Antifungal Cream [OTC]
Mentax®
Micatin® Topical [OTC]
miconazole
Mitrazol® [OTC]
Monazole-7® (Can)
Monistat-Derm™ Topical
Monistat i.v.™ Injection
Monistat™ Vaginal
Mycelex®
Mycelex®-7
Mycelex®-G
Myclo-Derm (Can)
Myclo-Gyne (Can)

M-Zole® 7 Dual Pack [OTC]
naftifine
Naftin®
Neo-Zol (Can)
Nizoral®
Nizoral® A-D Shampoo [OTC]
Novo-Ketoconazole (Can)
NP-27® [OTC]
Nu-Ketocon (Can)
Ony-Clear® Nail
Ony-Clear® Spray
oxiconazole
Oxistat® Topical
Pedi-Pro Topical [OTC]
Pitrex (Can)
Prescription Strength Desenex®
    [OTC]
Scholl Athlete's Foot Preparations
    (Can)
sodium thiosulfate
Spectazole™
sulconazole
terbinafine (topical)
Tinactin® [OTC]
Tinver® [OTC]
tolnaftate
triacetin
Tritin (Can)
Trivagizole 3™ [OTC]
undecylenic acid and derivatives
Versiclear™
Vioform® [OTC]
Whitfield's Ointment [OTC]
Zeasorb-AF® [OTC]
Zeasorb-AF® Powder [OTC]
Antifungal/Corticosteroid
  betamethasone and clotrimazole
  Lotriderm® (Can)
  Lotrisone®
Antiseborrheic Agent, Topical
  Exsel® Shampoo
  selenium sulfide

Selsun Blue® Shampoo [OTC]
Selsun® Shampoo
Versel (Can)
Disinfectant
  sodium hypochlorite solution

TOXOPLASMOSIS
Antibiotic, Miscellaneous
  Cleocin HCl® Oral
  Cleocin Pediatric® Oral
  Cleocin Phosphate® Injection
  Cleocin® Vaginal
  clindamycin
Folic Acid Antagonist (Antimalarial)
  Daraprim®
  pyrimethamine
Sulfonamide
  Coptin® (Can)
  SSD (Can)
  sulfadiazine

TUBERCULOSIS
Antibiotic, Aminoglycoside
  streptomycin
Antibiotic, Miscellaneous
  Capastat® Sulfate
  capreomycin
  cycloserine
  Rifadin® Injection
  Rifadin® Oral
  Rifamate®
  rifampin
  rifampin and isoniazid
  rifampin, isoniazid, and
      pyrazinamide
  Rifater®
  Rimactane® Oral
  Rofact® (Can)
  Seromycin® Pulvules®
Antimycobacterial Agent
  ethambutol
  ethionamide
  Etibi® (Can)

Myambutol®
Trecator®-SC
Antitubercular Agent
  isoniazid
  Isotamine (Can)
  Laniazid® Syrup
  PMS-Isoniazid (Can)
  PMS-Pyrazinamide (Can)
  pyrazinamide
  streptomycin
  Tebrazid (Can)
Biological Response Modulator
  BCG vaccine
  ImmuCyst (Can)
  OncoTICE (Can)
  Pacis (Can)
  TheraCys®
  TICE® BCG
Nonsteroidal Anti-inflammatory Drug
  (NSAID)
  aminosalicylate sodium
  Nemasol (Can)
  Tubasal® (Can)

TUBERCULOSIS (DIAGNOSTIC)

Diagnostic Agent
  Aplisol®
  Aplitest®
  Tine Test PPD
  tuberculin tests
  Tubersol®

TULAREMIA

Antibiotic, Aminoglycoside
  streptomycin

URINARY TRACT INFECTION

Antibiotic, Carbacephem
  Lorabid™
  loracarbef
Antibiotic, Miscellaneous

Apo®-Nitrofurantoin (Can)
Azactam®
aztreonam
Dehydral® (Can)
fosfomycin
Furadantin®
Furalan®
Furan®
Furanite®
Hiprex®
Lyphocin® Injection
Macrobid®
Macrodantin®
Mandelamine®
methenamine
Monurol™
Nephronex® (Can)
nitrofurantoin
Novo-Furan (Can)
Primsol®
Proloprim®
trimethoprim
Trimpex®
Urasal® (Can)
Urex®
Vancocin® CP (Can)
Vancocin® Injection
Vancocin® Oral
Vancoled® Injection
vancomycin
Antibiotic, Penicillin
  pivampicillin (Canada only)
  Pondocillin® (Can)
Antibiotic, Quinolone
  gatifloxacin
  Levaquin™
  levofloxacin
  Quixin™ Ophthalmic
  Tequin™
Antibiotic, Urinary Anti-infective
  Atrosept®
  Dolsed®

methenamine, phenyl salicylate,
   atropine, hyoscyamine, benzoic
   acid, and methylene blue
UAA®
Uridon Modified®
Urised®
Uritin®
Cephalosporin (First Generation)
   Ancef®
   Apo®-Cephalex (Can)
   Biocef®
   cefadroxil
   Cefadyl®
   Cefanex®
   cefazolin
   cephalexin
   cephalothin
   cephapirin
   cephradine
   Ceporacin (Can)
   Ceporex (Can)
   Duricef®
   Keflex®
   Keflin (Can)
   Keftab®
   Kefzol®
   Novo-Lexin (Can)
   Nu-Cephalex (Can)
   Velosef®
   Zartan®
   Zolicef®
Cephalosporin (Second Generation)
   Apo®-Cefaclor (Can)
   Ceclor®
   Ceclor® CD
   cefaclor
   cefamandole
   cefmetazole
   cefonicid
   Cefotan®
   cefotetan
   cefoxitin
   cefpodoxime

cefprozil
Ceftin® Oral
cefuroxime
Cefzil®
Kefurox® Injection
Mandol®
Mefoxin®
Monocid®
Novo-Cefaclor (Can)
Vantin®
Zefazone®
Zinacef® Injection
Cephalosporin (Third Generation)
   Cedax®
   cefixime
   Cefizox®
   Cefobid®
   cefoperazone
   cefotaxime
   ceftazidime
   ceftibuten
   ceftizoxime
   ceftriaxone
   Ceptaz™
   Claforan®
   Fortaz®
   Rocephin®
   Suprax®
   Tazicef®
   Tazidime®
Cephalosporin (Fourth Generation)
   cefepime
   Maxipime®
Genitourinary Irrigant
   neomycin and polymyxin B
   Neosporin® Cream [OTC]
   Neosporin® G.U. Irrigant
Irrigating Solution
   citric acid bladder mixture
   Renacidin®
Penicillin
   amoxicillin
   amoxicillin and clavulanate potassium

Amoxil®
ampicillin
ampicillin and sulbactam
Ampicin (Can)
Ampicin® Sodium (Can)
Ampilean (Can)
Apo®-Amoxi (Can)
Apo®-Ampi (Can)
Apo®-Cloxi (Can)
Apo®-Pen VK (Can)
Augmentin®
Ayercillin® (Can)
bacampicillin
Bactopen (Can)
Bicillin® C-R
Bicillin® C-R 900/300
Bicillin® L-A
carbenicillin
Clavulin® (Can)
cloxacillin
Cloxapen®
Crysticillin® A.S.
dicloxacillin
Dycill®
Dynapen®
Gen-Amoxicillin (Can)
Geocillin®
Geopen® (Can)
Jaa Amp® (Can)
Marcillin®
Megacillin (Can)
Mezlin®
mezlocillin
Nadopen-V® (Can)
nafcillin
Nallpen®
Novamoxin® (Can)
Novo-Cloxin (Can)
Novo-Pen-VK® (Can)
Nu-Amoxi (Can)
Nu-Ampi (Can)
Nu-Cloxi (Can)
Nu-Pen-VK (Can)

Omnipen®
Omnipen®-N
Orbenin® (Can)
oxacillin
Pathocil®
Penglobe (Can)
penicillin G benzathine
penicillin G benzathine and procaine
   combined
penicillin G (parenteral/aqueous)
penicillin G procaine
penicillin V potassium
Permapen®
Pfizerpen®
piperacillin
piperacillin and tazobactam
   sodium
Pipracil®
Principen®
Pro-Amox® (Can)
Pyopen (Can)
Spectrobid® Tablet
Taro-Cloxacillin® (Can)
Tazocin (Can)
Tegopen (Can)
ticarcillin and clavulanate
   potassium
Timentin®
Totacillin®
Trimox®
Truxcillin®
Unasyn®
Unipen® (Can)
Veetids®
Wycillin®
Wymox®
Zosyn™
Quinolone
   Apo®-Norflox (Can)
   Apo®-Oflox (Can)
   Chibroxin™ Ophthalmic
   Cinobac® Pulvules®
   cinoxacin

enoxacin
Floxin®
lomefloxacin
Maxaquin®
nalidixic acid
NegGram®
norfloxacin
Noroxin® Oral
Novo-Norfloxacin (Can)
Ocuflox™ Ophthalmic
ofloxacin
Penetrex™
sparfloxacin
Zagam®
Sulfonamide
Apo®-Sulfamethoxazole (Can)
Apo®-Sulfatrim (Can)
Azo Gantrisin (Can)
Bactrim™
Bactrim™ DS
Coptin® (Can)
Cotrim®
Cotrim® DS
co-trimoxazole
Gantrisin®
Novo-Soxazole (Can)
Novo-Trimel (Can)
Nu-Cotrimox (Can)
Protrin (Can)
Renoquid®
Roubac® (Can)
Septra®
Septra® DS
SSD (Can)
sulfacytine
sulfadiazine
Sulfamethoprim®
sulfamethoxazole
Sulfatrim®
Sulfatrim® DS
sulfisoxazole
sulfisoxazole and phenazopyridine

Sulfizole® (Can)
Trisulfa® (Can)
Trisulfa-S® (Can)
Uroplus® DS
Uroplus® SS
Urinary Tract Product
acetohydroxamic acid
Atrosept®
Dolsed®
Lithostat®
methenamine, phenyl salicylate,
    atropine, hyoscyamine, benzoic
    acid, and methylene blue
UAA®
Uridon Modified®
Urised®
Uritin®

VAGINITIS

Antibiotic, Vaginal
Femguard®
Gyne-Sulf®
sulfabenzamide, sulfacetamide, and
    sulfathiazole
Sulfa-Gyn®
Sulfa-Trip®
Sultrin™
Trysul®
V.V.S.®
Estrogen and Progestin
Combination
estrogens and medroxyprogesterone
Premphase™
Prempro™
Estrogen Derivative
Alora® Transdermal
Aquest®
Cenestin™
C.E.S.® (Can)
chlorotrianisene
Climara® Transdermal
Congest (Can)

Delestrogen (Can)
depGynogen® Injection
Depo®-Estradiol Injection
Depogen® Injection
dienestrol
diethylstilbestrol
Dioval® Injection
DV® Vaginal Cream
Esclim® Transdermal
Estinyl®
Estrace® Oral
Estraderm® Transdermal
estradiol
Estra-L® Injection
Estring®
Estro-Cyp® Injection
Estrogel (Can)
estrogens (conjugated A/synthetic)
estrogens (conjugated/equine)
estrone
ethinyl estradiol
Femogen® (Can)
Femogen Forte (Can)
Femogex (Can)
Gynogen L.A.® Injection
Honvol® (Can)
Kestrone®
Neo-Estrone® (Can)
Oestrilin® (Can)
Ortho®-Dienestrol Vaginal
PMS-Conjugated Estrogens
   (Can)
Premarin®
Stilphostrol®
TACE®
Vagifem®
Vivelle™ Transdermal

VANCOMYCIN-RESISTANT ENTEROCOCCUS FAECIUM BACTEREMIA
Antibiotic, Oxozolidinone
   linezolid
   Zyvox™
Antibiotic, Streptogramin
   quinupristin and dalfopristin
   Synercid®

VARICELLA
Antiviral Agent
   acyclovir
   Avirax® (Can)
   foscarnet
   Foscavir®
   Zovirax®
Immune Globulin
   Gammabulin Immuno (Can)
   immune globulin (intramuscular)

VARICELLA-ZOSTER
Vaccine, Live Virus
   varicella virus vaccine
   Varivax®

WHIPWORMS
Anthelmintic
   mebendazole
   Vermox®

WORMS
Anthelmintic
   Biltricide®
   Mintezol®
   oxamniquine
   praziquantel
   thiabendazole
   Vansil™